MOLECULAR MECHANISMS IN HYPERTENSION

MOLECULAR MECHANISMS IN HYPERTENSION

Editors

Richard N Re MD FACP FAHA

Scientific Director, Division of Research
Head, Hypertension Division
Ochsner Clinic Foundation, New Orleans, LA, USA

Donald J DiPette MD FACP FAHA

Chairman and Professor, Department of Medicine and
Dr A. Ford Wolf & Brooksie Nell Boyd Wolf
Centennial Chair of Medicine
Scott and White
The Texas A&M University
System Health Science Center College of Medicine
Temple, TX, USA

Ernesto L Schiffrin MD PhD FRCPC FACP FAHA

Physician-in-Chief and Chair, Department of Medicine,
Sir Mortimer B. Davis Jewish General Hospital and
Canada Research Chair and Director, Vascular and
Hypertension Research Unit, Lady Davis Institute for Medical Research,
Professor, Department of Medicine, McGill University
Montréal, Quebec, Canada

James R Sowers MD FACP FACE FAHA

Associate Dean, Clinical Research
Director, MU Diabetes and Cardiovascular Center
Professor, Internal Medicine, Physiology and Pharmacology
Department of Internal Medicine
University of Missouri
Columbia, MO, USA

informa
healthcare

New York London

First published in 2006 by Taylor & Francis, an imprint of the Taylor & Francis Group
This edition published in 2011 by Informa Healthcare, Telephone House, 69-77 Paul Street, London EC2A 4LQ, UK.

Simultaneously published in the USA by Informa Healthcare, 52 Vanderbilt Avenue, 7th Floor, New York, NY 10017, USA.

Informa Healthcare is a trading division of Informa UK Ltd. Registered Office: 37–41 Mortimer Street, London W1T 3JH, UK. Registered in England and Wales number 1072954.

A CIP record for this book is available from the British Library.

ISBN-13: 9781842143049

Orders may be sent to: Informa Healthcare, Sheepen Place, Colchester, Essex CO3 3LP, UK
Telephone: +44 (0)20 7017 5540
Email: CSDhealthcarebooks@informa.com
Website: http://informahealthcarebooks.com/

For corporate sales please contact: CorporateBooksIHC@informa.com
For foreign rights please contact: RightsIHC@informa.com
For reprint permissions please contact: PermissionsIHC@informa.com

Typeset by C&M Digitals (P) Ltd, Chennai, India

Contents

PART III

Contributors

Alexei V Agapitov MD
General Clinical Research Center
Carver College of Medicine
University of Iowa
Iowa City, IA, USA

Natalia Alenina PhD
Max-Delbrück-Center for Molecular Medicine (MDC)
Berlin-Buch, Germany

R Wayne Alexander MD PhD
Division of Cardiology
Department of Medicine
Emory University School of Medicine
Atlanta, GA, USA

Surender Arora MD
Division of Endocrinology, Diabetes and Hypertension
SUNY-Downstate
Kings County Hospital and Woodhul Hospital
Brooklyn, New York, NY, USA

Michael Bader PhD
Max-Delbrück-Center for Molecular Medicine (MDC)
Berlin-Buch, Germany

Kenneth M Baker MD
Division of Molecular Cardiology
Cardiovascular Research Institute
The Texas A&M University System Health Science Center
College of Medicine
Temple, TX, USA

Ovidiu Baltatu MD PhD
Max-Delbrück-Center for Molecular Medicine (MDC)
Berlin-Buch, Germany

Bradford C Berk MD PhD
Chairman, Department of Medicine
Director, Cardiovascular Research Institute (CVRI)
University of Rochester
Rochester, NY, USA

Mariela Garcia Blanes BSc
Endothelial Cell Biology Research Unit
Clinical Research Institute of Montreal (IRCM)
Université de Montréal
Montréal, Quebec, Canada

Nick JR Brain PhD
British Heart Foundation Glasgow Cardiovascular Research Centre
University of Glasgow Western Infirmary
Glasgow, UK

Celine A Burckle MD
GN and CAB: Inserm U36
Collège de France
Paris, France

Duncan J Campbell MD PhD
St Vincent's Institute of Medical Research
Fitzroy, Victoria, Australia

Robert M Carey MD MACP
David A. Harrison III Distinguished Professor of Medicine
Dean, Emeritus, and University Professor
University of Virginia School of Medicine
University of Virginia Health System
Charlottesville, VA, USA

Fadi J Charchar PhD
British Heart Foundation Glasgow Cardiovascular Research Centre
University of Glasgow Western Infirmary
Glasgow, UK

Songcang Chen MD
Department of Medicine and Diabetes Center
University of California at San Francisco
San Francisco, CA, USA

Julia L Cook PhD
Co-Director of Molecular Genetics
Ochsner Clinic Foundation
Division of Research
New Orleans, LA, USA

Dalila B Corry MD
Chief Nephrology and Hypertension
Division Olive View-UCLA Medical Center
Professor of Clinical Medicine
David Geffen School of Medicine at UCLA
Los Angeles, CA, USA

AH Jan Danser PhD
Department of Pharmacology
Erasmus MC
Rotterdam, The Netherlands

Denis deBlois PhD
Department of Pharmacology
Faculté de Médecine
Université de Montréal
Montréal, Quebec, Canada

Walmor C De Mello MD PhD
Professor and Chairman
Pharmacology & Toxicology Department
School of Medicine University of Puerto Rico
San Juan, PR, USA

Javier Diez MD PhD
Área de Fisiopatología Cardiovascular
CIMA
Pamplona, Spain

Sergey Dikalov PhD
Cardiology Division
Department of Medicine
Emory University School of Medicine and
Atlanta Veterans Administration Hospital
Atlanta, GA, USA

Donald J DiPette MD FACP FAHA
Chairman and Professor, Department of Medicine and Dr A. Ford Wolf & Brooksie Nell Boyd Wolf
Centennial Chair of Medicine
Scott and White
The Texas A&M University System Health Science Center College of Medicine
Temple, TX, USA

Anna F Dominiczak OBE MD FRCP FRSE FMedSci
British Heart Foundation Professor of Cardiovascular Medicine
Director, BHF Glasgow Cardiovascular Research Centre
Division of Cardiovascular and Medical Sciences
Western Infirmary, Glasgow, UK

David Duguay BSc
Department of Pharmacology
Faculté de Médecine
Université de Montréal CP
Montréal, Quebec, Canada

Satoru Eguchi MD PhD
Department of Physiology
Cardiovascular Research Center
Temple University School of Medicine
Philadelphia, PA, USA

Robin A Felder PhD
Professor of Pathology
University of Virginia School of Medicine
University of Virginia Health System
Charlottesville, VA, USA

Carlos M Ferrario MD
The Hypertension and Vascular Disease Center
Wake Forest University School of Medicine
Medical Center Boulevard
Winston-Salem, NC, USA

Ryan S Friese MS
Graduate Student
Departments of Bioengineering and Medicine
University of California, San Diego
Palade Cellular and Molecular Medicine West
La Jolla, CA, USA

Edward D Frohlich MD
Ochsner Clinic Foundation
New Orleans, LA, USA

Toshiro Fujita MD PhD FAHA
University of Tokyo
Faculty of Medicine
Tokyo, Japan

Patricia E Gallagher PhD
Hypertension & Vascular Disease Center
Wake Forest University Health Science
Winston-Salem, NC, USA

David G Gardner MS MD
University of California at San Francisco
San Francisco, CA, USA

Marina Goikhberg MD
Primary Care Attending Physician
Central Medical Group
Brooklyn, New York, NY, USA

Celso E Gomez-Sanchez MD
Division of Endocrinology
G.V. (Sonny) Montgomery VA Hospital and The University of Mississippi Medical Center
Jackson, MS, USA

Elise P Gomez-Sanchez DVM PhD
Division of Endocrinology and Metabolism
University of Mississippi Medical Center
Jackson, MS, USA

Gurushankar Govindarajan MD
Research Scientist
Center for Diabetes and Cardiovascular Research
Department of Medicine
University of Missouri-Columbia
Columbia, MO, USA

Jean-Philippe Gratton PhD
Directeur, Laboratoire de Biologie des Cellules Endothéliales
Director, Laboratory of Endothelial Cell Biology
Institut de Recherches Cliniques de Montréal (IRCM)
Université de Montréal
Montréal, Quebec, Canada

Kathy K Griendling PhD
Division of Cardiology
Department of Medicine
Emory University School of Medicine
Atlanta, GA, USA

Taben M Hale PhD
Department of Pharmacology
Faculté de Médecine
Université de Montréal
Montréal, Quebecc, Canada

John M Hamlyn PhD
Department of Physiology
School of Medicine
University of Maryland Baltimore
Baltimore, MD, USA

David G Harrison MD
Bernard Marcus Professor of Medicine
Director of Cardiology
Woodruff Memorial Research Building
Emory University School of Medicine
Atlanta, GA, USA

Meredith Hay PhD
Vice President for Research
Professor of Physiology and Biophysics
Professor of Psychology
University of Iowa
Iowa City, IA, USA

William G Haynes MB ChB MRCP MRCP MD
General Clinical Research Center
Carver College of Medicine
University of Iowa
Iowa City, IA, USA

Ivonne Hernandez Schulman MD FASN
Assistant Professor of Clinical Medicine
Division of Nephrology and Hypertension
University of Miami Miller School of Medicine
Nephrology-Hypertension Section
Veterans Affairs Medical Center
Miami, FL, USA

Lula L Hilenski PhD
Assistant Professor, Division of Cardiology
Director, Internal Medicine Imaging Core
Emory University School of Medicine
Department of Medicine, Division of Cardiology
Woodruff Memorial Research Building
Atlanta, GA, USA

Norman K Hollenberg MD PhD
Brigham and Women's Hospital
Boston, MA, USA

Virginia Huxley PhD
Professor, Department of Medical Pharmacology & Physiology
Director, The National Center for Gender Physiology
Senior Investigator, Dalton Cardiovascular Research Center
Columbia, MO, USA

Pedro A Jose MD PhD
Professor of Pediatrics and Physiology and Biophysics
Georgetown University School of Medicine
Georgetown University Hospital
Physicians Healthcare Center
Department of Pediatrics
Washington, DC, USA

Henry L Keen
Departments of Internal Medicine and Physiology & Biophysics and
The 2 Center for Bioinformatics and Computational Biology
University of Iowa College of Medicine
Iowa City, IA, USA

Hiroyuki Kobori MD PhD FAHA
Department of Physiology and Hypertension and
Renal Center of Excellence
Tulane University Health Sciences Center
New Orleans, LA, USA

Tetsuya Matoba MD PhD
Cardiovascular Research Institute (CVRI)
University of Rochester School of Medicine and Density
Rochester, NY, USA

Samy I McFarlane MD MPH FACP FACE CCD
Associate Professor of Medicine
Interim Chief, Division of Endocrinology, Diabetes and Hypertension
Department of Medicine
State University of New York
Health Science Center at Brooklyn
Kings County Hospital Center
Brooklyn, New York, NY, USA

Jawahar L Mehta MD PhD
Director, Division of Cardiovascular Medicine
University of Arkansas for Medical Sciences (UAMS)
Little Rock, AR, USA

Dominik N Muller PhD
Max-Delbrück-Center for Molecular Medicine (MDC)
Berlin-Buch, Germany

L Gabriel Navar PhD
Department of Physiology
Tulane University Health Sciences Center
New Orleans, LA, USA

Geneviève Nguyen MD PhD
GN and CAB: Inserm U36
Collège de France
Paris, France

Daniel T O'Connor MD
Professor of Medicine
Department of Medicine
University of California at San Diego School of Medicine, and VASDHS
Palade Cellular and Molecular Medicine West
La Jolla, CA, USA

Haruhiko Ohtsu PhD
Cardiovascular Research Center
Temple University School of Medicine
Philadelphia, PA, USA

Keith Olsen AB
Department of Medicine and Diabetes Center
University of California at San Francisco
San Francisco, CA, USA

John Palmer DO
Endocrine Fellow
Department of Internal Medicine
University of Missouri-Columbia
Columbia, MO, USA

Jing Pan MD PhD
Division of Molecular Cardiology
Cardiovascular Research Institute
The Texas A&M University System Health Science Center
Temple, TX, USA

Brian S Pavey DO MS
Resident Physician
University of Missouri-Columbia
Department of Internal Medicine
Columbia, MO, USA

Achille Cesare Pessina MD PhD
DMCS-Internal Medicine 4
University Hospital
Padova, Italy

Jörg Peters MD
University of Greifswald
Department of Physiology
Karlsburg, Germany

Minolfa C Prieto-Carrasquero MD PhD
Department of Physiology and Hypertension and Renal Center of Excellence
Tulane University Health Sciences Center
New Orleans, LA, USA

Dolkun Rahmutula MD PhD
Department of Medicine and Diabetes Center
University of California at San Francisco
San Francisco, CA, USA

Leopoldo Raij MD
Chief, Nephrology-Hypertension Section
Veterans Affairs Medical Center
Miami, FL, USA

Fangwen Rao MD
Visiting Scholar
Department of Medicine
University of California at San Diego
La Jolla, CA, USA

Richard N Re MD FACP FAHA
Scientific Director, Division of Research
Head, Hypertension Division
Ochsner Clinic Foundation,
New Orleans, LA, USA

Ricardo Rocha MD
Novartis Pharmaceuticals Corporation
Cardiovascular and Metabolic Diseases
East Hanover, NJ, USA

Gian Paolo Rossi MD FACC
DMCS-Internal Medicine 4
University Hospital
Padova, Italy

Alan Sacerdote MD
Division of Endocrinology, Diabetes and Hypertension
SUNY-Downstate
Kings County Hospital and Woodhul Hospital
Brooklyn, New York, NY, USA

Ernesto L Schiffrin MD PhD FRCPC FACP FAHA
Physician-in-Chief and Chair, Department of Medicine,
Sir Mortimer B. Davis Jewish General Hospital and Canada Research Chair and Director
Vascular and Hypertension Research Unit
Lady Davis Institute for Medical Research, Professor, Department of Medicine
McGill University
Montréal, Quebec, Canada

Tatsuo Shimosawa MD PhD FAHA
University of Tokyo, Faculty of Medicine
Department of Clinical Laboratory Medicine
Bunkyoku Tokyo, Japan

Curt D Sigmund PhD
Departments of Internal Medicine and Physiology & Biophysics
Medical Education and Biomedical Research Facility (MEBRF)
Roy J. and Lucille A. Carver College of Medicine
University of Iowa
Iowa City, IA, USA

James R Sowers MD FACP FACE FAHA
Associate Dean, Clinical Research
Director, MU Diabetes and Cardiovascular Center
Professor, Internal Medicine, Physiology and Pharmacology
Department of Internal Medicine
University of Missouri
Columbia, MO, USA

Craig S Stump MD PhD
Assistant Professor of Medicine
University of Missouri-Columbia
Department of Internal Medicine
Division of Endocrinology, Diabetes and Metabolism and
Research Scientist, Diabetes and Cardiovascular Disease Research Center
Staff Physician, Harry S. Truman VA Hospital
Columbia, MO, USA

Scott Supowit BA MS PhD
Associate Professor
Texas A&M University System Health Science Center and
Scott & White Health System
Department of Medicine
Temple, TX, USA

E Ann Tallant PhD
The Hypertension and Vascular Disease Center
Wake Forest University School of Medicine
Medical Center Boulevard
Winston-Salem, NC, USA

Marc Thibonnier MD MSc FAHA
Division of Clinical and Molecular Endocrinology
Department of Medicine
Case Western Reserve University School of Medicine
Cleveland, OH, USA

Maciej Tomaszewski MD
British Heart Foundation Glasgow Cardiovascular Research Centre
University of Glasgow
Western Infirmary
Glasgow, UK

Rhian M Touyz, MD PhD
Kidney Research Centre
Ottawa Health Research Institute
University of Ottawa
Ottawa, Ontario, Canada

Tri Tran BS
Division of Endocrinology, Diabetes and Hypertension
SUNY-Downstate
Kings County Hospital and Woodhul Hospital, Brooklyn, New York, NY, USA

Michael L Tuck MD
Chief Endocrine and Metabolism
VA Medical Centre, Sepulveda, CA and
Professor of Medicine
David Geffen School of Medicine at UCLA
Los Angeles, CA, USA

Jasmina Varagic MD PhD
Alton Ochsner Distinguished Scientist
Ochsner Clinic Foundation
New Orleans, LA, USA

Feng Wang MD PhD
Department of Medicine and Diabetes Center
University of California at San Francisco
San Francisco, CA, USA

Ralph Watson MD
Michigan State University
Department of Medicine
East Lansing, MI USA

Karolina Weiss BA
New York College of Osteopathic Medicine
New York, NY, USA

Adam Whaley-Connell DO
Post-Doctoral Fellow, Division of Nephrology
Research Fellow, Diabetes and Cardiovascular Lab
Department of Internal Medicine
University of Missouri Health Sciences Center
Columbia, MO, USA

Gordon H Williams MD
Brigham and Women's Hospital and
Harvard Medical School
Boston, MA, USA

Nathaniel Winer MD
Professor of Medicine
Division of Endocrinology, Diabetes and Hypertension
State University of New York
Downstate Medical Center
Brooklyn, New York, NY, USA

William F Young Jr MD MSc
Mayo Clinic
Rochester, MN, USA

Ming-Sheng Zhou MD PhD
Veterans Affairs Medical Center
Miami, FL, USA

Preface

Hypertension is a common affliction of 21st century man, conveying risk for heart disease, stroke, renal failure, and other disorders. The realization that this is the case, however, is relatively recent; a full appreciation of hypertension-related risk has developed only over the last 60 or so years. With the understanding that arterial hypertension is a significant health problem came the desire to understand the mechanisms which caused it so as to develop ever more effective therapies. Early on, Irvine Page suggested that the pathogenesis of hypertension should be viewed as a mosaic of sorts, with any final blood pressure potentially the result of any of a variety of underlying mechanisms.[1] This formulation has, indeed, been proven correct. Although it has been argued that altered pressure naturesis relationships in renal handling of sodium are the *sine qua non* of hypertension, it remains the case that even if this schema is correct, a large number of mechanisms can independently alter renal pressure/naturesis – the mosaic resurfaces.[2] Indeed, much has been learned over the last quarter century regarding the various systems that regulate blood pressure in health and disease, as well as about the mechanisms by which raised pressure produces vascular disease of various sorts. Much more can be glimpsed just over the current experimental horizon. For example, the workings of the renin-angiotensin-aldosterone system (RAAS) have been explored in great detail and this system is now seen to operate in the circulating blood, in the walls of vessels, and in tissues. It affects pressure, sodium handling, vascular structure, and inflammation, among other parameters. Its complexities include alternative enzymes for processing RAAS components – for example, chymase and ACE2 – as well as novel intracellular signaling mechanisms and actions mediated by the generation of reactive oxygen species. And what is true for the RAAS is similarly true for a wide variety of other peptide, steroid, and lipid regulators of arterial hypertension. It is the aim of this volume to provide insights at the molecular level into the growing body of experimental data which collectively defines these mechanisms responsible for arterial hypertension.

To achieve this goal, the editors have invited leaders in the experimental study of arterial hypertension to discuss mechanisms operative in the pathogenesis of the disorder and of its sequelae. Emphasis has been placed on molecular mechanisms, although in many instances relevant clinical/physiological correlates are also reviewed. This has resulted in a collection of essays describing current opinion regarding the various mechanisms that produce raised arterial pressure as well as current experimental evidence in support of these views. The editors believe this format will be useful to both clinicians and experimentalists alike as they formulate their own views of the pathogenesis of human hypertension.

Molecular Mechanisms in Hypertension is divided into three parts. Part I centers on the components of the renin-angiotensin system (RAS) in hypertensive disorders. The seminal work of Tigerstedt and Bergman identifying a renal pressor substance, followed by the identification of angiotensin II as the active vasopressor produced in the Goldblatt model, and the subsequent elucidation of the renin-angiotensin cascade, including the identification of angiotensin converting enzyme and the angiotensin II AT_1 and AT_2 receptors, has greatly informed medicine's understanding of the regulation of intravascular volume, arterial pressure, and the pathogenesis of vascular disease. Pharmacological agents which interrupt this system at various points are in common use, and the physiological principles surrounding the activity of the RAS are used daily by clinicians in attempting to tailor drug therapies to individual patients. However, over recent years, the RAS has been found to be substantially more complex than heretofore believed, with the activity and generation of angiotensin II in tissues, the dimerization and heterodimerazation of angiotensin II receptors, the identification of angiotensin converting enzyme 2, and the recognition that angiotensin peptides such as angiotensin 1–7 play important roles in vascular homeostasis, all contributing to an enlarged understanding of the role of the RAS in normal and hypertensive man. In Part I, molecular mechanisms relating to the action of renin and angiotensin are discussed in detail.

In addition, it has been long recognized that angiotensin II is a secretogogue for the adrenal hormone aldosterone and this creates the well-known renin-angiotensin-aldosterone system (RAAS). The pressor effects of angiotensin II, the renin suppressing effects of angiotensin II, and the volume expanding effects of aldosterone, all collaborate to form the renin-angiotensin-aldosterone feedback system, with an important role in the regulation of blood pressure and intravascular volume. But just as recent investigations have expanded the view of the RAS *per se*, so too the role of aldosterone is now seen to be substantially greater in both health and disease than previously appreciated. Thus, newly described mechanisms related to aldosterone action are also included in Part I.

Part II begins by dealing with non-RAS peptides in hypertension. Recent evidence suggests that a variety of peptide hormones, operating either in the circulation or in the tissues, may impact blood pressure and the development of the sequelae of hypertension in important ways. Among these are vasopressin, calcitonin gene-related peptide, adrenomedullin, neuropeptide Y, growth hormone, endothelin, members of the atrial natriuretic peptide family, and others. Although the participation of these peptides in the pathogenesis of hypertension is not as well understood or appreciated as that of angiotensin, it is, nonetheless, clearly important as evidenced, for example, by the growing interest in the potential role of endothelin antagonists in the treatment of hypertension and in preventing the sequelae of hypertension. The first goal of Part II is to explore recent data related to molecular mechanisms by which these non-RAS peptides regulate blood pressure. Next, the role of the adrenal medulla and its products in hypertension is explored on both the molecular and clinical levels. Finally, a variety of new technologies which are currently being employed to further define the role of these and other factors in hypertension are discussed. Included among these are microarray studies of models of hypertension, and genetic approaches to identifying the causes of hypertension.

In addition to the peptinergic and adrenal systems described in Parts I and II, recent experimental evidence points to the role of non-peptides in the regulation of blood pressure and in the genesis of hypertension. Endogenous Na/K-ATPase inhibitors appear to have important implications for the development of high blood pressure and, conversely, non-peptides such as nitric oxide play a role in vascular dilatation and in protection from the sequelae of hypertension. In addition, recent information has greatly expanded current thinking regarding the genesis of the sequelae of hypertension. New insights into the interaction of angiotensin, blood pressure, and lipids in atherogenesis, and the role of apoptosis in hypertensive heart disease, are examples of this, as is an expanding view of the interrelation of blood pressure and dyslipidemia in the genesis of the sequelae of diabetes. It is the goal of Part III to explore these multiple mechanisms which regulate blood pressure on the one hand, and participate in the development of the sequelae of hypertension on the other.

Hypertension is a complex disorder and new insights into its pathogenesis are being developed almost daily. Although this volume cannot claim to be exhaustive, it covers the major themes in the area and, indeed, explores a variety of less appreciated molecular mechanisms as well. The editors and contributors hope it serves the reader well.

Richard N Re MD
New Orleans

1. Page IH. The mosaic theory 32 years later. Hypertension 1982; 4: 177.
2. Hall JE, Guyton AC, Brands MW. Pressure-volume regulation in hypertension. Kidney Int Suppl 1996; 55: S35–S41.

PART I

1

Molecular aspects of the renal renin-angiotensin system

L Gabriel Navar, Minolfa C Prieto-Carrasquero and Hiroyuki Kobori

INTRODUCTION

Various recent studies have enhanced our understanding of the intrarenal renin-angiotensin system (RAS) and of the intriguing mechanisms involved in the intrarenal regulation of the angiotensin (Ang) peptides. The multiple components of the RAS present in the kidney allow it to operate in autocrine and intracrine fashion rather independently of the circulating endocrine system. Recent developments have raised our awareness of distinct mechanisms regulating intratubular and interstitial, as well as intracellular, RAS. In this chapter, we briefly review our current understanding of the intrarenal RAS and discuss how inappropriate activation of the intrarenal RAS compromises the kidney's capability to maintain an optimum sodium and fluid balance at normal arterial pressures, thus setting the stage for the development of hypertension.

RENIN-ANGIOTENSIN SYSTEM AND REGULATION OF SODIUM BALANCE AND ARTERIAL BLOOD PRESSURE

The RAS plays a pivotal role in the regulation of renal sodium and water excretion, and therefore in maintaining body sodium and fluid balance.[1,2] It has generally been held that renin produced by the kidney cleaves liver-derived angiotensinogen (AGT) to form Ang I in the systemic circulation. Ang I is converted into Ang II, the main effector peptide of the RAS, by angiotensin converting enzyme (ACE) located on the luminal side of the endothelium in many tissues. Ang II exerts its effects via stimulation of Ang II receptors, of which at least two types have been described, AT_1 and AT_2. As shown in Figure 1.1, multiple enzymatic pathways form Ang I and Ang II as well as other Ang peptides that may also have significant biological actions. There are alternative pathways for Ang I conversion in the various tissues, such as chymase in cardiac tissue[3,4] and in the clipped kidney of the 2-kidney-1-clip (2K1C) Goldblatt hypertension model in dogs, which appears to have a marked up-regulation of chymase activity.[5] Chymase up-regulation has also been reported in human subjects with diabetic nephropathy.[6] Endopeptidases such as neprilysin and prolyl endopeptidase may bypass Ang II and convert Ang I directly to Ang 1-7.[7] Metabolism of Ang II to Ang III (2-8) and Ang IV (3-8) is catalyzed by the aminopeptidases A, N, and B and dipeptidylaminopeptidase II.[8] Ang I conversion to Ang II via chymase, kallikrein, trypsin as well as tonin and Cathepsin G provide non-renin, non-ACE pathways for Ang I and Ang II formation[7,9] (Figure 1.1). A recently described enzyme, termed ACE 2, cleaves a single amino acid from Ang I to form Ang 1-9 and from Ang II to form Ang 1-7.[7,10,11] Ang 1-7 exerts significant vasodilator and natriuretic actions that may partially counteract the effects of Ang II.[7,12] Thus, actions of ACE 2 could have a substantial impact on the balance of Ang peptides found in the kidney by diverting the RAS cascade from Ang II to Ang 1-7.

The systemic RAS regulates arterial pressure and sodium balance by controlling extracellular fluid volume and through the actions of Ang II and related peptides on vascular smooth muscle cells throughout the body. Ang II also enhances myocardial contractility, stimulates aldosterone release, stimulates release of catecholamines from the adrenal medulla and sympathetic nerve endings, increases sympathetic nervous system activity, stimulates thirst and salt appetite, and influences epithelial salt and water reabsorption in the intestine and kidney.[1,13] Ang II stimulates postganglionic sympathetic

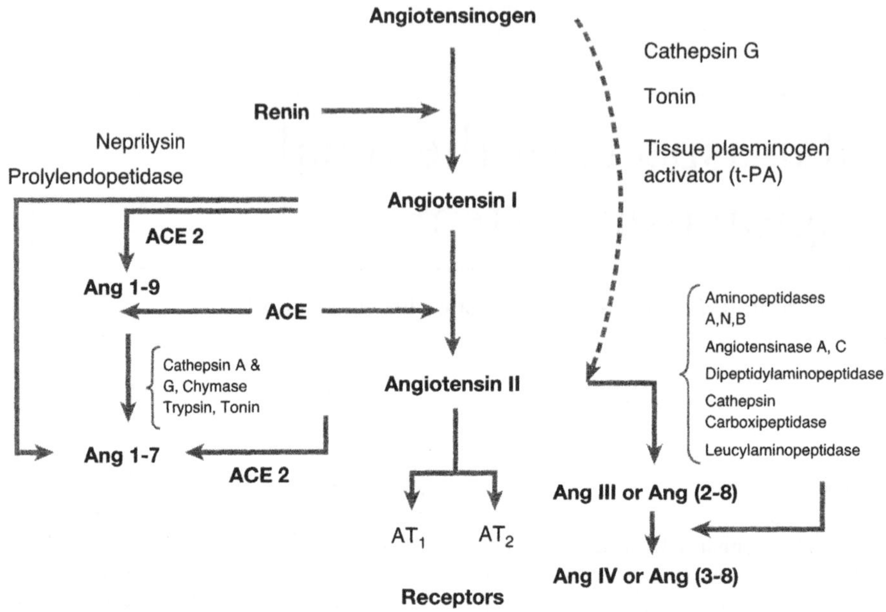

Figure 1.1 Known and postulated enzymatic pathways responsible for formation and metabolism of angiotensin peptides. Refer to text for further details and references

neurons by activating voltage-gated Ca^{2++} channels and increasing intracellular Ca^{2++}.[14] Ang II exerts long-term effects on growth and remodeling, development, vascular hypertrophy, and erythropoiesis. In pathological situations, Ang II exerts significant long-term proliferative effects leading to tissue injury due to activation of cytokines,[15–17] as well as alteration of the immune system with increases in gamma-interferon-secreting T cells.[18,19]

INTRARENAL RENIN-ANGIOTENSIN SYSTEM COMPONENTS AND LOCALLY FORMED ANGIOTENSIN PEPTIDES

Because the RAS serves endocrine, paracrine, autocrine, and intracrine functions,[20–24] it has been difficult to delineate the quantitative contributions of systemically delivered versus locally formed Ang peptides to the levels existing in any given tissue. Various studies have demonstrated the importance of locally generated Ang II in the brain, heart, adrenal glands, and vasculature, as well as in the kidney.[1,6,25–27] The kidneys are unique in having every component of the RAS along with compartmentalization in the tubular and interstitial networks. The kidneys, as well as the adrenal glands, have tissue concentrations of Ang II much greater than can be explained by the concentrations delivered by the arterial blood flow.[28–31] Accordingly, the major fraction of Ang II present in renal tissues is generated locally from AGT delivered to the kidney as well as from AGT produced locally by proximal tubule cells.

Renin

Renin, synthesized by the juxtaglomerular apparatus (JGA) cells, is the primary source of both circulating and intrarenal renin levels. Renin is secreted into the renal interstitium, as well as vascular compartments, providing a pathway for the local generation of Ang I.[32,33] Some strains of mice also produce substantial amounts of renin in the submandibular and submaxillary glands as expression of the duplicated renin gene, Ren-2.[34,35]

The secreted active form of renin contains 339–343 amino acid residues after proteolytic removal of the 43-amino acid residue at the N-terminus (prorenin). Although circulating active renin is derived mainly from the kidney, the kidneys and other tissues also secrete prorenin into the circulation and its concentration may exceed that of renin.[36] Besides serving as the precursor for active renin, circulating prorenin is taken up by some tissues where it may contribute to the local synthesis of angiotensin peptides.[37] The only well established role of renin is to act on AGT, a protein with a nonglycosylated weight of 52 KDa and synthesized primarily by the liver to form the decapeptide Ang I. It has also been suggested that renin or prorenin may directly elicit cellular effects, independent of the generation of Ang II. Recent reports support the existence of an actual renin receptor capable of initiating intracellular signaling to activate ERK1/ERK2.[38] In the heart and kidney the recently described renin receptor[38–41] binds renin and prorenin, leading to an increase in the catalytic efficiency of Ang I formation from AGT.

JGA cells are not the only intrarenal structures where renin has been localized. Kidneys from rats treated chronically with ACE inhibitors exhibit renin immunoreactivity on the afferent arteriole extending well beyond the JGA loci up towards the interlobular artery, suggesting that ACE inhibition induces a recruitment of cells that in the basal state were not expressing the renin gene.[42] Positive renin immunoreaction has also been observed in cells of glomeruli and in proximal and distal nephron segments.[43–46] Renin mRNA and protein expression are present in proximal and distal nephron segments, suggesting local formation.[44,46–50] In immunoblotting studies, renin was shown to be secreted by microdissected arcades of connecting tubule cells, indicating that renin is probably secreted into the distal tubular fluid.[50] Renin expression in principal cells of collecting ducts is further increased in Ang II-dependent hypertension.[46]

Angiotensin converting enzyme

The importance of ACE, in particular tissue-bound ACE in the kidney, has been impressively demonstrated by the numerous genetically modified mice with reduced ACE expression.[51] Intrarenal ACE is located on endothelial cells throughout the renal vasculature and on membranes of both proximal and distal nephron segments with the greatest abundance found on the brush border of proximal tubules.[52–54] Proximal tubules containing ACE are observed in the inner cortex and outer strip of the outer medulla corresponding primarily to the S3 segment.[54] Also, marked up-regulation of ACE in brush borders occurs in kidneys from Goldblatt hypertensive rats and Ang II-infused hypertensive rats.[54] There are some important differences between humans and commonly used experimental animals.[55] Kidneys from normal human subjects predominantly express ACE in the brush border of proximal tubular segments with very little ACE expression on vascular endothelial cells or in the vasculature of the glomerular tuft.[55] This finding contrasts with the intense labeling found on renal endothelial cells of rats. The lower renal vascular endothelial expression in humans helps to explain the much lower Ang I to Ang II conversion rates that have been reported for human kidneys as compared with other species. The reduced ACE on renal vascular endothelial cells in humans implies that the influence of intrarenal Ang II formed from circulating precursors may have less significance than in experimental animals.

The recently described ACE 2, which acts on Ang II to form Ang 1-7, is a membrane-associated and secreted enzyme expressed predominantly on endothelium, but highly restricted in humans to heart, kidneys, and testis. It has been suggested that Ang 1-7 acts on its own receptor, postulated to be the orphan Mas receptor.[56,57] Ang 1-7 may serve as an endogenous antagonist of the Ang II-induced actions mediated via AT_1 receptors.[58] Thus, differences in ACE 2 activity could have substantial impact on the balance of Ang peptides found in the kidney by shifting the balance from Ang II to Ang 1-7. This helps explain the elevated Ang II levels in the ACE 2 knockout mice.[57] Collectrin, a novel homolog of ACE 2, has been identified in mouse, rat, and human.[59,60] Both ACE 2 and collectrin have tissue-restricted expression in the kidney. Collectrin is localized on the luminal surface and in the cytoplasm of collecting duct cells and its mRNA is expressed in renal collecting duct cells[60] while ACE 2 is present throughout the endothelium and in proximal tubular epithelial cells. In contrast to ACE and ACE 2, collectrin does not contain dipeptidyl carboxypeptidase domains. Other peptides with reported biological activity formed as part of the Ang cascade include Ang 2-8 and Ang 3-8 as a consequence of action by aminopeptidases and other degrading enzymes.[61] While there is growing interest in the potential roles of these other Ang peptides, the bulk of the evidence continues to support the established premise that most of the vascular and transport actions attributed to the RAS that lead to vascular constriction, enhanced sodium transport and hypertension are due to the actions of Ang II and also Ang III (Ang 2-8) acting primarily on AT_1 receptors.[62–64] Nevertheless, Ang 1-7-, Ang IV-, and Ang II-mediated activation of AT_2 receptors may exert significant counteracting or protective actions, partially buffering the AT_1-mediated effects under certain circumstances.[7,65–68]

Angiotensinogen

Although most of the circulating AGT is produced and secreted by the liver, the kidneys produce substantial AGT. Intrarenal AGT mRNA and protein have been localized to proximal tubule cells, indicating that intratubular Ang II could be derived from locally formed and secreted AGT.[30,69–71] Furthermore, AGT is regulated by an amplification mechanism such that AGT mRNA and protein are stimulated by Ang II, which maintains or increases further the production of Ang II in Ang II-dependent hypertension.[69–72] The AGT produced in proximal tubule cells appears to be secreted directly into the tubular lumen in addition to producing its metabolites intracellularly and secreting them into the tubule lumen.[30,48,50,73,74] AGT formed in proximal tubule cells appears to be secreted primarily into the lumen.[50,75]

Proximal tubule AGT concentrations in anesthetized rats are in the range of 300 pmol/ml, which greatly exceed the free Ang I and Ang II tubular fluid concentrations.[76] Because of its molecular size, it seems unlikely that much of the plasma AGT filters across the glomerular membrane, further supporting the concept that proximal tubule cells secrete AGT directly into the tubule.[50,71,75,77] Human AGT infused into hypertensive rats was not detectable in the urine, suggesting that most of the AGT in the urine is of renal origin.[78] Formation of Ang I and II in the tubular lumen subsequent to AGT secretion may be possible because some renin is filtered and/or secreted from JGA cells. The identification of renin in distal nephron segments also indicates a possible pathway for Ang I generation from proximally delivered AGT.[46,50] Intact AGT in urine reflects its presence throughout the nephron and, to the extent that renin and ACE are available along the nephron, substrate availability supports continued Ang I generation and Ang II conversion in distal segments.[26,48,50,75]

Once Ang I is formed, conversion readily occurs because there are abundant amounts of ACE associated with the proximal tubule brush border. ACE activity is present in tubular fluid throughout the nephron except in the late distal tubule, being higher at the initial portion of the proximal tubule but then decreasing to the distal nephron and increasing again in the urine.[79] Therefore, intratubular Ang II formation may occur not only in the proximal tubule but also beyond the connecting tubule. Renal tissue ACE activity is critical to maintain the steady-state Ang II levels in the kidney.[51] Tissue-ACE (*tis*ACE–/–) knockout mice exhibit 80% lower intrarenal Ang II levels than wild-type mice.[80] In addition to the marked reduction of intrarenal Ang II levels, *tis*ACE–/– mice exhibited significant depletion of Ang I in renal tissue, which supports the concept that Ang II exerts a positive feedback loop on proximal AGT.[69,70,72] However, at present there are no data indicating what proportion of the Ang peptides are formed intracellularly and secreted and what proportion are formed in the tubule lumen from secreted substrate.

Intrarenal angiotensin II receptors

Ang II receptors are widely distributed in various regions and cell types of the kidney. Two major categories of Ang II receptors, AT_1 (subtypes AT_{1a} and AT_{1b}) and AT_2 have been described, pharmacologically characterized, and cloned.[81–86] Specific receptors for other Ang peptides remain controversial or unknown. As shown in Figure 1.2, however, most of the Ang II hypertensinogenic actions are generally attributed to the AT_1 receptor.[87–89] AT_1 receptor transcript has been localized to proximal tubules, thick ascending limb of the loop of Henle, glomeruli, arterial vasculature, vasa recta, arcuate arteries and juxtaglomerular cells.[90–92] In rodents, there are two AT_1 receptor subtypes, with AT_{1a} being the predominant subtype in all nephron segments, while AT_{1b} is more abundant than AT_{1a} only in the glomerulus.[93,94] The AT_{1a} receptor subtype has been found on ureteric bud derivatives as early as the embryonic day E11.5.[95] In mature kidneys, AT_{1a} receptors have been localized to the luminal and basolateral membranes of several segments of the nephron, as well as on the renal microvasculature in both cortex and medulla, smooth muscle cells of afferent and efferent arterioles, epithelial cells of the thick ascending limb of Henle, proximal tubular apical and basolateral membranes, mesangial cells, distal tubules, collecting ducts, and macula densa cells.[96–102] This evidence is consistent with the localization of the transcript for the AT_1 receptor subtypes in all of the renal tubular and vascular segments.[102] Interestingly, renal microvascular functional studies obtained from transgenic mice lacking the AT_{1a} receptor gene have shown that the afferent arteriole has both AT_{1a} and AT_{1b} receptors, whereas the efferent arteriole only expresses AT_{1a} receptors.[103] The essential role of the AT_{1a} receptor in mice is apparent from studies showing that 2K1C Goldblatt hypertension does not develop in AT_{1a}–/– mice.[104]

The regulation of intrarenal Ang II receptors in hypertensive conditions is complex because vascular and tubular receptors respond differently during high Ang II states.[2] High Ang II levels associated with a low salt diet decrease glomerular AT_1 receptor expression but increase tubular AT_1 receptor levels.[105] In 2K1C Goldblatt hypertensive rats, glomerular AT_1 receptors were decreased by 2 weeks after clipping but vascular receptors were not decreased until 16 weeks.[106] In the Ang II-infused rat model of hypertension, total kidney AT_1 mRNA levels and receptor protein were not significantly altered by 2 weeks of Ang II infusion

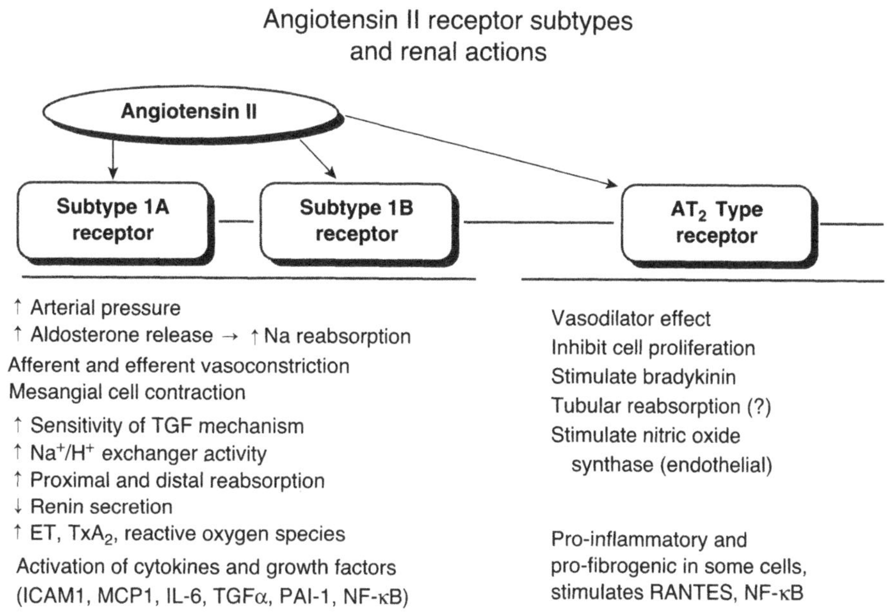

Figure 1.2 Major Ang II receptor subtypes and renal actions

sufficient to cause marked hypertension.[107] However, AT_{1a} receptor protein was reduced in both clipped and contralateral kidneys of 2K1C Goldblatt and two-kidney one-wrap hypertensive models and in kidneys of Ang II-infused rats.[108] AT_2 receptors were down-regulated only in ischemic kidneys. In the TGR (mRen2) harboring the mouse renin gene, AT_1 receptor binding was increased in vascular smooth muscle of afferent and efferent arterioles, JGA, glomerular mesangial cells, proximal tubular cells, and renomedullary interstitial cells, suggesting that up-regulation of AT_1 receptors may contribute to the pathogenesis of hypertension in these rats.[109] In Ang II-infused rats studied with in vitro autoradiography, there were differential responses with significant decreases in glomeruli and inner stripe but not in proximal tubules.[110] Furthermore, ACE abundance was significantly increased on brush borders of proximal tubules of Ang II-infused rats.[54] Thus, vascular and glomerular AT_1 receptors are down-regulated, but the proximal tubular receptors are either up-regulated or not significantly altered in Ang II-dependent hypertension.

The AT_2 receptor is highly expressed in human and rodent kidney mesenchyme during fetal life and decreases dramatically after birth.[111] AT_2 receptors have been localized to the glomerular epithelial cells, proximal tubules, collecting ducts, and parts of the renal vasculature of the adult rat.[102,108] AT_2 receptor activation is thought to counteract AT_1 receptor effects by stimulating formation of bradykinin and nitric oxide leading to increases in interstitial fluid concentration of cyclic guanosine monophosphate (cGMP).[112,113] AT_2 receptor activation appears to influence proximal tubule sodium reabsorption either by a cell membrane receptor-mediated mechanism or via an interstitial nitric oxide-cGMP pathway.[114] Ang II infusion into AT_2 knockout mice leads to exaggerated hypertension and reductions in renal function, probably due to decreased renal interstitial fluid levels of bradykinin and cyclic GMP available to counteract the direct effect of Ang II.[115] However, blocking AT_2 receptors does not seem to alter the course of the hypertension in 2K1C Goldblatt hypertensive rats.[104]

INTRARENAL LEVELS OF ANGIOTENSIN II

Interstitial and tubular angiotensin II

Intrarenal Ang II is not distributed in a homogeneous fashion but is compartmentalized in both a regional and segmental manner.[116] Earlier studies indicated that medullary Ang II levels are higher than the cortical levels in normal rats and increase further in

Ang II-infused hypertensive rats.[76] The combination of high Ang II levels in the medulla coupled with the high density of Ang II receptors suggests that Ang II exerts a major role in regulating hemodynamics and tubular function in the medulla.[2,110] However, recent studies indicate that Ang II levels in cortex and medulla are not very different and respond in a similar manner to alterations in dietary salt intake.[117]

Within the cortex, there is distribution of Ang II in the interstitial fluid, tubular fluid, and the intracellular compartments. The interstitial as well as the intratubular compartments contribute to the disproportionately high intrarenal Ang II levels. Ang II concentrations in interstitial fluid are much higher than the plasma concentrations, with recent results suggesting values in the range of 3–5 pmol/ml.[113,118–120] Interestingly, ACE inhibitors administered either directly into the renal artery or via microdialysis probe were not able to substantially suppress the renal interstitial fluid Ang II levels, suggesting that much of the Ang II in the renal interstitial compartment is formed by ACE not easily accessed by the ACE inhibitors or via non-ACE-dependent pathways.[119,120] Increases in renal interstitial fluid Ang II levels have been reported in the wrapped kidney of rats with Grollman hypertension and in rats infused with Ang II for 2 weeks.[113,121] The high renal interstitial values indicate local regulation of Ang II formation in the renal interstitial compartment and an enhancement of interstitial Ang II production in Ang II-dependent hypertension.

Proximal tubule fluid concentrations of Ang I and Ang II are also much greater than the plasma concentrations.[30,122–126] The finding that tubular fluid samples collected from perfused segments also had Ang II concentrations similar to those measured in nonperfused tubules indicates that the proximal tubule secretes Ang II or a precursor into the proximal tubule fluid.[122] In addition to AGT, proximal tubule cells also have renin mRNA that is stimulated by a low sodium diet, which may thus act on AGT to generate Ang I.[44] Distal nephron renin mRNA and protein[46,48,50] also provides a pathway for Ang I generation from proximally delivered AGT. Furthermore, distal nephron renin regulation by Ang II differs from that in JGA cells since chronic Ang II infusion in rats enhances renin protein in principal cells of collecting ducts while suppressing renin in JGA cells.[46] Ang II stimulatory effects on collecting duct renin could help to explain the marked impairment of sodium excretion and suppression of the pressure-natriuresis relationship observed in Ang II-infused hypertensive rats.[127] Because renal AGT mRNA and protein levels are up-regulated by increases in circulating Ang II levels,[69,70,128] renin from connecting tubule and collecting duct cells could be secreted into the tubular fluid to act on proximally delivered AGT to form Ang I in the luminal fluid. In turn, the presence of ACE in the distal nephron would lead to maintained renal Ang II-generating capacity that occurs in Ang II-dependent hypertension, leading to high intrarenal Ang II and the maintenance of high blood pressure.[79,129]

The Ang II concentrations in tubular fluid from the other segments of the nephron remain unknown. Several studies support an important role for Ang II in regulating reabsorptive function in distal nephron and collecting duct segments, as well as in proximal tubule segments, which activate the Ang II receptors on the luminal borders.[30,130] A direct action of Ang II on the luminal amiloride-sensitive sodium channel (ENaC) has been reported.[131] These data indicate that when luminal distal nephron Ang II concentrations are augmented, they could contribute directly to the regulation of distal tubule and collecting duct sodium reabsorption.

Intracellular angiotensin II

Ang II is internalized via AT_1 receptor-mediated endocytosis.[28,29,132,133] Endosomal accumulation of Ang II in intermicrovillar clefts and endosomes is increased further in Ang II-infused hypertensive rats.[134] AT_1 receptor blockade prevents the endosomal accumulation even though plasma Ang II increases. The presence of Ang II in renal endosomes indicates that some of the internalized Ang II remains intact and contributes to the total Ang II content measured in tissue homogenates.[28,133–136] As shown for proximal tubule cells, endocytosis of the Ang II-AT_1 receptor complex seems to be required for the full expression of functional responses coupled to the activation of signal transduction pathways.[137,138] In Ang II-dependent hypertension, a higher fraction of the total kidney Ang II is internalized into intracellular endosomes (light endosomes as well as intramicrovillar clefts) via an AT_1 receptor-mediated process.[134]

The possible functions of the internalized Ang II remain unresolved. Ang II could be recycled and secreted in order to exert further actions by binding to Ang II receptors on the cell membranes. Ang II may also act on cytosolic receptors to stimulate inositol 1,4,5-trisphosphate (IP3) as has been described for vascular smooth muscle cells.[139] A particularly intriguing hypothesis is that Ang II migrates to the nucleus to exert genomic effects.[136] Nuclear binding sites for Ang II in renal cells have been reported.[140] The nuclear receptors were primarily of the AT_1 subtype, since they were displaced by losartan as well as saralasin. Nuclear Ang II receptor density was not altered in Ang II-infused hypertension. In transfected Chinese hamster ovary cells with an AT_{1a} receptor fused with green fluorescent protein (GFP), Ang II increased colocalization of GFP fluorescence with nuclear markers, suggesting migration of the receptor complex to the nucleus.[136] Because Ang II exerts a positive stimulation on AGT mRNA and protein production, it is possible that the intracellular Ang II may have genomic actions to regulate AGT or renin mRNA expression in proximal tubule cells.

AUGMENTATION OF INTRARENAL ANGIOTENSINOGEN AND ANGIOTENSIN II IN HYPERTENSION

Although increased internalization of Ang II contributes to the increased intrarenal Ang II in the Ang II-infused model of hypertension, the overall Ang II levels are also due to additional Ang II formation as a consequence of enhanced AGT production. In vivo and in vitro studies have shown that Ang II stimulates intrarenal AGT mRNA localized in proximal tubule cells.[70,72,141] Recent studies have shown that Ang II-infused rats have increases in renal AGT mRNA[70] and protein,[69] and an enhancement of urinary excretion rate of AGT.[142] Chronic Ang II infusions to normal rats significantly increased the urinary excretion rate of AGT in a time- and dose-dependent manner.[78] This augmentation process may be responsible for sustained or enhanced generation of AGT leading to continued intrarenal production of Ang II under conditions of elevated circulating Ang II concentrations. The intrarenally produced Ang II would be additive with the Ang II that is internalized by the AT_1 receptors, leading to the overall increased intrarenal Ang II contents.

Urinary excretion rate of AGT is closely correlated with systolic blood pressure and kidney Ang II content, but not with plasma Ang II concentration.[78,142] This increase is not due to increased proteinuria or the development of hypertension since urinary protein excretion in volume-dependent hypertensive rats was significantly increased more than in Ang II-dependent hypertensive rats; however, urinary AGT excretion was significantly lower in volume-dependent hypertensive rats than in Ang II-dependent hypertensive rats.[78] The increased amounts of intact AGT in urine in Ang II-dependent hypertension suggests augmented levels throughout the nephron. To the extent that renin and ACE are available along the nephron, the AGT provides substrate for continued Ang I generation and Ang II conversion in segments beyond the proximal tubule.[26,50,75] Thus, urinary AGT excretion rates reflect the distal nephron spillover of AGT and, accordingly, provide an index of the magnitude of the enhanced intrarenal AGT production in angiotensin-dependent hypertension.

As mentioned earlier, renin has been demonstrated on the luminal side of connecting tubule cells in the mouse and human kidneys, suggesting that renin may be secreted into the distal tubular fluid.[50] The renin in distal nephron segments is localized specifically in principal cells of collecting tubule and collecting duct segments and colocalizes with aquaporin-2.[46] Regulation of renin in the principal cells is distinct from that in JGA cells since it is up-regulated by chronic Ang II infusions.[46] Ang II-dependent up-regulation of renin protein and renin mRNA is mediated by AT_1 receptor activation because AT_1 receptor blockade prevented the increases in renin protein and mRNA.[143] These data support the concept depicted in Figure 1.3 that, in Ang-dependent hypertension, there is increased AGT secretion by the proximal tubule cells, leading to greater spillover of intact AGT into distal nephron segments. Because there is increased renin and available ACE or other enzymes that can subserve similar functions, there would be enhanced distal tubular formation of Ang II and increased Ang II-dependent stimulation of distal sodium reabsorption rate.[79,131] This may help explain the markedly enhanced sodium reabsorption and suppression of pressure natriuresis that has been shown in Ang II-infused rats.[127] Ang I added to the luminal surface of collecting ducts can be converted to Ang II to activate ENaC, thus providing direct evidence of conversion of Ang I to Ang II in distal nephron segments.[129] These results add to the growing body of evidence that the intratubular RAS may be independently regulated and of substantial importance in regulating sodium reabsorption in both proximal and distal nephron segments. Inappropriate enhancement of the system may contribute to the progressive development of hypertension in high Ang II states.

Collectively, the experiments evaluating the regulation of urinary AGT excretion rates indicate that there is a quantitative relationship between urinary AGT and intrarenal AGT and Ang II production. When intrarenal AGT formation rate is increased, some of the increased AGT secreted into the tubular fluid spills over into the distal tubule and eventually into the urine. Renin from collecting tubule cells acts on AGT to form Ang I. Ang I can be converted to Ang II by ACE present in the tubular fluid of collecting ducts to allow activation of luminal AT_1 receptors and stimulation of sodium transport.[131] Further enhancement of this Ang II-mediated effect develops as a consequence of up-regulation of ENaC.[144]

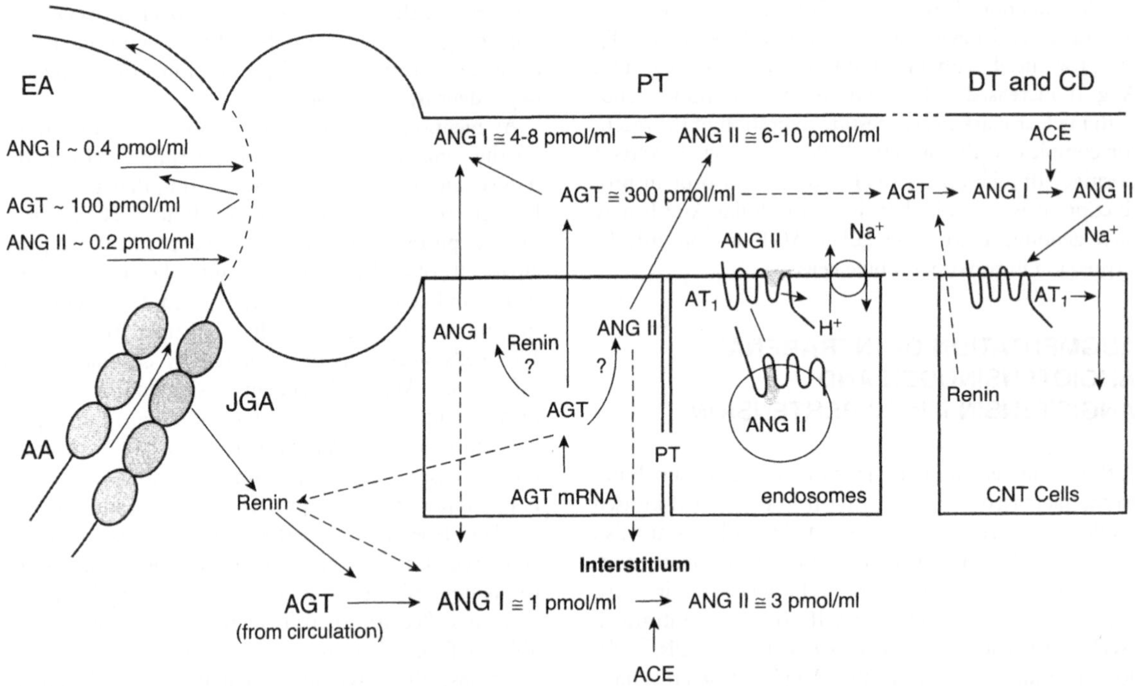

Figure 1.3 Intrarenal and intratubular processing of the renin-angiotensin system. All components of the renin-angiotensin system are present in the kidney providing multiple pathways for enhanced intrarenal Ang II formation. PT, proximal tubule; DT, distal tubule; CD, collecting duct; AGT, angiotensinogen; JGA, juxtaglomerular apparatus; AA, afferent arteriole; EA, efferent arteriole; ACE, angiotensin converting enzyme

CONCLUDING COMMENTS AND PERSPECTIVE

Recent findings have stimulated interest in the molecular mechanisms regulating the intrarenal and intratubular concentrations of Ang II and related peptides. It is becoming apparent that intratubular and interstitial Ang II are regulated independently from the circulating Ang II. The powerful actions of intrarenal Ang II acting via stimulation of AT_1 receptors on the vascular, glomerular, and tubular structures provide a synchronous cascade of effects contributing to the ability of the kidney to retain over 99% of the filtered sodium. From a functional perspective, the effects of Ang II not only on proximal nephron reabsorption but also on distal nephron transport function coupled with the associated actions of elevated aldosterone levels markedly increase the sodium-retaining capability of the kidney. When activated in a physiologically appropriate setting under conditions of volume contraction or salt-deficient states, these actions can be life-saving. When inappropriately maintained or augmented, however, these effects contribute to the development and maintenance of hypertension. Furthermore, the sustained increases in intrarenal Ang II in a setting of hypertension can lead to progressive renal injury, proliferation and fibrosis associated with activation of several major cytokines and growth factors.[16,17,145–147]

ACKNOWLEDGMENTS

The authors' studies cited in this article have been supported by grants from NHLBI, NCRR, Health Excellence Fund of the Louisiana Board of Regents and the American Heart Association. We acknowledge with appreciation the assistance of Debbie Olavarrieta for preparation of the manuscript and figures.

REFERENCES

1. Mitchell KD, Navar LG. Intrarenal actions of angiotensin II in the pathogenesis of experimental hypertension. In: Laragh JH, Brenner BM (eds). Hypertension: Pathophysiology, Diagnosis, and Management 2nd edn. New York: Raven Press, 1995; pp 1437–50.
2. Navar LG, Harrison-Bernard LM, Imig JD et al. Renal actions of angiotensin II at AT_1 receptor blockers. In: Epstein M, Brunner HR (eds). Angiotensin II Receptor Antagonists. Philadelphia: Hanley & Belfus, 2000; pp 189–214.
3. Urata H, Nishimura H, Ganten D. Chymase-dependent angiotensin II forming system in humans. Am J Hypertens 1996; 9: 277–84.
4. Chen LY, Li P, He Q et al. Transgenic study of the function of chymase in heart remodeling. J Hypertens 2002; 20: 2047–55.
5. Tokuyama H, Hayashi K, Matsuda H et al. Differential regulation of elevated renal angiotensin II in chronic renal ischemia. Hypertension 2002; 40: 34–40.
6. Huang XR, Chen WY, Truong LD et al. Chymase is upregulated in diabetic nephropathy: implications for an alternative pathway of angiotensin II-mediated diabetic renal and vascular disease. J Am Soc Nephrol 2003; 14: 1738–47.
7. Chappell MC, Tallant EA, Diz DI et al. The renin-angiotensin system and cardiovascular homeostasis. In: Husain A, Graham RM (eds). Drugs, Enzymes and Receptors of the Renin-Angiotensin System: Celebrating a Century of Discovery. Reading: Harwood Academic Publishers, 2000; pp 3–22.
8. Ardaillou R, Chansel D. Synthesis and effects of active fragments of angiotensin II. Kidney Int 1997; 52: 1458–68.
9. Fukamizu A. Genomic expression systems on hierarchy and network leading to hypertension: long on history, short on facts. Hypertens Res 2000; 23: 545–52.
10. Donoghue M, Hsieh F, Baronas E et al. A novel angiotensin-converting enzyme-related carboxypeptidase (ACE2) converts angiotensin I to angiotensin 1-9. Circ Res 2000; 87: E1–E9.
11. Crackower MA, Sarao R, Oudit GY et al. Angiotensin-converting enzyme 2 is an essential regulator of heart function. Nature 2002; 417: 822–8.
12. Ferrario CM. Contribution of Angiotensin-(1-7) to cardiovascular physiology and pathology. Curr Hypertens Rep 2003; 5: 129–34.
13. Corvol P, Jeunemaitre X, Charru A et al. Role of the renin-angiotensin system in blood pressure regulation and in human hypertension: new insights from molecular genetics. Recent Prog Horm Res 1995; 50: 287–308.
14. Ma X, Chapleau MW, Whiteis CA et al. Angiotensin selectively activates a subpopulation of postganglionic sympathetic neurons in mice. Circ Res 2001; 88: 787–93.
15. Wolf G, Ziyadeh F. The role of angiotensin II in diabetic nephropathy: emphasis on nonhemodynamic mechanisms. Am Kidney Dis 1997; 29: 153–63.
16. Ruiz-Ortega M, Lorenzo O, Ruperez M et al. Angiotensin II activates nuclear transcription factor κB through AT_1 and AT_2 in vascular smooth muscle cells. Circ Res 2000; 86: 1266–72.
17. Wolf G. The Renin-angiotensin System and Progression of Renal Diseases, Vol. 135. Hamburg: Karger, 2002, pp 1–268.
18. Ruiz-Ortega M, Bustos C, Egido J et al. Angiotensin II participates in mononuclear cell recruitment in experimental immune complex nephritis through nuclear factor-KB activation and monocyte chemoattractant protein-1 synthesis. J Immunol 1998; 161: 430–9.
19. Shao J, Nangaku M, Miyata T et al. Imbalance of T-cell subsets in angiotensin II-infused hypertensive rats with kidney injury. Hypertension 2003; 42: 31–8.
20. Navar LG, Inscho EW, Majid SA et al. Paracrine regulation of the renal microcirculation. Physiol Rev 1996; 76: 425–536.
21. Carretero OA, Scicli AG. Local hormonal factors (intracrine, autocrine, and paracrine) in hypertension. Hypertension 1991; 18 (Suppl I): I-58–I-69.
22. Re RN. The intracrine hypothesis and intracellular peptide hormone action. Bioessays 2003; 25: 401–9.
23. Re RN. Intracellular renin and the nature of intracrine enzymes. Hypertension 2003; 42: 117–22.
24. Cook JL, Zhang Z, Re RN. In vitro evidence for an intracellular site of angiotensin action. Circ Res 2001; 89: 1138–46.
25. Campbell DJ, Kladis A, Skinner SL et al. Characterization of angitoensin peptides in plasma of anephric man. J Hypertens 1991; 9: 265–74.
26. Davisson RL, Ding Y, Stec DE et al. Novel mechanism of hypertension revealed by cell-specific targeting of human angiotensinogen in transgenic mice. Physiol Genomics 1999; 1: 3–9.
27. Baltatu O, Silva JA Jr, Ganten D et al. The brain renin-angiotensin system modulates angiotensin II-induced hypertension and cardiac hypertrophy. Hypertension 2000; 35: 409–12.
28. Imig JD, Navar GL, Zou LX et al. Renal endosomes contain angiotensin peptides, converting enzyme, and AT_{1A} receptors. Am J Physiol 1999; 277: F303–F311.
29. Ingert C, Grima M, Coquard C et al. Contribution of angiotensin II internalization to intrarenal angiotensin II levels in rats. Am J Physiol Renal Physiol 2002; 283: F1003–F1010.
30. Navar LG, Harrison-Bernard LM, Wang C-T et al. Concentrations and actions of intraluminal angiotensin II. J Am Soc Nephrol 1999; 10: S189–S195.
31. van Kats JP, Schalekamp MA, Verdouw PD et al. Intrarenal angiotensin II: interstitial and cellular levels and site of production. Kidney Int 2001; 60: 2311–17.
32. Wilcox CS, Peart WS. Release of renin and angiotensin II into plasma and lymph during hyperchloremia. Am J Physiol 1987; 253: F734–F741.
33. Dzau VJ, Wilcox CS, Sands K et al. Dog inactive renin: biochemical characterization and secretion into renal plasma and lymph. Am J Physiol 1986; 250: E55–E61.
34. Field LJ, McGowan RA, Dickinson DP et al. Tissue and gene specificity of mouse renin expression. Hypertension 1984; 6: 597–603.
35. Catanzaro DF, Mullins JJ, Morris BJ. The biosynthetic pathway of renin in mouse submandibular gland. J Biol Chem 1983; 258: 7364–8.
36. Sealey JE, Laragh JH. 'Prorenin' in human plasma? Circ Res 1975; 36: 10–16.
37. Prescott G, Silversides DW, Reudelhuber TL. Tissue activity of circulating prorenin. Am J Hypertens 2002; 15: 280–5.
38. Nguyen G, Delarue F, Burckle C et al. Pivotal role of the renin/prorenin receptor in angiotensin II production and cellular responses to renin. J Clin Invest 2002; 109: 1417–27.
39. Nguyen G, Delarue F, Berrou J et al. Specific receptor binding of renin on human mesangial cells in culture increases plasminogen activator inhibitor-1 antigen. Kidney Int 1996; 50: 1897–903.
40. Sealey JE, Catanzaro DF, Lavin TN et al. Specific prorenin/renin binding (ProBP). Identification and characterization of a novel membrane site. Am J Hypertens 1996; 9: 491–502.
41. Danser AHJ, Saris JJ. Prorenin uptake in the heart: a prerequisite for local angiotensin generation? J Mol Cell Cardiol 2002; 34: 1463–72.
42. Gomez RA, Lynch KR, Chevalier RL et al. Renin and angiotensinogen gene expression and intrarenal renin distribution during ACE inhibition. Am J Physiol 1988; 254: F900–F906.

43. Taugner R, Mannek E, Nobiling R et al. Coexistence of renin and angiotensin II in epitheloid cell secretory granules of rat kidney. Histochemistry 1984; 81: 39–45.
44. Tank JE, Henrich WL, Moe OW. Regulation of glomerular and proximal tubule renin mRNA by chronic changes in dietary NaCl. Am J Physiol 1997; 273: F892–F898.
45. Moe OW, Ujiie K, Star RA et al. Renin expression in renal proximal tubule. J Clin Invest 1993; 91: 774–9.
46. Prieto-Carrasquero MC, Harrison-Bernard LM, Kobori H et al. Enhancement of collecting duct renin in angiotensin II-dependent hypertensive rats. Hypertension 2004; 44: 223–9.
47. Henrich WL, McAllister EA, Eskue A et al. Renin regulation in cultured proximal tubular cells. Hypertension 1996; 27: 1337–40.
48. Lantelme P, Rohrwasser A, Gociman B et al. Effects of dietary sodium and genetic background on angiotensinogen and renin in mouse. Hypertension 2002; 39: 1007–14.
49. Gilbert RE, Wu LL, Kelly DJ et al. Pathological expression of renin and angiotensin II in the renal tubule after subtotal nephrectomy. Implications for the pathogenesis of tubulointerstitial fibrosis. Am J Pathol 1999; 155: 429–40.
50. Rohrwasser A, Morgan T, Dillon HF et al. Elements of a paracrine tubular renin-angiotensin system along the entire nephron. Hypertension 1999; 34: 1265–74.
51. Bernstein KE, Xiao HD, Adams JW et al. Establishing the role of angiotensin-converting enzyme in renal function and blood pressure control through the analysis of genetically modified mice. J Am Soc Nephrol 2005; 16: 583–91.
52. Schulz WW, Hagler HK, Buja LM et al. Ultrastructural localization of angiotensin I-converting enzyme (EC 3.4.15.1) and neutral metalloendopeptidase (EC 3.4.24.11) in the proximal tubule of the human kidney. Lab Invest 1988; 59: 789–97.
53. Erdos EG. Angiotensin I converting enzyme and the changes in our concepts through the years. Hypertension 1990; 16: 363–70.
54. Vio CP, Jeanneret VA. Local induction of angiotensin-converting enzyme in the kidney as a mechanism of progressive renal diseases. Kidney Int Suppl 2003; 57–63.
55. Metzger R, Bohle RM, Pauls K et al. Angiotensin-converting enzyme in non-neoplastic kidney diseases. Kidney Int 1999; 56: 1442–54.
56. Roks AJ, Henning RH. Angiotensin peptides: ready to re(de)fine the angiotensin system? J Hypertens 2003; 21: 1269–71.
57. Santos RA, Simoes e Silva AC, Maric C et al. Angiotensin-(1-7) is an endogenous ligand for the G protein-coupled receptor Mas. Proc Natl Acad Sci U S A 2003; 100: 8258–63.
58. Stegbauer J, Vonend O, Oberhauser V et al. Effects of angiotensin-(1-7) and other bioactive components of the renin-angiotensin system on vascular resistance and noradrenaline release in rat kidney. J Hypertens 2003; 21: 1391–9.
59. Tipnis SR, Hooper NM, Hyde R et al. A human homolog of angiotensin-converting enzyme. Cloning and functional expression as a captopril-insensitive carboxypeptidase. J Biol Chem 2000; 275: 33238–43.
60. Zhang H, Wada J, Hida K et al. Collectrin, a collecting duct-specific transmembrane glycoprotein, is a novel homolog of ACE2 and is developmentally regulated in embryonic kidneys. J Biol Chem 2001; 276: 17132–9.
61. Goodfriend TL. Angiotensinases. In: JIS, Nichols MG, (eds). Renin-Angiotensin System. (Robertson London: Gower Medical Publishers 1993, pp 1–5.
62. Tharaux P-L, Chatziantoniou C, Fakhouri F et al. Angiotensin II activates collagen I gene through a mechanism involving the MAP/ER kinase pathway. Hypertension 2000; 36: 330–6.
63. Opie LH, Sack MN. Enhanced angiotensin II activity in heart failure – reevaluation of the counterregulatory hypothesis of receptor subtypes. Circ Res 2001; 88: 654–8.
64. Touyz RM, Schiffrin EL. Signal transduction mechanisms mediating the physiological and pathophysiological actions of angiotensin II in vascular smooth muscle cells. Pharmacol Rev 2000; 52: 639–72.
65. Ferrario CM, Averill DB, Brosnihan KB et al. Vasopeptidase inhibition and Ang-(1-7) in the spontaneously hypertensive rat. Kidney Int 2002; 62: 1349–57.
66. Unger T, Sandmann S. Angiotensin receptor blocker selectivity at the AT_1- and AT_2-receptors: conceptual and clinical effects. JRAAS 2000; 1: 6–9.
67. Carey RM, Wang ZQ, Siragy HM. Role of the angiotensin type 2 receptor in the regulation of blood pressure and renal function. Hypertension 2000; 35: 155–63.
68. Carey RM, Siragy HM. The intrarenal renin-angiotensin system and diabetic nephropathy. Trends Endocrinol Metab 2003; 14: 274–81.
69. Kobori H, Harrison-Bernard LM, Navar LG. Enhancement of angiotensinogen expression in angiotensin II-dependent hypertension. Hypertension 2001; 37: 1329–35.
70. Kobori H, Harrison-Bernard LM, Navar LG. Expression of angiotensinogen mRNA and protein in angiotensin II-dependent hypertension. J Am Soc Nephrol 2001; 12: 431–9.
71. Darby IA, Sernia C. In situ hybridization and immunohistochemistry of renal angiotensinogen in neonatal and adult rat kidneys. Cell Tissue Res 1995; 281: 197–206.
72. Ingelfinger JR, Jung F, Diamant D et al. Rat proximal tubule cell line transformed with origin-defective SV40 DNA: autocrine ANG II feedback. Am J Physiol 1999; 276: F218–F227.
73. Lalouel J-M, Rohrwasser A, Terreros D et al. Angiotensinogen in essential hypertension: from genetics to nephrology. J Am Soc Nephrol 2001; 12: 606–15.
74. Loghman-Adham M, Rohrwasser A, Helin C et al. A conditionally immortalized cell line from murine proximal tubule. Kidney Int 1997; 52: 229–39.
75. Ding Y, Davisson RL, Hardy DO et al. The kidney androgen-regulated protein promoter confers renal proximal tubule cell-specific and highly androgen-responsive expression on the human angiotensinogen gene in transgenic mice. J Biol Chem 1997; 272: 28142–8.
76. Navar LG, Imig JD, Zou L et al. Intrarenal production of angiotensin II. Semin Nephrol 1997; 17: 412–22.
77. Jeunemaitre X, Ménard J, Clauser E et al. Angiotensinogen: molecular biology and genetics. In: Laragh JH, Brenner BM (eds). Hypertension: Pathophysiology, Diagnosis, and Management, 2nd edn, Vol. 1. New York: Raven Press, 2000; pp 1653–65.
78. Kobori H, Nishiyama A, Harrison-Bernard LM et al. Urinary angiotensinogen as an indicator of intrarenal angiotensin status in hypertension. Hypertension 2003; 41: 42–9.
79. Casarini DE, Boim MA, Stella RCR et al. Angiotensin I-converting enzyme activity in tubular fluid along the rat nephron. Am J Physiol 1997; 272: F405–F409.
80. Modrall JG, Sadjadi J, Brosnihan KB et al. Depletion of tissue angiotensin-converting enzyme differentially influences the intrarenal and urinary expression of angiotensin peptides. Hypertension 2004; 43: 849–53.
81. Iwai N, Inagami T. Identification of two subtypes in rat type I angiotensin II receptor. FEBS Lett 1992; 298: 257–60.
82. Sasamura H, Hein L, Krieger JE et al. Cloning, characterization, and expression of two angiotensin receptor (AT-1) isoforms from the mouse genome. Biochem Biophys Res Communi 1992; 185: 253–9.
83. Iwai N, Yamano Y, Chaki S et al. Rat angiotensin II receptor: cDNA sequence and regulation of the gene expression. Biochem Biophys Res Commun 1991; 177: 299–304.

84. Murphy TJ, Alexander RW, Griendling KK et al. Isolation of a cDNA encoding the vascular type-1 angiotensin II receptor. Nature (Lond) 1991; 351: 233–6.
85. Nakajima M, Mukoyama M, Pratt RE et al. Cloning of cDNA and analysis of the gene for mouse angiotensin II type 2 receptor. Biochem Biophys Res Commun 1993; 197: 393–9.
86. Tsuzuki S, Ichiki T, Nakakubo H et al. Molecular cloning and expression of the gene encoding human angiotensin II type 2 receptor. Biochem Biophys Res Commun 1994; 200: 1449–54.
87. Ito M, Oliverio MI, Mannon PJ et al. Regulation of blood pressure by the type 1A angiotensin II receptor gene. Proc Natl Acad Sci USA 1995; 92: 3521–5.
88. Cervenka L, Mitchell KD, Oliverio MI et al. Renal function in the AT_{1A} receptor knockout mouse during normal and volume-expanded conditions. Kidney Int 1999; 56: 1855–62.
89. Oliverio MI, Best CF, Smithies O et al. Regulation of sodium balance and blood pressure by the AT(1A) receptor for angiotensin II. Hypertension 2000; 35: 550–4.
90. Meister B, Lippoldt A, Bunnemann B et al. Cellular expression of angiotensin type-1 receptor mRNA in the kidney. Kidney Int 1993; 44: 331–6.
91. Tufro-McReddie A, Harrison JK, Everett AD et al. Ontogeny of type 1 angiotensin II receptor gene expression in the rat. J Clin Invest 1993; 91: 530–7.
92. Gasc J-M, Monnot C, Clauser E et al. Co-expression of type 1 angiotensin II receptor (AT_1R) and renin mRNAs in juxtaglomerular cells of the rat kidney. Endocrinology 1993; 132: 2723–5.
93. Bouby N, Hus-Citharel A, Marchetti J et al. Expression of type 1 angiotensin II receptor subytpes and angiotensin II-induced calcium mobilization along the rat nephron. J Am Soc Nephrol 1997; 8: 1658–67.
94. Ruan XP, Wagner C, Chatziantoniou C et al. Regulation of angiotensin II receptor AT_1 subtypes in renal afferent arterioles during chronic changes in sodium diet. J Clin Invest 1997; 99: 1072–81.
95. Prieto M, Dipp S, Meleg-Smith S et al. Ureteric bud derivatives express angiotensinogen and AT_1 receptors. Physiol Genomics 2001; 6: 29–37.
96. Douglas JG. Angiotensin receptor subtypes of the kidney cortex. Am J Physiol 1987; 253: F1–F7.
97. Mendelsohn FAO, Dunbar M, Allen A et al. Angiotensin II receptors in the kidney. Fed Proc 1986; 45: 1420–5.
98. Burns KD, Inagami T, Harris RC. Cloning of a rabbit kidney cortex AT_1 angiotensin II receptor that is present in proximal tubule epithelium. Am J Physiol 1993; 264: F645–F654.
99. Paxton WG, Runge M, Horaist C et al. Immunohistochemical localization of rat angiotensin II AT_1 receptor. Am J Physiol 1993; 264: F989–F995.
100. Zhuo J, Alcorn D, McCausland J et al. Localization and regulation of angiotensin II receptors in renomedullary interstitial cells. Kidney Int 1994; 46: 1483–5.
101. Harrison-Bernard LM, Navar LG, Ho MM et al. Immunohistochemical localization of ANG II AT_1 receptor in adult rat kidney using a monoclonal antibody. Am J Physiol 1997; 273: F170–F177.
102. Miyata N, Park F, Li XF et al. Distribution of angiotensin AT_1 and AT_2 receptor subtypes in the rat kidney. Am J Physiol 1999; 277: F437–F446.
103. Harrison-Bernard LM, Cook AK, Oliverio MI et al. Renal segmental microvascular responses to ANG II in AT1A receptor null mice. Am J Physiol Renal Physiol 2003; 284: F538–F545.
104. Cervenka L, Horacek V, Vaneckova I et al. Essential role of AT_{1A} receptor in the development of 2K1C hypertension. Hypertension 2002; 40: 735–41.
105. Cheng HF, Becker BN, Burns KD et al. Angiotensin II upregulates type-1 angiotensin II receptors in renal proximal tubule. J Clin Invest 1995; 95: 2012–19.
106. Amiri F, Garcia R. Renal angiotensin II receptor regulation in two-kidney, one clip hypertensive rats. Effect of ACE inhibition. Hypertension 1997; 30 (Part 1): 337–44.
107. Harrison-Bernard LM, El-Dahr SS, O'Leary DF et al. Regulation of angiotensin II type 1 receptor mRNA and protein in angiotensin II-induced hypertension. Hypertension 1999; 33 (Part II): 340–6.
108. Wang Z-Q, Millatt LJ, Heiderstadt NT et al. Differential regulation of renal angiotensin subtype AT_{1A} and AT_2 receptor protein in rats with angiotensin-dependent hypertension. Hypertension 1999; 33: 96–101.
109. Zhuo J, Ohishi M, Mendelsohn FAO. Roles of AT_1 and AT_2 receptors in the hypertensive Ren-2 gene transgenic rat kidney. Hypertension 1999; 33 [Part II]: 347–53.
110. Harrison-Bernard LM, Zhuo J, Kobori H et al. Intrarenal AT_1 receptor and ACE binding in angiotensin II-induced hypertensive rats. Am J Physiol Renal Physiol 2001; 281: F19–F25.
111. Norwood VF, Garmey M, Wolford J et al. Novel expression and regulation of the renin-angiotensin system in metanephric organ culture. Am J Physiol Regul Integr Comp Physiol 2000; 279: R522–R530.
112. Siragy HM, Jaffa AA, Margolius HS. Bradykinin B_2 receptor modulates renal prostaglandin E_2 and nitric oxide. Hypertension 1997; 29: 757–62.
113. Siragy HM, Carey RM. Protective role of the angiotensin AT_2 receptor in a renal wrap hypertension model. Hypertension 1999; 33: 1237–42.
114. Jin XH, Siragy HM, Carey RM. Renal interstitial cGMP mediates natriuresis by direct tubule mechanism. Hypertension 2001; 38: 309–16.
115. Siragy HM, Inagami T, Ichiki T et al. Sustained hypersensitivity to angiotensin II and its mechanism in mice lacking the subtype-2 (AT_2) angiotensin receptor. Proc.Natl Acad Sci USA 1999; 96: 6506–10.
116. Navar LG, Harrison-Bernard LM, Imig JD. Compartmentalization of intrarenal angiotensin II. In: Ulfendahl HR, Aurell M (eds). Renin-Angiotensin. London: Portland Press, 1998, 193–208.
117. Ingert C, Grima M, Coquard C et al. Effects of dietary salt changes on renal renin-angiotensin system in rats. Am J Physiol Renal Physiol 2002; 283: F995–F1002.
118. Siragy HM, Howell NL, Ragsdale NV et al. Renal interstitial fluid angiotensin: modulation by anesthesia, epinephrine, sodium depletion and renin inhibition. Hypertension 1995; 25: 1021–4.
119. Nishiyama A, Seth DM, Navar LG. Renal interstitial fluid concentrations of angiotensins I and II in anesthetized rats. Hypertension 2002; 39: 129–34.
120. Nishiyama A, Seth DM, Navar LG. Renal interstitial fluid angiotensin I and angiotensin II concentrations during local angiotensin-converting enzyme inhibition. J Am Soc Nephrol 2002; 13: 2207–12.
121. Nishiyama A, Seth DE, Navar LG. Renal interstitial concentrations of angiotensin I and angiotensin II in angiotensin II-infused hypertensive rats. J Am Soc Nephrol 2001; 12: 574A.
122. Braam B, Mitchell KD, Fox J et al. Proximal tubular secretion of angiotensin II in rats. Am J Physiol 1993; 264: F891–F898.
123. Navar LG, Lewis L, Hymel A et al. Tubular fluid concentrations and kidney contents of angiotensins I and II in anesthetized rats. J Am Soc Nephrol 1994; 5: 1153–8.
124. Mitchell KD, Jacinto SM, Mullins JJ. Proximal tubular fluid, kidney, and plasma levels of angiotensin II in hypertensive ren-2 transgenic rats. Am J Physiol 1997; 273: F246–F253.

125. Wang C-T, Navar LG, Mitchell KD. Proximal tubular fluid angiotensin II levels in angiotensin II-induced hypertensive rats. J Hypertens 2003; 21: 353–60.
126. Cervenka L, Wang C-T, Mitchell KD et al. Proximal tubular angiotensin II levels and renal functional responses to AT_1 receptor blockade in nonclipped kidneys of Goldblatt hypertensive rats. Hypertension 1999; 33: 102–7.
127. Wang C-T, Chin SY, Navar LG. Impairment of pressure-natriuresis and renal autoregulation in ANG II-infused hypertensive rats. Am J Physiol Renal Physiol 2000; 279: F319–F325.
128. Kobori H, Prieto-Carrasquero MC, Ozawa Y et al. AT_1 receptor-mediated augmentation of intrarenal angiotensinogen in angiotensin II-dependent hypertension. Hypertension 2004; 43: 1126–32.
129. Komlosi P, Fuson AL, Fintha A et al. Angiotensin I conversion to angiotensin II stimulates cortical collecting duct sodium transport. Hypertension 2003; 42: 195–9.
130. Wang T, Giebisch G. Effects of angiotensin II on electrolyte transport in the early and late distal tubule in rat kidney. Am J Physiol 1996; 271: F143–F149.
131. Peti-Peterdi J, Warnock DG, Bell PD. Angiotensin II directly stimulates ENaC activity in the cortical collecting duct via AT(1) receptors. J Am Soc Nephrol 2002; 13: 1131–5.
132. Zou L, Imig JD, Hymel A et al. Renal uptake of circulating angiotensin II in Val^5-angiotensin II infused rats is mediated by AT_1 receptor. Am J Hypertens 1998; 11: 570–8.
133. van Kats JP, de Lannoy LM, Danser AHJ et al. Angiotensin II type 1 (AT_1) receptor-mediated accumulation of angiotensin II in tissues and its intracellular half-life in vivo. Hypertension 1997; 30 (Part 1): 42–9.
134. Zhuo JL, Imig JD, Hammond TG et al. Ang II accumulation in rat renal endosomes during Ang II-induced hypertension: role of AT(1) receptor. Hypertension 2002; 39: 116–21.
135. Hein L, Meinel L, Pratt RE et al. Intracellular trafficking of angiotensin II and its AT_1 and AT_2 receptors: evidence for selective sorting of receptor and ligand. Mol Endocrinol 1997; 11: 1266–77.
136. Chen R, Mukhin YV, Garnovskaya MN et al. A functional angiotensin II receptor-GFP fusion protein: evidence for agonist-dependent nuclear translocation. Am J Physiol Renal Physiol 2000; 279: F440–F448.
137. Linas SL. Role of receptor mediated endocytosis in proximal tubule epithelial function. Kidney Int 1997; 52 (Suppl 61): S-18–S-21.
138. Becker BN, Cheng H-F, Harris RC. Apical ANG II-stimulated PLA_2 activity and Na^+ flux: a potential role for Ca^{2+}-independent PLA_2. Am J Physiol 1997; 273: F554–F562.
139. Haller H, Lindschau C, Erdmann B et al. Effects of intracellular angiotensin II in vascular smooth muscle cells. Circ Res 1996; 79: 765–72.
140. Licea H, Walters MR, Navar LG. Renal nuclear angiotensin II receptors in normal and hypertensive rats. Acta Physiol Hung 2002; 89: 427–38.
141. Schunkert H, Ingelfinger JR, Jacob H et al. Reciprocal feedback regulation of kidney angiotensinogen and renin mRNA expressions by angiotensin II. Am J Physiol 1992; 263: E863–E869.
142. Kobori H, Harrison-Bernard LM, Navar LG. Urinary excretion of angiotensinogen reflects intrarenal angiotensinogen production. Kidney Int 2002; 61: 579–85.
143. Prieto-Carrasquero MC, Kobori H, Ozawa Y et al. AT_1 receptor mediated enhancement of collecting duct renin in angiotensin II-dependent hypertensive rats. Am J Physiol Renal Physiol 2005; 289: F632–7.
144. Beutler KT, Masilamani S, Turban S et al. Long-term regulation of ENaC expression in kidney by angiotensin II. Hypertension 2003; 41: 1143–50.
145. Ma L-J, Nakamura S, Whitsitt JS et al. Regression of sclerosis in aging by an angiotensin inhibition-induced decrease in PAI-1. Kidney Int 2000; 58: 2425–36.
146. Nakamura S, Nakamura I, Ma L et al. Plasminogen activator inhibitor-1 expression is regulated by the angiotensin type 1 receptor in vivo. Kidney Int 2000; 58: 251–9.
147. Taal MW, Chertow GM, Rennke HG et al. Mechanisms underlying renoprotection during renin-angiotensin system blockade. Am J Physiol Renal Physiol 2001; 280: F343–F355.

2

Angiotensin signaling in hypertension

Jing Pan and Kenneth M Baker

INTRODUCTION

A major hemodynamic abnormality in hypertension is increased peripheral vascular resistance due to changes in vascular reactivity and structural remodeling. Both in vivo and in vitro data suggest that the vasoconstrictor peptide angiotensin II (Ang II) has an important role in these processes. It has been recently recognized that Ang II, in addition to having a role in the regulation of salt–fluid homeostasis, is also a growth factor and contributes to the regulation of cellular hypertrophy or proliferation and extracellular matrix formation. At the cellular level, Ang II stimulates vascular smooth muscle cell growth, increases collagen deposition, induces inflammation, increases contractility, and decreases dilation. Molecular mechanisms associated with these changes in hypertension include up-regulation of many signaling pathways, which include the following: tyrosine kinases, mitogen-activated protein kinases, RhoA/Rho kinase, and increased generation of reactive oxygen species. In mammalian cells, Ang II mediates effects by at least two high-affinity, plasma membrane receptors, AT_1 and AT_2.[1,2] Two other Ang II receptors have been described, AT_3 and AT_4. In this chapter, we will focus on the signaling pathways mediated by AT_1 and AT_2.

AT_1-MEDIATED INTRACELLULAR SIGNALING

AT_1 receptor

AT_1, which was first cloned in 1991,[1,3] consists of 359 amino acids and has a molecular mass of 41 kDa. Two AT_1 receptor subtypes have been described in rodents, AT_{1a} and AT_{1b}, with greater than 94% amino acid sequence identity,[4] and which have similar pharmacological properties and tissue distribution patterns. The human AT_1 gene was mapped to chromosome 3.[5] AT_1 receptors are present at high levels in smooth muscle cells and relatively low levels in the adventitia in the human vasculature. It has been demonstrated that all of the known biological actions of Ang II, including elevation of blood pressure, vasoconstriction, increase in cardiac contractility, release of aldosterone and vasopressin, renal tubular sodium reabsorption, stimulation of sympathetic transmission and cellular growth, are mediated by AT_1.[6] Thus, the molecular and cellular actions of Ang II in cardiovascular diseases are almost exclusively mediated by AT_1. AT_1 belongs to the 7-transmembrane class of G protein-coupled receptors. Four cysteine residues are located in the extracellular domain, which represent sites of disulfide bridge formation and are critical tertiary structure determinants. The transmembrane domain and the extracellular loop have an important role in Ang II binding.[7] Like most G protein-coupled receptors, AT_1 is also subject to internalization when stimulated by Ang II, a process dependent on specific residues located on the cytoplasmic tail.[8] AT_1 receptors interact with various heterotrimeric G proteins including Gq/11, Gi, Gα12 and Gα13. The different G protein isoforms couple to distinct signaling cascades.

Classical signal transduction events

There are five classical signal transduction mechanisms for AT_1: activation of phospholipase A_2, phospholipase C, phospholipase D, and L-type Ca^{2+} channels, and inhibition of adenylyl cyclase. AT_1 couples to $G_{q/11}$ protein, and induces activation of phospholipase C-β, resulting in the generation of two secondary messengers, Ins(1,4,5)P_3 (IP3) and diacylglycerol (DAG). IP3 stimulates the release of Ca^{2+} from intracellular stores, and DAG activates protein kinase C (PKC), both of which are involved in vasoconstriction, cardiomyocyte protection, and cardiac hypertrophy.[9–12] Activation of phospholipases A_2 and D stimulates the release of arachidonic acid, the precursor molecule for the generation of prostaglandins, and is involved in the Ang II-induced growth of vascular smooth muscle cells (VSMC) and cardiac hypertrophy.[13] AT_1 couples to $G_{i/o}$ protein inhibiting adenylyl cyclase in several target tissues, thereby attenuating the production of the second messenger cAMP.[14] cAMP is a vasodilator and when production is decreased due to AT_1 activation, there is resulting vasoconstriction. Moreover, AT_1 is also involved in the opening of Ca^{2+} channels and influx of extracellular Ca^{2+} into cells,[15,16] and the activation of L-channels is mediated by AT_1 coupled to $G^{12/13}$ proteins.[17]

Mitogen-activated protein kinases

Mitogen-activated protein kinases (MAPK), found in all eukaryotes, are common participants in signal transduction pathways extending from the membrane to the nucleus. MAPK activity is regulated through a three-tiered cascade composed of a MAPK, MAPK kinase (MKK or MEK), and a MEK kinase (MAPKKK or MEKK).[18] At least four distinctly regulated groups of MAPKs are expressed in mammals, extracellular signal-related kinases (ERK)-1/2, c-Jun N-terminal kinases (JNK1/2/3), p38 proteins (p38α/β/γ/δ) and ERK5, that are activated by specific MKKs: MEK1/2 for ERK1/2, MKK3/6 for the p38, MKK4/7 for the JNKs, and MEK5 for ERK5. Each MKK, however, can be activated by more than one MEKK, increasing the complexity and diversity of MAPK signaling.[19] MAPKs have a central role in cellular responses by various stress stimuli, such as cell proliferation, apoptosis, migration, or gene expression.[20] Ang II induces phosphorylation of Ras, Raf and Shc, leading to the activation of MEKKs and MEKs, resulting in tyrosine and threonine phosphorylation of ERK1/2, JNK2 and p38.[21] Ang II-induced activation of ERK1/2 is associated with increased expression of the early response genes *c-fos*, *c-myc* and *c-jun*, DNA/protein synthesis, cell growth and differentiation and cytoskeletal organization in cardiovascular cells.[22] In addition to ERKs, Ang II activates JNKs, which regulate cardiomyocyte and VSMC growth.[23,24] Ang II induces activation of JNK via p21-activated kinase (PAK), which is dependent on intracellular Ca^{2+} mobilization and PKC activation.[25] Ang II-activated ERK1/2 and JNK have opposite growth effects in VSMC, with ERK1/2 being promoting and JNK inhibitory. Ang II also induces phosphorylation of p38, which has an important role in inflammatory responses, apoptosis, and regulation of cell growth.[26] The p38 pathway has been implicated in various pathological conditions, such as cardiac ischemia, ischemia/reperfusion injury, cardiac hypertrophy, progression of atherosclerosis, and vascular remodeling in hypertension.[26,27] Recent studies have shown that vascular gene transfer of each dominant negative mutant of MAP kinases or c-Jun, prevents intimal hyperplasia after balloon injury, which is associated with the inhibition of smooth muscle cell proliferation in the intima and the media and probably is also associated with inhibition of smooth muscle cell migration.[23] These data suggest that MAP kinases may be a promising therapeutic target for vascular remodeling.

AT_1-mediated tyrosine phosphorylation

Recent studies have shown that various tyrosine kinases play important roles in Ang II-stimulated cell proliferation and hypertrophy. Ang II stimulates phosphorylation of many receptor tyrosine kinases (RTK), such as epidermal growth factor receptor (EGFR), platelet-derived growth factor receptor (PDGFR), and insulin-like growth factor receptor (IGFR), and non-receptor tyrosine kinases including the Src family kinases, Janus kinases (JAKs), focal adhesion kinase (FAK), Ca^{2+}-dependent tyrosine kinases (e.g. Pyk2), p130Cas, and phosphoinositide 3-OH kinase (PI3K)[13,28–30] (Figure 2.1).

Src family kinases

To date at least 14 Src kinase family members have been identified, of which the 60 kDa c-Src is a prototype of the cellular members of the Src family kinases (Src, Fyn, Yes, Fgr, Lck, Lyn, Hck, Blk, and Yrk). All Src family members share common functional domains, including an N-terminal myristoylation sequence for membrane targeting, SH2 and SH3 domains for protein binding, a kinase domain, and a C-terminal noncatalytic domain.[31] c-Src is abundantly expressed in vascular smooth muscle cells and cardiomyocytes, and rapidly activated by Ang II.[32] Src has an important role in Ang II-induced phosphorylation of PLC-γ and IP_3 formation. Src, intracellular Ca^{2+}, and PKC regulate Ang II-induced phosphorylation of p130Cas, a signaling molecule involved in integrin-mediated cell adhesion. Src has also been associated with Ang II-induced activation of Pyk2 and ERKs, as well as activation of other downstream proteins including Fak, paxillin, JAK2, STAT1, caveolin, and the adapter protein, Shc.[33] Activation of c-Src is required for cytoskeletal reorganization, focal adhesion formation, cell migration, and growth. Increased activation of c-Src by Ang II may be an important mediator of cardiac hypertrophy and altered VSMC function in hypertension.

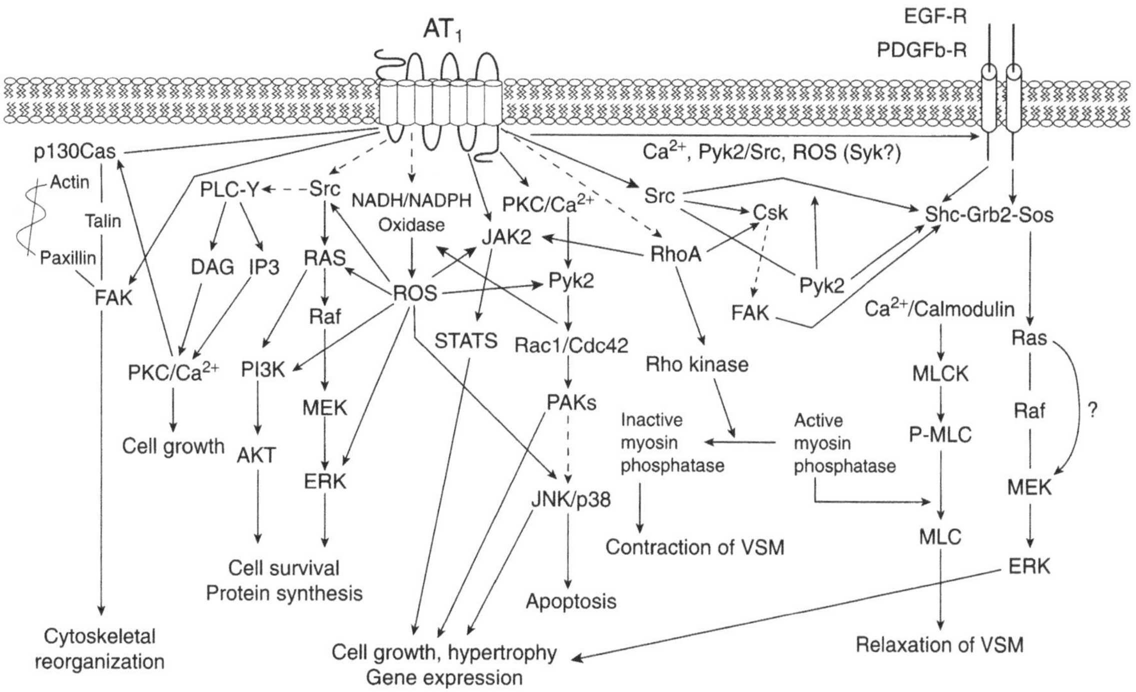

Figure 2.1 Novel signal transduction mechanisms mediated by AT_1. Ang II phosphorylates multiple tyrosine kinases, such as JAK, FAK, Pyk2, p130Cas, and PI3K. Activated tyrosine kinases phosphorylate many downstream targets including the MAPK cascade. Src associates with the adapter protein complex, Shc-GRB_2-Sos, that induces guanine nucleotide exchange on the small G protein Ras-GDP/GTP. Activated Ras interacts with Raf, resulting in phosphorylation of MEK, which in turn phosphorylates MAPKs. RhoA/Rho kinase is also activated through AT_1 receptors. In addition, Ang II influences activity of receptor tyrosine kinases (RTK), such as EGFR, and PDGFR. The transactivated EGFR serves as a scaffold for downstream adapters, leading to activation of MAP kinases. Intracellular reactive oxygen species (ROS) modify the activity of tyrosine kinases, such as Src, Ras, JAK2, Pyk2, PI3K, and EGFR, as well as MAPKs, particularly p38 and JNK

JAK/STAT activation

There are four JAK proteins in mammalian cells, JAK1, JAK2, JAK3, and TYK2.[34] JAKs bind specifically to intracellular domains of cytokine receptor signaling chains and catalyze ligand-induced phosphorylation of themselves and of intracellular tyrosine residues on the receptor, creating tyrosine-phosphorylated docking sites for signal transducers and activators of transcription (STATs). Tyrosine phosphorylation of STATs leads to STAT homo- and heterodimerization. STAT dimers are rapidly transported from the cytoplasm to the nucleus, where they activate gene transcription. AT_1 activates JAK2 and TYK2 in the cardiovascular system.[35] In VSMCs, JAKs apparently phosphorylate STAT proteins p91/84 (STAT1a/β), p113 (STAT2), and p92 (STAT3) in response to Ang II, suggesting a possible role for this pathway in the activation of early growth response genes by Ang II. The JAK/STAT signaling pathway activates early growth response genes, and may be a mechanism whereby Ang II influences vascular and cardiac growth, remodeling, and repair.[36,37] STATs also have an important role in angiotensinogen gene expression in cardiac myocytes. Ang II-induced angiotensinogen gene up-regulation by STAT3 and STAT6 activation may constitute part of an autocrine, positive feedback loop that contributes to cardiac hypertrophy in vivo.[35]

FAK and PYK 2 activation

FAK is a cytoplasmic protein tyrosine kinase localized to regions called focal adhesions. Many stimuli can induce tyrosine phosphorylation and activation of FAK, including integrins and growth factors. The major site of autophosphorylation, tyrosine 397, is a docking site for the SH2 domains of Src family proteins. The other sites are phosphorylated by Src kinases.[38] As a consequence of association with c-Src, FAK undergoes further tyrosine phosphorylation, which results in FAK binding to Grb2, Sos, and Ras. This in turn leads to ERK1/2 activation. Ang II-induced activation of FAK causes translocation to sites of focal adhesions within the extracellular matrix and phosphorylation of paxillin and talin, which may be involved in the regulation of cell morphology and movement.[39] AT_1-induced FAK activation also has an important role in Ang II-mediated hypertrophic responses in cardiomyocytes and VSMC.[40] The link between the AT_1 receptor and FAK is unknown, but the Rho family of GTPases are likely important.

Another FAK family member, Pyk2, also called cell adhesion kinase-β, related adhesion focal tyrosine kinase and calcium-dependent, nonreceptor, proline-rich tyrosine kinase (the rat homolog of Pyk2), is activated by AT_1 and is dependent on increased intracellular Ca^{2+} and PKC.[39,41] Since Pyk2 is a candidate to regulate c-Src and to link G protein-coupled vasoconstrictor receptors with protein tyrosine kinase-mediated contractile, migratory and growth responses, it may represent a potential point of convergence between Ca^{2+}-dependent signaling pathways and protein tyrosine kinase pathways in cardiovascular cells.

p130Cas

p130Cas is a tyrosine kinase that has a role in cell migration and actin filament reorganization. p130Cas serves as an adapter molecule because it contains proline-rich domains, an SH3 domain, and binding motifs for the SH2 domains of Crk and Src. p130Cas is important for integrin-mediated cell adhesion, by recruitment of cytoskeletal signaling molecules such as FAK, paxillin, and tensin to the focal adhesions.[42] The phosphorylation of p130Cas is dependent on Ca^{2+}, c-Src, and PKC, and requires an intact cytoskeletal network. Other studies reported that Ang II-induced activation of p130Cas is Ca^{2+} and PKC independent.[43] It has recently been demonstrated that Ang II-induced tyrosine phosphorylation of Src and p130Cas are essential, but differentially involved in Ang II-stimulated migration of VSMC through the activation of ERK1/2 and JNK. p130cas is involved in Ang II-induced migration of VSMC, via the JNK pathway.[44] Although the exact functional significance of Ang II-induced activation of p130Cas is unclear, it might regulate α-actin expression, cellular proliferation, migration, and cell adhesion.

PI3K

Phosphoinositide 3-OH kinase (PI3K)-dependent signaling is involved in the control of cell growth, proliferation, and survival, and has recently been identified as having an important role in the regulation of cardiomyocyte and VSMC growth.[45–47] PI3K is a heterodimeric enzyme composed of a p85 adapter and a p110 catalytic subunit.[48] Class I PI3K can be activated by either receptor tyrosine kinase (RTK)/cytokine receptor activation (class I_A) or G protein-coupled receptors (GPCR) (class I_B). PI3Kα, which is activated by RTK, appears to have a critical role in the induction of physiological cardiac growth, but not pathological growth, and it appears essential for maintaining contractile function in response to pathological stimuli.[49] In contrast, PI3Kγ, which is activated by GPCR, appears to negatively control cardiac contractility through different signaling mechanisms.[50] In SHR VSMC, PI3K has a role in augmented Ang II-induced ERK1/2 phosphorylation, and may contribute to vascular remodeling in SHR.[51] PI3K is also involved in Ang II-stimulated release of AA, which stimulates MAPK to phosphorylate cPLA(2) and enhance AA release. This mechanism may have an important role in Ang II-induced growth of VSMC.[52] Akt/PKB has been identified as an important downstream target of PI3K in Ang II-activated cardiomyocytes and VSMC.[53] It regulates protein synthesis by activating p70 S6-kinase and modulates Ang II-mediated Ca^{2+} responses by stimulating Ca^{2+} channel currents. Akt/PKB has also been implicated to promote cell survival by influencing Bcl-2 and c-Myc expression and by inhibiting caspases. Although the exact role of PI3K in Ang II signaling has not yet been established, it is possible that this complex pathway may control the balance between mitogenesis and apoptosis.

Receptor tyrosine kinases

Increasing evidence suggests that multiple levels of cross-talk exist between GPCR and RTK systems. In recent years, it has become apparent that transactivation of RTKs by GPCR agonists is a general phenomenon that has been demonstrated for many unrelated GPCRs and RTKs. GPCRs utilize signaling pathways downstream of RTKs to effect cellular responses. AT_1-mediated mitogenic responses may be regulated by activation of RTKs. This process of transactivation has been demonstrated for EGFR, PDGFR, and IGFR.[54] Ca^{2+}, Pyk2, Src, and redox-sensitive processes are involved in Ang II-induced transactivation of RTKs. AT_1-induced EGFR transactivation is important for some of the trophic effects of Ang II. Studies have demonstrated that EGFR activation is involved in Ang II-induced vascular contraction, cell growth, cardiac hypertrophy and hypertension.[55] It has recently been shown that Ang II-induced transactivation of the IGF-I receptor is a critical mediator of PI3K activation by Ang II, but is not required for stimulation of the MAPK cascade in VSMC.[56] Transactivation of the PDGFR in vivo contributes to vascular remodeling and growth factor-like effects of Ang II.[57,58]

Small G proteins

The small G protein superfamily is structurally classified into at least five families including the following: Ras, Rho/Rac/cdc42, Rab, Sar1/Arf, and Ran. The Ras family regulates gene expression, the Rho GTPases (Rho/Rac/cdc42) regulate cytoskeletal reorganization and gene expression, the Rab and Sar1/Arf families regulate vesicle trafficking, and the Ran family regulates nucleocytoplasmic transport and microtubule organization.[59] There is cross-talk between GPCRs and small G proteins. Studies have demonstrated that GPCR signaling through heterotrimeric G proteins can lead to the activation of Ras and Rho GTPases[59] (Figure 2.1). It has been demonstrated that Rho/Rho kinase-mediated signaling is involved in AT_1-stimulated cardiovascular cell growth, remodeling, atherosclerosis, and vascular contraction.[60] Inhibition of Rho or Rho kinase, inhibited Ang II-induced hypertrophy of VSMC and expression of monocyte chemoattractant protein-1 and plasminogen activator inhibitor protein-1. Ang II also activates Rac1, another Rho GTPase, which is an upstream regulator of p21-activated kinase and JNK. Rac1 participates in cytoskeletal organization, cell growth, and inflammation.[61] Rac1 also plays a role in Ang II-induced gene transcription and regulation of NAD(P)H oxidase, and the activation of JAK/STAT.[62] Rac1 controls superoxide production in both phagocytes and nonphagocytic cells, by regulating the activity of NADPH oxidase. NADPH oxidase-produced superoxide is an essential mediator of the hypertensive response to Ang II. These data suggest that Rac1 is likely an important regulatory target in hypertension. It has been demonstrated that Rac-derived superoxide in the cardiovascular system has a diverse array of functions.[63]

Generation of reactive oxygen species

Reactive oxygen species (ROS) are important both physiologically and in the pathogenesis of many cardiovascular disorders. Growing evidence indicates that production of ROS and activation of reduction-oxidation (redox)-dependent signaling cascades are critically involved in Ang II-induced actions.[64,65] All vascular cell types (endothelial cells, smooth muscle cells, adventitial fibroblasts, and resident macrophages) produce ROS. The major source of ROS in the vascular wall is nonphagocytic NADPH oxidase, which is regulated by vasoactive agents (Ang II, thrombin, serotonin), cytokines, and growth factors.[64] Ang II has been shown to activate vascular NAD(P)H oxidase(s), which results in the production of ROS, namely superoxide and hydrogen peroxide (H_2O_2). ROS function as important intracellular and intercellular second messengers to modulate downstream signaling molecules (Figure 2.1), such as protein tyrosine phosphatases, protein tyrosine kinases, transcription factors, MAPKs, and ion channels, and have a physiological role in vascular tone and cell growth, and a pathophysiological role in inflammation, ischemia-reperfusion, hypertension, and atherosclerosis.[66,67]

AT_2-MEDIATED INTRACELLULAR SIGNALING

AT_2 receptor

AT_2, the second major isoform of the Ang II receptor, has been cloned in a variety of species, including human,[68] rat,[69] and mouse.[2] AT_2 is also a 7-transmembrane glycoprotein, and shares only 34% sequence identity with AT_1.[70] AT_2 is normally expressed at high levels in developing fetal tissues, and is decreased rapidly after birth.[71] AT_2 is re-expressed in adults after vascular and cardiac injury and during wound healing and renal obstruction.[72–75] Using transgenic mice, studies have shown that AT_2 signals antiproliferative and antifibrotic effects, which results in lower blood pressures and diminished responses in secondary forms of hypertension.[76] In blood vessels, in addition to its vasodilatory actions, AT_2 exerts antiproliferative and apoptotic effects in vascular smooth muscle cells and decreases neointimal formation in response to injury, by counteracting Ang II actions at the AT_1 receptor.[77] In the heart, AT_2 inhibits growth and remodeling, induces vasodilation, and is up-regulated in pathological states.[78] After myocardial infarction, AT_2 overexpression resulted in preservation of left ventricular global and regional function, indicating a beneficial role for AT_2 in volume overload states, including post-myocardial infarction remodeling.[79,80]

AT_2-mediated signaling pathways

Signaling pathways through which AT_2 mediates cardiovascular actions have recently been elucidated (Figure 2.2). Three major cascades are involved.

1. Activation of protein phosphatases and protein dephosphorylation. Numerous studies have shown that Ang II rapidly induces activation of protein tyrosine phosphatase (PTPase), resulting in dephosphorylation and inactivation of corresponding tyrosine kinases.[81] Ang II stimulation activates MAPK phosphatase 1 (MKP-1), SH2 domain-containing phosphatase 1 (SHP-1) and PP2A, thereby inhibiting AT_1-mediated MAPK activation. In vivo and in vitro studies have indicated that ERK inactivation by AT_2 may have a physiological role in vivo, in relation to cardiac and vascular growth.[75,82,83] AT_2-stimulated tyrosine and serine/threonine phosphatases, serve to reverse, or counter-regulate the cell proliferative- and growth-promoting effects mediated by the various protein kinases in response to AT_1 activation.
2. Regulation of the nitric oxide-cyclic GMP system. Recent studies have shown that activation of AT_2 by Ang II results in a bradykinin-dependent stimulation of aortic NO release with subsequent generation of cGMP.[84,85] These data indicate that the AT_2-activated nitric oxide/cGMP system in the cardiovascular and renal systems is involved in AT_2-mediated cardioprotection, vasodilation, and pressure natriuresis.
3. Sphingolipid-derived ceramide. Ceramide belongs to a family of lipids known as sphingolipids, characterized by a sphingoid backbone and distinct head groups.[86] AT_2 activation has been demonstrated to increase intracellular concentrations of ceramide.[87,88] This suggests that AT_2 receptor-stimulated ceramide production may contribute to some of the physiological effects of Ang II. Recent studies have implicated ceramide as a possible vasodilatory second messenger.[89] In vitro and in vivo studies have shown that ceramide inhibits VSMC proliferation.[90,91] This study represents the first step toward utilizing ceramide signaling components as a therapeutic intervention for cardiovascular disease.

In contrast to extensive data on the molecular and cellular functions and pathophysiological significance of

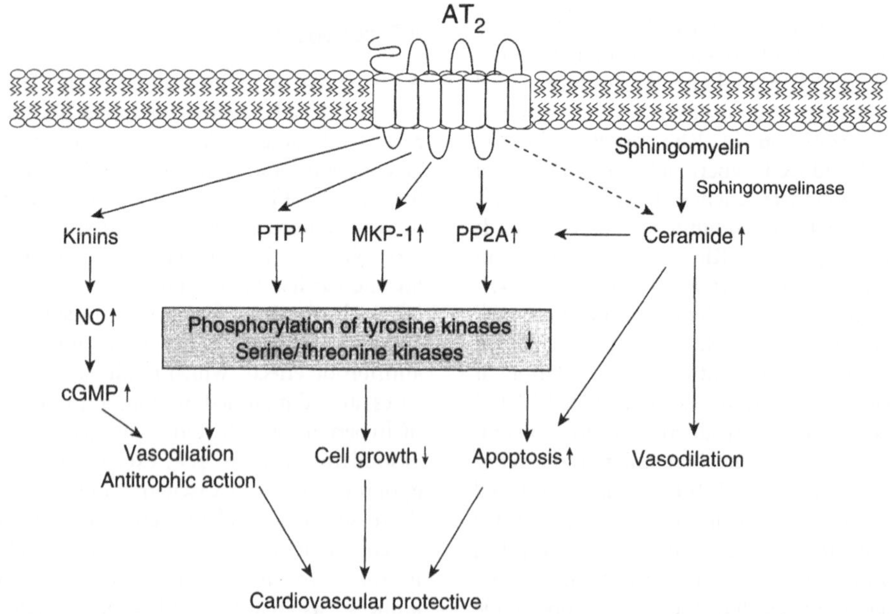

Figure 2.2 AT_2-mediated intracellular signaling. Three major cascades are involved, including (1) activation of protein phosphatases and protein dephosphorylation, (2) regulation of the nitric oxide-cGMP system, and (3) sphingolipid-derived ceramide

AT_1, the role of AT_2 in cardiovascular diseases remains to be defined.

CONCLUSIONS

Ang II influences vascular structure and functions in hypertension by stimulating VSMC contraction, cell growth, increasing deposition of extracellular matrix, promoting inflammation and cell migration. The majority of Ang II actions are mediated via AT_1. Evidence has accumulated that AT_2 opposes AT_1, especially by inducing vasodilation instead of vasoconstriction. Molecular mechanisms associated with these cellular effects in hypertension include Ang II-stimulated G protein-coupled phospholipases, tyrosine kinases, MAPKs, and RhoA/Rho kinase, and increased generation of ROS. Although there has been significant progress in the last few years in the elucidation of aberrations in Ang II-induced signal transduction in hypertension, very little is known about the interaction within these signaling pathways under pathological conditions. Alternative methodologies may be applied to further understand the role of Ang II in the process of hypertension and associated cardiovascular diseases.

REFERENCES

1. Murphy TJ, Alexander RW, Griendling KK et al. Isolation of a cDNA encoding the vascular type-1 angiotensin II receptor. Nature 1991; 351: 233–6.
2. Nakajima M, Mukoyama M, Pratt RE et al. Cloning of cDNA and analysis of the gene for mouse angiotensin II type 2 receptor. Biochem Biophys Res Commun 1993; 197: 393–9.
3. Sasaki K, Yamano Y, Bardhan S et al. Cloning and expression of a complementary DNA encoding a bovine adrenal angiotensin II type-1 receptor. Nature 1991; 351: 230–3.
4. Iwai N, Inagami T. Identification of two subtypes in the rat type I angiotensin II receptor. FEBS Lett 1992; 298: 257–60.
5. Guo DF, Furuta H, Mizukoshi M et al. The genomic organization of human angiotensin II type 1 receptor. Biochem Biophys Res Commun 1994; 200: 313–19.
6. Timmermans PB, Wong PC, Chiu AT et al. Angiotensin II receptors and angiotensin II receptor antagonists. Pharmacol Rev 1993; 45: 205–51.
7. Hunyady L, Balla T, Catt KJ. The ligand binding site of the angiotensin AT1 receptor. Trends Pharmacol Sci 1996; 17: 135–40.
8. Thekkumkara TJ, Thomas WG, Motel TJ et al. Functional role for the angiotensin II receptor (AT1A) 3′-untranslated region in determining cellular responses to agonist: evidence for recognition by RNA binding proteins. Biochem J 1998; 329 (Pt 2): 255–64.
9. Griendling KK, Ushio-Fukai M, Lassegue B et al. Angiotensin II signaling in vascular smooth muscle. New concepts. Hypertension 1997; 29 (1 Pt 2): 366–73.
10. Capponi AM. Distribution and signal transduction of angiotensin II AT1 and AT2 receptors. Blood Press Suppl 1996; 2: 41–6.
11. Ruan X, Arendshorst WJ. Role of protein kinase C in angiotensin II-induced renal vasoconstriction in genetically hypertensive rats. Am J Physiol 1996; 270 (6 Pt 2): F945–F952.
12. Booz GW, Dostal DE, Singer HA et al. Involvement of protein kianse C and Ca2+ in angiotensin II-induced mitogenesis of cardiac fibroblasts. Am J Physiol 1994; 267 (5 Pt 1): C1308–C1318.
13. Touyz RM, Berry C. Recent advances in angiotensin II signaling. Braz J Med Biol Res 2002; 35: 1001–15.
14. Anand-Srivastava MB. Angiotensin II receptors negatively coupled to adenylate cyclase in rat aorta. Biochem Biophys Res Commun 1983; 117: 420–8.
15. Kem DC, Johnson EI, Capponi AM et al. Effect of angiotensin II on cytosolic free calcium in neonatal rat cardiomyocytes. Am J Physiol 1991; 261 (1 Pt 1): C77–C85.
16. Iversen BM, Arendshorst WJ. AT1 calcium signaling in renal vascular smooth muscle cells. J Am Soc Nephrol 1999; 10 (Suppl 11): S84–S89.
17. Macrez N, Morel JL, Kalkbrenner F et al. A betagamma dimer derived from G13 transduces the angiotensin AT1 receptor signal to stimulation of Ca2+ channels in rat portal vein myocytes. J Biol Chem 1997; 272: 23180–5.
18. English J, Pearson G, Wilsbacher J et al. New insights into the control of MAP kinase pathways. Exp Cell Res 1999; 253: 255–70.
19. Chang L, Karin M. Mammalian MAP kinase signalling cascades. Nature 2001; 410: 37–40.
20. Strniskova M, Barancik M, Ravingerova T. Mitogen-activated protein kinases and their role in regulation of cellular processes. Gen Physiol Biophys 2002; 21: 231–55.
21. Kim S, Iwao H. Activation of mitogen-activated protein kinases in cardiovascular hypertrophy and remodeling. Jpn J Pharmacol 1999; 80: 97–102.
22. Ravingerova T, Barancik M, Strniskova M. Mitogen-activated protein kinases: a new therapeutic target in cardiac pathology. Mol Cell Biochem 2003; 247: 127–38.
23. Kim S, Iwao H. Stress and vascular responses: mitogen-activated protein kinases and activator protein-1 as promising therapeutic targets of vascular remodeling. J Pharmacol Sci 2003; 91: 177–81.
24. Wang Y, Su B, Sah VP et al. Cardiac hypertrophy induced by mitogen-activated protein kinase kinase 7, a specific activator for c-Jun NH2-terminal kinase in ventricular muscle cells. J Biol Chem 1998; 273: 5423–6.
25. Schmitz U, Ishida T, Ishida M et al. Angiotensin II stimulates p21-activated kinase in vascular smooth muscle cells: role in activation of JNK. Circ Res 1998; 82: 1272–8.
26. Behr TM, Berova M, Doe CP et al. p38 mitogen-activated protein kinase inhibitors for the treatment of chronic cardiovascular disease. Curr Opin Investig Drugs 2003; 4: 1059–64.
27. Liang Q, Molkentin JD. Redefining the roles of p38 and JNK signaling in cardiac hypertrophy: dichotomy between cultured myocytes and animal models. J Mol Cell Cardiol 2003; 35: 1385–94.
28. Kim S, Iwao H. Molecular and cellular mechanisms of angiotensin II-mediated cardiovascular and renal diseases. Pharmacol Rev 2000; 52: 11–34.
29. Yin G, Yan C, Berk BC. Angiotensin II signaling pathways mediated by tyrosine kinases. Int J Biochem Cell Biol 2003; 35: 780–3.
30. Haendeler J, Berk BC. Angiotensin II mediated signal transduction. Important role of tyrosine kinases. Regul Pept 2000; 95: 1–7.

31. Tatosyan AG, Mizenina OA. Kinases of the Src family: structure and functions. Biochemistry (Mosc) 2000; 65: 49–58.
32. Thomas SM, Brugge JS. Cellular functions regulated by Src family kinases. Annu Rev Cell Dev Biol 1997; 13: 513–609.
33. Erpel T, Courtneidge SA. Src family protein tyrosine kinases and cellular signal transduction pathways. Curr Opin Cell Biol 1995; 7: 176–82.
34. Aaronson DS, Horvath CM. A road map for those who don't know JAK-STAT. Science 2002; 296: 1653–5.
35. Booz GW, Day JN, Baker KM. Interplay between the cardiac renin angiotensin system and JAK-STAT signaling: role in cardiac hypertrophy, ischemia/reperfusion dysfunction, and heart failure. J Mol Cell Cardiol 2002; 34: 1443–53.
36. Bolli R, Dawn B, Xuan YT. Role of the JAK-STAT pathway in protection against myocardial ischemia/reperfusion injury. Trends Cardiovasc Med 2003; 13: 72–9.
37. Mascareno E, Siddiqui MA. The role of Jak/STAT signaling in heart tissue renin-angiotensin system. Mol Cell Biochem 2000; 212: 171–5.
38. Parsons JT. Focal adhesion kinase: the first ten years. J Cell Sci 2003; 116 (Pt 8): 1409–16.
39. Guan JL. Role of focal adhesion kinase in integrin signaling. Int J Biochem Cell Biol 1997; 29: 1085–96.
40. Schnee JM, Hsueh WA. Angiotensin II, adhesion, and cardiac fibrosis. Cardiovasc Res 2000; 46: 264–8.
41. Sabri A, Govindarajan G, Griffin TM et al. Calcium- and protein kinase C-dependent activation of the tyrosine kinase PYK2 by angiotensin II in vascular smooth muscle. Circ Res 1998; 83: 841–51.
42. O'Neill GM, Fashena SJ, Golemis EA. Integrin signalling: a new Cas(t) of characters enters the stage. Trends Cell Biol 2000; 10: 111–19.
43. Takahashi T, Kawahara Y, Taniguchi T et al. Tyrosine phosphorylation and association of p130Cas and c-Crk II by ANG II in vascular smooth muscle cells. Am J Physiol 1998; 274 (4 Pt 2): H1059–H1065.
44. Kyaw M, Yoshizumi M, Tsuchiya K et al. Src and Cas are essentially but differentially involved in angiotensin II-stimulated migration of vascular smooth muscle cells via extracellular signal-regulated kinase 1/2 and c-Jun NH2-terminal kinase activation. Mol Pharmacol 2004; 65: 832–41.
45. Prasad SV, Perrino C, Rockman HA. Role of phosphoinositide 3-kinase in cardiac function and heart failure. Trends Cardiovasc Med 2003; 13: 206–12.
46. Saward L, Zahradka P. Angiotensin II activates phosphatidylinositol 3-kinase in vascular smooth muscle cells. Circ Res 1997; 81: 249–57.
47. Oudit GY, Sun H, Kerfant BG et al. The role of phosphoinositide-3 kinase and PTEN in cardiovascular physiology and disease. J Mol Cell Cardiol 2004; 37: 449–71.
48. Cantley LC. The phosphoinositide 3-kinase pathway. Science 2002; 296: 1655–7.
49. McMullen JR, Shioi T, Zhang L et al. Phosphoinositide 3-kinase (p110alpha) plays a critical role for the induction of physiological, but not pathological, cardiac hypertrophy. Proc Natl Acad Sci U S A 2003; 100: 12355–60.
50. Alloatti G, Montrucchio G, Lembo G et al. Phosphoinositide 3-kinase gamma: kinase-dependent and -independent activities in cardiovascular function and disease. Biochem Soc Trans 2004; 32 (Pt 2): 383–6.
51. El Mabrouk M, Touyz RM, Schiffrin EL. Differential ANG II-induced growth activation pathways in mesenteric artery smooth muscle cells from SHR. Am J Physiol Heart Circ Physiol 2001; 281: H30–H39.
52. Silfani TN, Freeman EJ. Phosphatidylinositide 3-kinase regulates angiotensin II-induced cytosolic phospholipase A2 activity and growth in vascular smooth muscle cells. Arch Biochem Biophys 2002; 402: 84–93.
53. Chen QM, Tu VC, Purdon S et al. Molecular mechanisms of cardiac hypertrophy induced by toxicants. Cardiovasc Toxicol 2001; 1: 267–83.
54. Saito Y, Berk BC. Transactivation: a novel signaling pathway from angiotensin II to tyrosine kinase receptors. J Mol Cell Cardiol 2001; 33: 3–7.
55. Shah BH, Catt KJ. A central role of EGF receptor transactivation in angiotensin II-induced cardiac hypertrophy. Trends Pharmacol Sci 2003; 24: 239–44.
56. Zahradka P, Litchie B, Storie B et al. Transactivation of the insulin-like growth factor-I receptor by angiotensin II mediates downstream signaling from the angiotensin II type 1 receptor to phosphatidylinositol 3-kinase. Endocrinology 2004; 145: 2978–87.
57. Kelly DJ, Cox AJ, Gow RM et al. Platelet-derived growth factor receptor transactivation mediates the trophic effects of angiotensin II in vivo. Hypertension 2004; 44: 195–202.
58. Kim S, Zhan Y, Izumi Y et al. In vivo activation of rat aortic platelet-derived growth factor and epidermal growth factor receptors by angiotensin II and hypertension. Arterioscler Thromb Vasc Biol 2000; 20: 2539–45.
59. Bhattacharya M, Babwah AV, Ferguson SS. Small GTP-binding protein-coupled receptors. Biochem Soc Trans 2004; 32 (Pt 6): 1040–4.
60. Yamakawa T, Tanaka S, Numaguchi K et al. Involvement of Rho-kinase in angiotensin II-induced hypertrophy of rat vascular smooth muscle cells. Hypertension 2000; 35 (1 Pt 2): 313–18.
61. Laufs U, Liao JK. Targeting Rho in cardiovascular disease. Circ Res 2000; 87: 526–8.
62. Pelletier S, Duhamel F, Coulombe P et al. Rho family GTPases are required for activation of Jak/STAT signaling by G protein-coupled receptors. Mol Cell Biol 2003; 23: 1316–33.
63. Gregg D, Rauscher FM, Goldschmidt-Clermont PJ. Rac regulates cardiovascular superoxide through diverse molecular interactions: more than a binary GTP switch. Am J Physiol Cell Physiol 2003; 285: C723–C734.
64. Griendling KK, Sorescu D, Ushio-Fukai M. NAD(P)H oxidase: role in cardiovascular biology and disease. Circ Res 2000; 86: 494–501.
65. Griendling KK, Ushio-Fukai M. Reactive oxygen species as mediators of angiotensin II signaling. Regul Pept 2000; 91: 21–7.
66. Hanna IR, Taniyama Y, Szocs K et al. NAD(P)H oxidase-derived reactive oxygen species as mediators of angiotensin II signaling. Antioxid Redox Signal 2002; 4: 899–914.
67. Cai H, Griendling KK, Harrison DG. The vascular NAD(P)H oxidases as therapeutic targets in cardiovascular diseases. Trends Pharmacol Sci 2003; 24: 471–8.
68. Koike G, Horiuchi M, Yamada T et al. Human type 2 angiotensin II receptor gene: cloned, mapped to the X chromosome, and its mRNA is expressed in the human lung. Biochem Biophys Res Commun 1994; 203: 1842–50.
69. Koike G, Winer ES, Horiuchi M et al. Cloning, characterization, and genetic mapping of the rat type 2 angiotensin II receptor gene. Hypertension 1995; 26 (6 Pt 1): 998–1002.
70. Mukoyama M, Nakajima M, Horiuchi M et al. Expression cloning of type 2 angiotensin II receptor reveals a unique class of seven-transmembrane receptors. J Biol Chem 1993; 268: 24539–42.
71. Nahmias C, Strosberg AD. The angiotensin AT2 receptor: searching for signal-transduction pathways and physiological function. Trends Pharmacol Sci 1995; 16: 223–5.

72. Tsutsumi Y, Matsubara H, Ohkubo N et al. Angiotensin II type 2 receptor is upregulated in human heart with interstitial fibrosis, and cardiac fibroblasts are the major cell type for its expression. Circ Res 1998; 83: 1035–46.
73. Kimura B, Sumners C, Phillips MI. Changes in skin angiotensin II receptors in rats during wound healing. Biochem Biophys Res Commun 1992; 187: 1083–90.
74. Nio Y, Matsubara H, Murasawa S et al. Regulation of gene transcription of angiotensin II receptor subtypes in myocardial infarction. J Clin Invest 1995; 95: 46–54.
75. Nakajima M, Hutchinson HG, Fujinaga M et al. The angiotensin II type 2 (AT2) receptor antagonizes the growth effects of the AT1 receptor: gain-of-function study using gene transfer. Proc Natl Acad Sci U S A 1995; 92: 10663–7.
76. Gross V, Obst M, Luft FC. Insights into angiotensin II receptor function through AT2 receptor knockout mice. Acta Physiol Scand 2004; 181: 487–94.
77. Suzuki J, Iwai M, Nakagami H et al. Role of angiotensin II-regulated apoptosis through distinct AT1 and AT2 receptors in neointimal formation. Circulation 2002; 106: 847–53.
78. Schneider MD, Lorell BH. AT(2), judgment day: which angiotensin receptor is the culprit in cardiac hypertrophy? Circulation 2001; 104: 247–8.
79. Yang Z, Bove CM, French BA et al. Angiotensin II type 2 receptor overexpression preserves left ventricular function after myocardial infarction. Circulation 2002; 106: 106–11.
80. Oishi Y, Ozono R, Yano Y et al. Cardioprotective role of AT2 receptor in postinfarction left ventricular remodeling. Hypertension 2003; 41 (3 Pt 2): 814–18.
81. Bottari SP, King IN, Reichlin S et al. The angiotensin AT2 receptor stimulates protein tyrosine phosphatase activity and mediates inhibition of particulate guanylate cyclase. Biochem Biophys Res Commun 1992; 183: 206–11.
82. Masaki H, Kurihara T, Yamaki A et al. Cardiac-specific overexpression of angiotensin II AT2 receptor causes attenuated response to AT1 receptor-mediated pressor and chronotropic effects. J Clin Invest 1998; 101: 527–35.
83. Akishita M, Ito M, Lehtonen JY et al. Expression of the AT2 receptor developmentally programs extracellular signal-regulated kinase activity and influences fetal vascular growth. J Clin Invest 1999; 103: 63–71.
84. Searles CD, Harrison DG. The interaction of nitric oxide, bradykinin, and the angiotensin II type 2 receptor: lessons learned from transgenic mice. J Clin Invest 1999; 104: 1013–14.
85. Moore AF, Heiderstadt NT, Huang E et al. Selective inhibition of the renal angiotensin type 2 receptor increases blood pressure in conscious rats. Hypertension 2001; 37: 1285–91.
86. Hannun YA, Bell RM. Functions of sphingolipids and sphingolipid breakdown products in cellular regulation. Science 1989; 243: 500–7.
87. Lehtonen JY, Horiuchi M, Daviet L et al. Activation of the de novo biosynthesis of sphingolipids mediates angiotensin II type 2 receptor-induced apoptosis. J Biol Chem 1999; 274: 16901–6.
88. Gallinat S, Busche S, Schutze S et al. AT2 receptor stimulation induces generation of ceramides in PC12W cells. FEBS Lett 1999; 443: 75–9.
89. Johns DG, Osborn H, Webb RC. Ceramide: a novel cell signaling mechanism for vasodilation. Biochem Biophys Res Commun 1997; 237: 95–7.
90. Johns DG, Webb RC, Charpie JR. Impaired ceramide signalling in spontaneously hypertensive rat vascular smooth muscle: a possible mechanism for augmented cell proliferation. J Hypertens 2001; 19: 63–70.
91. Charles R, Sandirasegarane L, Yun J et al. Ceramide-coated balloon catheters limit neointimal hyperplasia after stretch injury in carotid arteries. Circ Res 2000; 87: 282–8.

3

Angiotensin AT_1 receptors

Lula L Hilenski, Kathy K Griendling and R Wayne Alexander

INTRODUCTION

The etiology of hypertension is complex, involving both neuronal and hormone systems acting upon multiple organs.[1] The octapeptide hormone angiotensin II (Ang II), the effector molecule of the renin-angiotensin system (RAS) which controls blood pressure, targets virtually all of these organs, including the heart, kidney, vasculature, and brain.[2] In addition to the 'classical' endocrine function of Ang II in circulating blood, the essential components of RAS (except for renin) have been identified in the brain, lung, heart, kidney, pancreas, and blood vessels, providing evidence for paracrine, autocrine, and intracrine[3] effects of Ang II acting locally in tissues.[4–6] These local RAS, by acting independently of the circulating Ang II, provide tissue-specific regulatory mechanisms and multiple functional responses within individual organs and/or tissues.[7]

Whether in the circulating blood or in tissues, the multiple physiological actions of Ang II are mediated by Ang II binding to two distinct plasma membrane receptors, angiotensin type 1 (AT_1R) or type 2 (AT_2R) receptors. The major pressor and trophic responses to Ang II are mediated through AT_1Rs,[2,8–11] and result in both short- and long-term effects. Acute effects of Ang II – vasoconstriction, increased aldosterone secretion for salt retention, and increased myocardial contraction to maintain cardiac output – provide a protective mechanism to increase blood pressure when blood volume decreases.[12] In contrast to these beneficial effects, chronic, long-term effects of elevated Ang II, which include cardiac hypertrophy, vascular remodeling and renal fibrosis, have been implicated in cardiovascular diseases, including hypertension.[13–17]

In order to understand how one hormone, Ang II, can have both beneficial and pathological effects, it is necessary to understand how Ang II interacts with and regulates AT_1Rs. The pro-hypertensive effects of Ang II can occur at many different levels, including increases in AT_1R mRNA expression and cell surface AT_1R density, differences in receptor structural modification or receptor/ligand affinity, alterations in upstream/downstream signaling events mediated by Ang II/AT_1R binding, or altered ligand and receptor routes in intracellular desensitization/internalization/trafficking patterns. This chapter examines these different levels of AT_1R structure/function, with emphasis on alterations that may affect hypertension.

STRUCTURE AND STRUCTURAL MODIFICATIONS OF AT_1R

Structure

Cloning of the AT_1R from rat aortic smooth muscle and bovine adrenal cells[18,19] indicated that it is a 41 kDa protein, consisting of 359 amino acids. In rodents, two isoforms of AT_1R, designated $AT_{1A}R$ and $AT_{1B}R$, are located at two different loci, chromosome 17 and 2, respectively, and share 95% amino acid sequence identity.[20] Studies using gene targeting showed that the $AT_{1A}R$ isoform is more important than $AT_{1B}R$ in blood pressure regulation: mice lacking the $AT_{1A}R$ gene exhibit a significant reduction in blood pressure,[21] while mice lacking the $AT_{1B}R$ gene have no significant difference in blood pressure from wild-type mice.[22]

The AT_1R belongs to the superfamily of seven-transmembrane guanine-nucleotide-binding regulatory protein (G protein)-coupled receptors (GPCRs).[23] The extracellular N-terminus, the seven α helical transmembrane domains (TM-1-6) and a cytoplasmic C-terminus are linked by three extracellular and three intracellular loops.[2] Functional sites within the receptor for glycosylation, phosphorylation, Ang II binding, G protein coupling, membrane tethering and ligand/receptor internalization have been identified within more than 40 residues in the receptor.[24–26] Modifications within these functional sites may be responsible for altered receptor function in cardiovascular diseases. Two types of receptor structural modifications, polymorphisms and receptor oligomerization, have recently been implicated in hypertension.

Polymorphisms

There is abundant evidence for a strong genetic component to hypertension.[27,28] Identification of single nucleotide polymorphisms (SNPs) in the AT_1R gene[29–32] has led to numerous studies showing associations between polymorphisms at A1166C in the 3′ untranslated region,[29] at C535T in the 5′ noncoding region[32] and at A44221G in exon 5[33] and increased risk for hypertension and its related disorders in various ethnic[33–35] and gender groups.[36] However, other association studies have produced conflicting results[37–41] or have suggested that single AT_1R gene polymorphisms have only a minor effect on hypertension.[42,43] The limitation of these studies is that few have attempted to relate polymorphisms in AT_1Rs to physiological outcomes.[41]

While the impact of single AT_1R polymorphisms on hypertension has been controversial, more recent studies, examining the AT_1R A1166C polymorphism in combination with other RAS gene variants,[44] have shown associations with hypertension[43,45] and renal failure.[46] These promising studies, using multiple gene approaches, together with studies using intermediate phenotypes and dense mapping of candidate genes,[47] need to be expanded to establish the importance of these linkages.[44]

Oligomerization

The AT_1R has been reported to engage in both homo-[48,49] and hetero-oligomerization with other GPCRs, including the AT_2R,[50] the bradykinin B_2 receptor,[51] the β_2-adrenergic receptor (β_2AR)[52] and the dopamine D_1 receptor.[53] These associations result in unique phenotypes of altered Ang II sensitivity and/or signaling, thus increasing the repertoire of multifunctional AT_1R signaling responses.[51,54,55]

The physiological relevance and clinical significance of AT_1R homo- and hetero-oligomerization in hypertension have been shown in recent studies. In clinical studies, increased levels of heterodimers between the AT_1R receptor for the vasopressor Ang II and the B_2 receptor for the vasodepressor bradykinin were found on platelets and vessels in women with preeclampsia, a pregnancy-specific condition characterized by elevated blood pressure and increased Ang II sensitivity.[56,57] Importantly, these AT_1R/B_2 heterodimers, which enhanced Ang II-stimulated signaling while decreasing the bradykinin response, represented the first association between GPCR oligomerization and a clinical disorder. In another study, Ang II-induced AT_1R homodimers, covalently cross-linked by factor XIIIA transglutaminase, also showed enhanced signaling and desensitization in vitro and in vivo.[49] The levels of AT_1R homodimers were significantly higher on monocytes from hypertensive patients and correlated with increased Ang II-induced monocyte sensitization and adhesiveness.

Further evidence suggests that AT_1R oligomerization may affect signaling and cross-talk with other pathways that regulate cardiovascular function. In mouse cardiomyocytes, blockade of either the β_2AR or the AT_1R inhibited signaling and trafficking of both receptors simultaneously, suggesting that AT_1R/β_2ARs heterodimerize.[52] This transinhibition has important implications in clinical drug treatments utilizing both β_2AR and AT_1R receptor blockers.[52] Additionally, AT_1R mutants defective in signaling or binding when coexpressed with wild-type AT_1Rs inhibited $G_{\alpha q}$ protein signaling without affecting ERK activation or β-arrestin recruitment,[48] demonstrating that AT_1R oligomers may differentially couple active Ang II/AT_1R binding conformations to specific signaling proteins.[58] Thus there is emerging evidence that AT_1R homo- or hetero-oligomer modifications can confer unique functional and pharmacological properties altering surface expression, desensitization, and coupling to G proteins, resulting in enhanced sensitivity (AT_1R/B_2)[51] or antagonism (AT_1R/AT_2R)[50] to Ang II, and leading to alterations in blood pressure, monocyte sensitivity and downstream signaling associated with vascular disease.

REGULATION OF AT_1R GENE EXPRESSION

Because the effects of Ang II in hypertension are limited by the extent of AT_1R expression, factors regulating AT_1R mRNA and protein expression are important in blood pressure control. These factors include cytokines, hormones, vasorelaxants, growth factors, and LDL cholesterol (Table 3.1).[59–74] In general, inflammatory cytokines up-regulate AT_1R expression, while individual growth factors and hormones have specific modes of regulation depending upon their physiological role. Thus, regulation of AT_1R expression may contribute to hypertensive disease associated with metabolic disorders such as hypercholesterolemia,[75] hyperinsulinemia and insulin resistance[65] and stress-related disorders.[67]

Table 3.1 Factors regulating AT_1R expression

Factor	*AT_1R expression*	*Reference*
Growth factors		
EGF	↓	59
PDGF-BB	↓	59
FGF	↓	59
Hormones		
Angiotensin II	↓	60
Estrogen	↓	61, 62
Progesterone	↑	62
Thyroid hormone	↓	63
Growth hormone	↑	64
Insulin	↑	65
Insulin-like growth factor	↑	66
Glucocorticoids	↑	67
Cytokines		
IL-6	↑	68
IL-1β	↑	69
TNF-α	↑	69
Vasorelaxants		
Nitric oxide	↓	70, 71
Retinoids	↓	72
LDL cholesterol	↑	73, 74

EGF, epidermal growth factor; PDGF-BB, platelet-derived growth factor; FGF, fibroblast growth factor, IL-6, interleukin-6; IL-1β, interleukin-1β; TNF-α, tumor necrosis factor-α; LDL, low density lipoprotein.

Evidence from cultured cells, animal and human studies shows that low-density lipoproteins (LDL) affect AT_1R expression, thus influencing Ang II-mediated changes associated with hypertension. Native LDL cholesterol up-regulates AT_1R expression by increasing mRNA stability in cultured vascular smooth muscle cells.[73] In hypercholesterolemic animals, elevated serum cholesterol levels are associated with increased Ang II-induced vasoconstriction and increased density of cell surface AT_1R receptors.[76] In hypercholesterolemic men, AT_1R is overexpressed on platelets and Ang II-induced vasoconstriction is enhanced.[77] These effects are prevented by 3-hydroxy-3-methylglutaryl-coenzyme A (HMG-CoA) reductase inhibitors (statins).[75,77] This evidence for cross-talk between two pathophysiologically important pathways – RAS and cholesterol metabolism – offers a potential explanation for the strong association of hypercholesterolemia with hypertension as cardiovascular disease risk factors and for the observed antihypertensive effects and decreases in progression of atherosclerosis with statins.[78,79]

ANG II/AT_1R SIGNALING PATHWAYS

Many of the myriad Ang II-induced signaling pathways are enhanced in hypertension and these alterations occur primarily downstream of the AT_1R. Alterations in these signaling pathways contribute to both functional and structural changes in the vasculature associated with hypertension[14,17,80,81] and are the result of AT_1R coupling to temporally and physically distinct signaling pathways.[82] Acute functional responses, such as vasoconstriction, are the result of Ang II-induced AT_1R activation of 'classical' GPCR signaling leading to Ca^{2+}-dependent smooth muscle contraction (Figure 3.1), while chronic responses, leading to structural vascular remodeling, including growth, migration, fibrosis and inflammation, appear to involve activation of both nonreceptor and receptor-type tyrosine kinases and inflammatory pathways[83] (Figure 3.2).

G protein-dependent pathways

Ang II affects vasoconstriction by coupling to G proteins and phospholipids and activating multiphasic, diverse signaling pathways.[84] In the 'classical' G protein-dependent signaling pathway, Ang II binding to the AT_1R[25] induces conformational changes in the AT_1R that promote its coupling to and activation of heterotrimeric G proteins through exchange of GTP for GDP, resulting in the release of G_α-GTP and $G_{\beta\gamma}$ complexes. The G_α and $G_{\beta\gamma}$ subunits dissociate, each possessing the capacity to activate or inhibit different effector molecules in downstream events. The intracellular downstream events are dependent upon the identity of the G proteins. Receptor coupling to $G_{\alpha q/11}$ or $G_{\alpha 12/13}$[85–87] leads to activation of phospholipase C (PLC), while coupling to $G_{\beta\gamma}$ subunit activates tyrosine kinases such as c-Src and is involved in phospholipase D (PLD) activation.[88]

The duration and intensity of signaling by the $G_{\alpha q}$ subunit of AT_1Rs is mediated by RGS2, a member of a class of regulators of G protein signaling (RGS) that function as GTPase activating proteins (GAPs) to terminate $G_{\alpha q}$/effector interactions.[89] In mice deficient for RGS2, blood pressure levels are increased due to chronic constriction of the peripheral vasculature,[90] while in patients with Bartter's/Gitelman's syndrome characterized by increased RGS2 expression, blood pressure is reduced.[91] These results demonstrate a

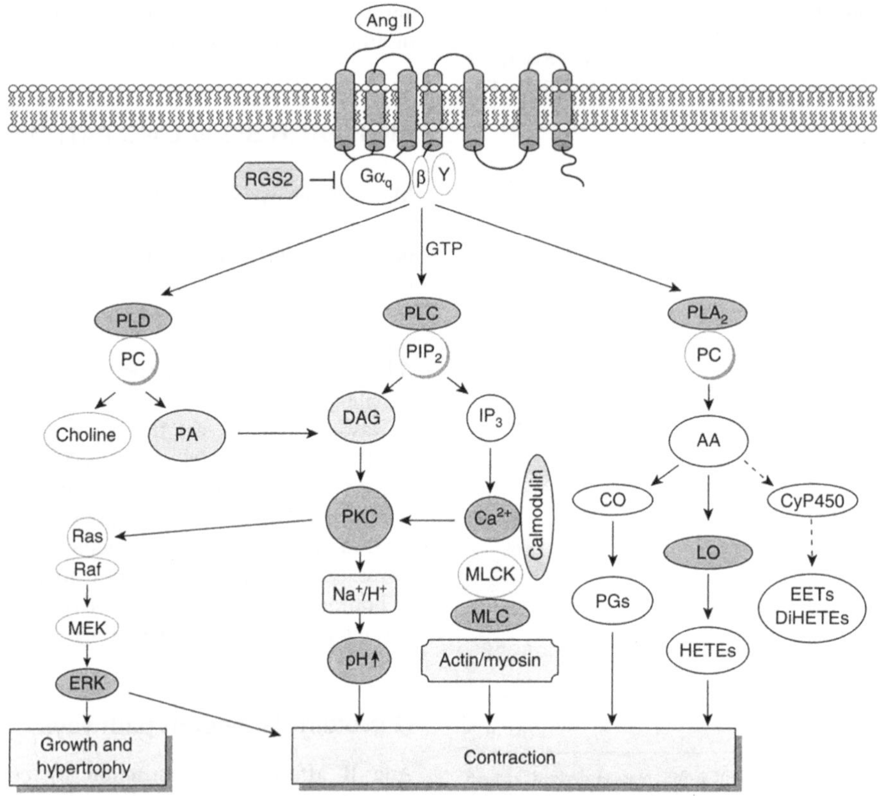

Figure 3.1 In hypertension, the Ang II-stimulated, heterotrimeric G protein-dependent activation of multiple phospholipases, including phospholipases C, D, and A_2, is increased, leading to enhanced contraction, growth and hypertrophy. Activation of these pathways is countered by RGS2, which serves to terminate signaling proximally. Phospholipase C (PLC) hydrolysis of phosphatidylinositol 4,5-bisphosphate (PIP_2) generates increased inositol trisphosphate (IP_3) and diacylglycerol (DAG), leading to augmented Ca^{2+} mobilization and activation of protein kinase C (PKC), respectively. Increased Ca^{2+} combines with calmodulin and activates myosin light chain kinase (MLCK), resulting in phosphorylated MLC which, together with actin, initiates contraction. PKC activates the Na^+/H^+ exchanger resulting in increased alkalinization. In addition, Ang II-induced increased activation of phospholipase D (PLD), which hydrolyzes phosphatidylcholine (PC) to choline and phosphatidic acid (PA), leads to enhanced contraction via the DAG-PKC-dependent pathway. Furthermore, Ang II-induced activation of phospholipase A_2 (PLA_2) generates arachidonic acid (AA), leading to the cyclooxygenase (CO)- and/or lipoxygenase (LO)-derived eicosanoids prostaglandins (PG) and hydroxyeicosatetraenoic acid (HETEs), respectively, which are pro-hypertensive. In contrast, the AA-derived cytochrome P450 metabolites epoxyeicosatrienoic acid (EETs) and dihydroxyeicosatetraenoic acid (DiHETEs) are antihypertensive (dashed lines). All of these early signaling pathways culminate in enhanced vascular contraction. The sustained phase of contraction is due to PKC stimulation of the Ras/Raf/MEK/ERK pathway, which also induces growth and hypertrophy.

central role for RGS2 in Ang II/AT_1R signaling and control of vascular tone in hypertension.

Second messengers generated by PLC, PLD, and PLA_2

In vascular smooth muscle cells, Ang II-induced PLC activation is rapid (within 5 seconds) but transient and produces two potent second messengers from the membrane lipid phosphatidylinositol 4,5-bisphosphate (PIP_2): inositol 1,4,5-trisphosphate (IP_3) and diacylglycerol (DAG)[92,93] (Figure 3.1). IP_3 binds to receptors on the sarcoplasmic reticulum, releasing intracellular Ca^{2+} which, by combining with calmodulin, activates myosin light chain (MLC) kinase to phosphorylate MLC. Phosphorylated MLC in conjunction with actin

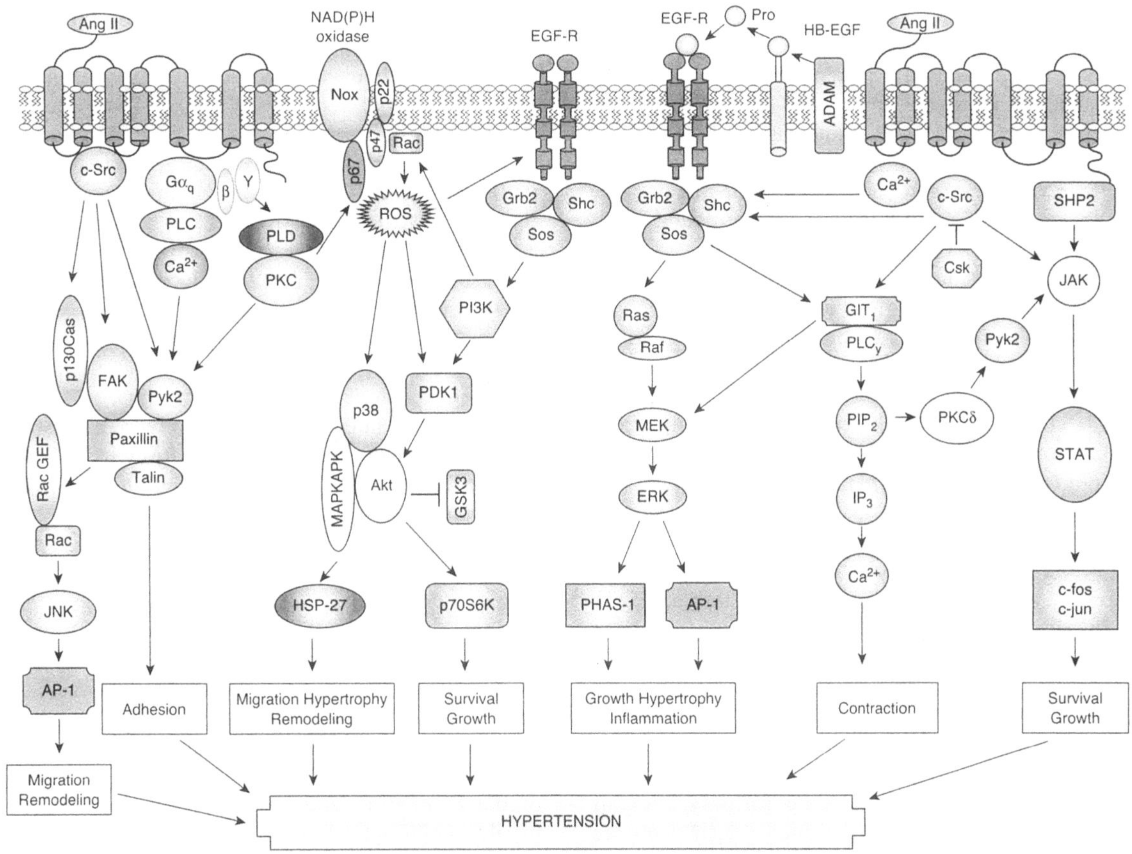

Figure 3.2 Ang II via AT$_1$R activation stimulates multiple kinase and enzyme pathways that are extensively interconnected in networks. One of the most important is Src and Src substrates in focal adhesions, including focal adhesion kinase (FAK) and proline-rich tyrosine kinase (Pyk2), which form multiprotein complexes with paxillin, tensin, and p130Cas. Ang II also stimulates the mitogen-activated protein (MAP) kinases ERK1/2, JNK, and p38MAPK; the phosphatidylinositol 3-kinase (PI3K) and protein kinase B (Akt) pathway; receptor kinases, including transactivation of epidermal growth factor receptor (EGFR) by reactive oxygen species (ROS) and the metalloprotease ADAM (a disintegrin and metalloprotease); inflammatory pathways (janus-activating kinase and signal transducers and activators of transcription: JAK/STAT); and oxidative stress pathways through NAD(P)H oxidase. These networks are regulated and coordinated by receptor activation, feedback loops, scaffolding proteins, subcellular compartmentalization, and cross-talk among the different pathways. Alterations in many of these signaling networks cause hypertension, the details of which are outlined in the text.

initiates contraction. Simultaneously, diacylglycerol, along with Ca^{2+}, activates protein kinase C (PKC), which in turn sensitizes the contractile machinery to Ca^{2+},[94] and enhances the activity of the Na^+/H^+ exchanger, resulting in increased alkalinization.[95] The sustained phase of contraction is due to PKC stimulation of the Ras/Raf/MEK/ERK pathway, which also induces growth and hypertrophy (discussed below). Ang II-mediated contraction via PLC activation is of particular relevance to hypertension.[96] Vascular PLC activity is enhanced in aortic walls[97] and smooth muscle cells[98] of hypertensive rats and in skin fibroblasts from patients with essential hypertension.[99]

Subsequent to activation of PLC, Ang II couples to PLD, hydrolyzing phosphatidylcholine (PC) to choline and phosphatidic acid (PA), which is then rapidly converted to DAG.[100,101] PLD activation first occurs within 1–2 minutes, but remains sustained for at least 1 hour and is responsible for prolonged PKC activation. PLD activity and Ang II-induced responses are increased in cells and tissues from hypertensive rats[102–104] and humans.[105] In spontaneously hypertensive rats (SHR), Ang II-induced activation of the PLC-IP_3-PLD-DAG pathway, release of Ca^{2+} and changes in pHi are augmented compared with normotensive controls.[80,106,107] Because DAG-PKC-dependent pathways are involved in both vasoconstriction and cell growth, alterations of PLD signaling in hypertension can have profound effects on hypertensive vasculopathy.[80,101,108]

Ang II also rapidly (within minutes) phosphorylates and stimulates phospholipase A_2 (PLA_2) to produce arachidonic acid (AA),[109] which is then converted via cyclooxygenase (CO) to prostaglandins (PGs), via lipoxygenase (LO) to a series of hydroxyeicosatetraenoic acids (HETES) and leukotrienes or via cytochrome P450 to epoxyeicosatrienoic acids (EETs) and dihydroxyeicosatetrienoic acids (DiHETEs).[110,111] Cytochrome P450 metabolites of AA, which influence renal function, vascular tone[112] and VSMC NAD(P)H oxidase activation,[113] thus play a role in the regulation of blood pressure and vascular hypertrophy. In addition, Ang II-induced activation of NAD(P)H oxidases produces superoxide,[114] which reduces the bioavailability of NO, leading to impaired vasorelaxation.

Activation of kinase pathways

In addition to classical signaling pathways, Ang II activates nonreceptor tyrosine kinases, such as the Src family kinases Src and Fyn, focal adhesion kinases, and the Ca^{2+}-dependent kinase Pyk2, as well as serine/threonine kinases such as the mitogen activated protein (MAP) kinases (Figure 3.2). Moreover, it transactivates receptor kinases such as epidermal growth factor receptor (EGFR), platelet-derived growth factor receptor (PDGFR), and insulin-like growth factor receptor (IGFR).[24,80,84,115]

Src family kinases

A major signaling pathway stimulated by Ang II begins with activation of the tyrosine kinase c-Src.[116,117] There is some evidence that Src is activated by $G_{\beta\gamma}$, but the precise coupling of Src to the AT_1R remains unclear.[88] Src, in turn, via its tyrosine kinase activity, is a major signal integrator for a variety of downstream pathways, including activation of PLC-γ via GPCR kinase-interacting protein-1 (GIT1)[118] and sustained Ca^{2+} release,[119,120] activation of the Ras pathway through Ras GAPs,[121] complex formation and phosphorylation of p130 Cas,[122,123] Pyk2[124,125] and phosphoinositide-dependent kinase-1 (PDK1),[126] regulation of focal adhesions via focal adhesion kinase (FAK)[127,128] and paxillin,[129] activation of the janus kinase/signal transducers and activators of transcription (JAK/STAT) nuclear signaling pathway,[130] as well as regulation of caveolin[131] and Shc.[127] Shc associates with Grb2,[132] thus activating the Sos/Ras-Raf/mitogen extracellular signal regulated kinase kinase (MEK) pathway, ultimately phosphorylating extracellular signal regulated kinase (ERK1/2).[133–135] In addition, Src-activated GIT1 serves as a scaffold for MEK1/ERK1/2 activation.[136] Ang II-induced Src-mediated growth of smooth muscle cells from resistance arteries of hypertensive patients is due to enhanced ERK1/2 signaling pathways.[137] Moreover, in smooth muscle cells from spontaneously hypertensive rats, activity of C-terminal Src kinase (Csk), a negative regulator of Src, is decreased, leading to increased Ang II-mediated Src signaling via EGFR transactivation.[138] These studies demonstrate a central role for Ang II-induced Src-dependent vascular growth signaling in hypertension.

AT_1R transactivation of EGFR

The growth promoting effects of Ang II, important in vascular and cardiac hypertrophic responses in hypertension, are in large part due to the cross-communication between AT_1R and tyrosine kinase receptor signaling pathways. AT_1R transactivation of the EGFR[139,140] and its signaling pathways, primarily MAPK activation, is redox-sensitive,[141] occurs through both Ca^{2+}-dependent and independent pathways,[141,142] and requires Ang II-induced phosphorylation of tyrosine 319 in the AT_1R.[143]

Ang II-induced EGFR activation occurs via the sequential activation of PLC, leading to Ca^{2+}-dependent activation of Pyk2,[144] and ROS-dependent activation of Src.[141] These pathways converge to activate ADAMs (a disintegrin and metalloprotease), transmembrane metalloproteases[145] that lead to ectodomain shedding of heparin-binding EGF (HB-EGF).[146,147] Free HB-EGF binds to the EGFR, leading to homodimerization and autophosphorylation on tyrosine. Interestingly, although addition of exogenous EGF leads to phosphorylation of five tyrosines in the cytoplasmic domain of the receptor, Ang II only phosphorylates two of these, Tyr 1068 and Tyr 1173, in a redox-sensitive manner.[141] Ang II induces tyrosine phosphorylation of EGFR with SHP-2 tyrosine phosphatase acting as a scaffold for AT_1R/EGFR association.[143] The transactivated EGFR recruits adaptor and signaling molecules including Shc, Grb2, Sos, Ras, and Raf that initiate phosphatidylinositol-3-kinase (PI3-K) pathways[148] and two MAPKs, ERK1/2 and p38MAPK.[149] In contrast, another member of the MAPK family, the c-Jun

NH_2-terminal kinase (JNK), is activated by Ang II without involvement of EGFR transactivation.[149]

The 'hijacking' of the EGFR by Ang II may explain the myriad effects – including growth, remodeling, and vasoconstriction – of Ang II-induced signaling in hypertension and cardiac hypertrophy.[150] Ang II-mediated increases in Src phosphorylation augment ERK1/2 signaling via transactivation of the EGFR in VSMCs from hypertensive rats compared with normal controls.[138] Blockade of EGFR transactivation by metalloprotease inhibition reduces blood pressure and HB-EGF shedding in hypertensive rats.[151] Additionally, inhibition of HB-EGFR shedding by dominant-negative ADAM12[152] or inhibition of EGFR by antisense[153] attenuates cardiac hypertrophy, suggesting a crucial role for EGFR transactivation in Ang II-induced growth and vasoconstriction in hypertension and cardiac hypertrophy.[154,155]

MAP kinases and Akt

Many of the pleiotrophic activities of AT$_1$R activation are due to the MAPK family, including ERK1/2,[156] JNK, and the p38 enzymes.[157,158] These Ang II-induced pathways promote growth, survival, migration, inflammation and fibrosis, processes important in vascular remodeling in hypertension.[16,80,83,159]

ERK1/2 activation occurs by two parallel independent pathways: a G protein-dependent pathway involving Src and PKC activation which is rapid and transient[160] and a G protein-independent pathway mediated by β-arrestin which is slow but sustained (see below).[160–162] One of the most important ERK1/2-mediated events is activation of the activator protein-1 (AP-1) transcription factor complex, which in turn regulates gene expression.[163–165] ERK1/2 also phosphorylates PHAS-1, which is a critical regulator of the translation initiation complex and protein synthesis.[166,167] Ang II stimulation of ERK1/2 in vascular smooth muscle cells[168] has been shown to be increased in VSMCs from SHR compared with WKY rats[169–171] and in arteries from Ang II-infused rats.[172] Furthermore, Ang II-induced ERK1/2 activity is increased and sustained in VSMCs from resistance arteries of hypertensive patients via a Src-mediated mechanism.[137] These in vivo and in vitro results implicate Ang II/AT$_1$R-induced enhanced ERK1/2 activation in hypertensive and cardiovascular disease models.

In addition to activation of the ERK1/2 MAP kinase, Ang II also activates other MAPKs, including p38 MAPK[173] and JNK.[174,175] While ERK1/2 and p38 MAPK have been shown to be important in hypertrophy in the vasculature,[173] JNK is more important in mediating inflammatory responses.[176,177] In rat models of acute[172] and chronic[178] hypertension, JNK pathways are activated in vascular and renal tissues and are involved in the development of vascular remodeling.[80,165] Furthermore, in relation to ERK1/2, JNK is preferentially activated in rat hearts by Ang II-induced hypertension, suggesting that JNK activation, mediated by the AT$_1$R, plays an important role in the Ang II-induced cardiac hypertrophic response.[179]

A major function of p38MAPK is stimulation of MAPKAPK-2, which phosphorylates the small mammalian heat-shock protein HSP-27[180] and the cell survival kinase Akt.[181] Ang II, via the AT$_1$R, activates Akt in VSMCs.[182] Akt is a serine kinase that has multiple downstream targets: Akt phosphorylation inactivates glycogen synthase kinase 3 (GSK3)[183] and activates p70S6 kinase.[184,185] In addition to cell survival, Akt mediates redox-sensitive stimulation of protein synthesis by Ang II in VSMCs.[186] Furthermore, Akt is up-regulated in aortas from stroke-prone spontaneously hypertensive rats, suggesting that Akt, via AT$_1$R-mediated ROS, is a determinant of the VSMC phenotype in hypertension.[187]

Focal adhesion kinase and Pyk2

Ang II has been shown to have profound effects both on focal adhesion formation and on enzymes/cytoskeletal associated components found within these cell-matrix signaling domains.[188] Ang II stimulates phosphorylation of the focal adhesion tyrosine kinases FAK[189] and Pyk2[190] and the cytoskeletal proteins paxillin[129] and talin.[191] Importantly, Ang II-mediated increases in phosphorylation of Pyk2 and FAK are greater in spontaneously hypertensive rats than in normotensive controls.[138] Pyk2, in association with Src,[124] leads to tyrosine phosphorylation of PDK1, which plays a role in focal adhesion assembly by conversion of focal adhesion complexes to mature focal adhesions.[126,192] Because focal adhesion assembly/disassembly is an important step in cell migration, the ability of Ang II to initiate cytoskeletal rearrangement has important potential implications in hypertensive vascular remodeling.

JAK/STAT pathway

Another important signaling pathway activated by Ang II is the JAK/STAT nuclear signaling pathway.[130,193,194] Phosphorylation of the AT$_1$R on the YIPP sequence within the C-terminus of the receptor,[195] which is facilitated by the SHP family of SH2 domain-containing tyrosine phosphatases, leads to complex formation with and activation of JAK2, indicating that SHP proteins act as adaptors for JAK phosphorylation and activation.[196] In vascular smooth muscle cells, AT_1R-derived second messengers Ca^{2+} and PKCδ signal to Pyk2, activating JAK2.[197] Ang II-induced activation of JAK results in phosphorylation of the STAT family of transcription factors.[194,198] Upon phosphorylation, STATs form dimers that are translocated to the nucleus[199] where they activate gene transcription, including the 'early growth response genes' *c-fos* and *c-jun*,[200] *c-myc*, α_2-macroglobulin and tissue inhibitor metalloproteinases 1 (TIMP-1) by binding to the sis-inducible element (SIE) of gene promoters.[201,202] Increases in the Ang II-induced JAK/STAT signaling pathway, leading to enhanced expression of growth genes, influence vascular and cardiac growth, hypertrophy and remodeling in hypertension.[80,203]

ROS pathway

In addition to the phospholipase activation and kinase signaling, Ang II also tonically activates NAD(P)H oxidases[204] to produce ROS (superoxide and hydrogen peroxide), which also serve as signaling molecules. The NAD(P)H oxidase is activated in a biphasic manner, first through PLD/PKC-mediated phosphorylation of one of its subunits (p47phox),[205] and then via Src/EGFR/PI3-K-mediated activation of Rac-1.[206] The resulting ROS mediate numerous redox-sensitive pathways implicated in Ang II-mediated hypertension,[16,207,208] including VSMC proliferation, hypertrophy and survival via activation of p38MAPK and Akt/PKB pathways.[173,186] Further discussions of AT_1R and NAD(P)H oxidase-induced redox signaling can be found in Chapter 6, and have been reviewed elsewhere.[14,17,80,81,159,207,209]

REGULATION OF AT_1R FUNCTION

In addition to the biochemical signals generated by AT_1R activation, intracellular events that control localization, trafficking routes and fates, recycling and degradation of the Ang II/AT_1R complex must be precisely regulated. This regulation can occur at multiple levels and has implications in understanding the pathogenesis of hypertension.

Desensitization

As discussed previously, Ang II-induced conformational changes in the AT_1R lead to recruitment of activated $G_{\alpha q/11}$/$G_{\beta\gamma}$ proteins which then separate and modulate a variety of downstream effectors such as PLC and PLD.[84] The $G_{\beta\gamma}$ subunit complex binds to different isoforms of G protein-coupled receptor kinases (GRK),[210,211] leading to phosphorylation of the C-terminus of the AT_1R with various functional consequences.[212] GRK2/3 phosphorylation of AT_1Rs results in recruitment and high-affinity binding of the multifunctional adaptor protein β-arrestin,[212,213] leading to receptor internalization via clathrin-coated pits or caveolae.[214] β-Arrestin binding blocks reassociation of the G proteins with the receptor, resulting in desensitization, a mechanism by which the receptor rapidly becomes less responsive to an agonist and is associated with removal of the receptors from the cell surface into intracellular compartments.[215–217] Alternatively, GRK5/6 phosphorylation of AT_1Rs results in β-arrestin-mediated ERK activation by a G protein-independent process.[212] Thus, β-arrestins have dual roles in regulating AT_1R signaling by desensitization or by serving as scaffolds for ERK cascades in G protein-independent signaling.[218,219]

Defects in the GRK-mediated AT_1R desensitization process have been postulated to alter Ang II responsiveness in Ang II-infused hypertensive rats. In these rats, vascular GRK5 expression is increased compared with normal rats[220] and could account for alterations in AT_1R phosphorylation and coupling to G proteins, resulting in long-term desensitization of receptor signaling or, inferentially, in increased growth responses due to enhanced ERK1/2 signaling via GRK5/6-induced AT_1R phosphorylation.

Internalization and trafficking

Internalization and trafficking of AT_1Rs play an important role in AT_1R activity by determining whether the receptor is recycled back to the membrane to continue signaling (resensitization)[221,222] or is degraded in lysosomes to terminate signaling (down-regulated).[223] Agonist-dependent endocytosis of AT_1Rs requires Ser and Thr phosphorylation by GRKs within the C-terminus of the receptor, which then binds to β-arrestin.[224,225] Internalization of AT_1Rs into endosomes differs according to agonist concentrations.[226] At physiological Ang II concentrations, agonist-induced internalization of the AT_1R occurs via clathrin-coated pits or caveolae by a dynamin (GTPase) and β-arrestin-dependent mechanism,[226,227] while at saturating Ang II concentrations, agonist-induced internalization is dynamin and β-arrestin independent.[226,228] AT_1R endocytosis is dependent upon the ADP-ribosylation factor 6 (Arf6),[229,230] is facilitated by PLD_2[231] and is regulated by ubiquitination of lysines 11 and 12 on β-arrestin which stabilizes AT_1R/β-arrestin complexes.[232] Stable AT_1R/β-arrestin complexes regulate trafficking of endocytosed AT_1Rs[227,233] and target the 'signalosomes' to endosomes for sustained ERK activation,[232] thus providing a molecular link between β-arrestin-induced endocytosis and signaling. Furthermore, the β-arrestin-mediated ERK activation requires AT_1R phosphorylation by GRK5/6.[212] Surface re-expression of AT_1Rs is mediated by a PI3 kinase-dependent rapid recycling route,[234] slow recycling, *de novo* receptor synthesis or recruitment of a reserve pool of intracellular receptors.[227]

Sorting and trafficking are also dependent upon budding and fusion of membrane compartments, processes that are regulated by Rab GTPases.[235] Like other GTPases, Rab proteins cycle between an active, GTP-bound and an inactive, GDP-bound state, and are regulated by GAPs that accelerate the intrinsic rate of hydrolysis of bound GTP to GDP, guanine nucleotide exchange factors (GEFs) that catalyze the exchange of bound GDP for GTP, and inhibitors of GDP dissociation (GDIs).[236]

Rab1 is required for AT_1R transport from the endoplasmic reticulum through the Golgi to the cell surface.[237] Overexpression of Rab1 in the hearts of transgenic mice results in abnormal protein trafficking associated with cardiomyopathy,[238] implicating an important role for Rab GTPase-regulated vesicle trafficking in the myocardium. Other Rab family members affect endocytosis and trafficking. Rab5 binds to the C-terminus of the AT_1R along with β-arrestin, and the Rab5/AT_1R/β-arrestin complex is specifically internalized via clathrin-coated pits to large Rab5 positive endosomes.[239] Rab5 and β-arrestin together mediate the retention of AT_1Rs in early endosomes. The activities of two other Rab proteins, Rab7 and Rab11, route the AT_1R to Rab7-positive multivesicular bodies (late endosomes) or to Rab11-positive perinuclear recycling vesicles.[223] Thus, the Rab proteins function to map the intracellular trafficking patterns of AT_1Rs and to control the timing and surface association of the AT_1R.

Ang II-induced transactivation of the EGFR occurs in cell surface signaling domains called caveolae.[240–242] Caveolae are morphologically defined as flask-shaped invaginations of the plasma membrane,[243] biochemically defined as a subset of lipid rafts enriched in cholesterol and sphingolipids,[244] and functionally defined as signaling domains due to the binding of caveolin-1, the signature protein of caveolae, to signaling proteins through a caveolin scaffolding domain (CSD).[245] The C-terminus of the AT_1R contains a CSD binding sequence, mediating AT_1R/caveolin interactions.[246] Ang II induces the translocation of a portion of AT_1Rs into caveolin-enriched/lipid raft fractions of the plasma membrane,[247] where AT_1R transactivation of EGFRs and assembly of signaling complexes are dependent upon intact microtubules.[240,248] Ang II-activated EGFRs are also localized with phosphorylated caveolin in focal adhesions.[240] These data implicate caveolae/lipid rafts and focal adhesions as important compartments for the spatial and temporal organization of Ang II-induced signaling via the AT_1R.[240,241]

Alterations in these AT_1R/caveolin signaling/trafficking pathways may contribute to cardiovascular changes observed in caveolin-deficient mice,[249] including smooth muscle hyperplasia,[250] pulmonary hyperproliferation and fibrosis[251] and cardiac hypertrophy due to hyperactivation of the ERK1/2 cascade.[242,252–254] Selective blockade of the pathological growth effects of AT_1Rs might be mitigated by antagonists to the EGFR or its signaling pathways, or by interfering with metalloproteases involved in HB-EGF shedding.[152,255] In clinical trials using Herceptin, a blocking antibody against the EGFR subtype ErbB2 used to improve survival in breast cancer patients, cardiomyopathy was a side effect, indicating an important role for ErbB2 in maintenance of normal heart function.[255,256]

The mechanisms by which AT_1R internalization occurs in caveolae are not well described. As noted above, the AT_1R can bind to caveolin-1, which also interacts with the EGFR.[240,248] Thus caveolin-1 may act as a scaffold facilitating the assembly of interacting signaling molecules in microdomains in which it is localized. In addition, there is evidence that caveolin may act as a chaperone in trafficking of AT_1Rs through the exocytic pathway to the cell surface.[257] The potential significance of Ang II signaling through caveolin-dependent mechanisms in hypertension awaits future studies in caveolin-1 null mice.[249,251]

CONCLUDING REMARKS AND FUTURE PERSPECTIVES

Ang II binding to AT_1Rs initiates a diverse range of cellular responses, many of which are important in the etiology of hypertension. The regulation of these diverse responses occurs at multiple levels, starting with polymorphic variants in the AT_1R gene and AT_1R transcriptional control by hormones, growth factors, cytokines, vasorelaxants, vitamins, and blood lipids. AT_1R-associated proteins provide additional levels of regulation: kinases (GRK, Src, PKC) can alter receptor structure or conformations with different affinities for binding proteins; G proteins ($G_{\alpha q}$) can directly mediate signaling; and scaffolds (β-arrestins, caveolin, SHP2) can physically link the receptor to effectors and can control receptor localization and/or trafficking, which determines receptor accessibility for activation. Finally, at the post-receptor level, activation of various second messenger systems and signal transduction pathways, including signaling cross-talk with growth factors, inflammatory cytokines and oxidative stress pathways, can provide diversity of responses. Modifications of AT_1R function at any of these levels can affect vascular structural and functional changes leading to blood pressure elevation.[80] Newer insights from basic science research into AT_1R functioning within the single cell may lead to therapeutic strategies to inhibit transactivation (by inhibiting EGFR subtypes such as HER2/ErbB2),[255] desensitization (with GRK inhibitors) or internalization (with β-arrestin inhibitors).[216]

REFERENCES

1. Carretero OA, Oparil S. Essential hypertension: part I: definition and etiology. Circulation 2000; 101: 329–35.
2. de Gasparo M, Catt KJ, Inagami T et al. International union of pharmacology. XXIII. The angiotensin II receptors. Pharmacol Rev 2000; 52: 415–72.
3. Re RN. Intracellular renin and the nature of intracrine enzymes. Hypertension 2003; 42: 117–22.
4. Bader M, Peters J, Baltatu O et al. Tissue renin-angiotensin systems: new insights from experimental animal models in hypertension research. J Mol Med 2001; 79: 76–102.
5. Jan Danser AH. Local renin-angiotensin systems: the unanswered questions. Int J Biochem Cell Biol 2003; 35: 759–68.
6. Re RN. Tissue renin angiotensin systems. Med Clin North Am 2004; 88: 19–38.
7. Leung PS. The peptide hormone angiotensin II: its new functions in tissues and organs. Curr Protein Pept Sci 2004; 5: 267–73.
8. Peach M. Renin-angiotensin system: biochemistry and mechanisms of action. Physiol Rev 1977; 57: 313–70.
9. Timmermans PB, Wong PC, Chiu AT et al. Angiotensin II receptors and angiotensin II receptor antagonists. Pharmacol Rev 1993; 45: 205–51.
10. Sadoshima J. Versatility of the angiotensin II type 1 receptor. Circ Res 1998; 82: 1352–5.
11. Miura S, Saku K, Karnik S. Molecular analysis of the structure and function of the angiotensin II type 1 receptor. Hypertens Res 2003; 26: 937–43.
12. Ruggenenti P, Remuzzi G. Seminars in nephrology: introduction. Semin Nephrol 2004; 24: 91–2.
13. Kim S, Iwao H. Molecular and cellular mechanisms of angiotensin II-mediated cardiovascular and renal diseases. Pharmacol Rev 2000; 52: 11–34.
14. Touyz RM. The role of angiotensin II in regulating vascular structural and functional changes in hypertension. Curr Hypertens Rep 2003; 5: 155–64.
15. Ruiz-Ortega M, Ruperez M, Esteban V et al. Molecular mechanisms of angiotensin II-induced vascular injury. Curr Hypertens Rep 2003; 5: 73–9.
16. Schiffrin EL, Touyz RM. From bedside to bench to bedside: role of renin-angiotensin-aldosterone system in remodeling of resistance arteries in hypertension. Am J Physiol Heart Circ Physiol 2004; 287: H435–H46.
17. Touyz RM. Molecular and cellular mechanisms in vascular injury in hypertension: role of angiotensin II – editorial review. Curr Opin Nephrol Hypertens 2005; 14: 125–31.
18. Murphy TJ, Alexander RW, Griendling KK et al. Isolation of a cDNA encoding the vascular type-1 angiotensin receptor. Nature 1991; 351: 233–6.
19. Sasaki K, Yamano Y, Bardhan S et al. Cloning and expression of a complementary DNA encoding a bovine adrenal angiotensin II type-1 receptor. Nature 1991; 351: 230–3.
20. Iwai N, Inagami T. Identification of two subtypes in the type 1 angiotensin II receptor. FEBS Lett 1992; 298: 257–60.
21. Ito M, Oliverio M, Mannon P et al. Regulation of blood pressure by the type 1A angiotensin II receptor gene. Proc Natl Acad Sci U S A 1995; 92: 3521–5.
22. Chen X, Li W, Yoshida H et al. Targeting deletion of angiotensin type 1B receptor gene in the mouse. Am J Physiol 1997; 272: F299–F304.
23. Pierce KL, Premont RT, Lefkowitz RJ. Seven-transmembrane receptors. Nat Rev Mol Cell Biol 2002; 3: 639–50.
24. Sayeski PP, Ali MS, Semeniuk DJ et al. Angiotensin II signal transduction pathways. Regul Pept 1998; 78: 19–29.
25. Tzakos AG, Gerothanassis IP, Troganis AN. On the structural basis of the hypertensive properties of angiotensin II: a solved mystery or a controversial issue? Curr Top Med Chem 2004; 4: 431–44.
26. Hunyady L, Gaborik Z, Shah BH et al. Structural determinants of agonist-induced signaling and regulation of the angiotensin AT1 receptor. Mol Cell Endocrinol 2004; 217: 89–100.
27. Lifton RP, Gharavi AG, Geller DS. Molecular mechanisms of human hypertension. Cell 2001; 104: 545–56.
28. Luft FC. Present status of genetic mechanisms in hypertension. Med Clin North Am 2004; 88: 1–18.
29. Bonnardeaux A, Davies E, Jeunemaitre X et al. Angiotensin II type 1 receptor gene polymorphisms in human essential hypertension. Hypertension 1994; 24: 63–9.
30. Erdmann J, Riedel K, Rohde K et al. Characterization of polymorphisms in the promoter of the human angiotensin II subtype 1 (AT1) receptor gene. Ann Hum Genet 1999; 63: 369–74.
31. Halushka MK, Fan JB, Bentley K et al. Patterns of single-nucleotide polymorphisms in candidate genes for blood-pressure homeostasis. Nat Genet 1999; 22: 239–47.
32. Takahashi N, Muakami H, Kodama K et al. Association of a polymorphism at the 5′-region of the angiotensin II type 1 receptor with hypertension. Ann Hum Genet 2000; 64: 197–205.
33. Zhu X, Chang Y-PC, Yan D et al. Associations between hypertension and genes in the renin-angiotensin system. Hypertension 2003; 41: 1027–34.
34. Miller JA, Thai K, Scholey JW. Angiotensin II type 1 receptor gene polymorphism predicts response to losartan and angiotensin II. Kidney Int 1999; 56: 2173–80.
35. Henderson S, Haiman C, Mack W. Multiple polymorphisms in the renin-angiotensin-aldosterone system (ACE, CYP11B2, AGTR1) and their contribution to hypertension in African Americans and Latinos in the multiethnic cohort. Am J Med Sci 2004; 328: 266–73.
36. Reich H, Duncan JA, Weinstein J et al. Interactions between gender and the angiotensin type 1 receptor gene polymorphism. Kidney Int 2003; 63: 1443–9.
37. Schmidt S, Beige J, Walla-Friedel M et al. A polymorphism in the gene for the angiotensin II type 1 receptor is not associated with hypertension. J Hypertens 1997; 15: 1385–8.
38. Hilgers KF, Langenfeld MRW, Schlaich M et al. 1166 A/C polymorphism of the angiotensin II type 1 receptor gene and the response to short-term infusion of angiotensin II. Circulation 1999; 100: 1394–9.

39. Baudin B. Angiotensin II receptor polymorphisms in hypertension. Pharmacogenomic considerations. Pharmacogenomics 2002; 3: 65–73.
40. Luft FC. Geneticism of essential hypertension. Hypertension 2004; 43: 1155–9.
41. Miller JA, Scholey JW. The impact of renin-angiotensin system polymorphisms on physiological and pathophysiological processes in humans. Curr Opin Nephrol Hypertens 2004; 13: 101–6.
42. Duncan JA, Scholey JW, Miller JA. Angiotensin II type 1 receptor gene polymorphisms in humans: physiology and pathophysiology of the genotypes. Curr Opin Nephrol Hypertens 2001; 10: 111–16.
43. Castellano M, Glorioso N, Cusi D et al. Genetic polymorphism of the renin-angiotensin-aldosterone system and arterial hypertension in the Italian population: the GENIPER Project. J Hypertens 2003; 21: 1853–60.
44. Michel MC, Hahntow I, Koopmans RP. Multiple gene approaches to delineate the role of the renin-angiotensin-aldosterone system in nephropathy. J Hypertens 2005; 23: 269–72.
45. Siani A, Russo P, Paolo Cappuccio F et al. Combination of renin-angiotensin system polymorphisms is associated with altered renal sodium handling and hypertension. Hypertension 2004; 43: 598–602.
46. Fabris B, Bortoletto M, Candido R et al. Genetic polymorphisms of the renin-angiotensin-aldosterone system and renal insufficiency in essential hypertension. J Hypertens 2005; 23: 309–16.
47. Agarwal A, Williams GH, Fisher NDL. Genetics of human hypertension. Trends Endocrinol Metab 2005; 16: 127–33.
48. Hansen JL, Theilade J, Haunso S et al. Oligomerization of wild type and nonfunctional mutant angiotensin II type I receptors inhibits $G_{\alpha q}$ protein signaling but not ERK activation. J Biol Chem 2004; 279: 24108–15.
49. AbdAlla S, Lother H, Langer A et al. Factor XIIIA transglutaminase crosslinks AT1 receptor dimers of monocytes at the onset of atherosclerosis. Cell 2004; 119: 343–54.
50. AbdAlla S, Lother H, Abdel-tawab AM et al. The angiotensin II AT2 receptor is an AT1 receptor antagonist. J Biol Chem 2001; 276: 39721–6.
51. AbdAlla S, Lother H, Quitterer U. AT1-receptor heterodimers show enhanced G-protein activation and altered receptor sequestration. Nature 2000; 407: 94–8.
52. Barki-Harrington L, Luttrell LM, Rockman HA. Dual inhibition of β-adrenergic and angiotensin II receptors by a single antagonist: a functional role for receptor-receptor interaction in vivo. Circulation 2003; 108: 1611–18.
53. Zeng C, Luo Y, Asico LD et al. Perturbation of D1 dopamine and AT1 receptor interaction in spontaneously hypertensive rats. Hypertension 2003; 42: 787–92.
54. Rashid AJ, O'Dowd BF, George SR. Minireview: Diversity and complexity of signaling through peptidergic G protein-coupled receptors. Endocrinology 2004; 145: 2645–52.
55. Barki-Harrington L. Oligomerisation of angiotensin receptors: novel aspects in disease and drug therapy. J Renin Angiotensin Aldosterone Syst 2004; 5: 49–52.
56. AbdAlla S, Lother H, Massiery AE et al. Increased AT1 receptor heterodimers in preeclampsia mediate enhanced angiotensin II responsiveness. Nat Med 2001; 7: 1003–9.
57. Quitterer U, Lother H, Abdalla S. AT1 receptor heterodimers and angiotensin II responsiveness in preeclampsia. Semin Nephrol 2004; 24: 115–19.
58. Terrillon S, Bouvier M. Roles of G-protein-coupled receptor dimerization. EMBO Rep 2004; 5: 30–4.
59. Nickenig G, Murphy TJ. Down-regulation by growth factors of vascular smooth muscle angiotensin receptor gene expression. Mol Pharmacol 1994; 46: 653–9.
60. Lassegue B, Alexander RW, Nickenig G et al. Angiotensin II down-regulates the vascular smooth muscle AT1 receptor by transcriptional and post-transcriptional mechanisms: evidence for homologous and heterologous regulation. Mol Pharmacol 1995; 48: 601–9.
61. Nickenig G, Baumer AT, Grohe C et al. Estrogen modulates AT1 receptor gene expression in vitro and in vivo. Circulation 1998; 97: 2197–201.
62. Nickenig G, Strehlow K, Wassmann S et al. Differential effects of estrogen and progesterone on AT1 receptor gene expression in vascular smooth muscle cells. Circulation 2000; 102: 1828–33.
63. Fukuyama K, Ichiki T, Takeda K et al. Downregulation of vascular angiotensin II type 1 receptor by thyroid hormone. Hypertension 2003; 41: 598–603.
64. Wyse B, Linas S, Thekkumkara T. Functional role of a novel cis-acting element (GAGA box) in human type-1 angiotensin II receptor gene transcription. J Mol Endocrinol 2000; 25: 97–108.
65. Nickenig G, Roling J, Strehlow K et al. Insulin induces upregulation of vascular AT1 receptor gene expression by posttranscriptional mechanisms. Circulation 1998; 98: 2453–60.
66. Muller C, Reddert A, Wassmann S et al. Insulin-like growth factor induces up-regulation of AT(1)-receptor gene expression in vascular smooth muscle cells. J Renin Angiotensin Aldosterone Syst 2000; 1: 273–7.
67. Saavedra JM, Ando H, Armando I et al. Brain angiotensin II, an important stress hormone: regulatory sites and therapeutic opportunities. Ann N Y Acad Sci 2004; 1018: 76–84.
68. Wassmann S, Stumpf M, Strehlow K et al. Interleukin-6 induces oxidative stress and endothelial dysfunction by overexpression of the angiotensin II type 1 receptor. Circ Res 2004; 94: 534–41.
69. Cowling RT, Gurantz D, Peng J et al. Transcription factor NF-κB is necessary for up-regulation of type 1 angiotensin II receptor mRNA in rat cardiac fibroblasts treated with tumor necrosis factor-α or interleukin-1β. J Biol Chem 2002; 277: 5719–24.
70. Ichiki T, Usui M, Kato M et al. Downregulation of angiotensin II type 1 receptor gene transcription by nitric oxide. Hypertension 1998; 31: 342–6.
71. Nithipatikom K, Holmes BB, McCoy MJ et al. Chronic administration of nitric oxide reduces angiotensin II receptor type 1 expression and aldosterone synthesis in zona glomerulosa cells. Am J Physiol Endocrinol Metab 2004; 287: E820–E827.
72. Haxsen V, Adam-Stitah S, Ritz E et al. Retinoids inhibit the actions of angiotensin II on vascular smooth muscle cells. Circ Res 2001; 88: 637–44.
73. Nickenig G, Sachinidis A, Michaelsen F et al. Upregulation of vascular angiotensin II receptor gene expression by low-density lipoprotein in vascular smooth muscle cells. Circulation 1997; 95: 473–8.
74. Yang BC, Phillips MI, Mohuczy D et al. Increased angiotensin II type 1 receptor expression in hypercholesterolemic atherosclerosis in rabbits. Arterioscler Thromb Vasc Biol 1998; 18: 1433–9.
75. Strehlow K, Wassmann S, Bohm M et al. Angiotensin AT1 receptor over-expression in hypercholesterolaemia. Ann Med 2000; 32: 386–9.
76. Nickenig G, Jung O, Strehlow K et al. Hypercholesterolemia is associated with enhanced angiotensin AT1-receptor expression. Am J Physiol 1997; 272: H2701–H2707.
77. Nickenig G, Baumer AT, Temur Y et al. Statin-sensitive dysregulated AT1 receptor function and density in hypercholesterolemic men. Circulation 1999; 100: 2131–4.
78. Glorioso N, Troffa C, Filigheddu F et al. Effect of the HMG-CoA reductase inhibitors on blood pressure in patients with essential hypertension and primary hypercholesterolemia. Hypertension 1999; 34: 1281–6.

79. Nickenig G. Should angiotensin II receptor blockers and statins be combined? Circulation 2004; 110: 1013–20.
80. Touyz RM, Schiffrin EL. Signal transduction mechanisms mediating the physiological and pathophysiological actions of angiotensin II in vascular smooth muscle cells. Pharmacol Rev 2000; 52: 639–72.
81. Berry C, Touyz R, Dominiczak AF et al. Angiotensin receptors: signaling, vascular pathophysiology, and interactions with ceramide. Am J Physiol Heart Circ Physiol 2001; 281: H2337–H2365.
82. Hunyady L, Vauquelin G, Vanderheyden P. Agonist induction and conformational selection during activation of a G-protein-coupled receptor. Trends Pharmacol Sci 2003; 24: 81–6.
83. Touyz RM. Recent advances in intracellular signalling in hypertension. Curr Opin Nephrol Hypertens 2003; 12: 165–74.
84. Griendling KK, Ushio-Fukai M, Lassegue B et al. Angiotensin II signaling in vascular smooth muscle: new concepts. Hypertension 1997; 29: 366–70.
85. Macrez-Lepretre N, Kalkbrenner F, Morel J-L et al. G protein heterotrimer $G\alpha_{13}\beta_1\gamma_3$ couples the angiotensin AT1A receptor to increases in cytoplasmic Ca^{2+} in rat portal vein myocytes. J Biol Chem 1997; 272: 10095–102.
86. Kai H, Alexander RW, Ushio-Fukai M et al. G-Protein binding domains of the angiotensin II AT1A receptors mapped with synthetic peptides selected from the receptor sequence. Biochem J 1998; 332 (Pt 3): 781–7.
87. Ushio-Fukai M, Griendling KK, Akers M et al. Temporal dispersion of activation of phospholipase C-β1 and -γ isoforms by angiotensin II in vascular smooth muscle cells: role of $\alpha_{q/11}$, α_{12}, and βγ G protein subunits. J Biol Chem 1998; 273: 19772–7.
88. Ushio-Fukai M, Alexander RW, Akers M et al. Angiotensin II receptor coupling to phospholipase D is mediated by the βγ subunits of heterotrimeric G proteins in vascular smooth muscle cells. Mol Pharmacol 1999; 55: 142–9.
89. Grant SL, Lassegue B, Griendling KK et al. Specific regulation of RGS2 messenger RNA by angiotensin II in cultured vascular smooth muscle cells. Mol Pharmacol 2000; 57: 460–7.
90. Heximer SP, Knutsen RH, Sun X et al. Hypertension and prolonged vasoconstrictor signaling in RGS2-deficient mice. J Clin Invest 2003; 111: 445–52.
91. Calo LA, Pagnin E, Davis PA et al. Increased expression of regulator of G protein signaling-2 (RGS-2) in Bartter's/Gitelman's syndrome. A role in the control of vascular tone and implication for hypertension. J Clin Endocrinol Metab 2004; 89: 4153–7.
92. Alexander RW, Brock TA, Gimbrone MA Jr et al. Angiotensin increases inositol trisphosphate and calcium in vascular smooth muscle. Hypertension 1985; 7: 447–51.
93. Griendling K, Rittenhouse S, Brock T et al. Sustained diacylglycerol formation from inositol phospholipids in angiotensin II-stimulated vascular smooth muscle cells. J Biol Chem 1986; 261: 5901–6.
94. Morgan K, Leinweber B. PKC-dependent signalling mechanisms in differentiated smooth muscle. Acta Physiol Scand 1998; 164: 495–505.
95. Vallega GA, Canessa ML, Berk BC et al. Vascular smooth muscle Na+-H+ exchanger kinetics and its activation by angiotensin II. Am J Physiol Cell Physiol 1988; 254: C751–C758.
96. Deinum J. Second messengers in primary hypertension. J Hypertens 2003; 21: 497–9.
97. Uehara Y, Ishii M, Ishimitsu T et al. Enhanced phospholipase C activity in the vascular wall of spontaneously hypertensive rats. Hypertension 1988; 11: 28–33.
98. Osanai T, Dunn MJ. Phospholipase C responses in cells from spontaneously hypertensive rats. Hypertension 1992; 19: 446–55.
99. Kosugi T, Osanai T, Kamada T et al. Phospholipase C activity is enhanced in skin fibroblasts obtained from patients with essential hypertension. J Hypertens 2003; 21: 538–90.
100. Lassegue B, Alexander RW, Clark M et al. Phosphatidylcholine is a major source of phosphatidic acid and diacylglycerol in angiotensin II-stimulated vascular smooth-muscle cells. Biochem J 1993; 292: 509–17.
101. Freeman EJ, Chisolm GM, Tallant EA. Role of calcium and protein kinase C in the activation of phospholipase D by angiotensin II in vascular smooth muscle cells. Arch Biochem Biophys 1995; 319: 84–92.
102. Freeman EJ, Ferrario CM, Tallant EA. Angiotensins differentially activate phospholipase D in vascular smooth muscle cells from spontaneously hypertensive and Wistar-Kyoto rats. Am J Hypertens 1995; 8: 1105–11.
103. Min DS, Lee K-H, Chang J-S et al. Altered expression of phospholipase D1 in spontaneously hypertensive rats. Mol Cells 2001; 11: 386–91.
104. Andresen BT, Jackson EK, Romero GG. Angiotensin II signaling to phospholipase D in renal microvascular smooth muscle cells in SHR. Hypertension 2001; 37: 635–9.
105. Touyz RM, Schiffrin EL. Increased generation of superoxide by angiotensin II in smooth muscle cells from resistance arteries of hypertensive patients: role of phospholipase D-dependent NAD(P)H oxidase-sensitive pathways. J Hypertens 2001; 19: 1245–54.
106. Touyz R, Tolloczko B, Schiffrin E. Mesenteric vascular smooth muscle cells from spontaneously hypertensive rats display increased calcium reponses to angiotensin II but not to endothelin-1. J Hypertens 1994; 12: 663–73.
107. Baines RJ, Brown C, Ng LL et al. Angiotensin II-stimulated phospholipase C responses of two vascular smooth muscle-derived cell lines: role of cyclic GMP. Hypertension 1996; 28: 772–8.
108. Gomez-Cambronero J, Keire P. Phospholipase D: a novel major player in signal transduction. Cell Signal 1998; 10: 387–97.
109. Rao GN, Lassegue B, Alexander RW et al. Angiotensin II stimulates phosphorylation of high-molecular-mass cytosolic phospholipase A2 in vascular smooth-muscle cells. Biochem J 1994; 299 (Pt 1): 197–201.
110. Roman RJ. P-450 metabolites of arachidonic acid in the control of cardiovascular function. Physiol Rev 2002; 82: 131–85.
111. Sarkis A, Lopez B, Roman RJ. Role of 20-hydroxyeicosatetraenoic acid and epoxyeicosatrienoic acids in hypertension. Curr Opin Nephrol Hypertens 2004; 13: 205–14.
112. Zhao X, Imig JD. Kidney CYP450 enzymes: biological actions beyond drug metabolism. Curr Drug Metab 2003; 4: 73–84.
113. Zafari A, Ushio-Fukai M, Minieri C et al. Arachidonic acid metabolites mediate angiotensin II-induced NADH/NADPH oxdiase activity and hypertrophy in vascular smooth muscle cells. Antioxid Redox Signal 1999; 1: 167–79.
114. Rajagopalan S, Kurz S, Munzel T et al. Angiotensin II-mediated hypertension in the rat increases vascular superoxide production via membrane NADH/NADPH oxidase activation: contribution to alterations of vasomotor tone. J Clin Invest 1996; 97: 1916–23.
115. Thomas WG, Qian H, Smith NJ. What's new in the renin-angiotensin system?: When 6 is 9: 'Uncoupled' AT1 receptors turn signalling on its head. Cell Mol Life Sci 2004; 61: 2687–94.
116. Linseman DA, Benjamin CW, Jones DA. Convergence of angiotensin II and platelet-derived growth factor receptor signaling cascades in vascular smooth muscle cells. J Biol Chem 1995; 270: 12563–8.
117. Thomas SM, Brugge JS. Cellular functions regulated by Src family kinases. Annu Rev Cell Dev Biol 1997; 13: 513–609.
118. Haendeler J, Yin G, Hojo Y et al. GIT1 mediates Src-dependent activation of phospholipase Cγ by angiotensin II and epidermal growth factor. J Biol Chem 2003; 278: 49936–44.

119. Marrero M, Paxton W, Duff J et al. Angiotensin II stimulates tyrosine phosphorylation of phospholipase Cγ1 in vascular smooth muscle cells. J Biol Chem 1994; 269: 10935–9.
120. Marrero MB, Schieffer B, Paxton WG et al. Electroporation of pp60c-src antibodies inhibits the angiotensin II activation of phospholipase C-γ1 in rat aortic smooth muscle cells. J Biol Chem 1995; 270: 15734–8.
121. Schieffer B, Paxton WG, Chai Q et al. Angiotensin II controls $p21^{ras}$ activity via $pp60^{c\text{-}src}$. J Biol Chem 1996; 271: 10329–33.
122. Sayeski PP, Ali MS, Harp JB et al. Phosphorylation of p130Cas by angiotensin II is dependent on c-Src, intracellular Ca2+, and protein kinase C. Circ Res 1998; 82: 1279–88.
123. Kyaw M, Yoshizumi M, Tsuchiya K et al. Src and Cas are essentially but differentially involved in angiotensin II-stimulated migration of vascular smooth muscle cells via extracellular signal-regulated kinase 1/2 and c-Jun NH2-terminal kinase activation. Mol Pharmacol 2004; 65: 832–41.
124. Dikic I, Tokiwa G, Lev S et al. A role for Pyk2 and Src in linking G-protein-coupled receptors with MAP kinase activation. Nature 1996; 383: 547–50.
125. Sabri A, Govindarajan G, Griffin T et al. Calcium-and protein kinase C-dependent activation of the tyrosine kinase PYK2 by angiotensin II in vascular smooth muscle. Circ Res 1998; 83: 841–51.
126. Taniyama Y, Weber DS, Rocic P et al. Pyk2- and Src-dependent tyrosine phosphorylation of PDK1 regulates focal adhesions. Mol Cell Biol 2003; 23: 8019–29.
127. Schorb W, Peeler T, Madigan N et al. Angiotensin II-induced protein tyrosine phosphorylation in neonatal rat cardiac fibroblasts. J Biol Chem 1994; 269: 19626–32.
128. Chaudhary A, Brugge JS, Cooper JA. Direct phosphorylation of focal adhesion kinase by c-src: evidence using a modified nucleotide pocket kinase and ATP analog. Biochem Biophys Res Commun 2002; 294: 293–300.
129. Leduc I, Meloche S. Angiotensin II stimulates tyrosine phosphorylation of the focal adhesion-associated protein paxillin in aortic smooth muscle cells. J Biol Chem 1995; 270: 4401–4.
130. Venema RC, Venema VJ, Eaton DC et al. Angiotensin II-induced tyrosine phosphorylation of signal transducers and activators of transcription 1 is regulated by Janus-activated kinase 2 and Fyn kinases and mitogen-activated protein kinase phosphatase 1. J Biol Chem 1998; 273: 30795–800.
131. Li S, Seitz R, Lisanti M. Phosphorylation of caveolin by Src tyrosine kinases: the α-isoform of caveolin is selectively phosphorylated by v-Src in vivo. J Biol Chem 1996; 271: 3863–8.
132. Skolnik EY, Lee CH, Batzer A et al. The SH2/SH3 domain-containing protein GRB2 interacts with tyrosine-phosphorylated IRS1 and Shc: implications for insulin control of ras signalling. EMBO J 1993; 12: 1929–36.
133. Eguchi S, Matsumoto T, Motley ED et al. Identification of an essential signaling cascade for mitogen-activated protein kinase activation by angiotensin II in cultured rat vascular smooth muscle cells. Possible requirement of G_q-mediated p21ras activation coupled to a Ca^{2+}/calmodulin-sensitive tyrosine kinase. J Biol Chem 1996; 271: 14169–75.
134. Inagami T, Eguchi S. Angiotensin II-mediated vascular smooth muscle cell growth signaling. Braz J Med Biol Res 2000; 33: 619–24.
135. Sayeski PP, Ali MS. The critical role of c-Src and the Shc/Grb2/ERK2 signaling pathway in angiotensin II-dependent VSMC proliferation. Exp Cell Res 2003; 287: 339–49.
136. Yin G, Haendeler J, Yan C et al. GIT1 functions as a scaffold for MEK1-extracellular signal-regulated kinase 1 and 2 activation by angiotensin II and epidermal growth factor. Mol Cell Biol 2004; 24: 875–85.
137. Touyz RM, He G, Wu X-H et al. Src is an important mediator of extracellular signal-regulated kinase 1/2-dependent growth signaling by angiotensin II in smooth muscle cells from resistance arteries of hypertensive patients. Hypertension 2001; 38: 56–64.
138. Touyz RM, Wu X-H, He G et al. Increased angiotensin II-mediated Src signaling via epidermal growth factor receptor transactivation is associated with decreased C-terminal Src kinase activity in vascular smooth muscle cells from spontaneously hypertensive rats. Hypertension 2002; 39: 479–85.
139. Eguchi S, Numaguchi K, Iwasaki H et al. Calcium-dependent epidermal growth factor receptor transactivation mediates the angiotensin II-induced mitogen-activated protein kinase activation in vascular smooth muscle cells. J Biol Chem 1998; 273: 8890–6.
140. Murasawa S, Mori Y, Nozawa Y et al. Angiotensin II type 1 receptor-induced extracellular signal-regulated protein kinase activation is mediated by Ca^{2+}/calmodulin-dependent transactivation of epidermal growth factor receptor. Circ Res 1998; 82: 1338–48.
141. Ushio-Fukai M, Griendling KK, Becker P et al. Epidermal growth factor receptor transactivation by angiotensin II requires reactive oxygen species in vascular smooth muscle cells. Arterioscler Thromb Vasc Biol 2001; 21: 489–95.
142. Saito Y, Berk BC. Transactivation: a novel signaling pathway from angiotensin II to tyrosine kinase receptors. J Mol Cell Cardiol 2001; 33: 3–7.
143. Seta K, Sadoshima J. Phosphorylation of tyrosine 319 of the angiotensin II type 1 receptor mediates angiotensin II-induced trans-activation of the epidermal growth factor receptor. J Biol Chem 2003; 278: 9019–26.
144. Andreev J, Galisteo ML, Kranenburg O et al. Src and Pyk2 mediate G-protein-coupled receptor activation of epidermal growth factor receptor (EGFR) but are not required for coupling to the mitogen-activated protein (MAP) kinase signaling cascade. J Biol Chem 2001; 276: 20130–5.
145. Blobel CP. ADAMS: key components in EGFR signalling and development. Nat Rev Mol Cell Biol 2005; 6: 32–43.
146. Prenzel N, Zwick E, Daub H et al. EGF receptor transactivation by G-protein-coupled receptors requires metalloproteinase cleavage of proHB-EGF. Nature 1999; 402: 884–8.
147. Shah BH, Yesilkaya A, Olivares-Reyes JA et al. Differential pathways of angiotensin II-induced extracellularly regulated kinase 1/2 phosphorylation in specific cell types: role of heparin-binding epidermal growth factor. Mol Endocrinol 2004; 18: 2035–48.
148. Bokemeyer D, Schmitz U, Kramer HJ. Angiotensin II-induced growth of vascular smooth muscle cells requires an Src-dependent activation of the epidermal growth factor receptor. Kidney Int 2000; 58: 549–58.
149. Eguchi S, Dempsey PJ, Frank GD et al. Activation of MAPKs by angiotensin II in vascular smooth muscle cells. Metalloprotease-dependent EGF receptor activations is required for activation of ERK and p38 MAPK but not for JNK. J Biol Chem 2001; 276: 7957–62.
150. Smith AI, Turner AJ. What's new in the renin-angiotensin system? Cell Mol Life Sci 2004; 61: 2675–6.
151. Hao L, Du M, Lopez-Campistrous A et al. Agonist-induced activation of matrix metalloproteinase-7 promotes vasoconstriction through the epidermal growth factor-receptor pathway. Circ Res 2004; 94: 68–76.
152. Asakura M, Kitakaze M, Takashima S et al. Cardiac hypertrophy is inhibited by antagonism of ADAM12 processing of HB-EGF: metalloproteinase inhibitors as a new therapy. Nat Med 2002; 8: 35–40.

153. Kagiyama S, Eguchi S, Frank GD et al. Angiotensin II-induced cardiac hypertrophy and hypertension are attenuated by epidermal growth factor receptor antisense. Circulation 2002; 106: 909–12.
154. Shah BH, Catt KJ. A central role of EGF receptor transactivation in angiotensin II-induced cardiac hypertrophy. Trends Pharmacol Sci 2003; 24: 239–44.
155. Shah BH, Catt KJ. Matrix metalloproteinase-dependent EGF receptor activation in hypertension and left ventricular hypertrophy. Trends Endocrinol Metab 2004; 15: 241–3.
156. Sasagawa S, Ozaki Y-i, Fujita K et al. Prediction and validation of the distinct dynamics of transient and sustained ERK activation. Nat Cell Biol 2005; 7: 365–73.
157. Widmann C, Gibson S, Jarpe MB et al. Mitogen-activated protein kinase: conservation of a three-kinase module from yeast to human. Physiol Rev 1999; 79: 143–80.
158. Johnson GL, Lapadat R. Mitogen-activated protein kinase pathways mediated by ERK, JNK, and p38 protein kinases. Science 2002; 298: 1911–12.
159. Intengan HD, Schiffrin EL. Vascular remodeling in hypertension: roles of apoptosis, inflammation, and fibrosis. Hypertension 2001; 38: 581–7.
160. Ahn S, Shenoy SK, Wei H et al. Differential kinetic and spatial patterns of β-arrestin and G protein-mediated ERK activation by the angiotensin II receptor. J Biol Chem 2004; 279: 35518–25.
161. Wei H, Ahn S, Shenoy SK et al. Independent β-arrestin 2 and G protein-mediated pathways for angiotensin II activation of extracellular signal-regulated kinases 1 and 2. Proc Natl Acad Sci U S A 2003; 100: 10782–7.
162. Wei H, Ahn S, Barnes WG et al. Stable interaction between β-arrestin 2 and angiotensin type 1A receptor is required for β-arrestin 2-mediated activation of extracellular signal-regulated kinases 1 and 2. J Biol Chem 2004; 279: 48255–61.
163. Karin M. The regulation of AP-1 activity by mitogen-activated protein kinases. J Biol Chem 1995; 270: 16483–6.
164. Kim S, Iwao H. Activation of mitogen-activated protein kinases in cardiovascular hypertrophy and remodeling. Jpn J Pharmacol 1999; 80: 97–102.
165. Kim S, Iwao H. Stress and vascular responses: mitogen-activated protein kinases and activator protein-1 as promising therapeutic targets of vascular remodeling. J Pharmacol Sci 2003; 91: 177–81.
166. Lin T, Kong X, Haystead T et al. PHAS-1 as a link between mitogen-activated protein kinase and translation initiation. Science 1994; 266: 653–6.
167. Rocic P, Seshiah P, Griendling KK. Reactive oxygen species sensitivity of angiotensin II-dependent translation initiation in vascular smooth muscle cells. J Biol Chem 2003; 278: 36973–9.
168. Duff JL, Berk BC, Corson MA. Angiotensin II stimulates the pp44 and pp42 mitogen-activated protein kinases in cultured rat aortic smooth muscle cells. Biochem Biophys Res Commun 1992; 188: 257–64.
169. Lucchesi PA, Bell JM, Willis LS et al. Ca^{2+}-dependent mitogen-activated protein kinase activation in spontaneously hypertensive rat vascular smooth muscle defines a hypertensive signal transduction phenotype. Circ Res 1996; 78: 962–70.
170. Wilkie N, Ng LL, Boarder MR. Angiotensin II responses of vascular smooth muscle cells from hypertensive rats: enhancement at the level of p42 and p44 mitogen activated protein kinase. Br J Pharmacol 1997; 122: 209–16.
171. Touyz RM, He G, El Mabrouk M et al. Differential activation of extracellular signal-regulated protein kinase 1/2 and p38 mitogen activated-protein kinase by AT1 receptors in vascular smooth muscle cells from Wistar-Kyoto rats and spontaneously hypertensive rats. J Hypertens 2001; 19: 553–9.
172. Xu Q, Liu Y, Gorospe M et al. Acute hypertension activates mitogen-activated protein kinases in arterial wall. J Clin Invest 1996; 97: 508–14.
173. Ushio-Fukai M, Alexander W, Akers M et al. p38 mitogen-activated protein kinase is a critical component of the redox-sensitive signaling pathways activated by angiotensin II: role in vascular smooth muscle cell hypertrophy. J Biol Chem 1998; 273: 15022–9.
174. Zohn I, Yu H, Li X et al. Angiotensin II stimulates calcium-dependent activation of c-Jun N-terminal kinase. Mol Cell Biol 1995; 15: 6160–8.
175. Kudoh S, Komuro I, Mizuno T et al. Angiotensin II stimulates c-Jun NH2-terminal kinase in cultured cardiac myocytes of neonatal rats. Circ Res 1997; 80: 139–46.
176. Force T, Pombo CM, Avruch JA et al. Stress-activated protein kinases in cardiovascular disease. Circ Res 1996; 78: 947–53.
177. Ip Y, Davis R. Signal transduction by the c-Jun N-terminal kinase (JNK) – from inflammation to development. Curr Opin Cell Biol 1998; 10: 205–19.
178. Kim S, Murakami T, Izumi Y et al. Extracellular signal-regulated kinase and c-Jun NH2-terminal kinase activities are continuously and differentially increased in aorta of hypertensive rats. Biochem Biophys Res Commun 1997; 236: 199–204.
179. Yano M, Kim S, Izumi Y et al. Differential activation of cardiac c-Jun amino-terminal kinase and extracellular signal-regulated kinase in angiotensin II–mediated hypertension. Circ Res 1998; 83: 752–60.
180. Stokoe D, Engel K, Campbell D et al. Identification of MAPKAP kinase 2 as a major enzyme responsible for the phosphorylation of the small mammalian heat shock proteins. FEBS Lett 1992; 313: 307–13.
181. Taniyama Y, Ushio-Fukai M, Hitomi H et al. Role of p38-MAPK and MAPKAPK-2 in angiotensin II-induced Akt activation in vascular smooth muscle cells. Am J Physiol Cell Physiol 2004; 287: C494–C499.
182. Takahashi T, Taniguchi T, Konishi H et al. Activation of Akt/protein kinase B after stimulation with angiotensin II in vascular smooth muscle cells. Am J Physiol Heart Circ Physiol 1999; 276: H1927–H1934.
183. Cross DA, Alessi DR, Cohen P et al. Inhibition of glycogen synthase kinase-3 by insulin mediated by protein kinase B. Nature 1995; 378: 785–9.
184. Burgering BM, Coffer PJ. Protein kinase B (c-Akt) in phosphatidylinositol-3-OH kinase signal transduction. Nature 1995; 376: 599–602.
185. Marte BM, Downward J. PKB/Akt: connecting phosphoinositide 3-kinase to cell survival and beyond. Trends Biochem Sci 1997; 22: 355–8.
186. Ushio-Fukai M, Alexander RW, Akers M et al. Reactive oxygen species mediate the activation of Akt-protein kinase B by angiotensin II in vascular smooth muscle cells. J Biol Chem 1999; 274: 22699–704.
187. Kawahara S, Umemoto S, Tanaka M et al. Up-regulation of Akt and eNOS induces vascular smooth muscle cell differentiation in hypertension in vivo. J Cardiovasc Pharmacol 2005; 45: 367–74.
188. Burridge K, Chrzanowska-Wodnicka M. Focal adhesions, contractility and signaling. Annu Rev Cell Dev Biol 1996; 12: 463–519.
189. Okuda M, Kawahara Y, Nakayama I et al. Angiotensin II transduces its signal to focal adhesions via angiotensin II type 1 receptors in vascular smooth muscle cells. FEBS Lett 1995; 368: 343–7.
190. Eguchi S, Iwasaki H, Inagami T et al. Involvement of PYK2 in angiotensin II signaling of vascular smooth muscle cells. Hypertension 1999; 33: 201–6.

191. Sabe H, Hamaguchi M, Hanafusa H. Cell to substratum adhesion is involved in v-Src-induced cellular protein tyrosine phosphorylation: implication for the adhesion-regulated protein tyrosine phosphatase activity. Oncogene 1997; 14: 1779–88.
192. Ishida T, Ishida M, Suero J et al. Agonist-stimulated cytoskeletal reorganization and signal transduction at focal adhesions in vascular smooth muscle cells require c-Src. J Clin Invest 1999; 103: 789–97.
193. Bhat G, Thekkumkara T, Thomas W et al. Angiotensin II stimulates sis-inducing factor-like DNA binding activity. Evidence that the AT1A receptor activates transcription factor-Stat91 and/or a related protein. J Biol Chem 1994; 269: 31443–9.
194. Marrero M, Schieffer B, Paxton W et al. Direct stimulation of Jak/STAT pathway by the angiotensin II AT1 receptor. Nature 1995; 375: 247–50.
195. Ali MS, Sayeski PP, Dirksen LB et al. Dependence on the motif YIPP for the physical association of Jak2 kinase with the intracellular carboxyl tail of the angiotensin II AT1 receptor. J Biol Chem 1997; 272: 23382–8.
196. Marrero MB, Venema VJ, Ju H et al. Regulation of angiotensin II-induced JAK2 tyrosine phosphorylation: roles of SHP-1 and SHP-2. Am J Physiol 1998; 275: C1216–C1223.
197. Frank GD, Saito S, Motley ED et al. Requirement of Ca^{2+} and PKCδ for Janus kinase 2 activation by angiotensin II: involvement of PYK2. Mol Endocrinol 2002; 16: 367–77.
198. McWhinney CD, Hunt RA, Conrad KM et al. The type I angiotensin II receptor couples to Stat1 and Stat3 activation through Jak2 kinase in neonatal rat cardiac myocytes. J Mol Cell Cardiol 1997; 29: 2513–24.
199. Liang H, Venema V, Wang X et al. Regulation of angiotensin II-induced phosphorylation of STAT3 in vascular smooth muscle cells. J Biol Chem 1999; 274: 19846–51.
200. Ihle JN. STATs: signal transducers and activators of transcription. Cell 1996; 84: 331–4.
201. Dostal DE, Hunt RA, Kule CE et al. Molecular mechanisms of angiotensin II in modulating cardiac function: intracardiac effects and signal transduction pathways. J Mol Cell Cardiol 1997; 29: 2893–902.
202. Dostal D. The cardiac renin-angiotensin system: novel signaling mechanisms related to cardiac growth and function. Regul Pept 2000; 91: 1–11.
203. Berk B, Corson M. Angiotensin II signal transduction in vascular smooth muscle: role of tyrosine kinases. Circ Res 1997; 80: 607–16.
204. Griendling KK, Minieri CA, Ollerenshaw JD et al. Angiotensin II stimulates NADH and NADPH oxidase activity in cultured vascular smooth muscle cells. Circ Res 1994; 74: 1141–8.
205. Touyz RM, Yao G, Quinn MT et al. p47phox associates with the cytoskeleton through cortactin in human vascular smooth muscle cells: role in NAD(P)H oxidase regulation by angiotensin II. Arterioscler Thromb Vasc Biol 2005; 25: 512–18.
206. Seshiah P, Weber D, Rocic P et al. Angiotensin II stimulation of NAD(P)H oxidase activity: upstream mediators. Circ Res 2002; 91: 406–13.
207. Touyz RM, Tabet F, Schiffrin EL. Redox-dependent signalling by angiotensin II and vascular remodelling in hypertension. Clin Exp Pharmacol Physiol 2003; 30: 860–6.
208. Lassègue B, Griendling KK. Reactive oxygen species in hypertension: an update. Am J Hypertens 2004; 17: 852–60.
209. Touyz RM, Schiffrin EL. Reactive oxygen species in vascular biology: implications in hypertension. Histochem Cell Biol 2004; 122: 339–52.
210. Inglese J, Freedman N, Koch W et al. Structure and mechanism of the G protein-coupled receptor kinases. J Biol Chem 1993; 268: 23735–8.
211. Pitcher J, Freedman N, Lefkowitz R. G protein-coupled receptor kinases. Annu Rev Biochem 1998; 67: 653–92.
212. Kim J, Ahn S, Ren X-R et al. Functional antagonism of different G protein-coupled receptor kinases for β-arrestin-mediated angiotensin II receptor signaling. Proc Natl Acad Sci U S A 2005; 102: 1442–7.
213. Lefkowitz RJ, Whalen EJ. β-arrestins: traffic cops of cell signaling. Curr Opin Cell Biol 2004; 16: 162–8.
214. Gaborik Z, Hunyady L. Intracellular trafficking of hormone receptors. Trends Endocrinol Metab 2004; 15: 286–93.
215. Lefkowitz RJ. G protein-coupled receptors. III. new roles for receptor kinases and β-arrestins in receptor signaling and desensitization. J Biol Chem 1998; 273: 18677–80.
216. Ferguson SSG. Evolving concepts in G protein-coupled receptor endocytosis: the role in receptor desensitization and signaling. Pharmacol Rev 2001; 53: 1–24.
217. Marchese A, Chen C, Kim Y-M et al. The ins and outs of G protein-coupled receptor trafficking. Trends Biochem Sci 2003; 28: 369–76.
218. Miller W, Lefkowitz R. Expanding roles for beta-arrestins as scaffolds and adapters in GPCR signaling and trafficking. Curr Opin Cell Biol 2001; 13: 139–45.
219. Perry S, Lefkowitz R. Arresting developments in heptahelical receptor signaling and regulation. Trends Cell Biol 2002; 12: 130–8.
220. Ishizaka N, Alexander RW, Laursen JB et al. G protein-coupled receptor kinase 5 in cultured vascular smooth muscle cells and rat aorta. Regulation by angiotensin II and hypertension. J Biol Chem 1997; 272: 32482–8.
221. Richard D, Chretien L, Caron M et al. Stimulation of the angiotensin II type 1 receptor on bovine adrenal glomerulosa cells activates a temperature-sensitive internalization-recycling pathway. Mol Cell Endocrinol 1997; 129: 209–18.
222. Hein L, Meinel L, Pratt R et al. Intracellular trafficking of angiotensin II and its AT_1 and AT_2 receptors: evidence for selective sorting of receptor and ligand. Mol Endocrinol 1997; 11: 1266–77.
223. Dale LB, Seachrist JL, Babwah AV et al. Regulation of angiotensin II type 1A receptor intracellular retention, degradation, and recycling by Rab5, Rab7, and Rab11 GTPases. J Biol Chem 2004; 279: 13110–18.
224. Thomas WG, Motel TJ, Kule CE et al. Phosphorylation of the angiotensin II (AT1A) receptor carboxyl terminus: a role in receptor endocytosis. Mol Endocrinol 1998; 12: 1513–24.
225. Kule CE, Karoor V, Day JNE et al. Agonist-dependent internalization of the angiotensin II type one receptor (AT1): role of C-terminus phosphorylation in recruitment of β-arrestins. Regul Pept 2004; 120: 141–8.
226. Gaborik Z, Szaszak M, Szidonya L et al. β-arrestin- and dynamin-dependent endocytosis of the AT_1 angiotensin receptor. Mol Pharmacol 2001; 59: 239–47.
227. Anborgh PH, Seachrist JL, Dale LB et al. Receptor/β-arrestin complex formation and the differential trafficking and resensitization of $β_2$-adrenergic and angiotensin II type 1A receptors. Mol Endocrinol 2000; 14: 2040–53.
228. Zhang J, Ferguson S, Barak L et al. Dynamin and β-arrestin reveal distinct mechanisms for G protein-coupled receptor internalization. J Biol Chem 1996; 271: 18302–5.
229. Claing A. Regulation of G protein-coupled receptor endocytosis by ARF6 GTP-binding proteins. Biochem Cell Biol 2004; 82: 610–17.
230. Houndolo T, Boulay P-L, Claing A. G protein-coupled receptor endocytosis in ADP-ribosylation factor 6-depleted cells. J Biol Chem 2005; 280: 5598–604.

231. Du G, Huang P, Liang BT et al. Phospholipase D2 localizes to the plasma membrane and regulates angiotensin II receptor endocytosis. Mol Biol Cell 2004; 15: 1024–30.
232. Shenoy SK, Lefkowitz RJ. Receptor-specific ubiquitination of β-arrestin directs assembly and targeting of seven-transmembrane receptor signalosomes. J Biol Chem 2005; 280: 15315–24.
233. Zhang J, Barak L, Anborgh P et al. Cellular trafficking of G protein-coupled receptor/β-arrestin endocytic complexes. J Biol Chem 1999; 274: 10999–1006.
234. Hunyady L, Baukal A, Gaborik Z et al. Differential PI3-kinase dependence of early and late phases of recycling of the internalized AT1 angiotensin receptor. J Cell Biol 2002; 157: 1211–22.
235. Takai Y, Sasaki T, Matozaki T. Small GTP-binding proteins. Physiol Rev 2001; 81: 153–208.
236. Seachrist JL, Ferguson SSG. Regulation of G protein-coupled receptor endocytosis and trafficking by Rab GTPases. Life Sci 2003; 74: 225–35.
237. Wu G, Zhao G, He Y. Distinct pathways for the trafficking of angiotensin II and adrenergic receptors from the endoplasmic reticulum to the cell surface: Rab1-independent transport of a G protein-coupled receptor. J Biol Chem 2003; 278: 47062–9.
238. Wu G, Yussman MG, Barrett TJ et al. Increased myocardial Rab GTPase expression: a consequence and cause of cardiomyopathy. Circ Res 2001; 89: 1130–7.
239. Seachrist JL, Laporte SA, Dale LB et al. Rab5 association with the angiotensin II type 1A receptor promotes Rab5 GTP binding and vesicular fusion. J Biol Chem 2002; 277: 679–85.
240. Ushio-Fukai M, Hilenski L, Santanam N et al. Cholesterol depletion inhibits epidermal growth factor receptor transactivation by angiotensin II in vascular smooth muscle cells: role of cholesterol-rich microdomains and focal adhesions in angiotensin II signaling. J Biol Chem 2001; 276: 48269–75.
241. Shah BH. Epidermal growth factor receptor transactivation in angiotensin II-induced signaling: role of cholesterol-rich microdomains. Trends Endocrinol Metab 2002; 13: 1–2.
242. Gratton J-P, Bernatchez P, Sessa WC. Caveolae and caveolins in the cardiovascular system. Circ Res 2004; 94: 1408–17.
243. Palade G. Fine structure of blood capillaries. J Appl Phys 1953; 24: 1424.
244. Simons K, Toomre D. Lipid rafts and signal transduction. Nat Rev Mol Cell Biol 2000; 1: 31–9.
245. Li S, Couet J, Lisanti M. Src tyrosine kinases, G_α subunits, and H-ras share a common membrane-anchored scaffolding protein, caveolin: caveolin binding negatively regulates the auto-activation of src tyrosine kinases. J Biol Chem 1996; 271: 29182–90.
246. Leclerc PC, Auger-Messier M, Lanctot PM et al. A polyaromatic caveolin-binding-like motif in the cytoplasmic tail of the type 1 receptor for angiotensin II plays an important role in receptor trafficking and signaling. Endocrinology 2002; 143: 4702–10.
247. Ishizaka N, Griendling K, Lassègue B et al. Angiotensin II type 1 receptor: relationship with caveolae and caveolin after initial agonist stimulation. Hypertension 1998; 32: 459–66.
248. Zuo L, Ushio-Fukai M, Hilenski LL et al. Microtubules regulate angiotensin II type 1 receptor and Rac1 localization in caveolae/lipid rafts: role in redox signaling. Arterioscler Thromb Vasc Biol 2004; 24: 1223–8.
249. Razani B, Engelman J, Wang XB et al. Caveolin-1 null mice are viable but show evidence of hyperproliferative and vascular abnormalities. J Biol Chem 2001; 276: 38121–38.
250. Hassan G, Jasmin J-F, Schubert W et al. Caveolin-1 deficiency stimulates neointima formation during vascular injury. Biochemistry 2004; 43: 8312–21.
251. Drab M, Verkade P, Elger M et al. Loss of caveolae, vascular dysfunction, and pulmonary defects in caveolin-1 gene-disrupted mice. Science 2001; 293: 2449–52.
252. Cohen AW, Park DS, Woodman SE et al. Caveolin-1 null mice develop cardiac hypertrophy with hyperactivation of p42/44 MAP kinase in cardiac fibroblasts. Am J Physiol Cell Physiol 2003; 284: C457–C474.
253. Cohen AW, Hnasko R, Schubert W et al. Role of caveolae and caveolins in health and disease. Physiol Rev 2004; 84: 1341–79.
254. Williams TM, Lisanti MP. The caveolin genes: from cell biology to medicine. Ann Med 2004; 36: 584–95.
255. Thomas WG, Mendelsohn FAO. Angiotensin receptors: form and function and distribution. Int J Biochem Cell Biol 2003; 35: 774–9.
256. Crone S, Zhao Y-Y, Fan L et al. ErbB2 is essential in the prevention of dilated cardiomyopathy. Nat Med 2002; 8: 459–65.
257. Wyse BD, Prior IA, Qian H et al. Caveolin interacts with the angiotensin II type 1 receptor during exocytic transport but not at the plasma membrane. J Biol Chem 2003; 278: 23738–46.

4

The angiotensin type 2 (AT_2) receptor in cardiovascular and renal regulation

Robert M Carey

INTRODUCTION

The renin-angiotensin system (RAS) is a coordinated hormonal cascade of major physiological and pathophysiological importance in the regulation of body fluid volume, electrolyte balance, and blood pressure.[1] The principal effector peptide of the RAS is angiotensin II (Ang II) which acts at two different cell membrane receptors, AT_1 and AT_2.[2] The vast majority of the actions of Ang II are mediated via the AT_1 receptor, including growth promotion, vasoconstriction, aldosterone secretion, salt appetite, thirst, sympathetic outflow, antinatriuresis, and inhibition of renin biosynthesis and secretion.[3] The AT_2 receptor has been much less well understood. However, past studies have demonstrated clearly that the AT_2 receptor mediates cellular differentiation and growth, thereby opposing the actions of Ang II to promote cellular dedifferentiation, proliferation and growth via the AT_1 receptor.[4] From a historical perspective, the biological actions of Ang II have been studied for decades and were thought to be mediated by a single Ang II receptor, which had not yet been cloned.[5,6] In the late 1980s, the development of highly specific non-peptide antagonists of angiotensin receptors opened the door to the identification, pharmacological characterization and molecular cloning of the two major angiotensin receptor subtypes, AT_1 and AT_2. AT_1 receptors were defined as those selectively blocked by biphenylimidazoles, the prototype of which is losartan, while AT_2 receptors were defined as those blocked by tetrahydromidazopyridines, the prototype of which is PD-123319 (PD).[7,8] The AT_1 receptor was cloned in 1991 and the AT_2 receptor in 1993.[9–12] Since that time, the signal transduction mechanisms for both the AT_1 and AT_2 receptors have been clarified,[2] and we now have a great deal of information concerning receptor genes, molecular and protein structures, sites and regulation of expression, and cellular mechanisms of action.

This chapter will focus upon the AT_2 receptor with particular emphasis on its molecular characteristics, cell signaling mechanisms, cellular expression and regulation of expression, physiological functions and possible pathophysiological role in the cardiovascular/renal systems with particular reference to hypertension. The physiological actions of Ang II that are mediated by the AT_2 receptor are just now beginning to be elucidated. It is now clear that most, but not all, of the identified actions mediated by the AT_2 receptor oppose those via the AT_1 receptor. Therefore, the AT_2 receptor is emerging as a mechanism for dampening AT_1 receptor-mediated events.

GENERAL CONSIDERATIONS OF THE AT_2 RECEPTOR

The molecular structure of the AT_2 receptor is similar to that of the superfamily of G protein-coupled receptors containing 7-transmembrane domains.[13] The cDNA for the AT_2 receptor encodes a 363 amino acid protein (Figure 4.1) with a molecular weight of 41 220 Da. The AT_2 receptor shares only about a 34% sequence homology with the AT_1 receptor.[14] The gene for the AT_2 receptor resides on the X chromosome and contains three exons with the entire coding region on the third exon.[14] In contrast, the gene for the AT_1 receptor is located on chromosome 3 in humans and on chromosomes 17 (AT_{1A}) and 2 (AT_{1B}) in the rat and on chromosomes 13 (AT_{1A}) and 3 (AT_{1B}) in the mouse.[2] Promoter activity of the rat AT_2 receptor gene is regulated by a number of *cis*-regulatory domains.[14] The AT_2 receptor protein contains five potential glycosylation

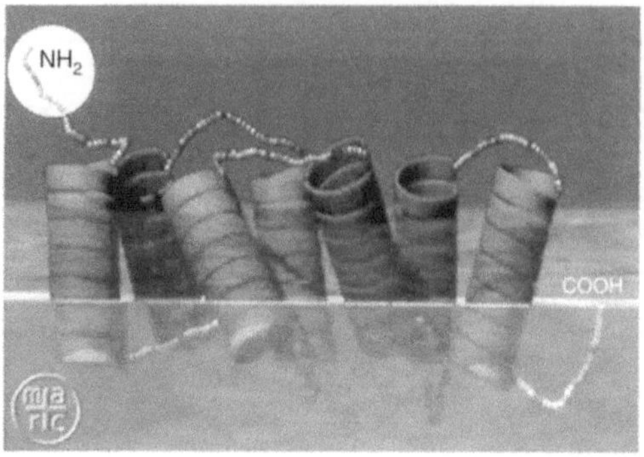
Proposed structure of the
AT_2 receptor
NH_2
COOH
• 7-Transmembrane G protein-coupled receptor
• Only 34% amino acid sequence homology with AT_1 receptor
• Single copy gene on X chromosome

Figure 4.1 Schematic representation of AT_2 receptor 7-trans-membrane structure

sites in its relatively long extracellular N-terminal tail. Among the several differences in the amino acid sequences, the AT_2 receptor but not the AT_1 receptor has a conserved LYS^{199}, which is important in ligand–receptor interactions. In addition, there is a potential protein kinase C phosphorylation site in the second intracellular loop and there are three consensus sequences for phosphorylation by protein kinase C and one phosphorylation site by cyclic AMP (cAMP)-dependent protein kinase in the C-terminal cytoplasmic tail of the receptor.[1,2] Interestingly, the AT_2 receptor amino acid sequences are 99% identical between the rat and mouse and 72% identical between the rat and human.[2] The differences between sequences in the rat and human occur mainly in the N-terminal region and not in the extracellular loops which would be important for agonist binding. Also, the homology between the AT_1 and AT_2 receptors is mainly localized in the trans-membrane hydrophobic regions of the molecule which form the seven transmembrane helical columns.[2] Almost complete divergence in the third intracellular loop is observed between AT_1 and AT_2 receptors.

SIGNALING MECHANISMS OF THE AT_2 RECEPTOR

The AT_2 receptor activates unconventional cell signaling pathways that in many cases appear not to involve coupling to classical regulatory G proteins.[2] In general, AT_2 receptor activation is associated with activation of tyrosine phosphatases and inhibition of protein kinases ultimately leading to inhibition of the phosphorylation of extracellular signal-related kinase 2 (ERK2). Recent evidence, however, indicates that the receptor can be G protein-coupled via $G_i\alpha_2$ and $G_i\alpha_3$.[15] Current evidence suggests that AT_2 receptor stimulation activates phosphotyrosine phosphatases, especially serine/threonine phosphatase 2A, protein kinase phosphatase and SHP-1 tyrosine phosphatase, resulting in inactivation of ERK2 (p42 and p44 MAP kinase).[2] There is also evidence that the AT_2 receptor opens the delayed rectifier K^+ channel, activates phospholipase A_2 and prostaglandin generation, and stimulates ceramide production.[2,4] Recently, it has been shown that the AT_2 receptor constitutively and physically associates with SHP-1. On stimulation by Ang II, SHP-1 becomes activated and physically dissociates from the receptor in a non-G protein-coupled manner.[16] However, the AT_2 receptor/SHP-1 association and SHP-1 activation require the presence of $G\alpha s$. Therefore, $G\alpha s$ alone, rather than $G\alpha\beta\gamma$ heterotrimer, may facilitate signal transduction for the AT_2 receptor.[16] Figure 4.2 depicts the aforementioned cell signaling pathways for the AT_2 receptor. Altogether, the evidence suggests that the AT_2 receptor may be coupled to G proteins in an unconventional manner and that the third intracellular loop is linked with a signaling pathway involving $G_i\alpha$ and ERK inactivation.

Recently, new signaling pathways have emerged for the AT_2 receptor. Firstly, AT_2 receptors were found to attenuate phospholipase D (PLD) activation, which is required for the ERK and NAD(P)H oxidase activation via the AT_1 receptor.[17] AT_2 receptors were observed to activate $G_i\alpha$ stimulating nitric oxide (NO) synthase and guanosine cyclic 3′,5′-monophosphate (cGMP) formation, in turn activating a protein kinase resulting in serine phophorylation of RhoA, thereby inhibiting RhoA activity. Secondly, an AT_2 receptor-interacting protein, termed ATIP-2, has been cloned and interacts with the C-terminal tail of the AT_2 receptor.[18] ATIP inhibits insulin-, basic fibroblast growth factor- and

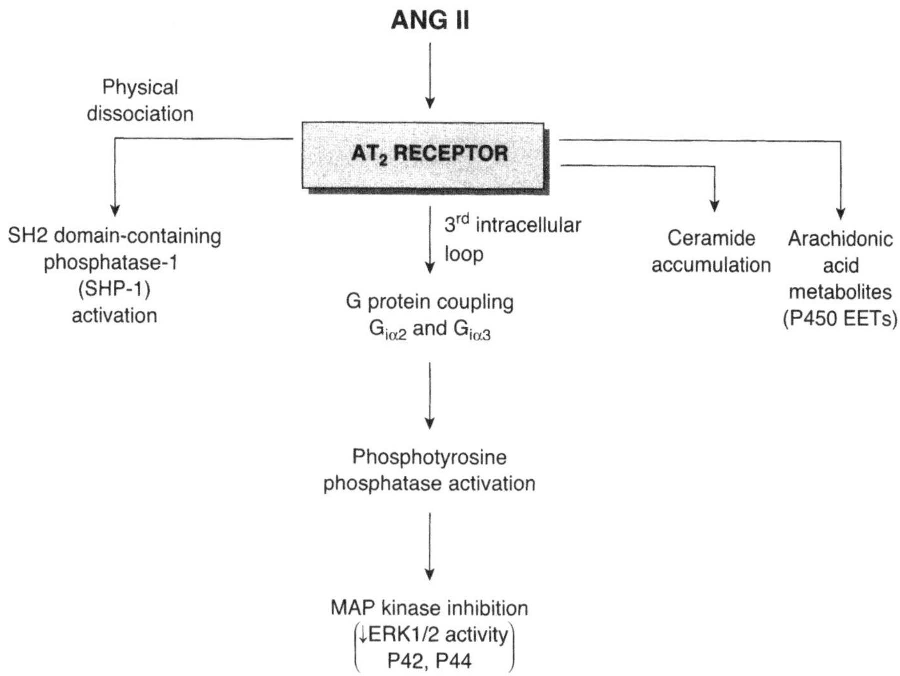

Figure 4.2 Schematic depiction of the cell signaling pathways whereby the AT$_2$ receptor is thought to carry out its biological functions

epidermal growth factor (EGF)-induced ERK2 activation and DNA synthesis and attenuates insulin receptor autophosphorylation in a similar manner to the AT$_2$ receptor.[18] These actions require the presence, but not the activation, of the AT$_2$ receptor.

A major cell-to-cell signaling complex of the AT$_2$ receptor is the bradykinin (BK)-NO-cGMP pathway as shown in Figure 4.3. This pathway, which is probably also involved in intracellular signaling, will be discussed later in the context of the renal and cardiovascular functions mediated by the AT$_2$ receptor.

AT$_2$ RECEPTOR EXPRESSION IN CELLS AND TISSUES

The AT$_2$ receptor is heavily expressed in fetal tissues, but in almost all tissues there is rapid regression to low levels or disappearance of expression early in the postnatal period.[19–29] Tissues in which the AT$_2$ receptor does not substantially regress and/or disappear in adulthood include brain, uterine myometrium and adrenal zona glomerulosa and medulla. In the fetus, the AT$_2$ receptor is expressed predominantly in areas of active mesenchymal differentiation, but the mRNA expression level decreases rapidly and disappears within days of birth.[21–24] AT$_2$ receptor mRNA is expressed in the fetal and neonatal rat kidney but regresses after the neonatal period and is expressed only in minute quantities in the adult.[21,22]

The AT$_2$ receptor is a low-copy receptor in most adult tissues, the mRNA being difficult to detect by methods other than quantitative real-time reverse-transcriptase polymerase chain reaction (RT-PCR). On the other hand, AT$_2$ receptor protein can be readily detected in the kidney, heart and vasculature using specific polyclonal antibodies in immunohistochemical and Western blot analyses.

In the adult kidney, the AT$_2$ receptor protein is detectable in proximal and distal tubules, glomeruli, renal vessels, juxtaglomerular (JG) cells, cortical and medullary collecting ducts, and cortical interstitial cells in a variety of studies.[26,30] Indeed, AT$_2$ receptor mRNA was detectable in the proximal tubule of adult rats by RT-PCR.[30]

In the vasculature, the AT$_2$ receptor has been more difficult to detect than in the kidney, but there is now substantial evidence for AT$_2$ receptor expression in various vascular beds including the aorta and coronary, mesenteric and uterine resistance arterioles, the main renal artery and renal arcuate and interlobular arteries.[30–38] AT$_2$ receptors are present in vascular smooth muscle cells as well as endothelial and adventitial cells in these vascular beds.[39]

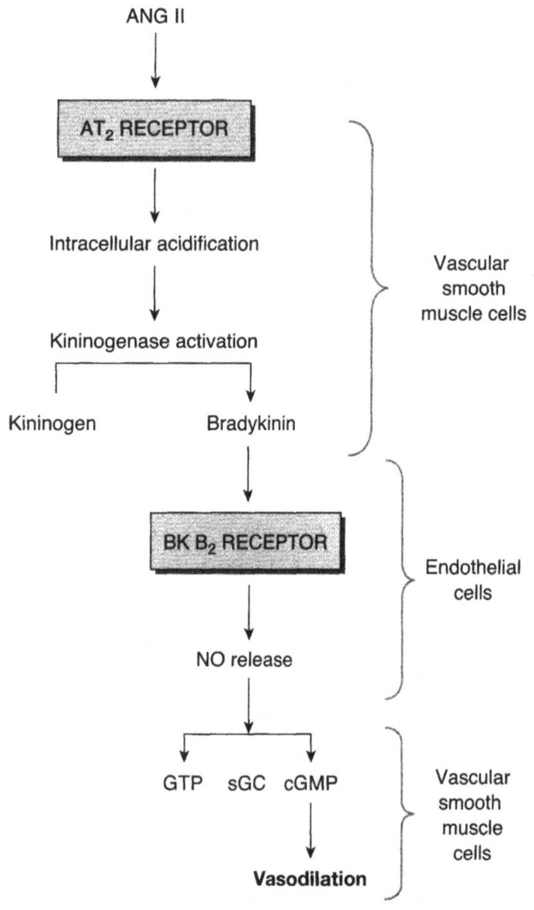

Figure 4.3 Schematic representation of the AT_2 receptor-mediated vasodilator pathway resulting in the generation of bradykinin, nitric oxide and cyclic GMP

In the heart, AT_2 receptors are expressed at low levels in adult rat cardiomyocytes[27,40] and fibroblasts[27] as well as in the coronary arteries[27,41] of rats and humans.

Interestingly, the AT_2 receptor is more highly expressed in human than in rodent tissues; for example, the receptor is highly expressed in the human kidney and heart.[41–44] In the human heart, available studies suggest an increased AT_2/AT_1 receptor ratio in which the AT_2 receptor is predominant.

REGULATION OF AT_2 RECEPTOR EXPRESSION

Although several factors are known to regulate AT_2 receptor expression, the control of this receptor is still largely unknown. Ang II, norepinephrine, insulin-like growth factor, basic fibroblast growth factor and transforming growth factor (TGF)-β decrease AT_2 receptor expression.[45–77] AT_2 receptor expression is up-regulated in experimental heart failure, myocardial infarction, vascular injury and during dietary sodium restriction.[26,48–53] An explanation for the discrepancy between Ang II-induced receptor down-regulation and sodium restriction-induced receptor up-regulation remains lacking, but may be tissue-, species- or model-specific. For example, in sheep uterine arteries Ang II decreases AT_2 receptor expression but in rat mesenterie arteries Ang II actually increases expression.[54,55] In addition, receptor cross-talk regulates AT_1 and AT_2 receptor expression. In mice lacking the AT_2 receptor (AT_2 null) the AT_1 receptor is up-regulated, but over-expression of the AT_2 receptor in the vasculature does not alter AT_2 receptor expression.[56,57] Much more work needs to be performed on the regulation of AT_2 receptor expression, especially in relation to AT_1 receptor expression.

GENERAL FUNCTIONS OF THE AT_2 RECEPTOR

The AT_2 receptor has well documented functions related to cell growth, differentiation, and ultimate disposal. In almost all studies, the AT_2 receptor inhibits cell growth and proliferation and promotes cell differentiation, opposing the growth effects of Ang II via the AT_1 receptor.[4,58–61] The antiproliferative actions of Ang II via the AT_2 receptor have been observed in several cell types, including endothelial cells, neonatal cardiomyocytes, cardiac fibroblasts, and vascular smooth muscle cells. Studies also suggest that the AT_2 receptor may inhibit angiogenesis.[1] In addition, the AT_2 receptor mediates apoptosis in certain cell systems.[1,5,6]

The AT_2 receptor has distinctive physiological actions in neuronal cells. Stimulation of AT_2 receptors promotes cell differentiation and regeneration in neuronal tissue.[62] Ang II-induced stimulation of AT_2 receptors causes neurite outgrowth in cultured neuronal cells, probably by a NO-dependent signaling pathway.[63] AT_2 receptors may contribute to Schwann cell-mediated myelinization and neuroregeneration of dorsal root ganglia after nerve transaction in adult rats.[64] Ang II also promotes neurite regeneration of retinal ganglion cells and dorsal root ganglia neurons in vitro as well as axonal regeneration of retinal ganglion cells following optic nerve crush in vivo via the AT_2 receptor.[62,65] Furthermore, recent evidence suggests that cerebral AT_2 receptors are neuroprotective in ischemia-induced neuronal injury, possibly by supporting neuronal survival and nitrite outgrowth in peri-ischemic areas of the brain.[66]

AT_2 receptors inhibit low-voltage T-type calcium channels in neuronal cells.[67,68] However, the role of AT_2 receptors, if any, in the pacemaker activity of neuronal cells is unclear. AT_2 receptors also activate the delayed rectifier K^+ channel leading to increased cellular polarization.[69] In sympathetic neurons, AT_2 receptors increase delayed K^+ rectifier current and inhibit norepinephrine release stimulated by AT_1 receptors.[69]

In the gastrointestinal tract, AT_2 receptors stimulate jejunal sodium and water absorption by a pathway involving stimulation of the sympathetic nervous system and NO production.[70] The final effector of this pathway is cGMP, which is released into the interstitial fluid on the serosal side of the jejunal transporting epithelial cells.[71] This pathway opposes the actions of Ang II via the AT_1 receptor to inhibit sodium and water absorption and/or to stimulate secretion through a prostaglandin E_2 and cAMP-dependent mechanism.[70]

ROLE OF THE AT_2 RECEPTOR IN CARDIOVASCULAR FUNCTION IN THE FETUS

The AT_2 receptor is highly expressed in the fetus, including both the aorta and small resistance arterioles, suggesting a potential role in vascular growth and remodeling. The AT_2 receptors expressed in the fetal aorta are functional and inhibit the development of contractile force.[72] However, the AT_2 receptor does not inhibit vascular smooth muscle proliferation during embryonic development, but rather may stimulate proliferation during late stages of development.[72] Further investigation needs to be performed on the functional role of AT_2 receptors in the fetus.

ROLE OF THE AT_2 RECEPTOR IN VASODILATION

A vasodilator role for the AT_2 receptor was initially suggested in 1992 because the vasodilator action of AT_1 receptor antagonists was prevented with concurrent AT_2 receptor blockade.[73] In 1995, two groups reported that AT_2 null mice have slightly increased blood pressure,[74,75] suggesting the possibility of a hypotensive action mediated by AT_2 receptors. These observations were followed rapidly in 1996 by the discovery that the AT_2 receptor stimulates BK, NO, and cGMP in the dog and rat kidney.[76–78] Subsequent studies strongly suggested that AT_2 receptor stimulation initiates a vasodilator cascade consisting of BK, NO, and cGMP;[79–82] this has been reviewed elsewhere.[3,42,83] Prior to 2003, evidence suggested that the AT_2 receptor induces a vasodilator response that opposes Ang II-mediated vasoconstriction via AT_1 receptors.[33,84–87] From several of these studies, it was apparent that at least some of the beneficial effects of AT_1 receptor blockade to lower blood pressure are attributable to stimulation of the unblocked AT_2 receptor.[82,86]

As indicated earlier, AT_2 receptor expression is relatively low in the adult vasculature compared with AT_1 receptor expression. The predominance of AT_1 receptor expression would predict that Ang II administration would induce net vasoconstriction and a rise in blood pressure, as is indeed the case. However, a very different result is obtained when Ang II is administered in the presence of AT_1 receptor blockade. Under these circumstances, Ang II induces a vasodilator response. Indeed, Ang II administration to AT_1 receptor-blocked animals induces a net hypotensive response that is attributable to increased generation of NO and is eliminated by concurrent inhibition of NO synthase.[87]

Recently, several convincing studies have confirmed the vasodilator action of the AT_2 receptor via a BK-NO-cGMP vasodilator signaling cascade. For example, AT_2 receptor blocker PD-123319 (PD) markedly potentiated Ang II-induced contraction in the rat uterine artery, and this action of PD was duplicated by both BK-B_2 receptor antagonist icatibant and NO synthase inhibitor N-nitro-L-arginine.[88] Since Ang II increased arterial wall content of cGMP, the AT_2 receptor inhibited Ang II-induced vasoconstriction via BK, NO, and cGMP.[88]

Nearly identical results were reported for mesenteric arterial segments studied under flow conditions.[89] In the presence of AT_1 receptor blockade, Ang II elicited a vasodilator response that was dependent upon endothelial AT_2 receptors and the BK-B_2 receptor. AT_2 receptor-induced vasodilation was substantially attenuated in kininogen-deficient Brown Norway Katholick rats compared with wild-type controls.[89] Thus, AT_2 receptors induce vasodilation via local BK production in mesenteric resistance vessels under flow conditions. Consistent with these observations, functional AT_2 receptors are necessary for kallekrein/kinin-induced flow-dependent vasodilation.[90] Flow-induced dilation was reduced by AT_2 receptor blockade in wild-type mice but not in mice lacking tissue kallekrein, and BK-B_2 receptor inhibition reduced the dilatory response to flow in wild-type mice but not in AT_2 null animals.[90] These studies constitute strong evidence that resistance microvessels are a major site of AT_2 receptor-mediated vasodilation.

On the other hand, recent evidence also suggests a role for AT_2 receptors in large capacitance vessels. AT_2 receptor mRNA was markedly unregulated in the pressure-overloaded thoracic aorta following super-renal aortic banding.[91] Ang II-induced vasoconstriction was attenuated in these aortas, but was restored by AT_2 receptor antagonist PD. Removal of the endothelium normalized these responses, indicating that endothelial AT_2 receptor up-regulation during pressure overload is a pathophysiological counter-regulatory mechanism that limits Ang II-induced constriction. Similar findings were observed in mice, wherein the reduced Ang II contractile response was restored with either AT_2 or BK-B_2 receptor blockade.[92] The ninefold Ang II-mediated increase in aortic cGMP was also abolished with AT_2 or BK-B_2 receptor blockade. These findings underscore the potential relevance of AT_2 receptor up-regulation initiating a counter-regulatory depressor response mediated by BK and NO.

As stated above, AT_2 receptor expression is relatively high in the coronary circulation, particularly in humans. In the normal or failing rat heart, chronic AT_1 receptor blockade induced coronary vasodilation that was abolished with AT_2 receptor or NO synthase blockade.[93] In bovine pulmonary endothelial cells AT_1 receptor blockade increased NO synthesis, which was abolished by AT_2 receptor blockade.[93] Thus, endothelium-dependent vasodilation with AT_1 receptor blockade may be due to AT_2 receptor stimulation. In the human coronary microarteries, Ang II-induced constriction was prevented by AT_2 receptor blockade, but this was not observed in the presence of NO synthase or BK-B_2 receptor inhibition or removal of the endothelium.[94] Also, in the presence of AT_1 receptor blockade, Ang II produced vasodilation that was eliminated with AT_2 receptor blockade.[94] These important studies demonstrate the presence of functional AT_2 vasodilator receptors in the coronary microcirculation that operate via BK, NO, and cGMP.

ROLE OF AT_2 RECEPTORS IN RENAL FUNCTION AND PROTECTION

As stated above, AT_2 receptor-mediated vasodilation opposes AT_1 receptor-induced vasoconstriction in several vascular beds. However, very few studies are available on the role of AT_2 receptors in the control of renal blood flow or regional perfusion. Recent studies have demonstrated that AT_2 receptors oppose AT_1 receptor-mediated vasoconstriction in the renal cortex.[95] In the renal medulla, however, AT_1 receptor stimulation dilated blood vessels and this effect also was opposed by AT_2 receptor activation.[95] These findings may be important in the pathogenesis of hypertension because in angiotensin-dependent forms of hypertension renal medullary blood flow is reduced.[96]

Regarding a potential role of AT_2 receptors in the control of renal sodium excretion, very little information is currently on hand. The only available cellular study suggests that renal proximal tubule sodium reabsorption is opposed by AT_2 receptors.[97] Most of the present knowledge comes from AT_2 null mice, which have exaggerated antinatriuretic responses to Ang II infusion and are not able to mount an effective pressure-natriuresis curve.[98,99] The difficulty with interpretation of the studies in AT_2 null mice, however, is that AT_1 receptors are chronically up-regulated in this model and it is uncertain whether the AT_1 receptor up-regulation can account for the antinatriuretic hypersensitivity of AT_2 null mice.

While the role of AT_2 receptors in natriuresis in normal animals is currently uncertain, one report suggests that obese Zucker rats may have functioning natriuretic AT_2 receptors. AT_1 receptor blockade with candesartan increased sodium excretion to a greater degree in Zucker rather than lean rats. Candesartan-induced natriuresis was abolished in the presence of AT_2 receptor blockade in the obese but not the lean rats.[100] Also, infusion of selective AT_2 receptor agonist CGP-42112A induced natriuresis to a greater extent in obese rather than lean rats.[100] AT_2 receptor protein was up-regulated in both basolateral membrane and brush border sites in renal proximal tubule cells of obese but not lean rats.[100] While these studies suggest that the AT_2 receptor may play a key role in renal proximal tubule sodium transport, especially under conditions wherein the receptor is up-regulated, the role of AT_2 receptors in sodium transport remains uncertain.

The AT_2 receptor has a protective role in the renal wrap model of angiotensin-dependent hypertension.[82] However, whether or not the AT_2 receptor has a more general renoprotective role is not well understood. AT_2 receptor transgenic (AT_2-Tg) and wild-type mice were subjected to 5/6 nephrectomy creating a model of ischemic renal injury.[101] In AT_2-Tg mice, AT_2 receptor expression in the glomerulus was increased and urinary albumin excretion was reduced by approximately one-third in 5/6-nephrectomized compared with wild-type mice. In response to 5/6 nephrectomy, AT_2-Tg mice had decreased TGF-β and platelet-derived growth factor, and urinary NO metabolite excretion was increased 2.5-fold.[101] The aforementioned responses were abolished by the AT_2 receptor antagonist PD, indicating that they were mediated by the AT_2 receptor.

The 5/6 nephrectomy model develops a time-dependent increase in AT_2 receptor expression at 7, 15, and 30 days following renal ablation.[102] Animals with renal ablation that were pretreated with AT_1 receptor anatagonist losartan demonstrated a further increase in AT_2 receptor expression. Treatment with AT_2 receptor antagonist PD down-regulated AT_2 receptor expression, increased blood pressure and provoked renal damage. These studies strongly suggest that the AT_2 receptor is protective in ischemic renal injury.[82,101,102]

ROLE OF THE AT_2 RECEPTOR IN RENIN BIOSYNTHESIS, PROCESSING, AND SECRETION

The AT_2 receptor is expressed in renal JG cells that are the exclusive source of circulating renin in the adult.[26] AT_1 receptors on JG cell membranes inhibit renin biosynthesis and secretion, providing a short-loop negative feedback mechanism to dampen Ang II production.[103] Angiotensin converting enzyme inhibition and/or AT_1 receptor blockade unmask(s) the short loop feedback of Ang II on renin secretion, resulting in increased plasma renin activity. AT_1 receptor blockade in cultured JG cells increases renin secretion rate and Ang II concentrations in the extracellular media and decreased cellular active, but not total, renin content.[104] The reduction in active renin content was abolished by AT_2 receptor blockade with PD. AT_2 receptor agonist CGP increased renin secretion rate and reduced active renin cellular content, and these CGP-related actions were blocked by PD.[104] Therefore, AT_1 receptor blockade may inhibit prorenin processing via AT_2 receptors in JG cells.

More recent studies strongly suggest that the AT_2 receptor, similar to the AT_1 receptor, inhibits renin biosynthesis and secretion.[105] In conscious rats, direct renal interstitial administration of either AT_1 receptor antagonist valsartan or AT_2 receptor antagonist PD increased plasma renin activity and intrarenal concentrations of Ang II.[105] Both receptor blockers independently up-regulated renin mRNA and renin tissue concentrations in the kidney. Both valsartan and PD increased renin immunoreactivity in both JG and tubule cells.[105] Therefore, renin biosynthesis and secretion are inhibited by either AT_1 or AT_2 receptor stimulation. These findings confirm that, while many of the AT_2 receptor functions oppose those of the AT_1 receptor, parallel functions also exist. The cellular mechanisms of AT_2 receptor suppression of renin need to be clarified.

CONCLUSIONS

The functions of AT_1 and AT_2 receptors are depicted in Figure 4.4. The AT_2 receptor is a relatively low copy receptor in the cardiovascular system. Nevertheless, the AT_2 receptor has been shown unequivocally to serve as a dilator of resistance microarteries as well as large capacitance vessels. The vasodilator action of the AT_2 receptor is mediated by BK, NO, and cGMP and physiologically opposes the vasoconstrictor action of Ang II via the AT_1 receptor. The role of the AT_2 receptor in the pathophysiology of hypertension requires further exploration. It is possible that down-regulation of AT_2 receptors contributes to the pathogenesis of hypertension and its accompanying tissue damage.

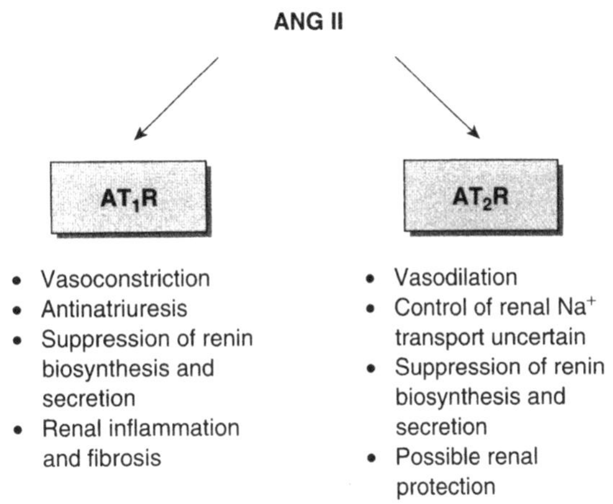
ANG II
AT_1R
AT_2R
• Vasoconstriction
• Antinatriuresis
• Suppression of renin biosynthesis and secretion
• Renal inflammation and fibrosis
• Vasodilation
• Control of renal Na^+ transport uncertain
• Suppression of renin biosynthesis and secretion
• Possible renal protection

Figure 4.4 Schematic representation of selected opposing functions of AT_1 and AT_2 receptors as currently understood and accepted

The role of the AT_2 receptor in renal function and particularly in natriuresis is less certain, and this is a major area of future investigation. Because the AT_2 receptor inhibits cell proliferation and growth, it is also possible that receptor up-regulation and/or stimulation may serve to protect tissues from damage, including inflammation and fibrosis, as suggested by the renoprotection studies described above. The AT_2 receptor also appears to work together with the AT_1 receptor in limiting renin biosynthesis and secretion.

REFERENCES

1. Matsusaka T, Ichikawa I. Biological functions of angiotensin and its receptors. Annu Rev Physiol 1997; 59: 395–412.
2. de Gasparo M, Catt KJ, Inagami T, Wright JW, Unger T. International union of pharmacology. XXIII. The angiotensin II receptors. Pharmacol Rev 2000; 52: 415–72.
3. Carey RM, Siragy HM. Newly recognized components of the renin-angiotensin system: potential roles in cardiovascular and renal regulation. Endocr Rev 2003; 24: 261–71.

4. Berry C, Touyz R, Dominiczak AF, Webb RC, Johns DG. Angiotensin receptors: signaling, vascular pathophysiology, and interactions with ceramide. Am J Physiol Heart Circ Physiol 2001; 281: H2337–H2365.
5. Goodfriend TL, Elliott ME, Catt KJ. Angiotensin receptors and their antagonists. N Engl J Med 1996; 334: 1649–54.
6. Griendling KK, Lassegue B, Alexander RW. Angiotensin receptors and their therapeutic implications. Annu Rev Pharmacol Toxicol 1996; 36: 281–306.
7. Chiu AT, McCall DE, Price WA et al. Nonpeptide angiotensin II receptor antagonists. VII. Cellular and biochemical pharmacology of DuP 753, an orally active antihypertensive agent. J Pharmacol Exp Ther 1990; 252: 711–18.
8. Timmermans PB, Wong PC, Chiu AT et al. Angiotensin II receptors and angiotensin II receptor antagonists. Pharmacol Rev 1993; 45: 205–51.
9. Murphy TJ, Alexander RW, Griendling KK, Runge MS, Bernstein KE. Isolation of a cDNA encoding the vascular type-1 angiotensin II receptor. Nature 1991; 351: 233–6.
10. Sasaki K, Yamano Y, Bardhan S et al. Cloning and expression of a complementary DNA encoding a bovine adrenal angiotensin II type-1 receptor. Nature 1991; 351: 230–3.
11. Kambayashi Y, Bardhan S, Takahashi et al. Molecular cloning of a novel angiotensin II receptor isoform involved in phosphotyrosine phosphatase inhibition. J Biol Chem 1993; 268: 24543–6.
12. Nakajima M, Mukoyama M, Pratt RE, Horiuchi M, Dzau VJ. Cloning of cDNA and analysis of the gene for mouse angiotensin II type 2 receptor. Biochem Biophys Res Commun 1993; 197: 393–9.
13. Inagami T. Molecular biology and signaling of angiotensin receptors: an overview. J Am Soc Nephrol 1999; 10 (Suppl 11): S2–S7.
14. Ichiki T, Inagami T. Expression, genomic organization, and transcription of the mouse angiotensin II type 2 receptor gene. Circ Res 1995; 76: 693–700.
15. Hansen JL, Servant G, Baranski TJ, Fujita T, Iiri T, Sheikh SP. Functional reconstitution of the angiotensin II type 2 receptor and G(i) activation. Circ Res 2000; 87: 753–9.
16. Feng YH, Sun Y, Douglas JG. Gβ-independent constitutive association of Gα s with SHP-1 and angiotensin II receptor AT_2 is essential in AT_2-mediated ITIM-independent activation of SHP-1. Proc Natl Acad Sci U S A 2002; 99: 12049–54.
17. Andresen BT, Shome K, Jackson EK, Romero GG. AT_2 receptors cross talk with AT_1 receptors through a nitric oxide- and RhoA-dependent mechanism resulting in decreased phospholipase D activity. Am J Physiol Renal Physiol 2005; 288: F763–F770.
18. Nouet S, Amzallag N, Li JM et al. Trans-inactivation of receptor tyrosine kinases by novel angiotensin II AT_2 receptor-interacting protein, ATIP. J Biol Chem 2004; 279: 28989–97.
19. Zhuo J, Song K, Harris PJ, Mendelsohn FA. In vitro autoradiography reveals predominantly AT_1 angiotensin II receptors in rat kidney. Renal Physiol Biochem 1992; 15: 231–9.
20. Zhuo J, Alcorn D, Harris PJ, Mendelsohn FA. Localization and properties of angiotensin II receptors in rat kidney. Kidney Int Suppl 1993; 42: S40–S46.
21. Shanmugam S, Llorens-Cortes C, Clauser E, Corvol P, Gasc JM. Expression of angiotensin II AT_2 receptor mRNA during development of rat kidney and adrenal gland. Am J Physiol 1995; 268: F922–F930.
22. Shanmugam S, Corvol P, Gasc JM. Angiotensin II type 2 receptor mRNA expression in the developing cardiopulmonary system of the rat. Hypertension 1996; 28: 91–7.
23. Kakuchi J, Ichiki T, Kiyama S et al. Developmental expression of renal angiotensin II receptor genes in the mouse. Kidney Int 1995; 47: 140–7.
24. Aguilera G, Kapur S, Feuillan P, Sunar-Akbasak B, Bathia AJ. Developmental changes in angiotensin II receptor subtypes and AT_1 receptor mRNA in rat kidney. Kidney Int 1994; 46: 973–9.
25. Sechi LA, Griffin CA, Grady EF, Kalinyak JE, Schambelan M. Characterization of angiotensin II receptor subtypes in rat heart. Circ Res 1992; 71: 1482–9.
26. Ozono R, Wang ZQ, Moore AF, Inagami T, Siragy HM, Carey RM. Expression of the subtype 2 angiotensin (AT_2) receptor protein in rat kidney. Hypertension 1997; 30: 1238–46.
27. Wang ZQ, Moore AF, Ozono R, Siragy HM, Carey RM. Immunolocalization of subtype 2 angiotensin II (AT_2) receptor protein in rat heart. Hypertension 1998; 32: 78–83.
28. Matsubara H, Sugaya T, Murasawa S et al. Tissue-specific expression of human angiotensin II AT_1 and AT_2 receptors and cellular localization of subtype mRNAs in adult human renal cortex using in situ hybridization. Nephron 1998; 80: 25–34.
29. Tsutsumi K, Saavedra JM. Characterization and development of angiotensin II receptor subtypes (AT_1 and AT_2) in rat brain. Am J Physiol 1991; 261: R209–R216.
30. Miyata N, Park F, Li XF, Cowley AW Jr. Distribution of angiotensin AT_1 and AT_2 receptor subtypes in the rat kidney. Am J Physiol 1999; 277: F437–F446.
31. Chang RS, Lotti VJ. Angiotensin receptor subtypes in rat, rabbit and monkey tissues: relative distribution and species dependency. Life Sci 1991; 49: 1485–90.
32. Viswanathan M, Tsutsumi K, Correa FM, Saavedra JM. Changes in expression of angiotensin receptor subtypes in the rat aorta during development. Biochem Biophys Res Commun 1991; 179: 1361–7.
33. Matrougui K, Loufrani L, Heymes C, Levy BI, Henrion D. Activation of AT_2 receptors by endogenous angiotensin II is involved in flow-induced dilation in rat resistance arteries. Hypertension 1999; 34: 659–65.
34. Matrougui K, Levy BI, Henrion D. Tissue angiotensin II and endothelin-1 modulate differently the response to flow in mesenteric resistance arteries of normotensive and spontaneously hypertensive rats. Br J Pharmacol 2000; 130: 521–6.
35. Touyz RM, Endemann D, He G, Li JS, Schiffrin EL. Role of AT_2 receptors in angiotensin II-stimulated contraction of small mesenteric arteries in young SHR. Hypertension 1999; 33: 366–72.
36. Burrell JH, Lumbers ER. Angiotensin receptor subtypes in the uterine artery during ovine pregnancy. Eur J Pharmacol 1997; 330: 257–67.
37. McMullen JR, Gibson KJ, Lumbers ER, Burrell JH, Wu J. Interactions between AT_1 and AT_2 receptors in uterine arteries from pregnant ewes. Eur J Pharmacol 1999; 378: 195–202.
38. Akishita M, Iwai M, Wu L et al. Inhibitory effect of angiotensin II type 2 receptor on coronary arterial remodeling after aortic banding in mice. Circulation 2000; 102: 1684–9.
39. Nora EH, Munzenmaier DH, Hansen-Smith FM, Lombard JH, Greene AS. Localization of the ANG II type 2 receptor in the microcirculation of skeletal muscle. Am J Physiol 1998; 275: H1395–H1403.
40. Busche S, Gallinat S, Bohle RM et al. Expression of angiotensin AT_1 and AT_2 receptors in adult rat cardiomyocytes after myocardial infarction. A single-cell reverse transcriptase-polymerase chain reaction study. Am J Pathol 2000; 157: 605–11.
41. Matsumoto T, Ozono R, Oshima T et al. Type 2 angiotensin II receptor is downregulated in cardiomyocytes of patients with heart failure. Cardiovasc Res 2000; 46: 73–81.
42. Carey RM, Wang ZQ, Siragy HM. Role of the angiotensin type 2 receptor in the regulation of blood pressure and renal function. Hypertension 2000; 35: 155–63.

43. Tsutsumi Y, Matsubara H, Ohkubo N et al. Angiotensin II type 2 receptor is upregulated in human heart with interstitial fibrosis, and cardiac fibroblasts are the major cell type for its expression. Circ Res 1998; 83: 1035–46.
44. Goette A, Arndt M, Rocken C et al. Regulation of angiotensin II receptor subtypes during atrial fibrillation in humans. Circulation 2000; 101: 2678–81.
45. Wang ZQ, Millatt LJ, Heiderstadt NT, Siragy HM, Johns RA, Carey RM. Differential regulation of renal angiotensin subtype AT_1A and AT_2 receptor protein in rats with angiotensin-dependent hypertension. Hypertension 1999; 33: 96–101.
46. Kijima K, Matsubara H, Murasawa S et el. Regulation of angiotensin II type 2 receptor gene by the protein kinase C-calcium pathway. Hypertension 1996; 27: 529–34.
47. Li JY, Avallet O, Berthelon MC, Langlois D, Saez JM. Effects of growth factors on cell proliferation and angiotensin II type 2 receptor number and mRNA in PC12W and R3T3 cells. Mol Cell Endocrinol 1998; 139: 61–9.
48. Ohkubo N, Matsubara H, Nozawa Y et al. Angiotensin type 2 receptors are reexpressed by cardiac fibroblasts from failing myopathic hamster hearts and inhibit cell growth and fibrillar collagen metabolism. Circulation 1997; 96: 3954–62.
49. Janiak P, Pillon A, Prost JF, Vilaine JP. Role of angiotensin subtype 2 receptor in neointima formation after vascular injury. Hypertension 1992; 20: 737–45.
50. Lopez JJ, Lorell BH, Ingelfinger JR et al. Distribution and function of cardiac angiotensin AT_1- and AT_2-receptor subtypes in hypertrophied rat hearts. Am J Physiol 1994; 267: H844–H852.
51. Ichiki T, Kambayashi Y, Inagami T. Multiple growth factors modulate mRNA expression of angiotensin II type-2 receptor in R3T3 cells. Circ Res 1995; 77: 1070–6.
52. Kambayashi Y, Nagata K, Ichiki T, Inagami T. Insulin and insulin-like growth factors induce expression of angiotensin type-2 receptor in vascular-smooth-muscle cells. Eur J Biochem 1996; 239: 558–65.
53. Horiuchi M, Yamada T, Hayashida W, Dzau VJ. Interferon regulatory factor-1 up-regulates angiotensin II type 2 receptor and induces apoptosis. J Biol Chem 1997; 272: 11952–8.
54. McMullen JR, Gibson KJ, Lumbers ER, Burrell JH. Selective down-regulation of AT_2 receptors in uterine arteries from pregnant ewes given 24-h intravenous infusions of angiotensin II. Regul Pept 2001; 99: 119–29.
55. Bonnet F, Cooper ME, Carey RM, Casley D, Cao Z. Vascular expression of angiotensin type 2 receptor in the adult rat: influence of angiotensin II infusion. J Hypertens 2001; 19: 1075–81.
56. Tanaka M, Tsuchida S, Imai T et al. Vascular response to angiotensin II is exaggerated through an upregulation of AT_1 receptor in AT_2 knockout mice. Biochem Biophys Res Commun 1999; 258: 194–8.
57. Tsutsumi YMH, Masaki H., Kurihara T et al. Vascular smooth muscle-targeted overexpression of angiotensin II type 2 receptor causes endothlium-dependent depressor and vasodilative effects via activation of the vascular kinin system. J Clin Invest 1999; 104: 855–64.
58. Meffert S, Stoll M, Steckelings UM, Bottari SP, Unger T. The angiotensin II AT_2 receptor inhibits proliferation and promotes differentiation in PC12W cells. Mol Cell Endocrinol 1996; 122: 59–67.
59. Stoll M, Steckelings UM, Paul M, Bottari SP, Metzger R, Unger T. The angiotensin AT_2-receptor mediates inhibition of cell proliferation in coronary endothelial cells. J Clin Invest 1995; 95: 651–7.
60. Maric C, Aldred GP, Harris PJ, Alcorn D. Angiotensin II inhibits growth of cultured embryonic renomedullary interstitial cells through the AT_2 receptor. Kidney Int 1998; 53: 92–9.
61. Kuizinga MC, Smits JF, Arends JW, Daemen M. AT_2 receptor blockade reduces cardiac interstitial cell DNA synthesis and cardiac function after rat myocardial infarction. J Mol Cell Cardiol 1998; 30: 425–34.
62. Reinecke K, Lucius R, Reinecke A, Rickert U, Herdegen T, Unger T. Angiotensin II accelerates functional recovery in the rat sciatic nerve in vivo: role of the AT_2 receptor and the transcription factor NF-kappaB. FASEB J 2003; 17: 2094–6.
63. Zhao Y, Biermann T, Luther C, Unger T, Culman J, Gohlke P. Contribution of bradykinin and nitric oxide to AT_2 receptor-mediated differentiation in PC12 W cells. J Neurochem 2003; 85: 759–67.
64. Gallinat S, Yu M, Dorst A, Unger T, Herdegen T. Sciatic nerve transection evokes lasting up-regulation of angiotensin AT_2 and AT_1 receptor mRNA in adult rat dorsal root ganglia and sciatic nerves. Brain Res Mol Brain Res 1998; 57: 111–22.
65. Lucius R, Gallinat S, Rosenstiel P, Herdegen T, Sievers J, Unger T. The angiotensin II type 2 (AT_2) receptor promotes axonal regeneration in the optic nerve of adult rats. J Exp Med 1998; 188: 661–70.
66. Li J, Culman J, Hortnagl H, Zhao Y et al. Angiotensin AT_2 receptor protects against cerebral ischemia-induced neuronal injury. FASEB J 2005; 19: 617–19.
67. Kang J, Sumners C, Posner P. Angiotensin II type 2 receptor-modulated changes in potassium currents in cultured neurons. Am J Physiol 1993; 265: C607–C616.
68. Buisson B, Laflamme L, Bottari SP, de Gasparo M, Gallo-Payet N, Payet MD. A G protein is involved in the angiotensin AT_2 receptor inhibition of the T-type calcium current in non-differentiated NG108–15 cells. J Biol Chem 1995; 270: 1670–4.
69. Kang J, Posner P, Sumners C. Angiotensin II type 2 receptor stimulation of neuronal K+ currents involves an inhibitory GTP binding protein. Am J Physiol 1994; 267: C1389–C1397.
70. Jin XH, Wang ZQ, Siragy HM, Guerrant RL, Carey RM. Regulation of jejunal sodium and water absorption by angiotensin subtype receptors. Am J Physiol 1998; 275: R515–R523.
71. Jin XH, Siragy HM, Guerrant RL, Carey RM. Compartmentalization of extracellular cGMP determines absorptive or secretory responses in the rat jejunum. J Clin Invest 1999; 103: 167–74.
72. Perlegas D, Xie H, Sinha S, Somlyo AV, Owens GK. ANG II type 2 receptor regulates smooth muscle growth and force generation in late fetal mouse development. Am J Physiol Heart Circ Physiol 2005; 288: H96–H102.
73. Widdop RE, Gardiner SM, Kemp PA, Bennett T. Inhibition of the haemodynamic effects of angiotensin II in conscious rats by AT_2-receptor antagonists given after the AT_1-receptor antagonist, EXP 3174. Br J Pharmacol 1992; 107: 873–80.
74. Hein L, Barsh GS, Pratt RE, Dzau VJ, Kobilka BK. Behavioural and cardiovascular effects of disrupting the angiotensin II type-2 receptor in mice. Nature 1995; 377: 744–7.
75. Ichiki T, Labosky PA, Shiota C et al. Effects on blood pressure and exploratory behaviour of mice lacking angiotensin II type-2 receptor. Nature 1995; 377: 748–50.
76. Siragy HM, Carey RM. The subtype-2 (AT_2) angiotensin receptor regulates renal cyclic guanosine 3′,5′-monophosphate and AT_1 receptor-mediated prostaglandin E2 production in conscious rats. J Clin Invest 1996; 97: 1978–82.
77. Siragy HM, Jaffa AA, Margolius HS, Carey RM. Renin-angiotensin system modulates renal bradykinin production. Am J Physiol 1996; 271: R1090–R1095.
78. Siragy HM, Carey RM. The subtype 2 (AT_2) angiotensin receptor mediates renal production of nitric oxide in conscious rats. J Clin Invest 1997; 100: 264–9.

79. Gohlke P, Pees C, Unger T. AT_2 receptor stimulation increases aortic cyclic GMP in SHRSP by a kinin-dependent mechanism. Hypertension 1998; 31: 349–55.
80. Barber MN, Sampey DB, Widdop RE. AT(2) receptor stimulation enhances antihypertensive effect of AT(1) receptor antagonist in hypertensive rats. Hypertension 1999; 34: 1112–16.
81. Tsutsumi Y, Matsubara H, Masaki H et al. Angiotensin II type 2 receptor overexpression activates the vascular kinin system and causes vasodilation. J Clin Invest 1999; 104: 925–35.
82. Siragy HM, Carey RM: Protective role of the angiotensin AT_2 receptor in a renal wrap hypertension model. Hypertension 1999; 33: 1237–42.
83. Widdop RE, Jones ES, Hannan RE. Gaspari TA. Angiotensin AT_2 receptors: cardiovascular hope or hype? Br J Pharmacol 2003; 140: 809–24.
84. Widdop RE, Matrougui K, Levy BI, Henrion D. AT_2 receptor-mediated relaxation is preserved after long-term AT_1 receptor blockade. Hypertension 2002; 40: 516–20.
85. Zwart AS, Davis EA, Widdop RE. Modulation of AT_1 receptor-mediated contraction of rat uterine artery by AT_2 receptors. Br J Pharmacol 1998; 125: 1429–36.
86. Siragy HM, de Gasparo M, Carey RM. Angiotensin type 2 receptor mediates valsartan-induced hypotension in conscious rats. Hypertension 2000; 35: 1074–7.
87. Carey RM, Howell NL, Jin XH, Siragy HM. Angiotensin type 2 receptor-mediated hypotension in angiotensin type-1 receptor-blocked rats. Hypertension 2001; 38: 1272–7.
88. Hannan RE, Davis EA, Widdop RE. Functional role of angiotensin II AT_2 receptor in modulation of AT_1 receptor-mediated contraction in rat uterine artery: involvement of bradykinin and nitric oxide. Br J Pharmacol 2003; 140: 987–95.
89. Katada J, Majima M. $AT(_2)$ receptor-dependent vasodilation is mediated by activation of vascular kinin generation under flow conditions. Br J Pharmacol 2002; 136: 484–91.
90. Bergaya S, Hilgers RH, Meneton P et al. Flow-dependent dilation mediated by endogenous kinins requires angiotensin AT_2 receptors. Circ Res 2004; 94: 1623–9.
91. Yayama K, Horii M, Hiyoshi H et al. Up-regulation of angiotensin II type 2 receptor in rat thoracic aorta by pressure-overload. J Pharmacol Exp Ther 2004; 308: 736–43.
92. Hiyoshi H, Yayama K, Takano M, Okamoto H. Stimulation of cyclic GMP production via AT_2 and B2 receptors in the pressure-overloaded aorta after banding. Hypertension 2004; 43: 1258–63.
93. Thai H, Wollmuth J, Goldman S, Gaballa M. Angiotensin subtype 1 receptor (AT_1) blockade improves vasorelaxation in heart failure by up-regulation of endothelial nitric-oxide synthase via activation of the AT_2 receptor. J Pharmacol Exp Ther 2003; 307: 1171–8.
94. Batenburg WW, Garrelds IM, Bernasconi CC et al. Angiotensin II type 2 receptor-mediated vasodilation in human coronary microarteries. Circulation 2004; 109: 2296–301.
95. Duke LM, Eppel GA, Widdop RE, Evans RG. Disparate roles of AT_2 receptors in the renal cortical and medullary circulations of anesthetized rabbits. Hypertension 2003; 42: 200–5.
96. Sarkis A, Liu KL, Lo M, Benzoni D. Angiotensin II and renal medullary blood flow in Lyon rats. Am J Physiol Renal Physiol 2003; 284: F365–F372.
97. Siragy HM, Inagami T, Ichiki T, Carey RM. Sustained hypersensitivity to angiotensin II and its mechanism in mice lacking the subtype-2 (AT_2) angiotensin receptor. Proc Natl Acad Sci U S A 1999; 96: 6506–10.
98. Gross V, Schunck WH, Honeck H et al. Inhibition of pressure natriuresis in mice lacking the AT_2 receptor. Kidney Int 2000; 57: 191–202.
99. Haithcock D, Jiao H, Cui XL, Hopfer U, Douglas JG. Renal proximal tubular AT_2 receptor: signaling and transport. J Am Soc Nephrol 1999; 10 (Suppl 11): S69–S74.
100. Hakan AC HT. Renal angiotensin II type-2 receptors are upregulated and mediate the candesartan-induced natriuresis/diuresis in obese Zucker rats. Hypertension 2004; 45: 1–7.
101. Hashimoto N, Maeshima Y, Satoh M et al. Overexpression of angiotensin type 2 receptor ameliorates glomerular injury in a mouse remnant kidney model. Am J Physiol Renal Physiol 2004; 286: F516–F525.
102. Vazquez E, Coronel I, Bautista R et al. Angiotensin II-dependent induction of AT(2) receptor expression after renal ablation. Am J Physiol Renal Physiol 2005; 288: F207–F213.
103. Johns DW, Peach MJ, Gomez RA, Inagami T, Carey RM. Angiotensin II regulates renin gene expression. Am J Physiol 1990; 259: F882–F887.
104. Ichihara A, Hayashi M, Hirota N et al. Angiotensin II type 2 receptor inhibits prorenin processing in juxtaglomerular cells. Hypertens Res 2003; 26: 915–21.
105. Siragy HM, Xue C, Abadir P, Carey RM. Angiotensin subtype-2 receptors inhibit renin biosynthesis and angiotensin II formation. Hypertension 2005; 45: 133–7.

5

Angiotensin converting enzyme 2: a potential target for cardiovascular therapy

Patricia E Gallagher, E Ann Tallant and Carlos M Ferrario

INTRODUCTION

Advances in the pharmacological management of patients with hypertension as well as other cardiac, renal, and vascular diseases have provided confirmatory evidence for a participation of the renin-angiotensin aldosterone system (RAAS) in the pathogenesis of heart disease, stroke, and renal failure. Both angiotensin converting enzyme (ACE) inhibitors, which block the action of the angiotensin II (Ang II) forming enzyme, and angiotensin type 1 (AT_1) receptor antagonists, which inhibit the interaction of Ang II and the AT_1 receptor, showed enhanced efficacy in numerous randomized clinical trials, such that these agents have become the standard of care for patients with hypertension, left ventricular dysfunction, post-myocardial infarction, diabetes mellitus, and renal disease.[1–5] The success of ACE inhibitors and AT_1 receptor antagonists as pharmacological treatments demonstrates the importance of RAAS regulation as a therapeutic target.

EXPANDING KNOWLEDGE ON THE BIOCHEMICAL PATHWAYS OF THE RAAS

The discovery of angiotensin-(1-7) (Ang-(1-7)) represented a critical step in the expansion of knowledge about the role of the RAAS in the regulation of cardiovascular function in terms of both physiology and pathology. Through a series of studies involving cellular, biochemical, and physiological approaches, we learned that Ang-(1-7) comprises a second arm of the RAAS functioning to oppose the actions of Ang II.[6,7] Knowledge of the mechanisms by which Ang II participates in the pathogenesis of cardiovascular disease was expanded by the recent emergence of angiotensin converting enzyme 2 (ACE2) as a critical regulator of the RAAS. This exciting breakthrough enhances our understanding of the factors that regulate the formation of Ang-(1-7) and the mechanisms by which this second arm of the system limits the actions of Ang II.[8] ACE2 was discovered by parallel, independent investigations using genome-based strategies to probe for either proteins with functions similar to that of ACE[9] or proteins involved in cardiac function.[10] ACE2 shares about 42% sequence homology and 61% similarity with the N-terminal catalytic domain of ACE. The human ACE2 gene, consisting of 18 exons, encodes an 805 amino acid single polypeptide containing an extracellular catalytic domain with two hydrophobic regions – a putative 18 amino acid signal sequence at the N-terminus and a 22 amino acid membrane anchor near the C-terminus. The extracellular domain contains a central zinc binding motif (HEXXH) with seven potential N-linked glycosylation sites. ACE2 migrates as a polypeptide of M_r 120 000, which is reduced to 85 000 by de-glycosylation.

It is of note that the ACE2 gene is localized on the X chromosome (Xp22). The importance of this gene location is illustrated by the recent work of Carrel and Willard showing extensive variability in X-linked gene expression.[11] In this study, the 'active' and 'inactive' X chromosomes of primary cultures of skin fibroblasts from 40 women were examined for the expression of 94 genes located throughout the chromosome. Limited gene expression was expected from the inactive X chromosome, based on the Lyon hypothesis stating that only one of the two X chromosomes is actively transcribed in female cells. In actuality, about 15% of the genes were actively transcribed from the supposedly 'inactive' X chromosome in all of the samples examined. An additional 20% of the genes escaped inactivation in some of the samples with only about 65% displaying total inactivation. More important, a wide variation in expression was observed in those genes escaping inactivation, indicating that a disparity in gene dosage exists in women. This incomplete X chromosome inactivation suggests that about 25% of the X chromosome, representing between 200 and 300 genes, is present at higher, and often variable, levels in females compared with males. ACE2 is located in the region of the X chromosome in which about 40% of the genes escaped X inactivation to some degree. It is of importance to determine whether ACE2 is among those genes, as an additive gene dosage might explain some of the cardioprotective effects observed in women, while a deletion in this region may result in a genetic predisposition to cardiovascular pathologies in men.

Similar to ACE, ACE2 is present in a wide variety of cells and tissues with high expression in the gut, heart, and kidney.[12] While both enzymes belong to the gluzincin family of zinc metalloproteinases, the substrate specificity of ACE and ACE2 is distinct, due to structural divergence. Amino acid substitutions in ACE2 result in changes in the substrate-binding subsite,[13] such that ACE2 is a carboxy monopeptidase with a preference for hydrolysis between a proline and carboxy-terminal hydrophobic or basic residues, differing from ACE which cleaves two amino acids from its substrate. Vickers et al. found that ACE2 exhibits a high catalytic efficiency for the conversion of several peptide substrates in vitro.[14] The hydrolysis of Ang II to Ang-(1-7) by ACE2 occurs with an almost 500-fold greater efficiency as compared with the breakdown of Ang I to Ang-(1-9). From an array of over 120 peptides, only dynorphin A and apelin-13 were hydrolyzed by the enzyme with comparable kinetics to the conversion of Ang II to Ang-(1-7).

ACE2 SUBSTRATES WITH CARDIOVASCULAR RELEVANCE

As shown in Figure 5.1, ACE2 provides a direct link between several regulatory systems involved in cardiovascular function – the RAAS, kinin, and apelin pathways. Ang II, a potent vasoconstrictor of the RAAS, stimulates thirst and aldosterone release, and inhibition of its production or effect using ACE inhibitors or AT_1 receptor antagonists reduces mean arterial pressure.[15] In contrast, Ang-(1-7) reduces the blood pressure of hypertensive dogs and rats,[16,17] alters renal fluid absorption,[18–21] causes vasodilation,[17,22–26] and participates in the antihypertensive responses to ACE inhibition or AT_1 receptor blockade in hypertensive rats.[27,28]

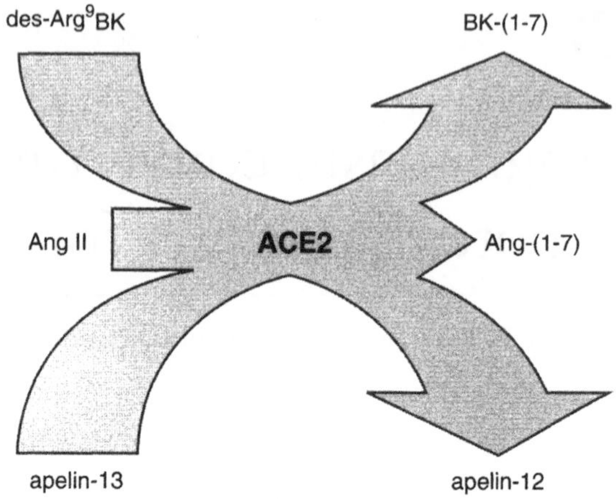

Figure 5.1 ACE2 substrates involved in cardiovascular function. des-arginine^9-bradykinin (des-Arg^9-BK), bradykinin-(1-7) (BK-(1-7)), angiotensin II (Ang II), angiotensin-(1-7) (Ang-(1-7)), and angiotensin converting enzyme 2 (ACE2)

Ang II is also a potent mitogen, stimulating vascular growth as well as hypertrophy in terminally differentiated cells.[29,30] In contrast, we showed that Ang-(1-7) inhibits the growth of vascular smooth muscle cells, cardiomyocytes, and cardiac fibroblasts.[31–33] Thus, a growing body of evidence indicates that Ang-(1-7) acts as a physiological modulator of Ang II, with opposing actions on body fluid volume, blood pressure, and cell growth. As illustrated in Figure 5.1, ACE2 serves as a regulatory connection between Ang II and Ang-(1-7), providing a means to maintain the balance between the pressor, mitogenic and depressor, growth inhibitory arms of the RAAS.

Decades of research have firmly established ACE as an enzymatic link between the RAAS and kinin pathway (Figure 5.2). ACE converts bradykinin to bradykinin-(1-7) which is further degraded to the inactive product, bradykinin-(1-5), while the vasoconstrictor Ang II is produced from Ang I.[34,35] Likewise, ACE cleaves Ang-(1-7) into the inactive fragment Ang-(1-5), a finding that provided evidence for a contribution of this peptide to the antihypertensive actions of ACE inhibitors.[36,37] ACE2 also bridges these two important regulatory pathways through the catalytic breakdown of [des-Arg^9]-bradykinin to bradykinin-(1-7) and the formation of the vasodilator and cell growth inhibitor, Ang-(1-7), from Ang II. Removal of the N-terminal arginine from bradykinin by a carboxypeptidase produces the ACE2 substrate, [des-Arg^9]-bradykinin, a ligand

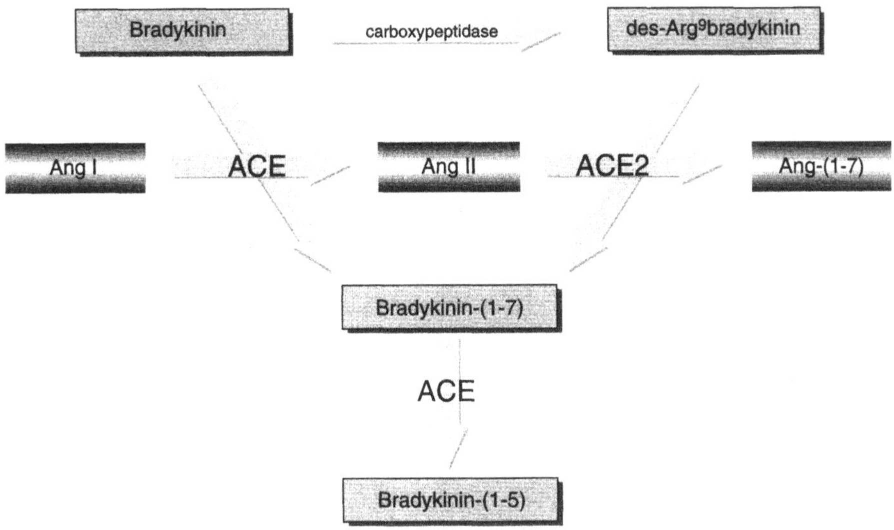

Figure 5.2 Enzymatic links between the RAAS and bradykinin pathway, angiotensin II (Ang II), angiotensin-(1-7) (Ang-(1-7)), angiotensin converting enzyme (ACE), and angiotensin converting enzyme 2 (ACE2)

for the B1 receptor which is up-regulated following inflammation or tissue injury. Unlike ACE, bradykinin is not a substrate for ACE2.[14] The enzymatic connections of the two systems underlie the therapeutic effectiveness of ACE inhibitors. Blockade of ACE activity prevents the formation of the vasoconstrictor Ang II and the degradation of the vasodilators bradykinin and Ang-(1-7), leading to a reduction in blood pressure as well as the myriad of beneficial effects attributed to ACE inhibition. While ACE inhibitors have no direct effect on ACE2 activity,[9,10] we found a marked up-regulation of ACE2 mRNA in Lewis rats treated with lisinopril[38] as well as an increase in cardiac ACE2 activity.[38] This study showed that ACE inhibitors indirectly affect ACE2 activity by a transcriptional regulatory mechanism and supports a role for Ang-(1-7) in the cardioprotective effects of ACE inhibitors. The actions of Ang-(1-7) may be mediated through interaction with its own receptor and activation of downstream signaling pathways, by bradykinin potentiation through the release of prostaglandins, nitric oxide or endothelium-derived hyperpolarizing factor,[7,39,40] or by the ability of the heptapeptide to also inhibit ACE activity.[41] The precise mechanism(s) will be dependent upon the species and the vascular bed.

ACE2 also serves to link the apelin pathway with the RAAS and the kinin pathway. Apelin, synthesized as a 77 amino acid preprohormone, is processed to a 36 amino acid peptide with further proteolytic cleavage to yield apelin-13, composed of the C-terminal active region.[42] The biological effects of the apelin peptides are mediated by the APJ receptor, a G protein-coupled, seven-transmembrane receptor, sharing sequence homology with the AT_1 receptor. A limited number of studies performed thus far indicate that apelin plays a role in cardiovascular physiology. Positive inotropic effects were observed in normal rodents as well as rats with heart failure following continuous infusion of apelin-16.[43–45] A dose response study showed that sub-nanomolar concentrations were sufficient to observe the effect on heart function. Intravenous bolus injection of apelin fragments decreased mean arterial pressure in rats[46–48] with apelin-12 as the most potent vasodilator.[46] The concurrent administration of a nitric oxide synthase inhibitor abolished the reduction, indicating that apelin lowers blood pressure through a nitric oxide-mediated mechanism.[46] The apelin-induced reduction in blood pressure was abolished in APJ-deficient mice and homozygous mice deficient in both the APJ and AT_{1a} receptor exhibited increased baseline blood pressure compared with the AT_{1a} knockout mice.[48] This indicates that apelin may counter-regulate the vasoconstrictor actions of Ang II.

As stated above, we showed that ACE2 mRNA was increased significantly in Lewis rat heart following administration of the ACE inhibitor, lisinopril.[38]

Additionally, treatment of the rats with the AT_1 receptor antagonist, losartan, caused a marked up-regulation of ACE2.[38] If apelin-12, the most potent of the apelin vasodilators, is increased following an up-regulation of ACE2, then this peptide hormone also may be involved in the cardioprotective effects observed following administration of ACE inhibitors or AT_1 receptor blockers. The role of apelin in cardiac function and blood pressure regulation, particularly following treatment with antihypertensive medications, requires further investigation.

A cursory examination of the known ACE2 substrates shows that an accurate view of the cellular and molecular mechanisms involved in regulation of blood pressure, homeostasis, electrolyte balance, and cell growth must include the contribution of numerous peptide hormones, their specific receptors, and the signaling pathways activated. It should be noted that the characterization of the ACE2 substrates identified thus far occurred primarily in vitro. Further investigations must corroborate these findings and determine which peptides serve as effective local and systemic substrates for ACE2 in vivo.

ACE2 AND HYPERTENSION

While the characterization of ACE2 in normal and pathologic states is still in its early stages, the substrate specificity of the enzyme suggests a role in blood pressure regulation. The importance of RAAS and kinin pathways in pressure homeostasis is well documented and research thus far demonstrates vasodilatory properties for the apelin fragments. Several genetic studies also support an ACE2 function in blood pressure control. Rat *ace2* maps to a quantitative trait locus with a significant logarithm-of-the-odds (lod) score for hypertension in three models of hypertension – the Sabra salt-sensitive rat, the spontaneously hypertensive rat (SHR), and the stroke-prone SHR (SHRSP). In these three rat strains, both ACE2 mRNA and protein were significantly reduced, suggesting that ACE2 is a candidate gene for this quantitative trait locus.[49] The elevated blood pressure in the three strains of rats may result from the increase in the vasoconstrictor Ang II and reduced vasodilators, Ang-(1-7) and apelin fragments, as a result of decreased ACE2 activity. Additionally, Allred et al.[50] reported a reduced tail-cuff pressure in a second line of ACE2 knockout mice as compared with controls in an abstract to the American Society of Nephrology. Infusion of Ang II at a dose that reduced heart rate without an effect on blood pressure in control mice markedly increased the blood pressure in the ACE2 knockout animals with diminished heart rate. These studies suggest that ACE2 maintains the delicate balance between the pressor and the depressor responses and pathophysiological conditions that alter ACE2 activity will tip this equilibrium, leading to hypertension or hypotension.

Two studies report conflicting results as to the role of ACE2 in regulation of pressure homeostasis. Crackower et al. did not observe increased blood pressure in male and female ACE2 knockout mice as compared to controls, even though increased concentrations of Ang II were found in both plasma and tissue.[49] The lack of effect on blood pressure may be due to a similar increase in Ang-(1-7) which could modulate the vasoconstrictor actions of Ang II. Additionally, the blood pressure result is confounded by the impaired heart function observed in this ACE2 knockout line. In contrast, Huang et al. stated that intravenous injection of DX512, a specific ACE2 inhibitor, caused a dose-dependent depressor response in SHRs with transient tachycardia.[51] There are no details of this experiment as the description is included in the discussion section of another paper, making it difficult to evaluate the study. Nevertheless, it is apparent that further investigations in both normotensive and hypertensive animals are required to definitively determine whether ACE2 plays a prominent role in the control of blood pressure. The generation of additional knockout and knockin models with both tissue-specific and time-controlled expression are needed to alleviate confounding developmental abnormalities as well as override the activation of compensatory mechanisms that may occur during embryonic growth and maturity. As discussed above, ACE2 action results in the degradation and synthesis of a variety of peptides involved in pressure homeostasis. It will be imperative to quantify circulating and tissue concentrations of these peptides to obtain a clear picture of the contribution of ACE2 and the molecular mechanisms involved in blood pressure regulation.

ACE2 AND CARDIAC FUNCTION

Two genetic studies suggest a role for ACE2 in cardiac function. Crackower et al.[49] observed severely impaired heart function in ACE2 knockout mice, including mild thinning of the left ventricle and a severe reduction in cardiac contractility. Loss of ACE2 was associated with an increase in the tissue and plasma Ang II, providing further evidence of a role for ACE2 in the hydrolysis of Ang II and the generation of

Ang-(1-7). No evidence of cardiac hypertrophy or fibrosis was observed in the 6-month-old ACE2-deficient mice, suggesting that compensatory mechanisms were activated during development or that more time may be needed for significant progression of these pathologies. Generation of double mutant *ace/ace2* knockout mice completely abolished the cardiac dysfunction of the ACE2 knockout mice and caused a decrease in blood pressure. In addition, disruption of ACER, the *Drosophila* ACE2 homolog, results in severe defects in heart morphogenesis.[49] These observations suggest that ACE2 counter-balances the function of ACE in the heart and provide strong support for the physiological interplay between the effector molecules, Ang II and Ang-(1-7).

In contrast, over-expression of a human ACE2 in mouse cardiac myocytes resulted in premature, sudden death, which was associated with ACE2 gene expression in a dose-dependent fashion.[52] In mice with moderate human ACE2 gene dosage, 50% of the animals succumbed to sudden death by 23 weeks of age, while 50% of the mice with higher expression (a 2.9-fold increase) were dead by 5 weeks of age. Although the hearts of these mice were normal on gross examination, they had severe and progressive conduction and rhythm disturbances which correlated with a loss of connexins 40 and 43. The effect of ACE2 over-expression on connexin 40 and 43 and the resulting abnormal heart function may result from increased production of Ang-(1-7) or decreased Ang II. Unfortunately, the circulating and tissue concentrations of these ACE2 peptide substrate and product were not measured. The results of these studies indicate that ACE2 is involved in cardiac function but that over-expression of the enzyme may not be a beneficial therapeutic treatment and in fact might contribute to cardiac pathology. It is important to note that the ACE2 concentration in the serum of these knockin animals was over 20-fold increased in the mice with the highest gene dosage and about 10-fold for the moderate expressing mice as compared with wild-type animals. The tissue levels of the enzyme were not reported. These recombinant mice were subjected to these extraordinarily high concentrations of ACE2 throughout development. The generation of additional knockout and knockin models with tissue-specific and time-controlled expression as well as the addition of regulatory elements to the promoter that limit the expression of ACE2 to more physiologically relevant concentrations is needed to determine the precise role of ACE2 as well as the roles that substrates and products of the enzyme play in cardiac development and function.

Several physiology studies also implicate ACE2 in cardiac function. We investigated the effect of coronary artery ligation on cardiac ACE2 in rats following a myocardial infarction (MI), to explore the role of the enzyme in heart function following injury.[53] Twenty-eight days after ligation, MI induced cardiac hypertrophy and left ventricular dysfunction, and increased plasma angiotensin peptide concentrations compared with sham-operated controls. Neither cardiac ACE2 nor ACE mRNA was altered by coronary artery ligation. In contrast, Burrell et al.[54] showed an up-regulation of both ACE and ACE2 mRNA in border/infarct area of Sprague-Dawley rat hearts 28 days after coronary artery ligation as well as increased ACE2 in the hearts of human subjects. As reviewed by Ferrario,[55] differences in strain and the use of ACE inhibitors may have contributed to the findings reported by Burrell et al.[54] As our report was the first to examine ACE2 following MI in Lewis rats, there are no other animal studies that lend support to one study or the other. However, similar conflicting results are found with respect to ACE regulation. Several studies report no change in ACE mRNA in rat left ventricle following coronary artery ligation as compared to sham-operated controls,[53,56–58] while Kobayashi et al.[59] observed an increase in ACE mRNA. Gaertner et al.[58] observed greater ACE mRNA in cardiac scar tissue with no change in ACE expression in the remaining viable left ventricular tissue, indicating that severity of damage might play a role in ACE regulation. Further study is required to determine whether ACE2 is similarly increased in the scar tissue with no change in ACE2 expression in the less damaged hypertrophied heart, not only to explain the discrepancy observed between our study[53] and the report of Burrell et al.[54] but also to further understand the molecular control of ACE2 following MI.

While ACE2 mRNA was not altered by coronary artery ligation in our studies, it was increased significantly in rats treated with losartan 28 days after ligation.[53] Cardiac ACE2 mRNA among all groups studied correlated directly with plasma levels of Ang-(1-7) and inversely with plasma Ang II. In addition, plasma Ang-(1-7)/Ang II ratios were significantly greater in the losartan-treated group, a finding that suggests increased formation of Ang-(1-7) from Ang II. Similarly, we found that treatment of normotensive Lewis rats with the ACE inhibitor lisinopril caused a significant up-regulation in cardiac ACE2 mRNA with a concomitant decrease in plasma Ang II and an increase in circulating Ang-(1-7).[38] AT_1 receptor blockade by losartan resulted in higher concentrations of plasma Ang II and Ang-(1-7) as well as cardiac ACE2 mRNA and activity in the normotensive Lewis rats. These results are in agreement with Goulter et al.,[60] who showed that ACE2 was up-regulated in the heart tissues from patients with idiopathic dilated cardiomyopathy (IDC) and ischemic cardiomyopathy (ICM) as compared with non-diseased controls. These cardiac patients received a variety of pharmacological therapies, including ACE inhibitors (9 of 11 IDC patients and 8 of 12 ICM patients) and an AT_1 receptor antagonist (1 of 11 IDC patients). Our data suggest that the cardioprotective effect of ACE inhibitors and AT_1 receptor blockers may be due, at least in part, to increased ACE2 which shifts the angiotensin peptide balance favoring metabolism of Ang II to produce increased Ang-(1-7).

The protective effects of the ACE2 product, Ang-(1-7), in the heart are supported by the following studies. First, an 8-week infusion of Ang-(1-7) following coronary artery ligation prevented the deterioration of cardiac function and was associated with a significant decrease in myocyte size.[61] Second, Ang-(1-7) treatment of isolated rat hearts following ischemia/reperfusion reduced the incidence and duration of arrhythmias; the effect was blocked by a selective $AT_{1\text{-}7}$ receptor antagonist or a cyclooxygenase inhibitor.[62] Finally, Zisman et al.[63] showed that Ang-(1-7) was made in the intact human heart of four transplant recipients, and that a decrease in Ang II by an ACE inhibitor reduced Ang-(1-7) formation, suggesting an Ang II-dependent pathway for synthesis of the heptapeptide. This production of Ang-(1-7) from Ang II was inhibited by the selective ACE2 inhibitor C16 (Millenium Corporation), decisively proving a role for ACE2 in Ang-(1-7) production in the heart.[63] In this same study, Ang-(1-7) was generated by the infusion of Ang I, which was reduced by the neprilysin inhibitor thiorphan, confirming our initial studies showing that neprilysin is an additional Ang-(1-7)-forming enzyme.[64] Both of the Ang-(1-7)-forming activities identified in the human heart were increased in failing human heart ventricles, providing evidence that Ang-(1-7) serves a cardioprotective role in heart failure.[63] Collectively, these data demonstrate that Ang-(1-7) and the enzymes that generate Ang-(1-7) are involved in the regulation of myocyte growth and in cardiac function.

Additional evidence for a role of ACE2 in Ang-(1-7) formation was derived from studies in which Lewis rats were medicated with lisinopril or losartan and plasma concentrations of angiotensin peptides and ACE2 activity were measured at the end of the 12-day treatment period. In these animals, the reduction of blood pressure associated with both treatment forms is accompanied by increased ACE2 activity in the kidney which correlated with both plasma Ang II and Ang-(1-7) (Figure 5.3).

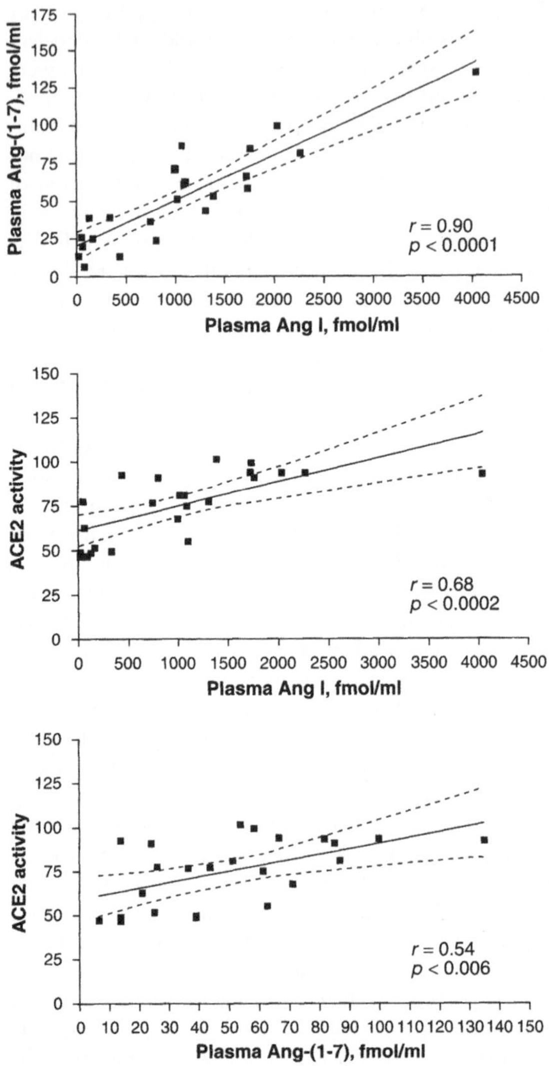

Figure 5.3 Evidence for a role of angiotensin converting enzyme 2 (ACE2) in the metabolism of angiotensin II (Ang II) and the formation of angiotensin-(1-7) (Ang-(1-7)) is illustrated in experiments in which Lewis normotensive rats were medicated with lisinopril or losartan for a 2-week period. Data were obtained on the twelfth day of the treatment regimen. ACE2 activity (in fmol/mg/min of generated Ang-(1-7) is measured as the rate of Ang-(1-7) formation from exogenous Ang II in isolated renal cortex membranes as described in reference 28 and unpublished observations

SUMMARY

In 1956, Skeggs et al. published an article entitled 'Preparation and function of the hypertensin-converting enzyme'.[65] This was the first description of the enzyme activity we now refer to as ACE. Fifty years later, new and exciting discoveries are still made about the enzymatic action of ACE, its function in vertebrate physiology, and its role in the pathophysiology of disease. Less than 5 years ago, the discovery of a novel ACE homolog, ACE2, was reported by Tipnis et al.[9] and Donahue et al.[10] While much has been learned about this novel enzyme in a short time, the study of ACE2 is still in its infancy. Little or no information exists on the role of ACE2 in development, gender differences, systemic and central control of blood pressure, heart and renal function or inflammation. More important, it is not clear whether ACE2 will be an effective therapeutic target. Intuitively, it seems likely since ACE2 provides a direct link between the RAAS, kinin, and apelin pathways, key systems involved in cardiovascular function. However, unlike ACE, in which inhibition of the enzyme activity causes a reduction of the vasoconstrictor and mitogen Ang II and an increase in Ang-(1-7) and bradykinin, vasodilators and growth inhibitors, initial studies indicate that an up-regulation of ACE2 will yield beneficial results. We showed that ACE inhibition or AT_1 receptor blockade caused a marked increase in ACE2 mRNA in the heart[38,53] and Zhong et al. reported a significant up-regulation of the enzyme in SHR following treatment with all-*trans*-retinoic acid.[66] These results may explain, in part, the beneficial effects of these agents. However, treatment of patients with these established medications will not exploit the potential advantage of enhancing ACE2 activity alone, thereby limiting added side effects. Such a novel therapy will require either precise control of ACE2 transcription or a means to effectively deliver ACE2 to the target tissue, such as the use of stem cells as a vector for gene delivery. Whatever the outcome, the discovery of ACE2 highlights the need to account for the action of multiple peptide hormones, including Ang-(1-7), [des-Arg^9]-bradykinin, and the apelin fragments when elucidating mechanisms of normal vascular and cardiac function as well as the development of drug regimes to combat cardiovascular pathologies.

ACKNOWLEDGMENTS

The authors gratefully acknowledge grant support in part provided by the National Institute of Health (HL51952) as well as Unifi, Inc., Greensboro, NC and Farley-Hudson Foundation, Jacksonville, NC, USA.

REFERENCES

1. Brenner BM, Cooper ME, de Zeeuw D et al. RENAAL Study Investigators. Effects of losartan on renal and cardiovascular outcomes in patients with type 2 diabetes and nephropathy. N Engl J Med 2001; 345: 861–9.
2. Dahlof B, Devereux RB, Kjeldsen SE et al. Cardiovascular morbidity and mortality in the losartan intervention for endpoint reduction in hypertension study (LIFE): a randomised trial against atenolol. Lancet 2002; 359: 995–1003.
3. HOPE Study. Effects of ramipril on cardiovascular and microvascular outcomes in people with diabetes mellitus: results of the HOPE study and MICRO-HOPE substudy. Lancet 2000; 355: 53–9.
4. Julius S, Kjeldsen SE, Weber M et al. Outcomes in hypertensive patients at high cardiovascular risk treated with regimens based on valsartan or amlodipine: the VALUE randomised trial. Lancet 2004; 363: 2022–31.
5. Lewis EJ, Hunsicker LG, Clarke WR et al. Renoprotective effect of the angiotensin-receptor antagonist irbesartan in patients with nephropathy due to type 2 diabetes. N Engl J Med 2001; 345: 851–60.
6. Ferrario CM, Chappell MC, Tallant EA, Brosnihan KB, Diz DI. Counterregulatory actions of angiotensin-(1-7). Hypertension 1997; 30 (Part 2): 535–41.
7. Ferrario CM, Averill DB, Brosnihan KB et al. Angiotensin-(1-7). It's contribution to arterial pressure control mechanisms. In: Unger T, Scholkens B (eds). Handbook of Experimental Pharmacology: Angiotensin, Vol. 1. Heidelberg: Springer Verlag, 2004, pp 478–518.
8. Ferrario CM, Chappell MC. Novel angiotensin peptides. Cell Mol Life Sci 2004; 61: 2720–7.
9. Tipnis SR, Hooper NM, Hyde R, Karran E, Christie G, Turner AJ. A human homolog of angiotensin-converting enzyme. Cloning and functional expression as a captopril-insensitive carboxypeptidase. J Biol Chem 2000; 275: 33238–43.
10. Donoghue M, Hsieh F, Baronas E et al. A novel angiotensin-converting enzyme-related carboxypeptidase (ACE2) converts angiotensin I to angiotensin 1-9. Circ Res 2000; 87: E1–E9.
11. Carrel L, Willard HF. X-inactivation profile reveals extensive variability in X-linked gene expression in females. Nature 2005; 434: 400–4.
12. Harmer D, Gilbert M, Borman R, Clark KL. Quantitative mRNA expression profiling of ACE2, a novel homologue of angiotensin converting enzyme. FEBS Lett 2002; 532: 107–10.
13. Towler P, Staker B, Prasad SG et al. ACE2 X-ray structures reveal a large hinge-bending motion important for inhibitor binding and catalysis. J Biol Chem 2004; 279: 17996–8007.
14. Vickers C, Hales P, Kaushik V et al. Hydrolysis of biological peptides by human angiotensin-converting enzyme-related carboxypeptidase. J Biol Chem 2002; 277: 14838–43.
15. Tallant EA, Ferrario CM. Biology of angiotensin II receptor inhibition with a focus on losartan: a new drug for the treatment of hypertension. Exp Opin Invest Drugs 1996; 5: 1201–14.
16. Nakamoto H, Ferrario CM, Fuller SB, Robaczwski DL, Winicov E, Dean RH. Angiotensin-(1-7) and nitric oxide interaction in renovascular hypertension. Hypertension 1995; 25: 796–802.
17. Benter IF, Ferrario CM, Morris M, Diz DI. Antihypertensive actions of angiotensin-(1-7) in spontaneously hypertensive rats. Am J Physiol Heart Circ Physiol 1995; 269: H313–H319.
18. DelliPizzi A, Hilchey SD, Bell-Quilley CP. Natriuretic action of angiotensin-(1-7). Br J Pharmacol 1994; 111: 1–3.

19. Hilchey SD, Bell-Quilley CP. Association between the natriuretic action of angiotensin-(1-7) and selective stimulation of renal prostaglandin I2 release. Hypertension 1995; 25: 1238–44.
20. Garcia NH, Garvin JL. Angiotensin-(1-7) has a biphasic effect on fluid absorption in the proximal straight tubule. J Am Soc Nephrol 1994; 5: 1133–8.
21. Handa RK, Ferrario CM, Strandhoy JW. Renal actions of angiotensin-(1-7) in vivo and in vitro studies. Am J Physiol 1996; 270: F141–F147.
22. Tran YL, Forster C. Angiotensin-(1-7) and the rat aorta: modulation by the endothelium. J Cardiovasc Pharmacol 1997; 30: 676–82.
23. Brosnihan KB, Li P, Ferrario CM. Angiotensin-(1-7) dilates canine coronary arteries through kinins and nitric oxide. Hypertension 1996; 27: 523–8.
24. Porsti I, Bara AT, Busse R, Hecker M. Release of nitric oxide by angiotensin-(1-7) from porcine coronary endothelium: implications for a novel angiotensin receptor. Br J Pharmacol 1994; 111: 652–4.
25. Meng W, Busija DW. Comparative effects of angiotensin-(1-7) and angiotensin II on piglet pial arterioles. Stroke 1993; 24: 2041–5.
26. Osei SY, Ahima RS, Minkes RK, Weaver JP, Khosla MC, Kadowitz PJ. Differential responses to angiotensin-(1-7) in the feline mesenteric and hindquarters vascular beds. Eur J Pharmacol 1993; 234: 35–42.
27. Iyer SN, Chappell MC, Averill DB, Diz DI, Ferrario CM. Vasodepressor actions of angiotensin-(1-7) unmasked during combined treatment with lisinopril and losartan. Hypertension 1998; 31: 699–705.
28. Iyer SN, Ferrario CM, Chappell CM. Angiotensin-(1-7) contributes to the antihypertensive effects of blockade of the renin-angiotensin system. Hypertension 1998; 31 (Part 2): 356–61.
29. Freeman EJ, Chisolm GM, Ferrario CM, Tallant EA. Angiotensin-(1-7) inhibits vascular smooth muscle cell growth. Hypertension 1996; 28: 104–8.
30. Sadoshima J, Izumo S. Molecular characterization of angiotensin II-induced hypertrophy of cardiac myocytes and hyperplasia of cardiac fibroblasts. Critical role of the AT1 receptor subtype. Circ Res 1993; 73: 413–23.
31. Strawn WB, Ferrario CM, Tallant EA. Angiotensin-(1-7) reduces smooth muscle growth after vascular injury. Hypertension 1999; 33 (Part II): 207–11.
32. Tallant EA, Diz DI, Ferrario CM. Antiproliferative actions of angiotensin-(1-7) in vascular smooth muscle. Hypertension 1999; 34 (Part 2): 950–7.
33. Tallant EA, Howard LT, Dancho B, Gallagher PE. Angiotensin-(1-7) reduces hypertrophy in cardiomyocytes and hyperplasia in cardiac fibroblasts. Hypertension 2003; 40: 389.
34. Tom B, Dendorfer A, Danser AHJ. Bradykinin, angiotensin-(1-7), and ACE inhibitors: how do they interact? Int J Biochem Cell Biol 2003; 35: 792–801.
35. Schmaier AH. The kallikrein-kinin and the renin-angiotensin systems have a multilayer interaction. Am J Physiol Regul Integr Comp Physiol 2003; 285: R1–R13.
36. Luque M, Martin P, Martell N, Fernandez C, Brosnihan KB, Ferrario CM. Effects of captopril related to increased levels of prostacyclin and angiotensin-(1-7) in essential hypertension. J Hypertens 1996; 14: 799–805.
37. Ferrario CM, Martell N, Yunis C et al. Characterization of angiotensin-(1-7) in the urine of normal and essential hypertensive subjects. Am J Hypertens 1998; 11: 137–46.
38. Ferrario CM, Jessup JA, Chappell MC et al. Effect of angiotensin converting enzyme inhibition and angiotensin II receptor blockers on cardiac angiotensin converting enzyme 2. Circulation 2005; 111: 2605–10.
39. Santos RA, Campagnole-Santos MJ, Andrade SP. Angiotensin-(1-7): an update. Regul Pept 2000; 91: 45–62.
40. Ueda S, Masumori-Maemoto S, Wada A, Ishii M, Brosnihan KB, Umemura S. Angiotensin-(1-7) potentiates bradykinin-induced vasodilatation in man. J Hypertens 2001; 19: 2001–9.
41. Chappell MC, Pirro NT, Sykes A, Ferrario CM. Metabolism of angiotensin-(1-7) by angiotensin-converting enzyme. Hypertension 1998; 31 (Part 2): 362–7.
42. Lee DK, Cheng R, Nguyen T et al. Characterization of apelin, the ligand for the APJ receptor. J Neurochem 2000; 74: 34–41.
43. Szokodi I, Tavi P, Foldes G et al. Apelin, the novel endogenous ligand of the orphan receptor APJ, regulates cardiac contractility. Circ Res 2002; 91: 434–40.
44. Berry MF, Pirolli TJ, Jayasankar V et al. Apelin has in vivo inotropic effects on normal and failing hearts. Circulation 2004; 110 (11 Suppl 1): II187–II193.
45. Ashley EA, Powers J, Chen M et al. The endogenous peptide apelin potently improves cardiac contractility and reduces cardiac loading in vivo. Cardiovasc Res 2005; 65: 73–82.
46. Tatemoto K, Takayama K, Zou MX et al. The novel peptide apelin lowers blood pressure via a nitric oxide-dependent mechanism. Regul Pept 2001; 99: 87–92.
47. Cheng X, Cheng XS, Pang CC. Venous dilator effect of apelin, an endogenous peptide ligand for the orphan APJ receptor, in conscious rats. Eur J Pharmacol 2003; 470: 171–5.
48. Ishida J, Hashimoto T, Hashimoto Y et al. Regulatory roles for APJ, a seven-transmembrane receptor related to angiotensin-type 1 receptor in blood pressure in vivo. J Biol Chem 2004; 279: 26274–9.
49. Crackower MA, Sarao ROG, Yagil C et al. Angiotensin-converting enzyme 2 is an essential regulator of heart function. Nature 2002; 417: 822–8.
50. Allred AJ, Donoghue M, Acton S, Coffman TM. Regulation of blood pressure by the angiotensin converting enzyme homologue ACE2. Proceedings of the American Society of Nephrology, 2002.
51. Huang L, Sexton DJ, Skogerson K et al. Novel peptide inhibitors of angiotensin-converting enzyme 2. J Biol Chem 2003; 278: 15532–40.
52. Donoghue M, Wakimoto H, Maguire CT et al. Heart block, ventricular tachycardia, and sudden death in ACE2 transgenic mice with downregulated connexins. J Mol Cell Cardiol 2003; 35: 1043–53.
53. Ishiyama Y, Gallagher PE, Averill DB, Tallant EA, Brosnihan KB, Ferrario CM. Up-regulation of angiotensin converting enzyme 2 after myocardial infarction by blockade of angiotensin II receptors. Hypertension 2004; 43: 1–7.
54. Burrell LM, Risvanis J, Kubota E et al. Myocardial infarction increases ACE2 expression in rat and humans. Eur Heart J 2005; 114: 1–7.
55. Ferrario CM. Myocardial infarction increases ACE2 expression in rat and humans. Eur Heart J 2005; 26: 1141.
56. Wollert KC, Studer R, von Bulow B, Drexler H. Survival after myocardial infarction in the rat. Role of tissue angiotensin-converting enzyme inhibition. Circulation 1994; 90: 2457–67.
57. Passier RCJJ, Smits JFM, Verluyten MJA, Studer R, Drexler H, Daemen JAP. Activation of angiotensin-converting enzyme expression in infarct zone following myocardial infarction. Am J Physiol Heart Circ Physiol 1995; 269: H1268–H1276.

58. Gaertner R, Prunier F, Philippe M, Louedec L, Mercadier J-J, Michel J-B. Scar and pulmonary expression and shedding of ACE in rat myocardial infarction. Am J Physiol Heart Circ Physiol 2002; 283: H156–H164.
59. Kobayashi T, Miyauchi T, Sakai S, Yamaguchi M, Goto K, Sugishita Y. Endothelin-converting enzyme and angiotensin-converting in failing hearts of rats with myocardial infarction. J Cardiovasc Pharmacol 1998; 31: S417–S420.
60. Goulter AB, Goddard MJ, Allen JC, Clark KL. ACE2 gene expression is up-regulated in the human failing heart. BMC Med 2004; 2: 19.
61. Loot AE, Roks AJ, Henning RH et al. Angiotensin-(1-7) attenuates the development of heart failure after myocardial infarction in rats. Circulation 2002; 105: 1548–50.
62. Ferreira AJ, Santos RA, Almeida AP. Angiotensin-(1-7): cardioprotective effect in myocardial ischemia/reperfusion. Hypertension 2001; 38 (3 Pt 2): 665–8.
63. Zisman LS, Meixell GE, Bristow MR, Canver CC. Angiotensin-(1-7) formation in the intact human heart: in vivo dependence on angiotensin II as substrate. Circulation 2003; 108: 1679–81.
64. Chappell MC, Tallant EA, Brosnihan KB, Ferrario CM. Conversion of angiotensin I to angiotensin-(1-7) by thimet oliogopeptidase (E.C.3.4.24.15) in vascular smooth muscle cells. J Vasc Biol Med 1995; 5: 129–37.
65. Skeggs LT Jr, Kahn JR, Shumway NP. The preparation and function of the hypertensin-converting enzyme. J Exp Med 1956; 103: 295–9.
66. Zhong JC, Huang DY, Yang YM et al. Upregulation of angiotensin-converting enzyme 2 by all-trans retinoic acid in spontaneously hypertensive rats. Hypertension 2004; 44: 907–12.

6

The biology of angiotensin II (formation, metabolism, fragments, measurement)

Duncan J Campbell

INTRODUCTION

Angiotensin (Ang) II is one of a family of bioactive angiotensin peptides that includes angiotensin 2-8 (Ang III), angiotensin 3-8 (Ang IV), and angiotensin 1-7 (Ang 1-7). Although long considered to be biologically inactive, a recent study suggests that Ang I may also be bioactive in the kidney, unrelated to its conversion to Ang II.[1] The nomenclature and sequences of angiotensin peptides referred to in this chapter are shown in Figure 6.1. The importance of Ang III, Ang IV, and Ang 1-7 lies in their potential to mediate some of the effects of Ang II, and to contribute to the effects of angiotensin converting enzyme (ACE) inhibitors and Ang II type 1 (AT_1) receptor blockers (ARBs). This chapter has a clinical focus, and will briefly review the formation, metabolism, and measurement of these peptides. Other aspects of the biology of these peptides are discussed elsewhere in this volume.

FORMATION OF ANGIOTENSIN PEPTIDES

All angiotensin peptides are derived from angiotensinogen. Angiotensinogen gene knockout mice have no detectable angiotensin peptides in blood or tissues.[2] In contrast to the essential role of angiotensinogen in angiotensin peptide formation, many different enzymes cleave angiotensinogen to release either Ang I or Ang II. The pathways of angiotensin peptide formation are shown in Figure 6.1.

In addition to renin, enzymes that release Ang I from angiotensinogen include cathepsin D,[3,4] pepsin,[5] and other aspartyl proteases and renin-like enzymes.[6–12] Moreover, serine proteases can release Ang II directly from angiotensinogen. These include tonin,[13] cathepsin,[14] trypsin,[15] and tissue kallikrein.[16] Enzymes other than ACE may convert Ang I to Ang II. These include tonin,[13] cathepsin G,[17] chymase,[17,18] and other serine proteases.[19,20]

Many of the enzymes that metabolize Ang I and Ang II are summarized in Figure 6.2. The levels of angiotensin peptides are as much dependent on their rate of metabolism as on their rate of formation. The half-life of Ang I and Ang II in arterial plasma in vivo is approximately one circulation time, with extensive conversion of Ang I to Ang II in all vascular beds and metabolism of Ang II in all vascular beds except the lung.[21]

Calculation of the ratio of the concentrations of two angiotensin peptides can provide an index of the rate of conversion of one peptide to the other. Thus, the plasma Ang II/Ang I ratio provides an index of plasma ACE activity, or the rate of Ang I conversion to Ang II.[22,23]

TISSUE ANGIOTENSIN SYSTEMS

Tissues are the main site of formation and metabolism of angiotensin peptides, and conversion of Ang I to Ang II.[24] Many different tissues synthesize angiotensinogen,[25,26] and adipose tissue may contribute to circulating angiotensinogen.[27] Renin is synthesized as the zymogen, prorenin. Although many tissues synthesize prorenin, the kidney is possibly the only site of active renin formation,[28] with the exception of the ovary and placenta.[29,30] Circulating levels of renin and angiotensin peptides are very low in anephric subjects.[28] Angiotensin peptide formation in non-renal tissues is thought to depend on tissue uptake of circulating renin.[24,31] In addition, the different abundance and proportions of angiotensin peptides in blood and tissues

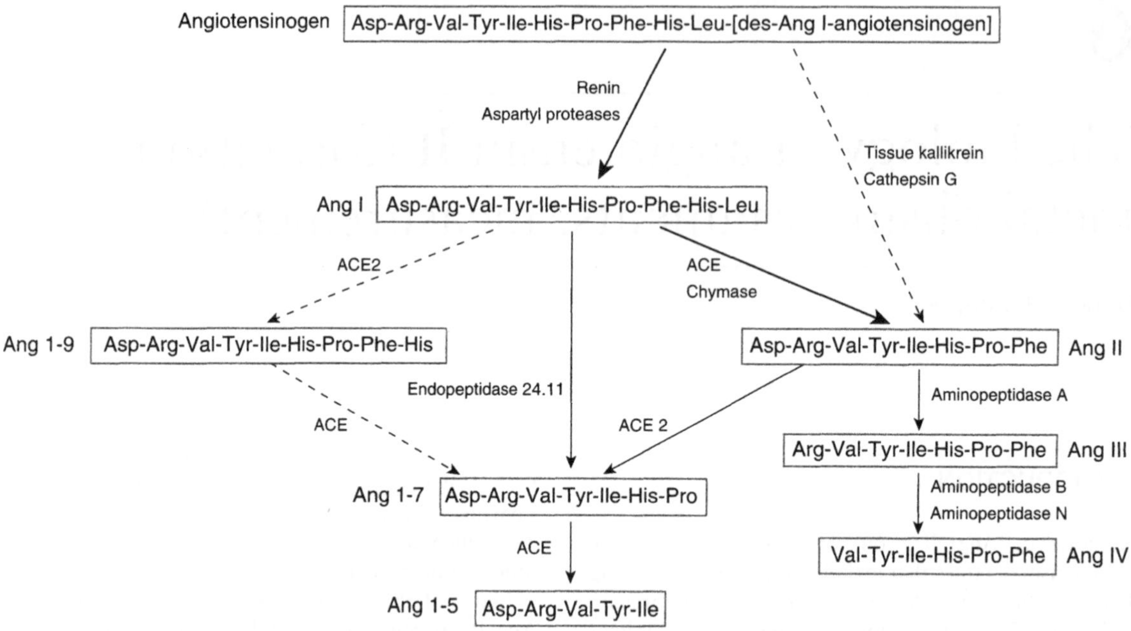

Figure 6.1 Pathways of formation of angiotensin peptides. Not all enzymes that may play a role are shown in this figure. Other enzymes are shown in Figure 6.2

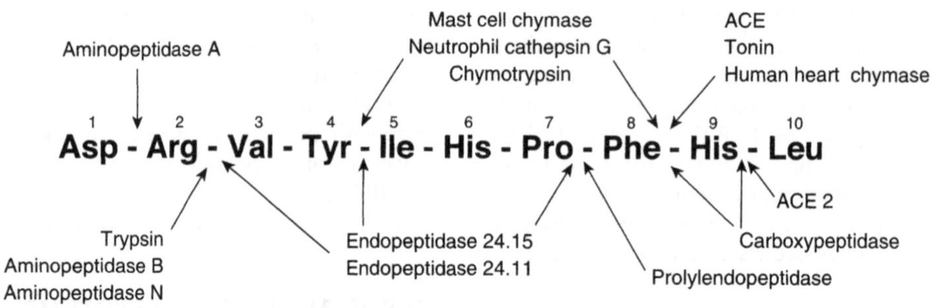

Figure 6.2 Enzymes that metabolize angiotensin peptides. The serine proteases mast cell chymase, neutrophil cathepsin G, and chymotrypsin all cleave between Tyr^4-Ile^5. ACE, tonin, and human heart chymase all cleave between Phe^8-His^9. Trypsin, aminopeptidase B, and aminopeptidase N all cleave between Arg^2-Val^3. Both endopeptidases 24.15 and 24.11 cleave between Tyr^4-Ile^5, and between Pro^7-Phe^8 and endopeptidase 24.11 also cleaves between Arg^2-Val^3

indicate tissue-specific differences in angiotensin peptide metabolism due to differences in peptidase activity.[32]

ALTERNATIVE PATHWAYS OF ANG II FORMATION AND METABOLISM

There are many unanswered questions concerning angiotensin peptide formation in tissues. It is possible, for example, that Ang II may be formed by processes, independent of renin, at sites of inflammation or coagulation where kallikrein and/or cathepsin G may be activated. In assessing the pathways of angiotensin peptide formation, it is important to distinguish between evidence obtained from studies of tissue homogenates, studies of isolated tissues, and studies performed in vivo. Whereas studies of tissue homogenates and isolated tissues suggest an important role for alternative pathways of angiotensin peptide formation and metabolism, studies in vivo indicate that the main pathway of Ang II formation is via renin and ACE.[33–35] Two enzymes that have received considerable recent attention with respect to angiotensin peptide formation and metabolism are chymase and ACE-related carboxypeptidase (ACE 2).

Chymase

Human heart chymase was initially discovered in homogenates of human heart and proposed to be the major pathway of conversion of Ang I to Ang II in the heart.[18] Given that chymase is not inhibited by ACE inhibitors, it represented a potential pathway of continued Ang II formation in patients taking ACE inhibitor therapy,[36] and thereby provided a rationale for a possible superiority of ARB therapy over ACE inhibitor therapy. Although studies of tissue homogenates and isolated tissues indicate that chymase may participate in Ang II formation,[18,37] studies in vivo show that the major pathway of Ang II formation involves ACE.[34,35,38] It is not possible to extrapolate from an enzyme's abundance in a tissue to its role in peptide metabolism in vivo. Chymase is reported to be more abundant than ACE in human lung;[39] however, the effects of ACE inhibition and ACE gene knockout on Ang I and Ang II levels in arterial blood and in lung indicate that ACE plays the dominant role in Ang II formation in lung.[2,35,38,40]

Dell'Italia and Husain offer three lines of physiological evidence for a chymase-Ang II system.[36] Firstly, they refer to the failure of ACE inhibitor therapy to completely suppress Ang II levels. Secondly, they refer to the report by Wei et al.[41] of similar Ang I and Ang II levels in kidney, heart, and lung of ACE gene knockout and wild-type mice. Thirdly, they refer to the failure of captopril to modify the high Ang II levels in microdialysate from dog cardiac ventricle.[42] Each of these three lines of evidence can be countered. Firstly, the failure of ACE inhibitor therapy to completely suppress Ang II levels is discussed below.

Secondly, in contrast to the findings of Wei et al.,[41] we found a marked suppression of Ang II levels in kidney, heart, and lung of ACE gene knockout mice.[2,38] We also showed that ACE inhibition produced a marked suppression of Ang II levels in blood and tissues of mice.[38] The differences between our results and those of Wei et al.[41] may have a methodological basis, in that by boiling frozen tissue in 1 mol/L acetic acid,[43] Wei et al.[41] may have permitted Ang I generation and conversion to Ang II by lysosomal enzymes released by the thawed tissue.

Thirdly, there is some doubt about the reliability of measurement of angiotensin peptide levels in microdialysate from dog cardiac ventricle in the experiments of Dell'Italia et al.[42] Dell'Italia et al.[42] reported Ang II levels in cardiac microdialysate (6333 fmol/ml) that were 200 times the levels in whole ventricular tissue (approximately 28 fmol/g).[44,45] This would require that the Ang II content of 1 g of cardiac ventricle be contained in a compartment with a total volume no greater than 5 μl, and that the investigators be able to place their microdialysis probe within this 5 μl compartment and collect microdialysate without dilution from other compartments within the heart. It is of note that Schuijt et al.[46] measured Ang II levels in pig cardiac tissue (approximately 22 fmol/g) similar to the levels reported for dog heart,[44,45] but Ang II levels in microdialysate from pig heart were below the limit of detection (<30 fmol/ml).[46] Further evidence against an important role for chymase in Ang II formation in the heart is the report by Kokkonen et al.[47] that interstitial fluid contains protease inhibitors that potently inhibit chymase activity.

Orally active chymase inhibitors are under development,[48] and it remains to be shown whether these drugs affect Ang II levels. These drugs may have effects independent of any influence on Ang II levels. Nishimoto et al.[49] reported that chymase inhibition reduced Ang II levels in the grafted jugular vein of dogs. However, there is uncertainty as to whether the reduced Ang II levels were due to inhibition of chymase-mediated Ang II formation, or due to inhibition of vascular proliferation by the chymase inhibitor.

ACE 2

ACE 2, like ACE, is a membrane-associated and secreted metalloprotease expressed predominantly on endothelium.[50,51] Initial reports were that ACE 2, unlike ACE, was restricted in humans to heart, kidney, and testis,[50–52] but subsequent studies found ACE 2 mRNA in all human tissues, with relatively high levels in renal and cardiovascular tissues, and also in the gut.[53] Immunocytochemical studies show that ACE 2 protein is present on arterial and venous endothelial cells in all tissues examined, including lung.[54] ACE 2 is a functional receptor for the SARS coronavirus.[55] ACE 2 is not inhibited by ACE inhibitors. In contrast to the dipeptidyl carboxypeptidase activity of ACE, ACE 2 cleaves Ang I to Ang 1-9 and also cleaves Ang II to Ang 1-7. Together with ACE and endopeptidases, ACE 2 may contribute to the metabolism of Ang I and Ang II, and to the formation of Ang 1-9 and Ang 1-7 (Figure 6.1). Both

ACE and ACE 2 are localized on the endothelium of coronary vessels.[50] However, recent studies indicate that ACE 2 has little role in angiotensin peptide metabolism in the human coronary circulation.[33]

To assess the role of ACE 2 on angiotensin metabolism in the coronary circulation, we measured Ang I, Ang II, Ang 1-9 and Ang 1-7 in arterial and coronary sinus blood of heart failure subjects receiving ACE inhibitor therapy, and of normal subjects not receiving ACE inhibitor therapy.[33] In comparison with normal subjects, heart failure subjects receiving ACE inhibitor therapy had greater than 40-fold increase in Ang I levels, but Ang 1-9 levels were low (1–2 fmol/ml), similar to those of normal subjects. Moreover, Ang 1-7 levels increased in parallel with Ang I levels. In a separate study, we measured Ang I, Ang II, and Ang 1-7 in arterial and coronary sinus blood of subjects with coronary artery disease, before, and at 2, 5, and 10 minutes after intravenous administration of a low dose of ACE inhibitor.[33] Intravenous administration of ACE inhibitor rapidly decreased Ang II levels by 54–58% and increased Ang I levels by 2.4–2.8-fold, but did not alter Ang 1-7 levels or net Ang 1-7 production across the myocardial vascular bed. In heart failure subjects receiving ACE inhibitor therapy, the failure of Ang 1-9 levels to increase in response to increased Ang I levels indicated little role for ACE 2 in Ang I metabolism. Additionally, the levels of Ang 1-7 were more linked to those of Ang I than Ang II, consistent with its formation by endopeptidase-mediated metabolism of Ang I rather than by ACE 2-mediated metabolism of Ang II.

Kinetic studies also suggest that ACE 2 has little role in Ang I metabolism.[52,56] ACE and ACE 2 have similar K_m for Ang I (16 and 6.9 µmol/L, respectively) but the K_{cat} for ACE (40 s^{-1}) is approximately 1000-fold higher than that for ACE 2 (0.034 s^{-1}), such that the K_{cat}/K_m ratio is approximately 500-fold higher for ACE (2.5×10^6 L/mol per s) than for ACE 2 (4.9×10^3 L/mol per s). By contrast, the K_m (2 µmol/L), K_{cat} (3.5 s^{-1}), and K_{cat}/K_m ratio (1.8×10^6 L/mol per s) of ACE 2 for Ang II[52] make it a more likely participant in Ang II metabolism. However, despite the expression of ACE 2 on endothelial cells of the pulmonary vasculature,[54] Ang II traverses the pulmonary circulation virtually intact,[21] indicating little role of ACE 2 in Ang II metabolism in the lung.

We must await the availability of specific ACE 2 inhibitors suitable for administration to humans before a more definitive assessment of the role of ACE 2 in angiotensin peptide metabolism can be performed. ACE 2 is discussed further in Chapter 5 by Gallagher et al in this volume.

EFFECT OF ACE INHIBITION ON ANGIOTENSIN PEPTIDE LEVELS

It is well recognized that ACE inhibition produces variable suppression of Ang II levels.[57] In a study using an ACE-resistant analog of Ang I, McDonald et al.[58] demonstrated the operation of a non-ACE enzymatic pathway of conversion of Ang I to Ang II in humans. However, there is no evidence that this non-ACE pathway makes a significant contribution to Ang I conversion to Ang II in vivo. Jorde et al.[59] showed that the persistent pressor effect of Ang I in heart failure subjects receiving ACE inhibitor therapy was largely due to a failure to produce complete ACE inhibition. The effect of ACE inhibition on angiotensin peptide levels is dependent on the responsiveness of renin secretion.[60] In situations where renin shows little increase in response to ACE inhibition, the levels of Ang II and its metabolites will show a marked fall, with little change in the levels of Ang I and its metabolites. By contrast, a large increase in renin levels in response to ACE inhibition will cause the levels of Ang I and its metabolites, such as Ang 1-7, to increase.

The increased Ang I levels that may accompany ACE inhibition serve to promote Ang II formation by residual uninhibited ACE and by serine protease pathways of Ang I conversion, thereby buffering any fall in Ang II levels during ACE inhibition.[22] The contribution of non-ACE enzymes or residual uninhibited ACE to Ang II formation during ACE inhibition depends on the prevailing Ang I levels, which are dependent on the levels of renin and angiotensinogen. A non-ACE enzymatic pathway that normally contributes to only 1% of Ang II formation, or 1% residual uninhibited ACE, may maintain Ang II levels at 30% of control if Ang I levels are increased 30-fold, as we have demonstrated in our studies of the effects of ACE inhibition on plasma angiotensin peptides in rats.[40] With the exception of lung, the increases in tissue Ang I levels during ACE inhibition are much less than the increase in plasma Ang I levels,[40] and are therefore less likely to drive Ang II formation in tissues during ACE inhibition. ACE inhibitor therapy effectively reduces Ang II levels and the Ang II/Ang I ratio in cardiac tissue from subjects undergoing coronary artery graft surgery.[34]

ACE inhibition is accompanied by increased levels of Ang 1-7. This is due in part to increase in the level of Ang I, with its subsequent conversion to Ang 1-7 by neutral endopeptidase.[61,62] Inhibition of neutral endopeptidase attenuates the increase in Ang 1-7 levels that accompanies ACE inhibition.[61,62] Another mechanism for the increase in Ang 1-7 levels during ACE inhibition is the inhibition of Ang 1-7 metabolism, given that ACE is an important pathway of Ang 1-7 metabolism.[63,64] Thus, ACE inhibition may produce a greater increase in Ang 1-7 levels than ARB therapy, for the same increase in Ang I levels.[65]

Neutral endopeptidase also has an important role in Ang II metabolism. Inhibition of neutral endopeptidase decreases Ang II clearance and increases Ang II levels and the pressor effect of administered Ang II.[61,66]

As mentioned above when discussing ACE 2, the parallel increase in Ang I and Ang 1-7 levels with ACE inhibition is evidence that the main pathway of Ang 1-7 formation is by endopeptidase-mediated cleavage of Ang I, and not by ACE 2-mediated cleavage of Ang II.[33] Ang 1-7 may also inhibit ACE,[67,68] but it is unlikely that Ang 1-7 levels are ever sufficient to have this effect in patients.[32]

EFFECTS OF ARB THERAPY ON ANGIOTENSIN PEPTIDE LEVELS

ARB therapy increases the levels of all angiotensin peptides in proportion to the increase in renin levels. Table 6.1 shows the effects of low doses of ARB on plasma angiotensin peptide levels in hypertensive humans.[69] Increased Ang II levels during ARB therapy counteract the effects of AT_1 receptor antagonism. In addition, stimulation of the AT_2 receptor by increased Ang II levels may contribute to the effects of ARB therapy.[70,71] Increased Ang IV and Ang 1-7 levels may also contribute to the effects of ARB therapy.

Angiotensin peptides respond differently to ACE inhibition and ARB therapy in different tissues.[40,72–74] The effects of these agents on angiotensin peptide levels suggest that of all tissues examined, angiotensin-mediated processes in the kidney are most sensitive to inhibition by ACE inhibition and ARB therapy.[74] Renal Ang II levels were reduced by lower doses of ACE inhibitor than were required to reduce Ang II levels in other tissues. Moreover, the kidney showed the smallest increase in Ang II levels in response to ARB therapy,[40,72,74] and was therefore most susceptible to AT_1 receptor blockade.

COMBINATION OF ACE INHIBITION AND ARB THERAPY

Combination of ACE inhibition and ARB therapy allows more complete blockade of the renin angiotensin system because ACE inhibition attenuates the increase in Ang II levels that would otherwise accompany ARB therapy.[65,75,76] However, it is noted that the effects of ACE inhibitors and ARBs on angiotensin peptide levels are very much dose-related, and different drugs have different potencies and durations of action.[22,75,77] These differences between drugs and drug combinations need to be taken into account when interpreting the effects of combination of ACE inhibitors and ARBs.[76]

Although the combination of ACE inhibition and ARB therapy may prevent the increase in Ang II and Ang IV levels in response to ARB therapy, it does not modify, and may potentiate, the increase in Ang I and Ang 1-7 levels.

MEASUREMENT OF ANGIOTENSIN PEPTIDES

Understanding of the role of angiotensin peptides in health and disease is dependent in large part on their accurate measurement. Measurement of angiotensin peptides presents a challenge because of their low levels in blood and tissues, their susceptibility to continued formation and metabolism during collection of blood and tissues for assay, and the lack of specificity of radioimmunoassays for these peptides.

Table 6.1 Plasma angiotensin peptide levels in hypertensive humans during treatment with placebo, or angiotensin receptor blockers losartan (50 mg OD) or eprosartan (600 mg OD)

Peptide (fmol/ml)	*Placebo*	*Losartan*	*Eprosartan*
Ang 1-7	1.5 (0.3–8.3)	1.8 (0.5–6.2)	1.8 (0.7–4.5)
Ang II	3.1 (1.0–9.5)	7.6 (1.3–44.5)*	6.5 (2.0–21.5)*
Ang 1-9	0.13 (0.02–0.75)	0.18 (0.03–1.19)	0.10 (0.03–0.43)
Ang I	1.8 (0.2–15.7)	6.6 (0.9–46.6)*	5.5 (0.9–34.4)*
Ang 2-8	0.24 (0.05–1.09)	0.53 (0.07–4.00)*	0.67 (0.09–4.94)*
Ang 3-8	0.34 (0.07–1.76)	0.58 (0.07–4.56)	0.76 (0.16–3.78)*

Data shown as geometric mean (95% confidence interval), $n = 19$. *$p < 0.01$ compared to placebo. Data from Campbell et al.[69]

Measurement of angiotensin peptides in blood requires the collection of blood into a cocktail of enzyme inhibitors that inhibit renin, ACE, and peptidases. After rapid centrifugation, the plasma is usually extracted to separate peptides from proteins, and the different angiotensin peptides are then separated by high performance liquid chromatography (HPLC) before radioimmunoassay.[78,79] The levels of some angiotensin peptides measured in plasma from hypertensive subjects receiving placebo therapy, and therapy with either of the two ARBs, losartan and eprosartan, are shown in Table 6.1.

An example of the importance of methodology in measurement of angiotensin peptides is an early report of relatively high levels of Ang II and Ang 1-7 in rat hypothalamus.[80] Much lower angiotensin peptide levels were measured in this tissue when precautions were taken to prevent thawing of frozen tissue, and artifactual generation of angiotensin peptides, during processing.[81,82] The use of HPLC cannot, by itself, provide assurance that angiotensin peptide measurements are reliable, because HPLC cannot correct for artifacts created during collection and processing of the sample.

SUMMARY AND CONCLUSIONS

In addition to Ang II, the truncated angiotensin peptides Ang III, Ang IV, and Ang 1-7 are also bioactive. Understanding of the role of different bioactive angiotensin peptides requires their accurate measurement. Less precise methodology may result in overestimation of peptide levels. The circulating levels of Ang IV and Ang 1-7 are in the low picomolar range, and whether these levels are sufficient to exert biological effects remains uncertain. Nevertheless, the potential contribution of these peptides to the effects of ACE inhibition and ARB therapy cannot be ignored. This is an active area of investigation and we can expect further insight into the role of these peptides in the near future.

REFERENCES

1. Marchetti J, Helou CM, Chollet C et al. ACE and non-ACE mediated effect of angiotensin I on intracellular calcium mobilization in rat glomerular arterioles. Am J Physiol 2003; 284: H1933–H1941.
2. Alexiou T, Boon WM, Denton DA et al. Angiotensinogen and angiotensin converting enzyme gene copy number and angiotensin and bradykinin peptide levels in mice. J Hypertens 2005; 23: 945–54.
3. Dorer FE, Lentz KE, Kahn JR et al. A comparison of the substrate specificities of cathepsin D and pseudorenin. J Biol Chem 1978; 253: 3140–2.
4. Hackenthal E, Hackenthal R, Hilgenfeldt U. Isorenin, pseudorenin, cathepsin D and renin: a comparative enzymatic study of angiotensin-forming enzymes. Biochim Biophys Acta 1978; 522: 574–88.
5. Franze de Fernandez MT, Paladini AC, Delius AE. Isolation and identification of a pepsitensin. Biochem J 1965; 97: 540–6.
6. Haas E, Lewis LV, Scipione P et al. Angiotensin-producing enzyme I of serum: formation by immunization with renin. J Hypertens 1984; 2: 131–40.
7. Haas E, Lewis LV, Scipione P et al. Angiotensin-producing serum enzyme II. Formation by inhibitor removal and proenzyme activation. Hypertension 1985; 7: 938–47.
8. Husain A, Smeby RR, Wilk D et al. Biochemical and immunological properties of dog brain isorenin. Endocrinology 1984; 114: 2210–15.
9. Deboben A, Inagami T, Ganten D. Tissue renin. In: Genest J, Kuchel O, Hamet P, Cantin M (eds). Hypertension, 2 edn. New York: McGraw Hill, 1983, pp 194–209.
10. Haber E, Slater EE. Purification of renin. A review. Circ Res 1977; 40 (Suppl I): I-36–I-40.
11. Menard J, Galen F-X, Devaux C et al. Immunochemical differences between angiotensin I-forming enzymes in man. Clin Sci 1980; 59 (Suppl 6): 41s–44s.
12. Dzau VJ, Brenner A, Emmett N et al. Identification of renin and renin-like enzymes in rat brain by a renin-specific antibody. Clin Sci 1980; 59 (Suppl 6): 45s–47s.
13. Boucher R, Demassieux S, Garcia R et al. Tonin, angiotensin II system. A review. Circ Res 1977; 41 (Suppl II): II-26–II-29.
14. Tonnesen MG, Klempner MS, Austen KF et al. Identification of a human neutrophil angiotensin II generating protease as cathepsin G. J Clin Invest 1982; 69: 25–30.
15. Arakawa K, Yuki M, Ikeda M. Chemical identity of tryptensin with angiotensin. Biochem J 1980; 187: 647–53.
16. Maruta H, Arakawa K. Confirmation of direct angiotensin formation by kallikrein. Biochem J 1983; 213: 193–200.
17. Reilly CF, Tewksbury DA, Schechter NM et al. Rapid conversion of angiotensin I to angiotensin II by neutrophil and mast cell proteinases. J Biol Chem 1982; 257: 8619–22.
18. Urata H, Kinoshita A, Misono KS et al. Identification of a highly specific chymase as the major angiotensin II-forming enzyme in the human heart. J Biol Chem 1990; 265: 22348–57.
19. Okunishi H, Miyazaki M, Toda N. Evidence for a putatively new angiotensin II-generating enzyme in the vascular wall. J Hypertens 1984; 2: 277–84.
20. Padmanabhan N, Jardine AG, McGrath JC et al. Angiotensin-converting enzyme-independent contraction to angiotensin I in human resistance arteries. Circulation 1999; 99: 2914–20.
21. Campbell DJ. Metabolism of prorenin, renin, angiotensinogen, and the angiotensins by tissues. In: Robertson JIS, Nicholls MG (eds). The Renin-Angiotensin System. London: Gower Medical Publishing, 1993, pp 23.21–23.23.
22. Juillerat L, Nussberger J, Ménard J et al. Determinants of angiotensin II generation during converting enzyme inhibition. Hypertension 1990; 16: 564–72.
23. Gorski TP, Campbell DJ. Angiotensin-converting enzyme determination in plasma during therapy with converting enzyme inhibitor: two methods compared. Clin Chem 1991; 37: 1390–3.
24. Campbell DJ. The site of angiotensin production. J Hypertens 1985; 3: 199–207.
25. Campbell DJ, Bouhnik J, Menard J et al. Identity of angiotensinogen precursors of rat brain and liver. Nature 1984; 308: 206–8.

26. Campbell DJ, Habener JF. Angiotensinogen gene is expressed and differentially regulated in multiple tissues of the rat. J Clin Invest 1986; 78: 31–9.
27. Engeli S, Bohnke J, Gorzelniak K et al. Weight loss and the renin-angiotensin-aldosterone system. Hypertension 2005; 45: 356–62.
28. Campbell DJ, Kladis A, Skinner SL et al. Characterization of angiotensin peptides in plasma of anephric man. J Hypertens 1991; 9: 265–74.
29. Skinner SL, Cran EJ, Gibson R et al. Angiotensins I and II, active and inactive renin, renin substrate, renin activity, and angiotensinase in human liquor amnii and plasma. Am J Obstet Gynecol 1975; 121: 626–30.
30. Delbaere A, Englert Y, Bergmann PJM et al. Bioactive angiotensin (1–8) is the main component of angiotensin II immunoreactivity in human follicular fluid. Peptides 1996; 17: 1135–8.
31. Schuijt MP, Danser AH. Cardiac angiotensin II: an intracrine hormone? Am J Hypertens 2002; 15: 1109–16.
32. Campbell DJ. Bioactive angiotensin peptides other than angiotensin II. In: Epstein M, Brunner HR (eds). Angiotensin II Receptor Antagonists. Philadelphia, PA: Hanley and Belfus, 2001, pp 9–27.
33. Campbell DJ, Zeitz CJ, Esler MD et al. Evidence against a major role for angiotensin converting enzyme-related carboxypeptidase (ACE 2) in angiotensin peptide metabolism in the human coronary circulation. J Hypertens 2004; 22: 1971–6.
34. Campbell DJ, Duncan A-M, Kladis A. Angiotensin converting enzyme inhibition modifies angiotensin, but not kinin peptide levels in human atrial tissue. Hypertension 1999; 34: 171–5.
35. Zeitz CJ, Campbell DJ, Horowitz JD. Myocardial uptake and biochemical and hemodynamic effects of ACE inhibitors in humans. Hypertension 2003; 41: 482–7.
36. Dell'Italia LJ, Husain A. Dissecting the role of chymase in angiotensin II formation and heart and blood vessel diseases. Curr Opin Cardiol 2002; 17: 374–9.
37. van Esch JH, Tom B, Dive V et al. Selective angiotensin-converting enzyme C-domain inhibition is sufficient to prevent angiotensin I-induced vasoconstriction. Hypertension 2005; 45: 120–5.
38. Campbell DJ, Alexiou T, Xiao HD et al. Effect of reduced angiotensin-converting enzyme gene expression and angiotensin-converting enzyme inhibition on angiotensin and bradykinin peptide levels in mice. Hypertension 2004; 43: 854–9.
39. Akasu M, Urata H, Kinoshita A et al. Differences in tissue angiotensin II-forming pathways by species and organs in vitro. Hypertension 1998; 32: 514–20.
40. Campbell DJ, Kladis A, Duncan A-M. Effects of converting enzyme inhibitors on angiotensin and bradykinin peptides. Hypertension 1994; 23: 439–49.
41. Wei CC, Tian B, Perry G et al. Differential ANG II generation in plasma and tissue of mice with decreased expression of the ACE gene. Am J Physiol 2002; 282: H2254–H2258.
42. Dell'Italia LJ, Meng QC, Balcells E et al. Compartmentalization of angiotensin II generation in the dog heart – evidence for independent mechanisms in intravascular and interstitial spaces. J Clin Invest 1997; 100: 253–8.
43. Meng QC, Durand J, Chen Y-F et al. Simplified method for quantitation of angiotensin peptides in tissue. J Chromatogr Biomed Appl 1993; 614: 19–25.
44. Dell'Italia LJ, Balcells E, Meng QC et al. Volume-overload cardiac hypertrophy is unaffected by ACE inhibitor treatment in dogs. Am J Physiol 1997; 273: H961–H970.
45. Dell'Italia LJ, Meng QC, Balcells E et al. Increased ACE and chymase-like activity in cardiac tissue of dogs with chronic mitral regurgitation. Am J Physiol 1995; 269: H2065–H2073.
46. Schuijt MP, van Kats JP, de Zeeuw S et al. Cardiac interstitial fluid levels of angiotensin I and II in the pig. J Hypertens 1999; 17: 1885–91.
47. Kokkonen JO, Saarinen J, Kovanen PT. Regulation of local angiotensin II formation in the human heart in the presence of interstitial fluid – inhibition of chymase by protease inhibitors of interstitial fluid and of angiotensin-converting enzyme by Ang-(1-9) formed by heart carboxypeptidase A-like activity. Circulation 1997; 95: 1455–63.
48. Sukenaga Y, Kamoshita K, Takai S et al. Development of the chymase inhibitor as an anti-tissue-remodeling drug: myocardial infarction and some other possibilities. Jpn J Pharmacol 2002; 90: 218–22.
49. Nishimoto M, Takai S, Kim S et al. Significance of chymase-dependent angiotensin II-forming pathway in the development of vascular proliferation. Circulation 2001; 104: 1274–9.
50. Donoghue M, Hsieh F, Baronas E et al. A novel angiotensin-converting enzyme-related carboxypeptidase (ACE 2) converts angiotensin I to angiotensin 1-9. Circ Res 2000; 87: E1–9.
51. Tipnis SR, Hooper NM, Hyde R et al. A human homolog of angiotensin-converting enzyme. Cloning and functional expression as a captopril-insensitive carboxypeptidase. J Biol Chem 2000; 275: 33238–43.
52. Vickers C, Hales P, Kaushik V et al. Hydrolysis of biological peptides by human angiotensin-converting enzyme-related carboxypeptidase. J Biol Chem 2002; 277: 14838–43.
53. Harmer D, Gilbert M, Borman R et al. Quantitative mRNA expression profiling of ACE 2, a novel homologue of angiotensin converting enzyme. FEBS Lett 2002; 532: 107–10.
54. Hamming I, Timens W, Bulthuis ML et al. Tissue distribution of ACE 2 protein, the functional receptor for SARS coronavirus. A first step in understanding SARS pathogenesis. J Pathol 2004; 203: 631–7.
55. Li W, Moore MJ, Vasilieva N et al. Angiotensin-converting enzyme 2 is a functional receptor for the SARS coronavirus. Nature 2003; 426: 450–4.
56. Jaspard E, Wei L, Alhenc-Gelas F. Differences in the properties and enzymatic specificities of the two active sites of angiotensin I-converting enzyme (kininase II). Studies with bradykinin and other natural peptides. J Biol Chem 1993; 268: 9496–503.
57. Campbell DJ, Aggarwal A, Esler M et al. β-blockers, angiotensin II, and ACE inhibitors in patients with heart failure. Lancet 2001; 358: 1609–10.
58. McDonald JE, Padmanabhan N, Petrie MC et al. Vasoconstrictor effect of the angiotensin-converting enzyme-resistant, chymase-specific substrate [$Pro^{11}{}_{D}$-Ala^{12}] angiotensin I in human dorsal hand veins: in vivo demonstration of non-ACE production of angiotensin II in humans. Circulation 2001; 104: 1805–8.
59. Jorde UP, Ennezat PV, Lisker J et al. Maximally recommended doses of angiotensin-converting enzyme (ACE) inhibitors do not completely prevent ACE-mediated formation of angiotensin II in chronic heart failure. Circulation 2000; 101: 844–6.
60. Mooser V, Nussberger J, Juillerat L et al. Reactive hyperreninemia is a major determinant of plasma angiotensin II during ACE inhibition. J Cardiovasc Pharmacol 1990; 15: 276–82.
61. Yamamoto K, Chappell MC, Brosnihan KB et al. In vivo metabolism of angiotensin I by neutral endopeptidase (EC 3.4. 24.11) in spontaneously hypertensive rats. Hypertension 1992; 19: 692–6.
62. Duncan AM, James GM, Anastasopoulos F et al. Interaction between neutral endopeptidase and angiotensin converting enzyme inhibition in rats with myocardial infarction: effects on cardiac hypertrophy and angiotensin and bradykinin peptide levels. J Pharmacol Exp Ther 1999; 289: 295–303.

63. Chappell MC, Pirro NT, Sykes A et al. Metabolism of angiotension-(1-7) by angiotensin-converting enzyme. Hypertension 1998; 31: 362–7.
64. Yamada K, Iyer SN, Chappell MC et al. Converting enzyme determines plasma clearance of angiotensin-(1-7). Hypertension 1998; 32: 496–502.
65. Ménard J, Campbell DJ, Azizi M et al. Synergistic effects of ACE inhibition and Ang II antagonism on blood pressure, cardiac weight, and renin in spontaneously hypertensive rats. Circulation 1997; 96: 3072–8.
66. Richards AM, Wittert GA, Espiner EA et al. Effect of inhibition of endopeptidase 24.11 on responses to angiotensin II in human volunteers. Circ Res 1992; 71: 1501–7.
67. Li P, Chappell MC, Ferrario CM et al. Angiotensin-(1-7) augments bradykinin-induced vasodilation by competing with ACE and releasing nitric oxide. Hypertension 1997; 29: 394–400.
68. Deddish PA, Marcic B, Jackman HL et al. N-domain-specific substrate and C-domain inhibitors of angiotensin-converting enzyme angiotensin-(1-7) and Keto-ACE. Hypertension 1998; 31: 912–17.
69. Campbell DJ, Krum H, Esler MD. Losartan increases bradykinin levels in hypertensive humans. Circulation 2005; 111: 315–20.
70. Volpe M, Musumeci B, De Paolis P et al. Angiotensin II AT2 receptor subtype: an uprising frontier in cardiovascular disease? J Hypertens 2003; 21: 1429–43.
71. Carey RM. Update on the role of the AT2 receptor. Curr Opin Nephrol Hypertens 2005; 14: 67–71.
72. Campbell DJ, Kladis A, Valentijn AJ. Effects of losartan on angiotensin and bradykinin peptides, and angiotensin converting enzyme. J Cardiovasc Pharmacol 1995; 26: 233–40.
73. Campbell DJ, Lawrence AC, Towrie A et al. Differential regulation of angiotensin peptide levels in plasma and kidney of the rat. Hypertension 1991; 18: 763–73.
74. Campbell DJ. Endogenous angiotensin II levels and the mechanism of action of angiotensin-converting enzyme inhibitors and angiotensin receptor type 1 antagonists. Clin Exp Pharmacol Physiol 1996; Suppl 3: S125–S131.
75. Forclaz A, Maillard M, Nussberger J et al. Angiotensin II receptor blockade. Is there truly a benefit of adding an ACE inhibitor? Hypertension 2003; 41: 31–6.
76. Azizi M, Menard J. Combined blockade of the renin-angiotensin system with angiotensin-converting enzyme inhibitors and angiotensin II type 1 receptor antagonists. Circulation 2004; 109: 2492–9.
77. Mazzolai L, Maillard M, Rossat J et al. Angiotensin II receptor blockade in normotensive subjects: a direct comparison of three AT1 receptor antagonists. Hypertension 1999; 33: 850–5.
78. Nussberger J, Brunner DB, Waeber B et al. Specific measurement of angiotensin metabolites and in vitro generated angiotensin II in plasma. Hypertension 1986; 8: 476–82.
79. Campbell DJ, Lawrence AC, Kladis A et al. Strategies for measurement of angiotensin and bradykinin peptides and their metabolites in central nervous system and other tissues. In: Smith AI (ed). Methods in Neurosciences, Vol 23: Peptidases and Neuropeptide Processing. Orlando: Academic Press, 1995, pp 328–43.
80. Chappell MC, Brosnihan KB, Diz DI et al. Identification of angiotensin-(1-7) in rat brain. Evidence for differential processing of angiotensin peptides. J Biol Chem 1989; 264: 16518–23.
81. Lawrence AC, Clarke IJ, Campbell DJ. Angiotensin peptides in brain and pituitary of rat and sheep. J Neuroendocrinol 1992; 4: 237–44.
82. Senanayake PD, Moriguchi A, Kumagai H et al. Increased expression of angiotensin peptides in the brain of transgenic hypertensive rats. Peptides 1994; 15: 919–26.

7

(Pro)renin receptors: their functional properties

Geneviève Nguyen, AH Jan Danser, Celine A Burckle, Michael Bader and Dominik N Muller

INTRODUCTION

In the last decade a variety of studies have shown that there are two separate renin-angiotensin systems (RAS), the classical RAS that plays a key role in the regulation of blood pressure and fluid and salt balance and the tissue RAS or 'local angiotensin (Ang) II generating system'. The components are identical except for the cell surface (pro)renin receptors that are probably only involved in the tissue RAS. These receptors may play a crucial role in determining (pro)renin catalytic activity, as well as in their contribution to (pro)renin-specific intracellular signaling and clearance.

Three (pro)renin receptors have been characterized to date (Figure 7.1).[1–4] One receptor specific for renin and prorenin, originally described on human mesangial cells, was cloned from a human kidney library. The ubiquitously present mannose-6-phosphate receptor (M6P-R) was shown to play a role in renin and prorenin binding, internalization, and degradation in neonatal rat cardiomyocytes, whereas in adult rat cardiomyocytes, a receptor distinct from the M6P-R was reported to be responsible for binding and internalizing unglycosylated renin and prorenin.

THE SPECIFIC RECEPTOR OF RENIN AND PRORENIN

A functional receptor of renin was first identified on human mesangial cells in culture. Renin binding was independent of the active site of renin and induced an increase of [^{3}H]thymidine incorporation and an increase of plasminogen activator inhibitor-1 synthesis. Renin bound to the receptor was not internalized or degraded.[5]

The receptor is a 350 amino acid protein with a single transmembrane domain. It also binds prorenin, the inactive precursor of renin. Interestingly, the receptor acts as a (pro)renin cofactor on the cell surface by enhancing renin catalytic activity and by unmasking catalytic activity of receptor-bound prorenin. The binding of (pro)renin to the receptor triggers intracellular signaling via the MAP kinases ERK1/2 pathway.

Immunofluorescence studies performed on frozen tissues have localized the receptor in glomerular mesangial cells and in vascular smooth muscle cells of renal cortical arteries and coronary arteries.[1] However, immunohistochemical studies performed on paraffin-embedded sections showed that the receptor can also be found in distal and collecting tubular cells of the kidney, and these results were confirmed by in situ hybridization (J-M Gasc and G Nguyen, unpublished data).

Potential significance of this functional receptor

The receptor provides a functional role for prorenin

In plasma, prorenin represents 70–90% of total circulating renin in normal subjects and up to 95% in diabetic patients.[6–9] Since the receptor binds prorenin and unmasks prorenin catalytic activity, prorenin binding to the receptor provides a mechanism by which prorenin may exert pathological effects. These effects may be due either to cell activation specific to prorenin–receptor interaction or to enhanced Ang II generation.[10,11] Indeed, experimental data suggest that the receptor may contribute to the pathogenic role of prorenin in diabetic nephropathy. Suzuki et al. have demonstrated the existence of a non-proteolytic

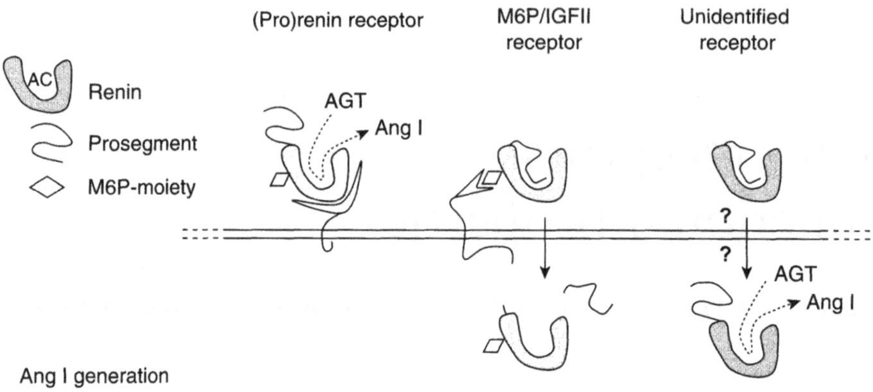

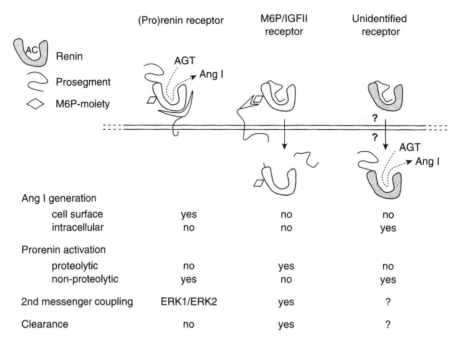

	(Pro)renin receptor	M6P/IGFII receptor	Unidentified receptor
Ang I generation			
cell surface	yes	no	no
intracellular	no	no	yes
Prorenin activation			
proteolytic	no	yes	no
non-proteolytic	yes	no	yes
2nd messenger coupling	ERK1/ERK2	yes	?
Clearance	no	yes	?

Figure 7.1 Current status of (pro)renin receptors, prorenin internalization and prorenin-induced effects. The (pro)renin receptor cloned by Nguyen et al.[1] facilitates cell surface angiotensin (Ang) generation from angiotensinogen (AGT), mannose 6-phosphate/insulin-like growth factor II (M6P/IGFII) receptor-induced internalization of M6P-containing prorenin results in prorenin clearance,[2,3] and an unknown mechanism allows non-glycosylated (i.e. non-M6P-containing) prorenin to internalize and to subsequently generate Ang I intracellularly.[4] AC, active center

activation mechanism of prorenin, due to a conformational change of the molecule when an antibody was bound to the 'handle' region of the prosegment.[12] In line with these findings, Ichihara et al.[13] have hypothesized that such non-proteolytic activation of prorenin could occur in vivo, especially in situations with high prorenin concentrations, like in diabetes. These authors showed that the infusion of a decoy peptide against the handle region of prorenin could completely prevent diabetic nephropathy assessed on morphological and functional data and that the improvement was associated with a normalization of the kidney content of Ang II. Since in vivo, no antibody to the handle region exists, they suggested that a renin receptor could account for non-proteolytic prorenin activation in the kidney.[13] If the pathogenic role of the receptor-activated prorenin in diabetic nephropathy can be confirmed, for example by using renin receptor-deficient animals, then these results would have major therapeutic consequences, implying that a prorenin and renin active site inhibitor or a compound able to inhibit both (pro)renin binding and activity would be beneficial in diabetic nephropathy.

There are common characteristics between diabetic retinopathy and nephropathy. Indeed, prorenin is abundant in the in the vitreous fluid[14,15] and its levels are increased in diabetic proliferative retinopathy.[16] Furthermore, both an ACE inhibitor and an Ang II type 1 receptor antagonist effectively prevent proliferative retinopathy.[17] It is therefore tempting to speculate that the interruption of prorenin activation or the inhibition of receptor-bound prorenin catalytic activity would also be effective in preventing diabetic retinopathy.

Signaling of the receptor via ERK1/2 activation may be important for cell function in the central nervous system and for cell metabolism

In the central nervous system (CNS), the role of the RAS includes the control of cell growth and death, of neuroendocrine regulation, of cognitive properties, in addition to its role as modulator of cardiovascular functions, like autonomic activity, salt intake and drinking.[18,19] We have recently found a specific role for the renin receptor in cognitive functions and brain development. A mutation in the renin receptor gene (ATP6AP2) was described in patients with X-linked mental retardation and epilepsy in the absence of cardiovascular and renal dysfunction. This mutation resulted in inefficient inclusion of exon 4 in 50% of renin receptor mRNA and functional studies showed that, although the mutated receptor could bind renin and increase renin catalytic activity as described for wild-type receptor, renin binding did not activate the MAP kinases ERK1/2.[20] The reason why the CNS is more sensitive to the lack of renin receptor is unclear. Our findings suggest that activation of the ERK1/2 system via the renin receptor system is important in brain development and to maintain normal neurological functions. Its impairment can apparently not be be compensated by other extracellular stimuli as might be the case for cardiac, vascular, and renal tissues. Furthermore, it is interesting to note that the renin receptor interaction that normally leads to ERK1/2 activation was recently reported to be essential for proliferation and survival of human glial cells.[21] The renin receptor has also been described in association with the vacuolar proton ATPase.[22] *In silico* research showed that the protein is highly homologous in human, mouse and rat, as well as in chicken, fish, xenopus and *C. elegans*.[23] Thus the renin receptor is a protein conserved among species. Taken together, the data indicate that the receptor has two types of function, one related to the RAS and one independent of the RAS and possibly related to the vacuolar proton ATPase.

THE MANNOSE-6-PHOSPHATE RECEPTOR

The mannose-6-phosphate receptor (M6P-R), which is also known as the insulin-like growth factor II receptor, is a ubiquitously present receptor that has been shown to bind renin and prorenin on neonatal rat cardiomyocytes[2,24,25] and human endothelial cells.[3,26] The M6P-R exclusively binds M6P-containing renin and prorenin. The binding of (pro)renin triggers the internalization of the M6P-R/(pro)renin complex, the proteolytic activation of prorenin and the subsequent degradation of renin. Most likely therefore, this receptor is a clearance receptor for (pro)renin. Co-incubation of prorenin and angiotensinogen with cardiomyocytes resulted in an increase of [^{3}H]thymidine incorporation.[27] This effect was not due to the binding of prorenin to the M6P-R, but to the intrinsic activity of prorenin, responsible for the generation of Ang I and, subsequently, Ang II on the cell surface. No intracellular Ang II was detected. A very interesting fact is that [^{3}H]thymidine incorporation provoked by 1 nM Ang II generated during co-incubation of prorenin plus angiotensinogen with cardiomyocytes could be reproduced only by the addition of a 100-fold higher concentration of exogenous Ang II (100 nM). This observation strongly suggests that formation of Ang II on the cell surface, in close vicinity of AT_1 receptors, is more efficient than in solution because it allows immediate binding to AT_1 receptors. Such cell surface angiotensin generation might in fact involve the renin receptor.

A RECEPTOR FOR UNGLYCOSYLATED (PRO)RENIN ON ADULT CARDIOMYOCYTES

A second (pro)renin receptor was described on adult rat cardiomyocytes, with properties different from the M6P-R in that it binds unglycosylated prorenin only, and that internalization of mouse *ren-2^d* (but not rat) prorenin is associated with intracellular angiotensin generation.

Rats transgenic for the mouse *ren-2^d* renin gene (coding for unglycosylated prorenin) develop extremely severe hypertension and cardiac damage.[28,29] Using this model, with an inducible expression of *ren-2^d* renin gene restricted to the liver, Peters et al. have shown that the increased synthesis of *ren-2^d* renin was associated with high levels of *ren-2^d* (pro)renin in plasma and within cardiac cells.[4] In addition, unglycosylated (pro)renin was bound in vitro by rat cardiomyocytes and internalized. Internalization was associated with an increased intrinsic activity of prorenin and with intracellular Ang I and Ang II generation. To date, this (pro)renin binding protein has not been identified, but these results revive the controversy as to the existence of an intracrine RAS, and the mitogenic effect of intracellular Ang II.[30–33]

CONCLUSION

In summary, two major facts have emerged from the characterization of the three receptors: (i) the importance of the cell surface generation of Ang II, which increases the efficiency of Ang II-AT_1 receptor binding and AT_1 receptor activation, and (ii) the demonstration of a functional role for prorenin.

The reasons for the contradictory results of (pro)-renin binding and effects in rat neonatal versus adult cardiomyocytes and human mesangial cells are still unclear. Nonetheless, the existence of receptors with different functions and possessing different characteristics may not be surprising, considering the heterogeneity in glycosylation and phosphomannosylation of circulating (pro)renin.[34] This heterogeneity also determines the in vivo half-life of (pro)renin.[35–37]

Overall, the renin receptors may have a high potential impact because the RAS and the renin receptor are not restricted to the cardiovascular field. Activation of the tissue RAS is also involved in many physiological and pathological processes such as tissue growth and remodeling,[38] organ development,[39] inflammation and cardiac hypertrophy,[40] vascular hypertrophy, obesity,[41] and learning and memory.[42] Further studies are needed to elucidate the exact physiological role of the different renin receptors.

REFERENCES

1. Nguyen G, Delarue F, Burcklé C et al. Pivotal role of the renin/prorenin receptor in angiotensin II production and cellular responses to renin. J Clin Invest 2002; 109: 1417–27.
2. Saris JJ, Derkx FHM, de Bruin RJA et al. High-affinity prorenin binding to cardiac man-6-P/IGF-II receptors precedes proteolytic activation to renin. Am J Physiol 2001; 280: H1706-H1715.
3. van den Eijnden MMED, Saris JJ, de Bruin RJA et al. Prorenin accumulation and activation in human endothelial cells. Importance of the mannose-6-phosphate receptors. Arterioscler Thromb Vasc Biol 2001; 21: 911–16.
4. Peters J, Farrenkopf R, Clausmeyer S et al. Functional significance of prorenin internalization in the rat heart. Circ Res 2002; 90: 1135–41.
5. Nguyen G, Delarue F, Berrou J et al. Specific receptor binding of renin on human mesangial cells in culture increases plasminogen activator inhibitor-1 antigen. Kidney Int 1996; 50: 1897–903.
6. Luetscher JA, Kraemer FB, Wilson DM, Schwarz HC, Bryer-Ash M. Increased plasma inactive renin in diabetes mellitus a marker of microvascular complications. N Engl J Med 1985; 312: 1412–17.
7. Price DA, Porter LE, Gordon M et al. The paradox of the low-renin state in diabetic nephropathy. J Am Soc Nephrol 1999; 10: 2382–91.
8. Deinum J, Ronn B, Mathiesen E, Derkx FHM, Hop WC, Schalekamp MADH. Increase in serum prorenin precedes onset of microalbuminuria in patients with insulin-dependent diabetes mellitus. Diabetologia 1999; 42: 1006–10.
9. Valabhji J, Donovan J, Kyd PA, Schachter M, Elkeles RS.The relationship between active renin concentration and plasma renin activity in Type 1 diabetes. Diabetic Med 2001; 18: 451–8.
10. Véniant M, Ménard J, Bruneval P et al. Vascular damage without hypertension in transgenic rats expressing prorenin exclusively in the liver. J Clin Invest 1996; 98: 1966–70.
11. Methot D, Silversides DW, Reudelhuber TL. In vivo enzymatic assay reveals catalytic activity of the human renin precursor in tissues. Circ Res 1999; 84: 1067–72.
12. Suzuki F, Hayakawa M, Nakagawa T et al. Human prorenin has 'gate and handle' regions for its non-proteolytic activation. J Biol Chem 2003; 278: 22217–22.
13. Ichihara A, Hayashi M, Kaneshiro Y et al. Inhibition of diabetic nephropathy by a decoy peptide corresponding to the 'handle' region for nonproteolytic activation of prorenin. J Clin Invest 2004; 114: 1128–35.
14. Deinum J, Derkx FHM, Danser AHJ, Schalekamp MADH. Identification and quantification of renin and prorenin in the bovine eye. Endocrinology 1990; 126: 1673–82.
15. Wagner J, Danser AHJ, Derkx FHM et al. Demonstration of renin mRNA, angiotensinogen mRNA, and angiotensin converting enzyme mRNA expression in the human eye: evidence for an intraocular renin-angiotensin system. Br J Ophthalmol 1996; 80: 159–63.
16. Danser AHJ, van den Dorpel MA, Deinum J et al. Renin, prorenin, and immunoreactive renin in vitreous fluid from eyes with and without diabetic retinopathy. J Clin Endocrinol Metab 1989; 68: 160–7.
17. Moravski CJ, Kelly DJ, Cooper ME et al. Retinal neovascularization is prevented by blockade of the renin-angiotensin system. Hypertension 2000; 36: 1099–104.
18. McKinley MJ, Albiston AL, Allen AM et al. The brain renin-angiotensin system: location and physiological roles. Int J Biochem Cell Biol 2003; 35: 901–18.
19. Bader M, Ganten D. It's renin in the brain: transgenic animals elucidate the brain renin angiotensin system. Circ Res 2002; 90: 8–10.
20. Ramser J, Abidi FE, Burckle CA et al. A unique exonic splice enhancer mutation in a family with X-linked mental retardation and epilepsy points to a novel role of the renin receptor. Hum Mol Genet 2005; 14: 1019–27.
21. Juillerat-Jeanneret L, Celerier J, Chapuis BC et al. Renin and angiotensinogen expression and functions in growth and apoptosis of human glioblastoma. Br J Cancer 2004; 90: 1059–68.
22. Ludwig J, Kersher S, Brandt U et al. Identification and characterization of a novel 9.2 kDa membrane sector-associated protein of vacuolar proton ATPase from chromaffin granules. J Biol Chem 1998; 273: 10939–47.
23. L'Huillier N, Sharp MGF, Dunbar DR, Mullins JJ. On the relationship between the renin receptor and the vacuolar proton ATPase membrane sector associated protein (M8-9). Mol Mech Hypertens 2005; in press.
24. van Kesteren CAM, Danser AHJ, Derkx FHM et al. Mannose-6-phosphate receptor mediated internalization and activation of prorenin by cardiac cells. Hypertension 1997; 30: 1389–96.
25. Saris JJ, Derkx FHM, Lamers JMJ et al. Cardiomyocytes bind and activate native human prorenin. Role of soluble mannose-6-phoshate receptor. Hypertension 2001; 37: 710–15.
26. Admiraal PJJ, van Kesteren CAM, Danser AHJ et al. Uptake and proteolytic activation of prorenin by cultured human endothelial cells. J Hypertens 1999; 17: 621–9.
27. Saris JJ, van den Eijnden MMED, Lamers JMJ et al. Prorenin-induced myocyte proliferation. No role for intracellular angiotensin II. Hypertension 2002; 39: 573–7.
28. Mullins JJ, Peters J, Ganten D. Fulminant hypertension in transgenic rats harbouring the mouse ren-2^d gene. Nature 1990; 344: 541–4.
29. Peters J, Munter K, Bader M, Hackenthal E, Mullins JJ, Ganten D. Increased adrenal renin in transgenic hypertensive rats, TGR(mREN2)27, and its regulation by cAMP, angiotensin II, and calcium. J Clin Invest 1993; 91: 742–7.
30. Sadoshima J, Xy Y, Slayter HS, Izumo S. Autocrine release of angiotensin II mediates stretch-induced hypertrophy of cardiac myocytes in vitro. Cell 1993; 75: 977–84.
31. De Mello WC, Danser AHJ. Angiotensin II and the heart. On the intracrine renin-angiotensin system. Hypertension 2000; 35: 1183–8.

32. Cook JL, Zhang Z, Re RN. In vitro evidence for intracellular site of angiotensin action. Circ Res 2001; 89: 1138–46.
33. Schuijt MP, Danser AHJ. Cardiac angiotensin II: an intracrine hormone? Am J Hypertens 2002; 15: 1109–16.
34. Kim S, Hososi M, Hiruma M et al. Heterogeneity in glycosylation of circulating active and inactive renin. Clin Exp Hypertens 1988; A10: 1203–11.
35. Kim S, Hiruma M, Ikemoto F, Yamamoto K. Importance of glycosylation for hepatic clearance of renal renin. Am J Physiol 1988; 255: E642–E651.
36. Danser AHJ, Admiraal PJJ, Derkx FHM et al. Changes in plasma renin and angiotensin run parallel after nephrectomy. J Hypertens 1993; 11 (Suppl 5): S238–S239.
37. Stubbs AJ, Skinner SL. Lectin chromatography of extrarenal renin protein in human plasma and tissues: potential endocrine function via the renin receptor. J Renin Angiotensin Aldosterone Syst 2004; 5: 189–96.
38. Tamura T, Said S, Harris J et al. Reverse modeling of cardiac myocyte hypertrophy in hypertension and failure by targeting of the renin-angiotensin system. Circulation 2000; 102: 253–9.
39. Guron G, Friberg P. An intact renin-angiotensin system is a prerequisite for renal development. J Hypertens 2000; 18: 123–37.
40. Schieffer B, Schieffer E, Hilfiker-Kleiner D et al. Expression of angiotensin II and interleukin 6 in human coronary atherosclerotic plaques. Potential implications for inflammation and plaque instability. Circulation 2000; 101: 1372–8.
41. Engeli S, Negrel R, Sharma AM. Physiology and pathophysiology of the adipose tissue renin-angiotensin system. Hypertension 2000; 35: 1270–7.
42. Wright JW, Harding JW. The brain angiotensin system and extracellular matrix molecules in neural plasticity, learning, and memory. Prog Neurobiol 2004; 72: 263–93.

8

Brain renin-angiotensin system: focus on transgenic animal models

Natalia Alenina, Ovidiu Baltatu and Michael Bader

INTRODUCTION

Due to the presence of the blood-brain barrier circulating angiotensin (Ang) II has no access to most brain areas.[1–3] Thus, the brain renin-angiotensin system (RAS) is autonomous concerning the generation and action of Ang peptides in contrast to most other tissue-specific RASs. Nevertheless, circulating Ang II transmits effects inside the brain through areas lacking the blood-brain barrier.[4] The brain RAS is involved in the modulation of cardiovascular and fluid–electrolyte homeostasis,[4] by modulating the activity of the autonomic nervous system,[5–7] the hypothalamic-pituitary axis, the release of vasopressin,[8] and baroreflex sensitivity[9] and stimulating thirst.[10,11] Moreover, the local RAS influences higher brain functions, such as memory, cognition, stress, and addiction.[12,13]

RAS COMPONENTS IN THE BRAIN

Angiotensinogen

Essential for a functional brain RAS is the presence of the only known precursor for Ang peptides, angiotensinogen (AOGEN), in the brain.[14–16] It is found throughout the brain with highest levels in areas of homeostatic control such as hypothalamus and brain stem. Astrocytes represent the main cell type synthesizing AOGEN.[17]

Angiotensin-generating enzymes

The classical enzymes responsible for the conversion of AOGEN into Ang peptides, renin and angiotensin converting enzyme (ACE), have both been located in the brain. However, despite the fact that there is high renin activity and immunoreactivity in several brain regions including hypothalamus and in pituitary and pineal glands, renin mRNA levels are very low or under the limit of detection.[4] On the other hand, when green fluorescent protein (GFP) is expressed under the control of the mouse renin promoter in transgenic mice, the marker gene is expressed in neurons of several brain regions including some with known function in cardiovascular control.[18] Furthermore, a human renin gene overexpressed under its own transcriptional control elements in transgenic mice leads to easily detectable human renin in different brain regions.[19,20] However, not only the classical secreted version of the protein is generated but even predominantly an intracellular renin isoform, called renin A, which has an unknown function and probably accumulates in mitochondria.[21–23] Interestingly, in this transgenic model human renin protein is mostly found in astrocytes. Thus, the role of renin in the brain is not yet completely solved. In particular, it remains to be clarified which isoform is generated in which cell type and how much of Ang peptide generation is dependent on renin in the brain.

ACE activity and its mRNA are high in different brain areas and in pituitary and pineal glands.[24–26] Biochemical experiments have indicated that enzymes other than renin and ACE can produce Ang II either from AOGEN or from Ang I. These include tonin, cathepsin G, tissue plasminogen activator, and chymase, all of which have been demonstrated in the brain.[27] However, the in vivo relevance of these enzymes for Ang peptide generation in the brain needs to be clarified.

Angiotensin metabolites

Besides Ang I and Ang II there are several other biologically active Ang peptides particularly but not exclusively in the brain. These include Ang 2-8 or Ang III[28] and Ang 3-8 or Ang IV,[29] both produced from Ang II by sequential aminopeptidase digestions, and Ang 1-7 generated from Ang I and Ang II by ACE 2.[4,30,31]

Angiotensin receptors

The distribution of Ang II receptors in the central nervous system has been comprehensively reviewed.[4,32,33] Most of the known effects of Ang II are attributed to the AT_1 receptor. Rodents have two AT_1 subtypes: AT_{1A} localized in brain areas involved in the control of blood pressure and fluid homeostasis, such as hypothalamus, area postrema, and medulla, and AT_{1B} predominating in glandular tissues, such as anterior pituitary, pineal and adrenal gland. The AT_2 receptor was found in very few and – depending on the species – different brain regions and in most cases causes opposite effects to that of the AT_1. Specific receptors for Ang IV and Ang 1-7 have been proposed. The Ang IV receptor (AT_4) may be the enzyme insulin-regulated membrane aminopeptidase (IRAP)[34] and Ang 1-7 is the ligand for the G protein-coupled receptor Mas,[35] which is predominantly expressed in the brain.[36]

TRANSGENIC ANIMAL MODELS FOR THE BRAIN RAS

Transgenic technology allows the systematic manipulation of a specific gene and has considerably furthered our understanding of the physiology and pathophysiology of tissue RAS and the brain RAS in particular.[31] In the following we will first delineate the technology used to develop transgenic and knockout animal models and then we will list and describe all animal models generated so far with targeted alterations in the brain RAS (Tables 8.1 and 8.2).

Transgenic technology

A transgenic animal is one whose genotype was modified by introduction of a foreign DNA (called

Table 8.1 Transgenic animal models relevant for the brain RAS

Model	*Species*	*Transgene*	*Promoter*	*Expressing tissue*	*Reference*
TGR(mREN2)27	Rat	Mouse renin *Ren-2*	Mouse renin *Ren-2*	Ubiquitous	
TGR(ASrAOGEN)	Rat	Mouse AOGEN antisense	GFAP	Astrocytes; leads to up to 90% decrease in AOGEN protein levels in the brain	74
Pac160 hRen	Mouse	Human renin	Human renin	Juxtaglomerular cells of kidney	79
hAGT	Mouse	Human AOGEN	1.2 kb of human AOGEN	Ubiquitous	115
hRen	Mouse	Human renin	900 bp of human renin	Ubiquitous	78
GFAP-hREN	Mouse	Human renin	GFAP	Astrocytes	80
SYN-hREN	Mouse	Human renin	Synapsin-1	Neurons	80
SYN-hAGT	Mouse	Human AOGEN	Synapsin-1	Neurons	116
GFAP-hAGT	Mouse	Human AOGEN	GFAP	Astrocytes	77
GFAP-Ang II	Mouse	Chimeric cDNA: hRen-IgG2b-furin cleavage site – Ang II	GFAP	Astrocytes	81
GFAP-Ang IV	Mouse	Chimeric cDNA: hRen-IgG2b-furin cleavage site – Ang IV	GFAP	Astrocytes	82
NSE-AT_{1A}	Mouse	Rat AT_{1A}	NSE	Neurons	83

Table 8.2 Knockout mice for the RAS

Gene	*Reference*
Mouse renin *Ren-1c*	109, 110
Mouse renin *Ren-1d*	120
Mouse renin *Ren-2*	121
AOGEN	104–106
ACE	107, 108
AT_{1A}	117
AT_{1B}	87
AT_2	118, 119
Mas	122

transgene), which is transmitted through the germ line. The term transgenic also refers to knockout animals, which carry a targeted gene deletion or other modifications in their genome.

Three different methodologies are currently used to generate transgenic animals:

1. Microinjection of DNA into the pronucleus of a fertilized oocyte.
2. Retrovirus-mediated gene transfer.
3. Gene targeting in embryonic stem cells.

Microinjection technique

Pronucleus microinjection of DNA (also traditionally called 'transgenic technology') was first successfully used in mice more than 20 years ago[37–41] and afterwards was extended to various other mammalian species such as rats, rabbits, sheep, cattle, pigs, and goats.[42–46]

To create transgenic animals, the exogenous DNA is injected directly into the male pronucleus of a fertilized egg (Figure 8.1B). The microinjected embryos are transplanted into the oviduct of a pseudopregnant female in which they develop to term (Figure 8.1C) (for detailed protocols see elsewhere[47,48]). The newborns, that have integrated the transgene into their genome (about 5–30% in rats and mice) are called founders and thereafter are mated with wild-type animals to establish transgenic lines (Figure 8.1D).

The mechanism of transgene integration is not fully understood. It includes concatemerization of the injected fragment (therefore usually multiple copies of the transgene are incorporated into a single site) and subsequent integration of concatemers into the double-stranded chromosomal breaks which are naturally occurring during replication in the S-phase of the cell cycle.[49] It is preferable if the integration occurs during the first zygotic replication, which takes place several hours after fertilization, before the male and female pronucleus are fused, since in this case all cells of the embryo, including the germ line, will contain the transgene. However, the injected DNA is quite stable and integration may occur also after the first or even the second cleavage of the embryo.[50] This late integration leads to mosaicism of the resulting founder, and therefore usually only about 70% of transgenic founders will transmit the transgene through the germ line.[51,52]

Mostly, the microinjection technique is applied either to overexpress the gene of interest (ubiquitously or in a time- or tissue-specific pattern), or to study transcription regulatory elements with a reporter gene, which can easily be visualized and quantitatively assessed (like luciferase, β-galactosidase (lacZ), GFP, or chloramphenicol acetyltransferase (CAT)).

In both cases, basic constructs for the microinjection should contain the following (Figure 8.1A).

1. The cDNA of the gene of interest or of a reporter gene, which may be altered by the addition of sequences encoding signaling peptides for subcellular localization, protease cleavage sites or a tag for detection or purification by specific antibodies.
2. A promoter 5′ of the cDNA. Depending on the purpose the promoter can be ubiquitously active (e.g. for the housekeeping genes β-actin and ubiquitin or viruses such as cytomegalovirus (CMV) and simian virus 40 (SV40)) or active in a time- and tissue-specific manner (e.g. promoter-enhancers such as the ones for neuron-specific enolase (NSE), synapsin-I (SYN), or glial fibrillary acidic protein (GFAP), which have been successfully used for brain-specific transgene expression).
3. A polyadenylation site 3′ of the cDNA for the accurate transcription termination – those from SV40 or the bovine growth hormone gene (BGH) are most commonly used.
4. Since the involvement of the splicing machinery in cotranscriptional processing of mRNA affects the efficiency of gene expression (recently reviewed elsewhere[53,54]), it is preferable to have an intron with donor and acceptor splicing sites in the construct.[55] In a lot of cases, the first untranslated exon of the gene, from which the promoter was taken, is an excellent candidate for this. The intron should not be 3′ of the cDNA, otherwise the resulting mRNA may be subject to nonsense-mediated mRNA decay.[56]

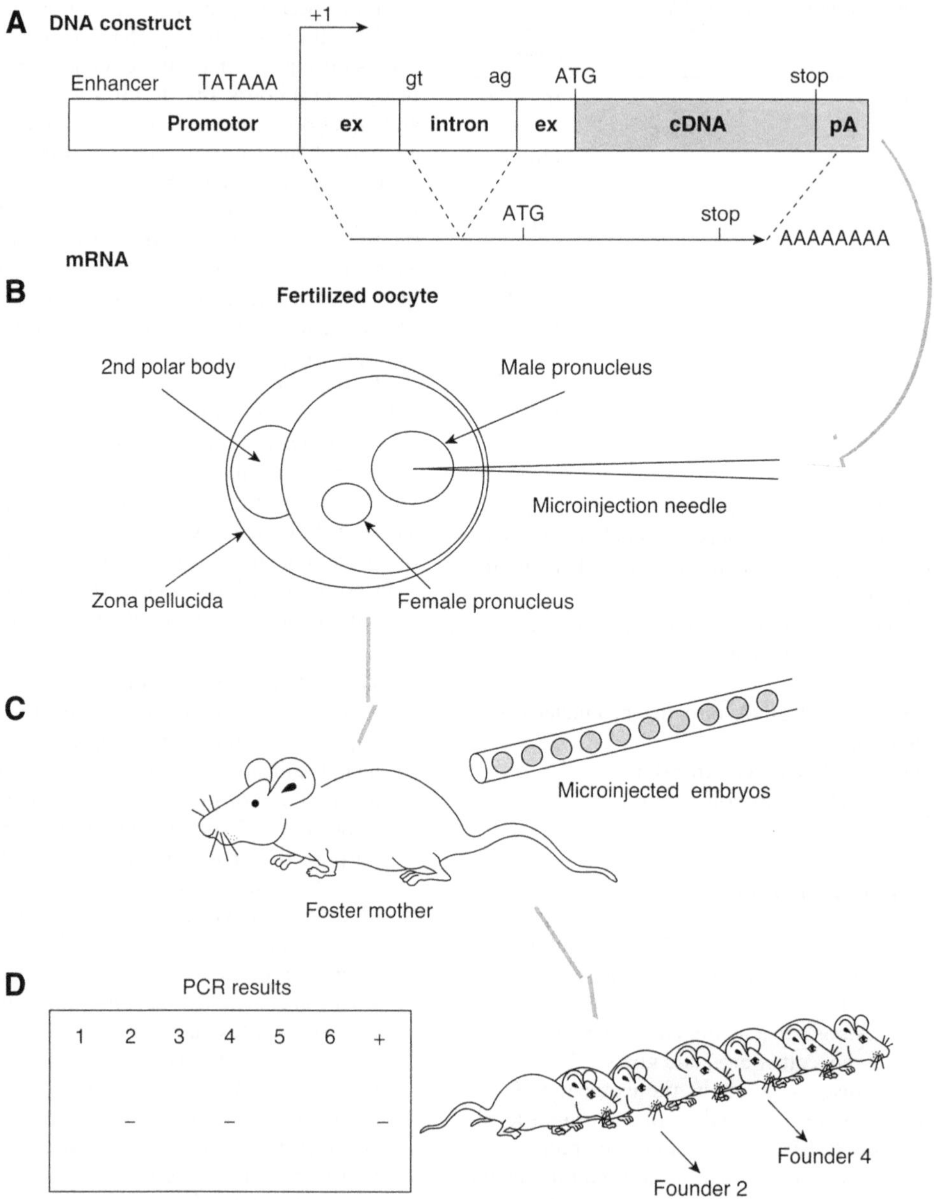

Figure 8.1 Generation of transgenic mice by microinjection. (A) A typical DNA construct consists of: a promoter (contains the basal promoter with the TATA-box and other regulatory elements, such as tissue-specific enhancers), +1 = transcriptional start site; an intron with splice donor (gt) and splice acceptor (ag) sites, surrounded by exon (ex) sequences; a cDNA for the gene of interest, ATG = start codon, stop = stop codon; a polyadenylation site (pA). The line 'mRNA' shows the resulting mRNA after transcription and processing of the DNA construct. (B) Fertilized eggs are harvested from superovulated females. Microinjection is performed early after fertilization, when the paternal and maternal genomes are still separated in two pronuclei. Several copies of the DNA construct are microinjected into the male pronucleus with a fine glass needle. (C) Microinjected embryos are transferred into the oviduct of a foster mother in which the embryos develop to term. (D) The offspring are analyzed by PCR; positive animals are called founders and give rise to a new transgenic line (lines 1–6, offspring, '+', positive PCR control)

However, the expression of the transgene does not only depend on the copy number and on the activity of the promoter. As the insertion of the transgene occurs at random, the integration site is not predictable and the transgene may come under the control of the genetic neighborhood, an effect known as positional variegation.[57] In this case, even tissue-specific promoters may lead to ectopic expression of the transgene because of integration into an active region of the chromatin. On the other hand, a high copy number of the transgene may lead to heterochromatization of the transgene locus and its transcriptional repression. Therefore, the expression level of the transgene should be always accurately proven before experiments are performed with newly established animal models. Furthermore, the generation of more than one founder and consequently more than one line of mice for each transgene is desirable. Only similar changes in phenotype of different transgenic lines can be attributed to transgene expression.

Sometimes the expression of the injected cassette in early embryos may lead to embryonic lethality due to toxic effects of the transgene expression. In this case, inducible promoters or the recently developed Cre-loxP system – a recombination system of the bacteriophage P1, which allows the tissue-specific or developmental stage-dependent switch-on of a transgene[58] – can be used.

Despite all these limitations, microinjection is still the most frequently used method to generate transgenic models in different mammalian species for the overexpression of a gene.

Retrovirus-mediated gene transfer

Historically the first successful attempt to generate transgenic animals was done by infection of preimplantation mouse embryos with retroviruses.[59,60] The method developed further comprises either injection of viruses into the perivitelline space of fertilized oocytes or incubation of defective viruses with zona pellucida-free embryos (the incubation of denuded zygotes with viruses seems to be practically easier, but results in a lower implantation rate). Subsequently, a single copy of the transgene is incorporated into genome in a site-unspecific manner by the virus integration machinery. The generation of transgenic animals with oncoretroviruses, such as the Moloney strain of murine leukemia virus (MMuLV), a highly leukemogenic replication-competent retrovirus, results in the efficient integration of proviral copies in germline cells;[61,62] however, the number of provirus integration sites in the genome varies substantially from animal to animal, ranging from 1 to more then 20. Furthermore, infection of preimplantation embryos leads to efficient *de novo* methylation of proviral sequences upon chromosomal integration, resulting in low to undetectable levels of transgene expression.[63,64]

A lentiviral technology (a retroviral vector system based on the human immunodeficiency virus, HIV), established for cultured cells[65,66] was recently shown to be a powerful tool to generate transgenic mice and rats, since they can infect nondividing cells and overcome the problem of epigenetic repression.[67,68]

Gene targeting in embryonic stem cells

The total ablation of genes was made possible by gene targeting in embryonic stem (ES) cells ('knockout' technology) developed about 15 years ago on the basis of two methods:

- The permanent culture of ES cells, which were derived from preimplantation mouse embryos and have retained their pluripotency in culture, thus they can participate in the generation of all cell lineages of a mouse (including germ cells) if transferred into an early mouse embryo.[69,70]
- The targeted disruption of a gene by homologous recombination.[71,72]

Gene targeting includes first the inactivation of the one allele of the gene of interest in ES cells by homologous recombination. Transfer of mutant ES cells into early mouse embryos then allows the transmission of the mutation in question into the mouse germ line. The resulting chimeras between the host embryo and the ES cells are recognized by coat color and are used to develop, after two subsequent generations, a line of homozygous (knockout) animals carrying the mutation in both alleles of the targeted gene. Despite the fact that a lot of effort has been put in the development of ES cells from other vertebrates,[73] for yet unknown reasons germ-line-competent ES cells could not be established from any species other than the mouse. Thus, this powerful transgenic technology is not available in rats, which have, therefore, lost ground as predominant species in cardiovascular research to the advantage of the mouse.

Transgenic rats

TGR(mREN2)27

One of the most characterized transgenic models in cardiovascular research is the TGR(mREN2)27 rat produced by introducing the mouse renin *Ren-2* gene into the rat germ line.[44] A significant degree of the fulminant hypertension that develops in TGR(mREN2)27 rats is attributed to an overactive brain RAS.[31] However, the overexpression of the transgene in a wide variety of tissue has precluded the use of this model to study the specific effects of the brain RAS. Therefore, tissue-specific targeted gene manipulation has been employed to develop transgenic models with alterations of the RAS solely in the brain.

TGR(ASrAOGEN)

Up to now no knockout mouse with brain-specific ablation of a RAS component has been published. We have used transgenic methodology to develop a rat model with brain-specific knockdown of AOGEN (TGR(ASrAOGEN)), in order to elucidate a causative role for the brain RAS and its relevance in different pathophysiological processes.[74] The TGR(ASrAOGEN) rat shows an inhibited production of AOGEN solely in the brain due the control of the transgene coding for antisense RNA against AOGEN by the astrocyte-specific GFAP promoter.[74] Consequently, TGR (ASrAOGEN) rats exhibit an up to 90% decrease in AOGEN protein and markedly reduced Ang peptides levels in the brain, while the plasma levels are not altered.[74,75] Furthermore, they are hyperresponsive to central injections of Ang II due to a compensatory up-regulation of the AT_1 receptor in several brain areas.[76]

Transgenic mice

Curt Sigmund's group has generated several mouse models with targeted overexpression of human RAS components in the brain. The first one was a mouse expressing the human AOGEN gene under the control of the GFAP promoter.[77] Cross-breeding these animals with mice transgenic for ubiquitously expressed human renin[78,79] or for a human renin gene under the control of the same GFAP promoter,[80] resulted in animals with elevated blood pressure due to astrocyte-selective Ang II generation. In parallel, the same group generated transgenic mice carrying the human renin and AOGEN genes under the control of the synapsin promoter leading to neuron-selective Ang II over-expression and also moderate hypertension.[80]

Timothy Reudelhuber's group generated mice which directly produce Ang II or Ang IV[81,82] in astrocytes using a chimeric cDNA under the control of the GFAP promoter. This cDNA codes for a protein consisting of parts of human renin and mouse immunoglobulin IgG2b linked by a furin cleavage site to an Ang II or Ang IV coding domain. When the resulting protein is passing through the secretory pathway the peptides are liberated without the action of any other RAS component and are released from the cells. These mice exhibit increased Ang peptide concentrations in the brain and consequently both models became hypertensive.

Robin Davisson's group has generated mice which overexpress the human AT_{1A} receptor under the control of the NSE promoter, leading to pan-neuronal over-expression of this gene.[83] These animals were normotensive but reactions were more pronounced on central Ang II injections and they more rapidly developed hypertension induced by clipping of one renal artery.[84]

FUNCTIONS OF THE BRAIN RAS

Fluid–electrolyte homeostasis

Ang II in the brain modulates thirst and salt appetite and regulates fluid–electrolyte homeostasis.[85,86] Accordingly, TGR(ASrAOGEN) rats excrete higher amounts of diluted urine and have lower plasma levels of vasopressin (AVP) than control rats, confirming the importance of Ang II in fluid–electrolyte homeostasis.[74] Double transgenic mice expressing the human renin gene and a GFAP-driven human AOGEN transgene have a greater preference for saline.[77] The same result was also observed in mice overexpressing the human renin and AOGEN genes either only in neurons or only in astrocytes.[80] In mice with targeted deletions of the AT_{1B} receptor[87] the drinking response evoked by central Ang II is blunted, demonstrating that AT_{1B} receptors are the primary mediators of the central dipsogenic actions of Ang II.[88] Taken together, these transgenic animal models demonstrated that the brain RAS is an important modulator of fluid–electrolyte homeostasis and AVP release.

Blood pressure control

TGR(ASrAOGEN) rats have low blood pressure.[74] In contrast, both the glia- and neuron-targeted double transgenic mice overexpressing human renin and human AOGEN as well as mice overexpressing an Ang II releasing protein become hypertensive.[80,81] These alterations in blood pressure may at least in part be due to an influence on the sympathetic outflow.[75,80,89] One possible site of Ang II action within the brain that may be affected in these transgenic animals is the rostral ventrolateral medulla (RVLM) which represents the main relay for sympathetic output.[90]

The brain RAS has been suggested to moderate baroreceptor reflex.[91] Indeed, the TGR(ASrAOGEN) rats have an exaggerated spontaneous baroreflex sensitivity[92] and an increase in Ang II responsiveness at the nucleus tractus solitarii, which is the first synaptic relay of the baroreflex in the brain.[93]

Infusing Ang II in rats at slow pressor doses[94] led to an inversion of the circadian rhythm of blood pressure.[92] The fact that this treatment inverted the day-night rhythm in control but not in TGR-(ASrAOGEN) rats indicates that the brain RAS is an important modulator of the 24-hour blood pressure rhythm. One may hypothesize that these effects are mediated through an action of Ang II within the suprachiasmatic nucleus (SCN), which is considered the master clock of mammals, also regulating circadian rhythmicity of cardiovascular parameters.[95,96] Also, it is well known that Ang II can act within the SCN[97] and induce differential effects in different neuronal populations.[98] On the other hand, the pineal gland is considered to regulate rhythmicity via its main hormone melatonin and therefore alterations in melatonin synthesis may also influence the circadian blood pressure rhythm.[99,100] Accordingly, we demonstrated the existence of a local RAS in the rat pineal gland[101] and observed that TGR-(ASrAOGEN) rats have low levels of pineal indoles (including melatonin).[102]

Cardiovascular diseases

Slow pressor Ang II-induced hypertension is attenuated in TGR(ASrAOGEN), indicating that increased Ang II mediates parts of its hypertensive actions by activating the central RAS.[94] Interestingly, cardiac damage after myocardial infarction is also blunted in TGR(ASrAOGEN).[103] Probably, sympathetic activation induced by the infarct is attenuated when central Ang II synthesis is decreased (see above). Lack of central Ang II may therefore have the same beneficial effect after myocardial infarction as the novel standard therapy with β-adrenoceptor blockers. Consequently, ACE inhibitors and AT_1 antagonists with known penetrance through the blood-brain barrier may be preferable to other substances for the treatment of infarct patients.

A very interesting effect of central Ang II on peripheral organs is observed in AOGEN-deficient mice expressing a transgenic protein which releases Ang II only in the brain.[81] These mice with brain-specific rescue of Ang II generation do not show the hydronephrosis normally observed in all mouse models lacking Ang II or its receptors, such as AOGEN-,[104–106] ACE-,[107,108] renin-,[109,110] or AT_{1A}/AT_{1B}-deficient animals.[87,111] The mechanism of this effect of central Ang II remains enigmatic but may also involve the sympathetic nervous system.

These data provide clear evidence for the implication of the brain RAS in different cardiovascular diseases. The brain RAS exerts these effects through several neuroendocrinological mechanisms including the sympathetic nervous system. In fact, a large amount of data supports the implication of neurohumoral systems in cardiovascular diseases, such as heart failure[112,113] or kidney disease.[7,114]

CONCLUSIONS

Transgenic animal models have substantially advanced our understanding of the brain RAS; however, much remains to be elucidated. In particular, the sites and metabolic pathways of Ang peptide generation in different brain areas are still enigmatic. Most interesting however, is the unexpected function of the brain RAS in cardiovascular diseases, which renders it a valid drug target. Thus, the brain penetrability of ACE or renin inhibitors or AT_1 antagonists will probably become of great therapeutic relevance.

REFERENCES

1. Volicer L, Loew CG. Penetration of angiotensin II into the brain. Neuropharmacology 1971; 10: 631–6.
2. Joy MD, Lowe RD. Evidence that the area postrema mediates the central cardiovascular response to angiotensin II. Nature 1970; 228: 1303–4.
3. Schelling P, Hutchinson JS, Ganten U et al. Impermeability of the blood-cerebrospinal fluid barrier for angiotensin II in rats. Clin Sci Mol Med 1976; 51: 399s–402s.
4. Bader M, Peters J, Baltatu O et al. Tissue renin-angiotensin systems: new insights from experimental animal models in hypertension research. J Mol Med 2001; 79: 76–102.
5. DiBona GF, Sawin LL. Effect of metoprolol administration on renal sodium handling in experimental congestive heart failure. Circulation 1999; 100: 82–6.
6. Gelband CH, Sumners C, Lu D et al. Angiotensin receptors and norepinephrine neuromodulation: implications of functional coupling. Regul Pept 1997; 72: 139–45.
7. Fink GD. Long-term sympatho-excitatory effect of angiotensin II: a mechanism of spontaneous and renovascular hypertension. Clin Exp Pharmacol Physiol 1997; 24: 91–5.
8. Aguilera G, Kiss A. Regulation of the hypothalamic-pituitary-adrenal axis and vasopressin secretion. Role of angiotensin II. Adv Exp Med Biol 1996; 396: 105–12.
9. Averill DB, Diz DI. Angiotensin peptides and baroreflex control of sympathetic outflow: pathways and mechanisms of the medulla oblongata. Brain Res Bull 2000; 51: 119–28.
10. Fitzsimons JT. Angiotensin, thirst, and sodium appetite. Physiol Rev 1998; 78: 583–686.

11. Denton DA, McKinley MJ, Weisinger RS. Hypothalamic integration of body fluid regulation. Proc Natl Acad Sci U S A 1996; 93: 7397–404.
12. Baltatu O, Bader M, Ganten D. Angiotensin. In: Fink G (ed). Encyclopedia of Stress. San Diego: Academic Press, 2000, pp 190–5.
13. Maul B, Siems WE, Hoehe MR et al. Alcohol consumption is controlled by angiotensin II. FASEB J 2001; 15: 1640–2.
14. Campbell DJ, Bouhnik J, Menard J et al. Identity of angiotensinogen precursors in rat brain and liver. Nature 1984; 308: 206–8.
15. Sernia C, Mowchanuk MD. Brain angiotensinogen: in vitro synthesis and chromatographic characterization. Brain Res 1983; 259: 275–83.
16. Ohkubo H, Nakayama K, Tanaka T et al. Tissue distribution of rat angiotensinogen mRNA and structural analysis of its heterogeneity. J Biol Chem 1986; 261: 319–23.
17. Deschepper CF, Bouhnik J, Ganong WF. Colocalization of angiotensinogen and glial fibrillary acidic protein in astrocytes in rat brain. Brain Res 1986; 374: 195–8.
18. Lavoie JL, Cassell MD, Gross KW et al. Localization of renin expressing cells in the brain, by use of a REN-eGFP transgenic model. Physiol Genomics 2004; 16: 240–6.
19. Morimoto S, Cassell MD, Sigmund CD. The brain renin-angiotensin system in transgenic mice carrying a highly regulated human renin transgene. Circ Res 2002; 90: 80–6.
20. Bader M, Ganten D. Editorial: It's renin in the brain. Circ Res 2002; 90: 8–10.
21. Lee-Kirsch MA, Gaudet F, Cardoso MC et al. Distinct renin isoforms generated by tissue-specific transcription initiation and alternative splicing. Circ Res 1999; 84: 240–6.
22. Clausmeyer S, Stürzebecher R, Peters J. An alternative transcript of the rat renin gene can result in a truncated prorenin that is transported into adrenal mitochondria. Circ Res 1999; 84: 337–44.
23. Bader M, Ganten D. Regulation of renin: new evidence from cultured cells and genetically modified mice. J Mol Med 2000; 78: 130–9.
24. Strittmatter SM, Lo MMS, Javitch JA et al. Autoradiographic visualization of angiotensin-converting enzyme in rat brain with [3H]captopril: localization to a striatonigral pathway. Proc Natl Acad Sci U S A 1984; 81: 1599–603.
25. Strittmatter SM, Snyder SH. Angiotensin converting enzyme immunohistochemistry in rat brain and pituitary gland: correlation of isozyme type with cellular localization. Neuroscience 1987; 21: 407–20.
26. Saavedra JM, Fernandez-Pardal J, Chevillard C. Angiotensin-converting enzyme in discrete areas of the rat forebrain and pituitary gland. Brain Res 1982; 245: 317–25.
27. Baltatu O, Bader M, Ganten D. Brain and renin-angiotensin system. In: Nicholls MG, Ikram H, Brunner H et al. (eds). 100 Years of Renin-Angiotensin System. Oxford: Hughes Associates, 1998, pp 167–70.
28. Reaux A, Fournie-Zaluski MC, Llorens-Cortes C. Angiotensin III: a central regulator of vasopressin release and blood pressure. Trends Endocrinol Metab 2001; 12: 157–62.
29. von Bohlen und Halbach O. Angiotensin IV in the central nervous system. Cell Tissue Res 2003; 311: 1–9.
30. Santos RA, Campagnole-Santos MJ, Andrade SP. Angiotensin-(1-7): an update. Regul Pept 2000; 91: 45–62.
31. Baltatu O, Bader M, Ganten D. Functional testing of components of the brain renin-angiotensin system in transgenic animals. In: Ulfendahl HR, Aurell M (eds). Renin-Angiotensin. London: Portland Press, 1998, pp 105–14.
32. Culman J, Blume A, Gohlke P et al. The renin-angiotensin system in the brain: possible therapeutic implications for AT(1)-receptor blockers. J Hum Hypertens 2002; 16 (Suppl 3): S64–S70.
33. Allen AM, MacGregor DP, McKinley MJ et al. Angiotensin II receptors in the human brain. Regul Pept 1999; 79: 1–7.
34. Albiston AL, McDowall SG, Matsacos D et al. Evidence that the angiotensin IV (AT(4)) receptor is the enzyme insulin-regulated aminopeptidase. J Biol Chem 2001; 276: 48623–6.
35. Santos RA, Simoes e Silva AC, Maric C et al. Angiotensin-(1-7) is an endogenous ligand for the G-protein coupled receptor Mas. Proc Natl Acad Sci U S A 2003; 100: 8258–63.
36. Metzger R, Bader M, Ludwig T et al. Expression of the mouse and rat mas proto-oncogene in the brain and peripheral tissues. FEBS Lett 1995; 357: 27–32.
37. Costantini F, Lacy E. Introduction of a rabbit β-globin gene into the mouse germ line. Nature 1981; 294: 92–4.
38. Gordon JW, Ruddle FH. Integration and stable germ line transmission of genes injected into the mouse pronucleus. Science 1981; 214: 1244–6.
39. Harbers K, Jähner D, Jaenisch R. Microinjection of cloned retroviral genomes into mouse zygotes: integration and expression in the animal. Nature 1981; 293: 540–2.
40. Wagner EF, Stewart TA, Mintz B. The human β-globin gene and a functional viral thymidine kinase gene in developing mice. Proc Natl Acad Sci U S A 1981; 78: 5016–20.
41. Wagner TE, Hoppe PC, Jollick JD et al. Microinjection of a rabbit beta-globin gene into zygotes and its subsequent expression in adult mice and their offspring. Proc Natl Acad Sci U S A 1981; 78: 6376–80.
42. Hammer RE, Pursel VG, Reynolds RC et al. Production of transgenic rabbits, sheep and pigs by microinjection. Nature 1985; 315: 680–3.
43. Hammer RE, Maika SD, Richardson JA et al. Spontaneous inflammatory disease in transgenic rats expressing HLA-B27 and human β2m: an animal model of HLA-B27-associated human disorders. Cell 1990; 63: 1099–112.
44. Mullins JJ, Peters J, Ganten D. Fulminant hypertension in transgenic rats harbouring the mouse Ren-2 gene. Nature 1990; 344: 541–4.
45. Ebert KM, Selgrath JP, DiTullio P et al. Transgenic production of a variant of human tissue-type plasminogen activator in goat milk: generation of transgenic goats and analysis of expression. Bio/Technology 1991; 9: 835–8.
46. Krimpenfort P, Rademakers A, Eyestone W et al. Generation of transgenic dairy cattle using 'in vitro' embryo production. Bio/Technology 1991; 9: 844–7.
47. Gordon JW. Production of transgenic mice. Methods Enzymol 1993; 225: 747–71.
48. Hogan B, Beddington F, Costantini F et al. Manipulating the Mouse Embryo. Cold Spring Harbor, NY: Cold Spring Harbor Laboratory, 1994.
49. Auerbach AB. Production of functional transgenic mice by DNA pronuclear microinjection. Acta Biochim Pol 2004; 51: 9–31.
50. Burdon TG, Wall RJ. Fate of microinjected genes in preimplantation mouse embryos. Mol Reprod Dev 1992; 33: 436–42.
51. Wilkie TM, Brinster RL, Palmiter RD. Germline and somatic mosaicism in transgenic mice. Dev Biol 1986; 118: 9–18.
52. Whitelaw CB, Springbett AJ, Webster J et al. The majority of G0 transgenic mice are derived from mosaic embryos. Transgenic Res 1993; 2: 29–32.
53. Bentley D. The mRNA assembly line: transcription and processing machines in the same factory. Curr Opin Cell Biol 2002; 14: 336–42.
54. Kornblihtt AR, de la MM, Fededa JP et al. Multiple links between transcription and splicing. RNA 2004; 10: 1489–98.

55. Choi T, Huang M, Gorman C et al. A generic intron increases gene expression in transgenic mice. Mol Cell Biol 1991; 11: 3070–4.
56. Hentze MW, Kulozik AE. A perfect message: RNA surveillance and nonsense-mediated decay. Cell 1999; 96: 307–10.
57. Wilson C, Bellen HJ, Gehring WJ. Position effects on eukaryotic gene expression. Annu Rev Cell Biol 1990; 6: 679–714.
58. Rajewsky K, Gu H, Kühn R et al. Conditional gene targeting. J Clin Invest 1996; 98: 600–3.
59. Jaenisch R, Mintz B. Simian virus 40 DNA sequences in DNA of healthy adult mice derived from preimplantation blastocysts injected with viral DNA. Proc Natl Acad Sci U S A 1974; 71: 1250–4.
60. Jaenisch R. Germ line integration and Mendelian transmission of the exogenous Moloney leukemia virus. Proc Natl Acad Sci U S A 1976; 73: 1260–4.
61. Jahner D, Jaenisch R. Integration of Moloney leukaemia virus into the germ line of mice: correlation between site of integration and virus activation. Nature 1980; 287: 456–8.
62. Jaenisch R, Jahner D, Nobis P et al. Chromosomal position and advance of retroviral genomes inserted into germ line of mice. Cell 1981; 24: 519.
63. Jahner D, Stuhlmann H, Stewart CL et al. De novo methylation and expression of retroviral genomes during mouse embryogenesis. Nature 1982; 298: 623–8.
64. Jahner D, Jaenisch R. Retrovirus-induced de novo methylation of flanking host sequences correlates with gene inactivity. Nature 1985; 315: 594–7.
65. Naldini L, Blomer U, Gallay P et al. In vivo gene delivery and stable transduction of nondividing cells by a lentiviral vector. Science 1996; 272: 263–7.
66. Miyoshi H, Blomer U, Takahashi M et al. Development of a self-inactivating lentivirus vector. J Virol 1998; 72: 8150–7.
67. Lois C, Hong EJ, Pease S et al. Germline transmission and tissue-specific expression of transgenes delivered by lentiviral vectors. Science 2002; 295: 868–72.
68. Pfeifer A, Ikawa M, Dayn Y et al. Transgenesis by lentiviral vectors: lack of gene silencing in mammalian embryonic stem cells and preimplantation embryos. Proc Natl Acad Sci U S A 2002; 99: 2140–5.
69. Bradley A, Evans M, Kaufman MH et al. Formation of germ-line chimaeras from embryo-derived teratocarcinoma cell lines. Nature 1984; 309: 255–6.
70. Evans MJ, Kaufman MH. Establishment in culture of pluripotential cells from mouse embryos. Nature 1981; 292: 154–6.
71. Capecchi MR. Altering the genome by homologous recombination. Science 1989; 244: 1288–92.
72. Bronson SK, Smithies O. Altering mice by homologous recombination using embryonic stem cells. J Biol Chem 1994; 269: 27155–8.
73. Brenin DR, Bader M, Hübner N et al. Rat embryonic stem cells: a progress report. Transplant Proc 1997; 29: 1761–5.
74. Schinke M, Baltatu O, Böhm M et al. Blood pressure reduction and diabetes insipidus in transgenic rats deficient in brain angiotensinogen. Proc Natl Acad Sci U S A 1999; 96: 3975–80.
75. Huang BS, Ganten D, Leenen FH. Responses to central Na(+) and ouabain are attenuated in transgenic rats deficient in brain angiotensinogen. Hypertension 2001; 37: 683–6.
76. Monti J, Schinke M, Böhm M et al. Glial angiotensinogen regulates brain angiotensin II receptors in transgenic rats TGR(ASrAOGEN). Am J Physiol 2001; 280: R233–R240.
77. Morimoto S, Cassell MD, Beltz TG et al. Elevated blood pressure in transgenic mice with brain-specific expression of human angiotensinogen driven by the glial fibrillary acidic protein promoter. Circ Res 2001; 89: 365–72.
78. Sigmund CD, Jones CA, Kane CM et al. Regulated tissue- and cell-specific expression of the human renin gene in transgenic mice. Circ Res 1992; 70: 1070–9.
79. Sinn PL, Davis DR, Sigmund CD. Highly regulated cell type-restricted expression of human renin in mice containing 140- or 160-kilobase pair P1 phage artificial chromosome transgenes. J Biol Chem 1999; 274: 35785–93.
80. Morimoto S, Cassell MD, Sigmund CD. Glia- and neuron-specific expression of the renin-angiotensin system in brain alters blood pressure, water intake, and salt preference. J Biol Chem 2002; 277: 33235–41.
81. Lochard N, Silversides DW, van Kats JP et al. Brain-specific restoration of angiotensin II corrects renal defects seen in angiotensinogen-deficient mice. J Biol Chem 2003; 278: 2184–9.
82. Lochard N, Thibault G, Silversides DW et al. Chronic production of angiotensin IV in the brain leads to hypertension that is reversible with an angiotensin II AT1 receptor antagonist. Circ Res 2004; 94: 1451–7.
83. Lazartigues E, Dunlay SM, Loihl AK et al. Brain-selective overexpression of angiotensin (AT1) receptors causes enhanced cardiovascular sensitivity in transgenic mice. Circ Res 2002; 90: 617–24.
84. Lazartigues E, Lawrence AJ, Lamb FS et al. Renovascular hypertension in mice with brain-selective overexpression of AT1a receptors is buffered by increased nitric oxide production in the periphery. Circ Res 2004; 95: 523–31.
85. Johnson AK, Thunhorst RL. The neuroendocrinology of thirst and salt appetite: visceral sensory signals and mechanisms of central integration. Front Neuroendocrinol 1997; 18: 292–353.
86. Phillips MI, Sumners C. Angiotensin II in central nervous system physiology. Regul Pept 1998; 78: 1–11.
87. Oliverio MI, Kim HS, Ito M et al. Reduced growth, abnormal kidney structure, and type 2 (AT2) angiotensin receptor-mediated blood pressure regulation in mice lacking both AT1A and AT1B receptors for angiotensin II. Proc Natl Acad Sci U S A 1998; 95: 15496–501.
88. Davisson RL, Oliverio MI, Coffman TM et al. Divergent functions of angiotensin II receptor isoforms in the brain. J Clin Invest 2000; 106: 103–6.
89. Baltatu O, Campos LA, Bader M. Genetic targeting of the brain renin-angiotensin system in transgenic rats. Impact on stress-induced renin release. Acta Physiol Scand 2004; 181: 579–84.
90. Baltatu O, Fontes MA, Campagnole-Santos MJ et al. Alterations of the renin-angiotensin system at the RVLM of transgenic rats with low brain angio-tensinogen. Am J Physiol Regul Integr Comp Physiol 2001; 280: R428–R433.
91. Head GA, Mayorov DN. Central angiotensin and baroreceptor control of circulation. Ann NY Acad Sci 2001; 940: 361–79.
92. Baltatu O, Janssen BJ, Bricca G et al. Alterations in blood pressure and heart rate variability in transgenic rats with low brain angiotensinogen. Hypertension 2001; 37: 408–13.
93. Couto AS, Baltatu O, Santos RA et al. Differential effects of angiotensin II and angiotensin-(1-7) at the nucleus tractus solitarii of transgenic rats with low brain angiotensinogen. J Hypertens 2002; 20: 919–25.
94. Baltatu O, Silva JA Jr, Ganten D et al. The brain renin-angiotensin system modulates angiotensin II-induced hypertension and cardiac hypertrophy. Hypertension 2000; 35: 409–12.
95. Janssen BJ, Tyssen CM, Duindam H et al. Suprachiasmatic lesions eliminate 24-h blood pressure variability in rats. Physiol Behav 1994; 55: 307–11.
96. Witte K, Schnecko A, Buijs RM et al. Effects of SCN lesions on circadian blood pressure rhythm in normotensive and transgenic hypertensive rats. Chronobiol Int 1998; 15: 135–45.

97. Mendelsohn FAO, Quirion R, Saavedra JM et al. Autoradiographic localization of angiotensin II receptors in rat brain. Proc Natl Acad Sci U S A 1984; 81: 1575–9.
98. Tang KC, Pan JT. Differential effects of angiotensin II on the activities of suprachiasmatic neurons in rat brain slices. Brain Res Bull 1995; 37: 529–32.
99. Pevet P. Melatonin and biological rhythms. Biol Signals Recept 2000; 9: 203–12.
100. Stehle JH, von Gall C, Korf HW. Melatonin: a clock-output, a clock-input. J Neuroendocrinol 2003; 15: 383–9.
101. Baltatu O, Lippoldt A, Hansson A et al. Local renin-angiotensin system in the pineal gland. Brain Res Mol Brain Res 1998; 54: 237–42.
102. Baltatu O, Afeche FC, Santos SHJ et al. Locally synthesized angiotensin modulates pineal melatonin generation. J Neurochem 2002; 80: 328–34.
103. Wang H, Huang BS, Ganten D et al. Prevention of sympathetic and cardiac dysfunction after myocardial infarction in transgenic rats deficient in brain angiotensinogen. Circ Res 2004; 94: 843.
104. Tanimoto K, Sugiyama F, Goto Y et al. Angiotensinogen-deficient mice with hypotension. J Biol Chem 1994; 269: 31334–7.
105. Kim H-S, Krege JH, Kluckman KD et al. Genetic control of blood pressure and the angiotensinogen locus. Proc Natl Acad Sci U S A 1995; 92: 2735–9.
106. Niimura F, Labosky PA, Kakuchi J et al. Gene targeting in mice reveals a requirement for angiotensin in the development and maintenance of kidney morphology and growth factor regulation. J Clin Invest 1995; 96: 2947–54.
107. Krege JH, John SW, Langenbach LL et al. Male-female differences in fertility and blood pressure in ACE-deficient mice. Nature 1995; 375: 146–8.
108. Esther CR Jr, Howard TE, Marino EM et al. Mice lacking angiotensin-converting enzyme have low blood pressure, renal pathology, and reduced male fertility. Lab Invest 1996; 74: 953–65.
109. Yanai K, Saito T, Kakinuma Y et al. Renin-dependent cardiovascular functions and renin-independent blood-brain barrier functions revealed by renin-deficient mice. J Biol Chem 2000; 275: 5–8.
110. Takahashi N, Lopez ML, Cowhig JE Jr et al. Ren1c homozygous null mice are hypotensive and polyuric, but heterozygotes are indistinguishable from wild-type. J Am Soc Nephrol 2005; 16: 125–32.
111. Tsuchida S, Matsusaka T, Chen X et al. Murine double nullizygotes of the angiotensin type 1A and 1B receptor genes duplicate severe abnormal phenotypes of angiotensinogen nullizygotes. J Clin Invest 1998; 101: 755–60.
112. Felder RB, Francis J, Zhang ZH et al. Heart failure and the brain: new perspectives. Am J Physiol Regul Integr Comp Physiol 2003; 284: R259–R276.
113. Weiss ML, Kenney MJ, Musch TI et al. Modifications to central neural circuitry during heart failure. Acta Physiol Scand 2003; 177: 57–67.
114. Campese VM, Krol E. Neurogenic factors in renal hypertension. Curr Hypertens Rep 2002; 4: 256–60.
115. Yang G, Merrill DC, Thompson MW et al. Functional expression of the human angiotensinogen gene in transgenic mice. J Biol Chem 1994; 269: 32497–502.
116. Morimoto S, Cassell MD, Sigmund CD. Neuron-specific expression of human angiotensinogen in brain causes increased salt appetite. Physiol Genomics 2002; 9: 113–20.
117. Ito M, Oliverio MI, Mannon PJ et al. Regulation of blood pressure by the type 1A angiotensin II receptor gene. Proc Natl Acad Sci U S A 1995; 92: 3521–5.
118. Hein L, Barsh GS, Pratt RE et al. Behavioural and cardiovascular effects of disrupting the angiotensin II type-2 receptor in mice. Nature 1995; 377: 744–7.
119. Ichiki T, Labosky PA, Shiota C et al. Effects on blood pressure and exploratory behaviour of mice lacking angiotensin II type-2 receptor. Nature 1995; 377: 748–50.
120. Clark AF, Sharp MGF, Morley SD et al. Renin-1 is essential for normal renal juxtaglomerular cell granulation and macula densa morphology. J Biol Chem 1997; 272: 18185–90.
121. Sharp MG, Fettes D, Brooker G et al. Targeted inactivation of the Ren-2 gene in mice. Hypertension 1996; 28: 1126–31.
122. Walther T, Balschun D, Voigt JP et al. Sustained long term potentiation and anxiety in mice lacking the Mas protooncogene. J Biol Chem 1998; 273: 11867–873.

9

The adrenal renin-angiotensin system

Jörg Peters

INTRODUCTION

A few years after the role of the circulating renin angiotensin system (RAS) in the regulation of aldosterone synthesis had been discovered[1–4] Ryan[5] and Ganten et al.[6] described the existence of a renin-like enzyme within the adrenal gland and proposed that the secretory function of the gland could be modulated by a local RAS.[5,7] Renin was further detected in human adrenal tissues and adrenal tumors.[8–10] Also angiotensinogen has been co-localized with renin in human adrenals.[11] Furthermore, in rat angiotensin (Ang) II remained detectable even 20 hours after bilateral nephrectomy, a procedure which removes the source for circulating renin.[12] This surely indicated local Ang production.

LOCALIZATION OF RENIN AND OTHER COMPONENTS OF THE RAS WITHIN THE ADRENAL GLAND

Renin and its mRNA are present predominantly within adrenocortical cells of the outer adrenal cortex in most species.[13–16] Interestingly, during fetal development in mice, the adrenal gland and not the kidney is the primary site of renin expression.[17] During further embryonic development and after birth renin expression is markedly reduced in the adrenal and at the same time specific expression becomes located to the afferent arterioles of the kidney.

All other components of the RAS, such as angiotensin converting enzyme (ACE), angiotensins, as well as the gene transcripts for ACE and angiotensinogen have been detected within the adrenal gland of several species including human.[18] A human adrenocortical tumor cell line (NCI-H295) was recently found to express angiotensinogen, renin, and AT_1 receptors, as well as ACE-like activity.[19]

REGULATION AND FUNCTION OF RENIN EXPRESSION WITHIN THE ADRENAL GLAND

Sodium depletion increases adrenal renin concentration similarly to its effect on renal and plasma renin concentrations.[13,20] A high potassium diet increases adrenal renin concentrations, while decreasing plasma renin concentrations.[13,21,22] ACTH increases adrenal but not circulating renin activity.[23] Bilateral nephrectomy markedly increases adrenal renin levels, while even eliminating circulating renin.[13,24]

Of particular interest is the fact that circulating Ang II inhibits adrenal renin expression in vivo.[16,22] This supports the view that the adrenal system is partially under control of the circulating system. The inhibitory effect of Ang II appears to be mediated by the AT_1 receptor, since AT_1 receptor antagonist potentiates the nephrectomy-induced increase of renin mRNA levels.[16]

The fact that all components of the RAS are present in the outer adrenal cortex suggests a physiological function for aldosterone biosynthesis and in regulation of glomerulosa size or growth processes. A number of in vitro studies indeed demonstrated inhibition of aldosterone production by using antagonists of the RAS.[18] In vivo, changes of adrenal renin expression in response to changes in electrolyte concentrations correlate with similar changes in aldosterone production. Importantly, under potassium loading or bilateral nephrectomy, aldosterone production correlates positively with adrenal renin, but even inversely with circulating renin levels.[13] In vivo the existence of a local intra-adrenal RAS is supported further by the fact that even after elimination of circulating renin inhibitors of the RAS still inhibit aldosterone production.[16] Unexpectedly, however, a nephrectomy-induced rise of plasma aldosterone levels was inhibited not only by AT_1 receptor antagonists, but also by the agonist,

Ang II. This was quite surprising, since Ang II is usually known to stimulate aldosterone production and usually agonists and antagonists exert opposite effects. The inhibitory effect of Ang II on aldosterone production, however, was associated with marked inhibition of adrenal renin expression.[16] Assuming a causal relationship between inhibition of aldosterone production and of adrenal renin expression by Ang II, one may wonder why the inhibitory effect of circulating Ang II on aldosterone production – through inhibition of adrenal renin expression – should overrule its known direct stimulatory effect on aldosterone production. A possible explanation could be that the intra-adrenal renin at least partially uses targets that are not accessible to extracellular Angs (see Figure 9.1 and text below).

THE ADRENAL RAS AND HYPERTENSION

It has been proposed that an intra-adrenal RAS is involved in the sodium dependency of the sensitivity of adrenocortical cells to Ang II. In a sodium-depleted state, glomerulosa cells respond more readily to Ang II and produce greater quantities of aldosterone. Sodium chloride load, on the other hand, inhibits aldosterone production and decreases the sensitivity of glomerulosa cells to Ang II.[25] This sodium modulation of adrenal sensitivity correlates well with intra-adrenal content of renin and Angs.[25–27] In some forms of primary hypertension the sodium dependency of adrenal responses to Ang II is pathologically altered in that the cells do not respond with increased sensitivity to a low salt diet or with decreased sensitivity to a high salt diet. Inhibitors of the RAS correct the pathological responses, supporting a causal link between sodium-dependent changes of adrenal sensitivity to Ang II and activity of the intra-adrenal RAS.[28]

A role for adrenal renin in hypertension is further indicated by studies with ten-2 transgenic rats, TGR(mREN2)27. These rats express particularly high levels of the renin transgene within the adrenal cortex. In this model, high intra-adrenal renin content is accompanied by elevated basal production of aldosterone and other adrenocortical steroids[29–32] and hypertension.

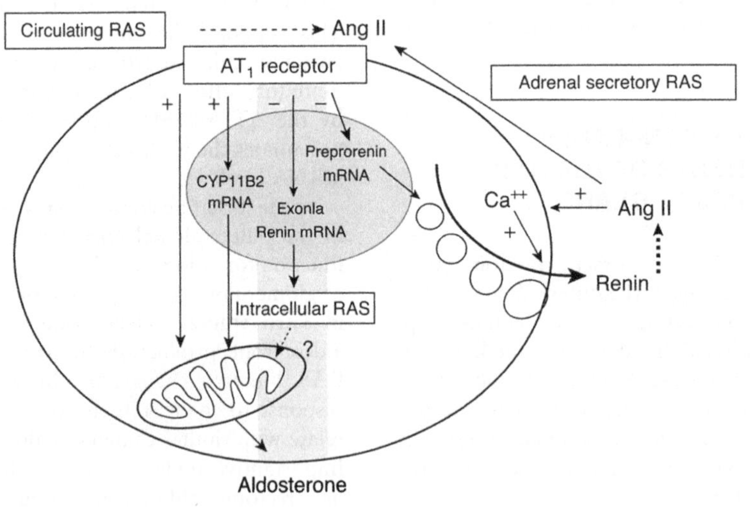

Figure 9.1 Two adrenal and one circulating renin-angiotensin system (RAS). The circulating RAS stimulates aldosterone biosynthesis via the AT_1 receptor. The stimulation involves increased availability of substrate, increased activity of steroidogenic enzymes and increased transcription of steroidogenic genes, such as *cyp11b2*. The circulating RAS further inhibits adrenal renin expression. The adrenal cells express two renin transcripts from the same renin gene. The preprorenin transcript encodes for renin which is sorted into the secretory pathway. Renin secretion is acutely stimulated by intracellular free calcium. Adrenal secretory renin is thus part of an intra-adrenal amplification system for circulating and locally produced ANG II. Another transcript encodes for a truncated prorenin, which cannot be secreted and may modulate adrenal function by so far unknown intracellular mechanisms

Interestingly, as in some forms of human hypertension, blood pressure in TGR(mREN2)27 is salt sensitive and the transgenic rats show virtually no decrease in the sensitivity of glomerulosa cells to Ang II under conditions of high sodium chloride intake.[33,34] This is associated with a failure of sodium load to sufficiently decrease adrenal renin expression.

MODES OF ACTION OF THE ADRENAL RAS

The adrenal RAS as a secretory system

The intracellular fate of renin in the adrenal is different from that in the kidney. Renin sorting as well as renin secretion is determined not only by specific features of the protein but also by specific features of the cell type expressing it. Glycosylated renin in kidney cells appears to be sorted to lysosomes, which thereby become modified to form renin-containing secretory storage granules.[35–37] When unglycosylated, renin is not transported into lysosomal-like storage granules, likely because it lacks the classical lysosomal sorting signal. In contrast to renin-producing cells of the kidney, which are modified smooth muscle cells, the majority of renin-producing cells in the adrenal cortex is endocrine in origin. Endocrine cells target both unglycosylated renin and glycosylated renin to the regulated secretory pathway and not to the lysosomal pathway.[38,39]

The cell-type specific difference of renin sorting has consequences on the regulation of renin secretion. Secretion of any hormone or transmitter via the regulated secretory pathway of neuroendocrine cells would be stimulated by intracellular calcium. Calcium initiates fusion of secretory granules with the plasma membrane and thus exocytosis. Renin secretion from lysosomal-like storage granules of the kidney, in contrast, is inhibited by calcium ('the calcium paradox'[40,41]) and also by Ang II, which increases intracellular free calcium. These inhibitory effects are crucial for the pressor-dependent regulation of the activity of the renal and thus circulating RAS.

Primary adrenal cells, in contrast, store unglycosylated renin and respond with increased secretion to Ang II or elevation of intracellular calcium levels.[42–45] Thus under conditions of normal and chronically high circulating angiotensins, acute increases of renin secretion by circulating Ang II may serve as an amplification system (Figure 9.1). There are two important implications of this scheme. First, the intra-adrenal amplification of the signal could conceivably minimize the demand on circulating Ang II for effective stimulation of aldosterone release. Second, immediate adrenal responses to circulating Ang II could be modulated by the intra-adrenal RAS. Since the intra-adrenal RAS itself is subject to regulation, aldosterone production is accessible to dual regulation, both by the circulating and local adrenal RAS. Indeed such a concept could help clarify the previously recognized salt dependency of adrenal sensitivity to Ang II.

The adrenal RAS as an intracellular system

To extend our studies on adrenal renin we characterized the intracellular distribution of renin on the subcellular levels by means of electron microscopy. As expected we found renin within secretory vesicles, supporting the secretory model.[43] Surprisingly, however, we additionally found immunoreactive renin within adrenal mitochondria, where it was located in electron-dense inclusion bodies.[24] Isolated mitochondria also exhibit renin activity. Most surprising then, was the fact that the known renin transcript encodes for a protein with a signal sequence for the endoplasmic reticulum (ER). Such a protein could be sorted to lysosomes or secretory vesicles, but not to mitochondria, because it will be unequivocally packed into vesicles. We thus searched for and discovered a transcript encoding a renin protein which is translated at free ribosomes.[46] This transcript, termed exon1a renin, lacks exon 1 and thus the coding sequence for the ER signal. Instead, a sequence derived from intron 1 precedes exon 2. The translation product of this transcript would be a truncated prorenin. This protein was further shown to be imported into isolated adrenal mitochondria in vitro.[46] Analysis of tissue-specific expression revealed that the kidney expresses exclusively the classical preprorenin transcript, in accordance with its secretory function. The adrenal gland expresses both the secretory and the intracellular renin transcript.[47] The functions of intracellular renin so far still remain speculative. However, the alternative renin transcript provides a molecular basis for an intracellular RAS, which has been proposed previously.[48–50]

CONCLUSIONS

In summary, there is considerable in vitro and in vivo evidence for the existence of an intra-adrenal RAS. There are conditions when activation of this system is of advantage. The adrenal RAS modulates adrenal sensitivity and appears to serve as an amplification system, reducing the need for high levels of circulating Ang.

Its mode of action is largely different from that of the renal system in terms of renin secretion, expression, and intracellular targeting. Regulation of electrolyte balance appears to be the result of subtle interactions between the circulating and local system. Overexpression of renin within the adrenal gland may lead to hypertension.

REFERENCES

1. Gross F. Renin und Hypertensin, physiologische und pathophysiologische Wirkstoffe. Klin Wochenschr 1958; 36: 693–705.
2. Genest J, Nowaczynski W, Koiw E, Sandor T, Biron P. Adrenocortical function in essential hypertension. In: Bock KD, Cottier PR (eds). Essential Hypertension. Heidelberg: Springer, 1960.
3. Laragh JH, Angers M, Kelly WG et al. Hypotensive agents and pressor substances. The effect of epinephrine, norepinephrine, ANGII and others on the secretory rate of aldosteron in man. JAMA 1960; 17: 234.
4. Ganong WF, Mulrow PJ. Evidence of secretion of an aldosterone-stimulating substance by the kidney. Nature 1961; 190: 1115.
5. Ryan JW. Renin-like enzyme in the adrenal gland. Science 1967; 158: 1589–90.
6. Ganten D, Ganten U, Kubo S et al. Influence of sodium, potassium, and pituitary hormones on iso-renin in rat adrenal glands. Am J Physiol 1974; 227: 224–9.
7. Ganten D, Ganten U, Kubo S et al. Proceedings: Iso-renin in adrenal glands of rats: a possible factor in steroid production. Naunyn Schmiedebergs Arch Pharmacol 1974; 282: (Suppl 282): R24.
8. Ganten D, Schelling P, Vecsei P et al. Iso-renin of extrarenal origin. 'The tissue angiotensinogenase systems'. Am J Med 1976; 60: 760–72.
9. Naruse M, Sussman CR, Naruse K et al. Renin exists in human adrenal tissue. J Clin Endocrinol Metab 1983; 57: 482–7.
10. Iimura O, Shimamoto K, Hotta D et al. A case of adrenal tumor producing renin, aldosterone, and sex steroid hormones. Hypertension 1986; 8: 951–6.
11. Racz K, Pinet F, Gasc JM et al. Coexpression of renin, angiotensinogen, and their messenger ribonucleic acids in adrenal tissues. J Clin Endocrinol Metab 1992; 75: 730–7.
12. Aguilera G, Schirar A, Baukal A et al. Circulating angiotensin II and adrenal receptors after nephrectomy. Nature 1981; 289: 507–9.
13. Doi Y, Atarashi K, Franco-Saenz R et al. Effect of changes in sodium or potassium balance, and nephrectomy, on adrenal renin and aldosterone concentrations. Hypertension 1984; 6: I124–I129.
14. Deschepper CF, Mellon SH, Cumin F et al. Analysis by immunocytochemistry and in situ hybridization of renin and its mRNA in kidney, testis, adrenal, and pituitary of the rat. Proc Natl Acad Sci U S A 1986; 83: 7552–6.
15. Doi Y, Atarashi K, Franco-Saenz R, Mulrow P. Adrenal renin: a possible regulator of aldosterone production. Clin Exp Hypertens A 1983; 5: 1119–26.
16. Peters J, Obermuller N, Woyth A et al. Losartan and angiotensin II inhibit aldosterone production in anephric rats via different actions on the intraadrenal renin-angiotensin system. Endocrinology 1999; 140: 675–82.
17. Jones CA, Sigmund CD, McGowan RA et al. Expression of murine renin genes during fetal development. Mol Endocrinol 1990; 4: 375–83.
18. Bader M, Peters J, Baltatu O et al. Tissue renin-angiotensin systems: new insights from experimental animal models in hypertension research. J Mol Med 2001; 79: 76–102.
19. Hilbers U, Peters J, Bornstein SR et al. Local renin-angiotensin system is involved in K+-induced aldosterone secretion from human adrenocortical NCI-H295 cells. Hypertension 1999; 33: 1025–30.
20. Brecher AS, Shier DN, Dene H et al. Regulation of adrenal renin messenger ribonucleic acid by dietary sodium chloride. Endocrinology 1989; 124: 2907–13.
21. Nakamaru M, Misono KS, Naruse M et al. A role for the adrenal renin-angiotensin system in the regulation of potassium-stimulated aldosterone production. Endocrinology 1985; 117: 1772–8.
22. Baba K, Doi Y, Franco-Saenz R et al. Mechanisms by which nephrectomy stimulates adrenal renin. Hypertension 1986; 8: 997–1002.
23. Yamaguchi T, Naito Z, Stoner GD et al. Role of the adrenal renin-angiotensin system on adrenocorticotropic hormone- and potassium-stimulated aldosterone production by rat adrenal glomerulosa cells in monolayer culture. Hypertension 1990; 16: 635–41.
24. Peters J, Kranzlin B, Schaeffer S et al. Presence of renin within intramitochondrial dense bodies of the rat adrenal cortex. Am J Physiol 1996; 271: E439–E450.
25. Hollenberg NK, Chenitz WR, Adams DF et al. Reciprocal influence of salt intake on adrenal glomerulosa and renal vascular responses to angiotensin II in normal man. J Clin Invest 1974; 54: 34–42.
26. Kifor I, Moore TJ, Fallo F et al. The effect of sodium intake on angiotensin content of the rat adrenal gland. Endocrinology 1991; 128: 1277–84.
27. Williams GH, Hollenberg NK. Functional derangements in the regulation of aldosterone secretion in hypertension. Hypertension 1991; 18: III143–III149.
28. Taylor T, Moore TJ, Hollenberg NK et al. Converting-enzyme inhibition corrects the altered adrenal response to angiotensin II in essential hypertension. Hypertension 1984; 6: 92–9.
29. Peters J, Ganten D. Adrenal renin expression and its role in ren-2 transgenic rats TGR(mREN2)27. Horm Metab Res 1998; 30: 350–4.
30. Sander M, Bader M, Djavidani B et al. The role of the adrenal gland in hypertensive transgenic rats TGR(mREN2)27. Endocrinology 1992; 131: 807–14.
31. Mullins JJ, Peters J, Ganten D. Fulminant hypertension in transgenic rats harbouring the mouse Ren-2 gene. Nature 1990; 344: 541–4.
32. Djavidani B, Sander M, Kreutz R et al. Chronic dexamethasone treatment suppress hypertension development in the transgenic rat TGR(mREN2)27. J Hypertens 1995; 13: 637–45.
33. Mortensen RM, Conlin PR, Menachery A et al. Abnormally increased adrenal sensitivity to ANG II in hypertensive transgenic rats (mREN2–27) with high salt diets and a paradoxical effect of low salt. Hypertension 1993; 22: 441.
34. Mortensen RM, Menachery A, Braley L et al. Unique salt sensitivity of adrenal phenotype and blood pressure in hypertensive rats carrying a murine renin transgene. Hypertension 1994; 21: 441.
35. Taugner R, Hackenthal E. The Juxtaglomerular Apparatus. Berlin: Springer, 1989.
36. Hackenthal E, Paul M, Ganten D et al. Morphology, physiology and molecular biology of renin secretion. Physiol Rev 1990; 70: 1067–116.

37. Clark AF, Sharp MG, Morley SD et al. Renin-1 is essential for normal renal juxtaglomerular cell granulation and macula densa morphology. J Biol Chem 1997; 272: 18185–90.
38. Paul M, Nakamura N, Pratt RE et al. Cell-dependent posttranslational processing and secretion of recombinant mouse renin-2. Am J Physiol 1992; 262: E224–E229.
39. Pratt RE, Flynn JA, Hobart PM et al. Different secretory pathways of renin from mouse cells transfected with human renin gene. J Biol Chem 1988; 263: 3137–41.
40. Schwertschlag U, Hackenthal E, Hackenthal R et al. The effects of calcium and calcium-ionophores (X 537 A and A 23187) on renin release in the isolated perfused rat kidney. Clin Sci Mol Med Suppl 1978; 4: 171s–174s.
41. Taugner R, Nobiling R, Metz R et al. Hypothetical interpretation of the calcium paradox in renin secretion. Cell Tissue Res 1988; 252: 687–90.
42. Yamaguchi T, Franco-Saenz R, Mulrow PJ. Effect of angiotensin II on renin production by rat adrenal glomerulosa cells in culture. Hypertension 1992; 19: 263–9.
43. Mizuno K, Hoffman LH, McKenzie JC et al. Presence of renin secretory granules in rat adrenal gland and stimulation of renin secretion by angiotensin II but not by adrenocorticotropin. J Clin Invest 1988; 82: 1007–16.
44. Hackenthal E, Münter K, Fritsch S. Kidney function and renin processing in transgenic rats, TGR(mREN2)27. In: Sassard, Montrouge J (eds). Genetic Hypertension. London: John Libbey Eurotext, 1992; pp 349–51.
45. Peters J, Münter K, Bader M et al. Increased adrenal renin in transgenic hypertensive rats, TGR(mREN2)27, and its regulation by cAMP, angiotensin II, and calcium. J Clin Invest 1993; 91: 742–7.
46. Clausmeyer S, Stürzebecher R, Peters J. An alternative transcript of the rat renin gene can result in a truncated prorenin that is transported into adrenal mitochondria. Circ Res 1999; 84: 337–44.
47. Clausmeyer S, Reinecke A, Farrenkopf R et al. Tissue-specific expression of a rat renin transcript lacking the coding sequence for the prefragment and its stimulation by myocardial infarction. Endocrinology 2000; 141: 2963–70.
48. Re RN. Intracellular renin and the nature of intracrine enzymes. Hypertension 2003; 42: 117–22.
49. Cook JL, Giardina JF, Zhang Z et al. Intracellular angiotensin II increases the long isoform of PDGF mRNA in rat hepatoma cells. J Mol Cell Cardiol 2002; 34: 1525–37.
50. Cook JL, Zhang Z, Re RN. In vitro evidence for an intracellular site of angiotensin action. Circ Res 2001; 89: 1138–46.

10

The cardiac renin-angiotensin-aldosterone system in hypertension and heart failure

Walmor C De Mello

INTRODUCTION

Evidence is available that the heart is a target for the renin-angiotensin system (RAS). Indeed, angiotensin II (Ang II) regulates heart contractility,[1] cell coupling, and impulse propagation,[2–5] and is responsible for remodeling and the induction of apoptosis.[6]

The heart is not only influenced by the plasma RAS but has its own system. The evidence that there is a local cardiac RAS gained strength with the demonstration that renin, angiotensinogen (AGT), Ang I, Ang II, and the angiotensin converting enzyme (ACE) are present in the heart.[7] Moreover, the beneficial effects of ACE inhibitors in the treatment of congestive heart failure, myocardial ischemia and, myocardial hypertrophy[8] at doses that do not change the arterial blood pressure support this view.

However, the synthesis of some of the RAS components inside the heart cell is controversial. The levels of cardiac renin are extremely low in nephrectomized animals,[9] suggesting that cardiac renin is dependent upon uptake from plasma, at least in the normal heart.[10,11] Moreover, the source of AGT in the heart, for instance, is not known. Although AGT is shown in the heart, no AGT is released from the perfused rat heart[12] and no AGT is present in the supernatant of serum-deprived neonatal cardiac cells,[13] which suggests that cardiac AGT is derived from the circulation. Similar observations have been published with respect to cardiac renin. Indeed, renin and renin mRNA levels in normal heart tissues are very low or even undetectable,[12,13] suggesting that, under normal conditions, cardiac renin is derived from plasma via two possible pathways: (a) diffusion in the interstitial space; (b) binding to receptors.[14]

The contribution of plasma renin to cardiac renin was tested by using transgenic mice expressing human renin in the liver (TTRhRen-A3), which were mated to mice expressing human AGT exclusively in the heart (MHChAgt-2). The results indicated low or undetectable angiotensin peptide in the heart of single transgenic animals while double transgenic mice showed a remarkable increase in cardiac levels of Ang I and Ang II, indicating that plasma renin is able to act on its substrate within the heart.[15]

However, this is not the whole history. It has been demonstrated that in some tissues a second renin gene transcription start site can be utilized leading to the synthesis of renin but lacking the secretory signal peptide. Initially found in the brain, the non-secreted transcript was also found in the myocardium, particularly during myocardial infarction,[16] when the cardiac RAS is activated. Indeed, the expression of exon1A-renin mRNA in the left ventricle was found to be stimulated four-fold during myocardial ischemia, supporting the view of an intracellular function of renin.[16]

More recently, it was shown that transgenic animal models used to investigate the role of the cardiac RAS provided important information. Overexpression of AGT gene in normal heart muscle cells of mice, for instance, caused an increase in Ang II concentration in the right and left ventricles and elicited hypertrophy of both ventricles without any change in arterial blood pressure.[17] These observations substantiate the notion of a cardiac RAS at the level of cardiac myocytes.

Up-regulation of cardiac ACE mRNA as well as protein has been reported in salt-sensitive types of hypertension, supporting the view that the cardiac RAS is in part responsible for the detrimental effects of salt overload.[18]

The concept of an intracrine RAS has been described previously[2,19,20] and is particularly important under pathological conditions when an increased expression of renin and AGT genes seems to occur in cardiac muscle. Evidence has been presented, for instance, that stretching of myocardial fibers enhanced the expression of these genes.[21,22] On the other hand, it is known that ACE and Ang II, at cardiac sites, are increased after myocardial infarction and ventricular hypertrophy induced by pressure overload.[23] Cardiac Ang II generation increases the expression of renin, AGT, AT_1 and AT_2, forming a positive feedback loop.[22] The left ventricular hypertrophy induced by aortic coarctation leads to an increase of renin and AGT mRNA in the left ventricle, while the renin levels in plasma are only transiently elevated.[24] The major question remains: what is the physiological or physiopathological significance of a cardiac RAS and particularly of an intracellular system?

RAS AND CELL-TO-CELL COMMUNICATION

Evidence is available that intercellular communication is impaired in the failing heart.[5] Indeed, the values of gap junction conductance measured in cell pairs isolated from the failing hearts of cardiomyopathic hamsters showed areas in which the gap junction conductance was extremely low (0.8–2.5 nS) and incompatible with impulse propagation.[3] Furthermore, measurements of transmembrane action potentials performed on isolated ventricles of the failing heart, at an advanced stage of the disease, showed some areas of the ventricular wall in which the impulse propagation was normal while in others block of impulse conduction occured. Histological studies revealed interstitial fibrosis, necrosis, and calcifications in the failing heart,[4] which explains, at least in part, the anisotropy and the impairment of impulse propagation. Moreover, the distribution of connexin 43, which is the main gap junction protein in mammals, is altered[25] in the failing heart, which might explain, at least in part, the abnormalities of impulse propagation.

The question as to whether the activation of the cardiac RAS is responsible for the changes in cell communication and impulse propagation in the failing heart is of seminal importance. It is known that activation of the plasma RAS during the process of heart failure is largely responsible for the impairment of heart function and the remodeling of the ventricle.[8,26] Furthermore, the activation of a local renin angiotensin in the failing heart,[19] might be implicated in cell abnormalities seen during this condition.

The mechanism by which the cardiac RAS is activated is not well known. Some hemodynamic changes or glucocorticoid treatment seem to increase the AGT mRNA levels in the heart.[26] Only local factors seem to be involved because stretching of the right ventricle activates the system in this ventricle but not in the left ventricle.[27]

Initial studies[3] demonstrated that in cardiomyopathic hamsters at an advanced stage of the disease with overt heart failure, Ang II (10^{-8} M) added to the extracellular medium caused cell uncoupling in cell pairs with very low values of junctional conductance (0.8–2.5 nS) and reduced gap junction conductance by $53 \pm 6.6\%$ in cell pairs with higher gap junction conductance values (7–35 nS).[3] The effect of the peptide is not related to a fall in surface membrane resistance (1.4 G Ω) which remained unchanged during the experiments. The decline or suppression of cell coupling elicited by extracellular Ang II administration requires the activation of protein kinase C (PKC), because PKC inhibitors abolished the effect of Ang II.[28] The activation of this kinase leads to phosphorylation of gap junction proteins with consequent decline of cell coupling. The effect of PKC activation on cell communication, however, seems to vary with the different states of phosphorylation of connexin 43 before the activation of PKC.[29]

It is known that tyrosine kinase represents a quite large family of molecules which play an important role in signal transduction and are involved in regulatory mechanisms such as growth and differentiation.[30] It has been shown that viral scr tyrosine protein kinase suppresses cell communication in fibroblasts.[31] Other studies showed that connexin 43 is a MAP kinase substrate in vivo and that phosphorylation of Ser 255, Ser 279, and Ser 282 initiates the down-regulation of junctional communication.[32] The levels of tyrosine-phosphorylated connexin 43 are increased in the heart of cardiomyopathic hamsters at an advanced stage of the disease.[33] These findings open the possibility that Ang II reduces the junctional conductance in the failing heart through tyrosine phosphorylation, an idea supported by the evidence that tyrosine phosphorylation is involved in Ang II-mediated signal transduction in different systems.[34]

Studies performed on neonatal heart cells indicated no Ang II generation, probably because of the lack of angiotensinogen or ACE in these cells.[13] However, in adult cardiomyocytes the situation is quite different because their incubation with ren-2^d prorenin led to the intracellular appearance of both Ang I and Ang II.[35] Although intracellular Ang II can be the result of synthesis or internalization, the presence of a RAS inside the cardiomyocyte (intracrine system) has been supported experimentally.[21] Similar observations were described in vascular smooth muscle cells in which intracellular Ang II promotes growth.[36–38] Indeed, when Ang I (10^{-9} M) was dialyzed inside myocytes isolated from the failing ventricle, the junctional conductance was greatly reduced,[3] an effect practically suppressed by enalaprilat given to the cytosol. This finding indicates that the effect of intracellular Ang I was related to its conversion to Ang II because intracellular Ang II, by itself, reduced or abolished cell coupling.[3] Furthermore, the decline in cell communication caused by intracellular dialysis of Ang II in isolated cell pairs of the failing heart was suppressed by intracellular administration of losartan (10^{-7} M) but not by the administration of the AT_1 blocker to the extracellular space. This finding might indicate that the peptide is acting intracellularly and that an intracellular Ang II receptor similar to AT_1 is involved in the decline of cell coupling. Indeed, evidence is available that there is an intracellular Ang II receptor.[39,40] Moreover, nuclear and chromatin Ang II receptors have been identified.[41] Immunochemical studies also indicated the presence of intracellular Ang II receptors in cardiomyocytes and fibroblasts,[42] an observation that contrasts with previous studies by Kato et al.,[43] which demonstrated that the porcine soluble Ang-binding protein is a microsomal endopeptidase.

The possible internalization of prorenin and the formation of renin inside the cardiac myocyte under pathological conditions might lead to two possible consequences: formation of Ang II inside the cell[35] with consequent intracellular action of the peptide or release of renin to the extracellular medium and formation of Ang II outside the cell with activation of AT_1 receptors. However, further studies are needed to characterize the possible intracellular role of renin.

As regards ACE, there is reliable evidence that the enzyme is synthesized at cardiac sites because ACE and ACE mRNA are detectable in the heart by autoradiography as well as in homogenate of cardiac muscle.[23,44] Is the ACE located intracellularly or at the surface cell membrane of cardiac myocytes? This is an important question because the uptake of renin by the heart might be followed by its release from the cardiomyocyte and consequent formation of Ang II at the level of the cell membrane. Previous observations indicated that in endothelial cells the enzyme is membrane-bound with the active site projecting into the extracellular space[45] and that the majority of its molecule is bound to the plasma membrane by a C-terminal transmembrane-spanning region.[45]

Recently, it was found that Ang I added to the extracellular fluid elicited an appreciable increase in cardiac excitability with the generation of spontaneous discharge of action potentials, a phenomenon suppressed by enalapril.[46] Evidence that Ang I is converted to Ang II at the cell membrane was provided by the change in inward calcium current elicited by Ang I in isolated cardiomyocytes – a change abolished by AT_1 blocker.[46] However, the question as to whether there is an intracellular ACE remains. It is known that there are tissue-bound and soluble forms of ACE[47] but no information is available as to whether there is a soluble form of the enzyme inside the cell.

ANG II, ALDOSTERONE, AND CARDIAC FIBROBLASTS

The persistent activation of the RAS and the increment in the cardiac levels of Ang II, however, lead to remodeling of the gap junctions and interstitial fibrosis. Studies by Booz and Baker[48] showed that chronic infusion of Ang II induces fibrosis, an effect reduced by AT_1 receptor antagonists or ACE inhibitors. The activation of AT_1 receptors in fibroblasts activates MAP kinases and the JAK/STAT pathways, with consequent increased expression of AGT and fibrosis-related proteins.[49]

The enhanced stiffness caused by abnormal collagen deposition seen in the failing heart is in part related to cytokines, particularly interleukin-6, tumor necrosis factor-α (TNF-α), and the transforming growth factor-β (TGF-β).[50] Fibroblast growth factor-2 (FGF-2), an endogenous growth-promoting protein, is involved in tyrosine-dependent phosphorylation of connexin 43 in cardiac myocytes[51] and represents an example of the role of fibroblasts in the regulation of metabolic coupling between cardiomyocytes. These findings not only indicate that Ang II elicits cellular sequestration through the generation of fibrosis but also that there is a cross-talk between fibroblasts and cardiac myocytes (see Figure 10.1).

The presence of aldosterone receptors in cardiac muscle[52,53] and the evidence that the heart can synthesize aldosterone, lead to the conclusion that aldosterone plays an important role in cardiac function. Adverse effects of aldosterone include interstitial fibrosis, congestive heart failure, and cardiac arrhythmias.

Aldosterone induces myocardial fibrosis independently of its effect on blood pressure because the hormone causes fibrosis in the right ventricle and pulmonary artery.[54]

The mechanisms involved in the profibrotic effect of aldosterone are: (1) an increase of AT_1 receptor density; (2) an increased expression of ACE; (3) and reactive oxygen species generation in which the RAS is

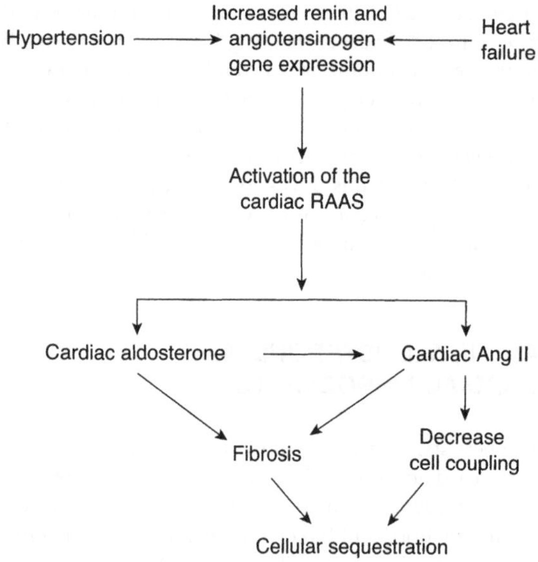

Figure 10.1 Diagram illustrating the role of the cardiac renin-angiotensin-aldosterone system (RAAS) on fibrosis, cell coupling, and cellular sequestration

involved.[55] These observations have important clinical implications because treatment with ACE inhibitors does not reliably suppress aldosterone production. This phenomenon of 'aldosterone escape' occurs in about 40% of patients with congestive heart failure.[56]

INTRACELLULAR AND EXTRACELLULAR ANG II MODULATE THE INWARD CALCIUM CURRENT IN THE FAILING HEART

The influence of intracellular and extracellular Ang II on the L-type calcium current of cardiomyocytes isolated from cardiomyopathic hamsters was investigated.[57] The results indicated that Ang II (10^{-8} mmol/L), added to the bath, increased the peak I_{Ca} density by $37 \pm 3.4\%$ ($p < 0.05$), an effect that depends on the activation of PKC. Intracellular administration of the same dose of Ang II (10^{-8} mmol/L) also elicited an increase of peak I_{Ca} density but enhanced the rate of I_{Ca} inactivation, an effect not seen with extracellular Ang II. Moreover, in control animals no change in the rate of I_{Ca} inactivation was seen with intracellular Ang II. Thapsigargin (1 μmol/L), a potent inhibitor of sarcoplasmic reticulum (SR) ATPase which depletes the SR, decreased the rate of I_{Ca} inactivation elicited by intracellular Ang II even though the cytoplasmic calcium concentration was highly buffered with 10 mmol/L EGTA. These findings might indicate that intracellular Ang II releases calcium from the SR and inactivates I_{Ca}. The effect of intracellular Ang II on peak I_{Ca} was not altered by extracellular losartan (10^{-7} mmol/L), supporting the notion that the peptide acted intracellularly.

Other studies showed that intracellular administration of Ang I (10^{-8} mmol/L) enhanced the peak I_{Ca} density and the rate of I_{Ca} inactivation, an effect that was reduced by intracellular enalaprilat (10^{-8} mmol/L). Moreover, intracellular enalaprilat, by itself, reduced the peak I_{Ca} density.[57] These observations might indicate that endogenous Ang II is contributing to the modulation of I_{Ca} in the failing heart.

CONCLUSION

The activation of the cardiac renin angiotensin aldosterone system (RAAS) during the process of heart failure and hypertension induces cellular sequestration by promoting remodeling of the gap junctions and interstitial fibrosis (see Figure 10.1). Therefore, the establishment of slow conduction pathways facilitates the generation of cardiac arrhythmias. The presence of aldosterone receptors and the enhanced production of the hormone in the failing heart indicates that aldosterone is an important factor in the formation of interstitial fibrosis. Evidence is available that there is a relationship between Ang II and aldosterone, which represents an important topic for further studies.

The beneficial effects of ACE inhibitors and AT_1 blockers seen in the failing heart are related to different effects of these drugs, including improvement of cell coupling and decrease of cardiac fibrosis with consequent decline of cellular sequestration.

REFERENCES

1. Koch Weser J. Nature of inotropic action of angiotensin on ventricular myocardium. Circ Res 1965; 16: 230–7.
2. De Mello WC. Is an intracellular renin angiotensin system involved in the control of cell communication in heart? J Cardiovasc Pharmacol 1994; 23: 640–6.
3. De Mello WC. Renin angiotensin system and cell communication in the failing heart. Hypertension 1996; 27: 1267–72.
4. De Mello WC, Cherry R, Manivannan S. Electrophysiologic and morphologic abnormalities in the failing heart; effect of enalapril on electrical properties. J Card Failure 1997; 3: 53–62.
5. De Mello WC. Cell coupling and impulse propagation in the failing heart: the possible role of the renin angiotensin system. In: De Mello WC, Janse M (eds). Heart Cell Coupling and Impulse Propagation in Health and Disease. Boston: Kluwer Academic, 2002, pp 283–320.

6. Horiuchi M, Hayashida W, Kambe T et al. Angiotensin type 2 receptor dephosphorylates Bcl-2 by activating mitigen-activated protein kinase phosphatase-1 and induces apoptosis. J Biol Chem 1997; 272: 19022–6.
7. Dzau VJ. Implications of local angiotensin production in cardiovascular physiology and pharmacology. Am J Cardiol 1987; 59 (Suppl A): 59A–65A.
8. Nicholls MG, Richards AM, Agarwal M. The importance of the renin angiotensin system in cardiovascular disease. J Hum Hypertens 1998; 12: 295–9.
9. Katz SA, Opsahl JA, Lunzer MM, Forbis LM, Hirsch AT. Effect of bilateral nephrectomy on active renin, angiotensinogen, and renin glycoforms in plasma and myocardium. Hypertension 1997; 30: 259–66.
10. Danser AHJ, van Katz JP, Admiraal PJJ et al. Cardiac renin and angiotensins. Uptake from plasma versus in situ synthesis. Hypertension 1994; 24: 37–48.
11. Campbell DJ, Valentin AJ. Identification of vascular renin-binding proteins by chemical cross-linking: inhibition of renin by renin inhibitors. J Hypertens 1994; 12: 879–90.
12. de Lannoy LM, Danser AHJ, van Katz JP et al. Renin angiotensin system components in the interstitial fluid of isolated perfused rat heart: local production of angiotensin I. Hypertension 1997; 29: 1240–51.
13. van Kesteren CAM, Saris JJ, Dekkers FHM et al. Cultured neonatal rat cardiac myocytes and fibroblasts do not synthesize renin or angiotensinogen: evidence for stretch-induced cardiomyocyte hypertrophy independent of angiotensin II. Cardiovasc Res 1999; 43: 148–56.
14 Nguyen G, Burckle C, Tremey B. The cardiac renin receptors. In: De Mello WC (ed). Renin Angiotensin System and the Heart. Chichester: John Wiley and Sons, 2004, pp 74–83.
15. Prescott G, Siversides DW, Chiu SML, Reudelhuber TL. Contribution of circulating renin to local synthesis of angiotensin peptides in the heart. Physiol Genomics 2000; 4: 67–73.
16. Clausmeyer S, Reinecke A, Farrenkoft R et al. Tissue-specific expression of a rat renin transcript lacking the coding sequence for the prefragment and its stimulation by myocardial infarction. Endocrinology 2000; 141: 2963–70.
17. Mazzolai L, Nussberger J, Aubert JF et al. Blood pressure-independent cardiac hypertrophy induced by local activated renin angiotensin system. Hypertension 1998; 31: 1324–30.
18. Zhao X, White R, Van Huysse L, Leenen FH. Cardiac hypertrophy and cardiac renin angiotensin system in Dahl rats on high salt uptake. J Hypertens 2000; 18: 1319–26.
19. De Mello WC, Danser AHJ. Angiotensin II and the heart. On the intracrine renin angiotensin system. Hypertension 2000; 35: 1183–8.
20. De Mello WC, Re RN. Is an intracrine renin angiotensin system involved in the control of cardiovascular function? In: Pawan K, Sigal I, Dixon MC, Lorrie A, Kirshenbaum, Dhalla S (eds). Cardiac Remodeling and Failure. Boston: Kluwer Academic, 2003, pp 365–75.
21. Malhotra R, Sadoshima J, Broscius FC, Izumo S. Mechanical stretch and angiotensin II differentially upregulated the renin angiotensin system in cardiac myocytes in vitro. Circ Res 1999; 85: 137–46.
22. Tamura K, Umemura S, Nyui N et al. Activation of angiotensinogen gene in cardiac myocytes by angiotensin II and mechanical stretch. Am J Physiol 1998; 44: R1–R9.
23. Yamada H, Fabris B, Allen AM, Jackson CI, Mendelsohn AO. Localization of angiotensin converting enzyme in rat heart. Circ Res 1991; 68: 141–9.
24. Baker K, Chermin M, Wixcon S, Aceto J. Renin angiotensin system involvement in pressure-overload cardiac hypertrophy in rats. Am J Physiol 1990; 259: H324–H332.
25. De Mello WC. Cell coupling and impulse propagation in the failing heart. J Cardiovasc Electrophysiol 1999; 10: 1409–20.
26. Lindpaintner K, Jin MW, Niedrmaier N, Wilhelm MJ, Ganten D. Cardiac angiotensinogen and its local activation in the isolated perfused beating heart. Circ Res 1990; 67: 564–73.
27. Lee YA, Liang CS, Lee HA, Lindpaintner K. Local stress, not systemic factors regulate gene expression of cardiac renin angiotensin system in vivo: a comprehensive study of all its components in the dog. Proc Natl Acad Sci U S A 1996; 93: 11035–40.
28. De Mello WC, Altieri P. The role of the renin angiotensin system in the control of cell communication in the heart; effects of angiotensin II and enalapril. J Cardiovasc Pharmacol 1992; 20: 643–51.
29. Imanaga I, Hirosawa N, Lin H et al. Phosphorylation of connexin 43 and regulation of cardiac gap junctions. In: De Mello WC, Janse M (eds). Heart Cell Coupling and Impulse Propagation in Health and Disease. Boston: Kluwer Academic, 2002, pp 185–205.
30. Hunter T. Tyrosine phosphorylation: past, present and future. Biochem Soc Trans Hopkins Medal Lecture 1996; 24: 307–27.
31. Atkinson MM, Menko AS, Johnson RG et al. Rapid and reversible reduction of junctional permeability in cells infected with a temperature-sensitive mutant of avian sarcome virus. J Cell Biol 1981; 91: 573–8.
32. Zhou L, Kasperek EM, Nicholson BJ. Dissection of the molecular basis of Pp60-src induced gating of connexin43 gap junctions. J Cell Biol 1999; 144: 1033–45.
33. Toyofuku T, Yabuki M, Otsu K, Kusaya T, Tada M, Hori M. Functional role of c-src in gap junctions of the cardiomyopathic hamster heart. Circ Res 1999; 85: 672–81.
34. Haendeler J, Berk B. Tyrosine phosphorylation is involved in Ang II-mediated signal transduction. Regul Pept 2000; 95: 1–7.
35. Peters J, Farrenkopf R, Clausmeyer S et al. Functional significance of prorenin internalization in the rat heart. Circ Res 2002; 90: 1135–41.
36. Filipenu CM, Henning RH, de Zeeuw D, Nelemans A. Intracellular angiotensin II and cell growth of vascular smooth muscle cells. Br J Pharmacol 2001; 132: 1590–6.
37. Eto K, Ohya Y, Nakamura Y, Abe I, Lida M. Intracellular angiotensin II stimulates voltage-operated Ca^{2+} channels in arterial myocytes. Hypertension 2002; 39: 474–8.
38. Cook JL, Zhung Z, Re RN. In vitro evidence for an intracellular site of angiotensin action. Circ Res 2001; 89: 1138–46.
39. Baker KM, Campanile MP, Trachte GJ, Peach MJ. Identification and characterization of the rabbit angiotensin II myocardial receptor. Circ Res 1984; 54: 286–93.
40. Sen I, Rajasekaran AK. Angiotensin II-binding protein in adult and neonatal rat heart. J Mol Cell Cardiol 1991; 23: 563–72.
41. Re RN, LaBiche RA, Bryan SE. Nuclear-hormone mediated changes in chromatin solubility. Biochem Biophys Res Commun 1983; 110: 61–8.
42. Fu ML, Schulze W, Wallukat G et al. Immunochemical localization of angiotensin II receptor (AT1) in the heart with anti-peptide antibody showing a positive chronotropic effect. Receptor Channels 1998; 6: 99–111.
43. Kato A, Sugiura N, Hagiwara H, Hirose S. Cloning, amino acid sequence and tissue distribution of porcine thimet oligopeptidase. A comparison with soluble angiotensin-binding protein. Eur J Biochem 1994; 221: 159–65.
44. De Mello WC, Crespo MJ. Correlation between changes in morphology, electrical properties and angiotensin converting enzyme activity in the failing heart. Eur J Pharmacol 1999; 378: 187–94.
45. Soubrier F, Alhenc-Gelas F, Hubert C et al. Two putative active centers in human angiotensin I-converting enzyme revealed by molecular cloning. Proc Natl Acad Sci U S A 1988; 85: 9386–90.

46. De Mello WC. Angiotensin converting enzyme and the arhythmogenic action of angiotensin I: cardiac cell membrane as a site of angiotensin I conversion. Regul Pept 2004; 121: 83–8.
47. Aersten WM, Schuijt MP, Danser AH, Daemen MJ, Smits JF. The role of locally expressed angiotensin converting enzyme in cardiac remodeling after myocardial infarction in mice. Cardiovasc Res 2002; 92: 651–8.
48. Booz GW, Baker KM. Molecular signaling mechanisms controlling growth and function of cardiac fibroblasts. Cardiovasc Res 1995; 30: 537–43.
49. Lijnen PJ, Petrov VV, Fagard RH. Angiotensin II-induced stimulation of collagen secretion and production in cardiac fibroblasts is mediated via angiotensin II subtype 1 receptors. Renin Angiotensin Aldosterone Syst 2001; 2: 117–22.
50. Sarkar S, Vellaichamy E, Young D, Sen S. Influence of cytokines and growth factors in Ang II-mediated collagen upregulation by fibroblasts in rats; role of myocytes. Am J Physiol Heart Circ Physiol 2004; 287: 107–17.
51. Doble BW, Chen Y, Bosc DG, Litchfield DW, Kardami E. Fibroblast growth factor-2 decreases metabolic coupling and stimulates phosphorylation as well as masking of connexin43 epitopes in cardiac myocytes. Circ Res 1996; 79: 647–58.
52. Bonvalet JP, Alfaidy N, Farman N, Lombes M. Aldosterone intracellular receptors in human heart. Eur Heart J 1995; 16 (Suppl N); 92–7.
53. Delcayre C, Swynghedauw B. Molecular mechanisms of myocardial remodeling. The role of aldosterone. J Mol Cell Cardiol 2002; 34: 1577–84.
54. Schmidt BM, Schmieder RE. Aldosterone-induced cardiac damage: focus on blood pressure independent effects. Am J Hypertens 2003; 16: 80–6.
55. Iglarz M, Touyz RM, Viel EC, Amiri F, Schiffrin EL. Involvement of oxidative stress in the profibrotic action of aldosterone: interaction with the renin-angiotensin system. Am J Hypertens 2004; 17: 597–603.
56. Struthers AD. The clinical implications of aldosterone escape in congestive heart failure. Eur J Heart Fail 2004; 6: 539–45.
57. De Mello WC, Monterrubio J. Intracellular and extracellular angiotensin II enhance the L-type calcium current in the failing heart. Hypertension 2004; 4: 1–5.

11

Intracrine mechanisms in hypertension

Julia L Cook and Richard N Re

INTRODUCTION

Although by definition arterial hypertension is a hemodynamic disease, the primary cause of the disorder in young and middle-aged individuals usually does not involve structural abnormalities in the arteries themselves. Rather the increased pressure found in the early hypertensive patient results from impaired pressure natriuresis associated with functional vasoconstriction, volume overload, or both, with fixed architectural changes in the vessels usually occurring later in the history of the disorder. Moreover, the causes of vasoconstriction and impaired natriuresis are multiple so that idiopathic (essential) hypertension can be considered a multifaceted disease process resulting from the abnormal elaboration of vasoconstricting and/or fluid-retaining physiological signals, be they neurotransmitters at nerve terminals abutting vascular smooth muscle cells in arteries, vasoconstricting peptides such as angiotensin (Ang), or sodium-retaining hormones such as aldosterone. Moreover, some heritable forms of hypertension have been shown to be associated with disorders of hormone-associated receptors and intracellular signaling cascades leading to abnormal signaling and hypertension. This formulation of the causation of hypertension has been extremely productive and has led to the understanding of the roles of signaling proteins like renin in the genesis and treatment of hypertension.[1,2]

Yet for all its success, the above schema may be incomplete in an important way because it is, in part, based on the tacit assumption that all peptide hormone signaling is mediated by cell surface receptors and that knowledge of the status of these hormones and their cognate receptors is sufficient to predict their effect on the physiologic state of a tissue. While this may be true in the example of dynamic vasoconstriction, there is reason to believe that it is not the case for longer-term growth abnormalities that are produced by hypertensinogenic hormones which lead to the sequelae of hypertension. The idea that some peptide/protein hormones can act within cells after internalization and even in cells which synthesize them (i.e. without benefit of secretion) is old but remains little appreciated.[1,3–6] Two decades ago we introduced the term *intracrine* for the intracellular action of a peptide hormone either after internalization or retention in the cell that synthesized it.[7,8] Thereafter, evidence was developed to support the association of intracrine functionality with many hormones and growth factors, as well as with some transcription factors and enzymes. For example, there are enzymes (such as phospholipase A2-I, acetyl cholinesterase R, and phosphoglucose isomerase) which, in addition to serving catalytic functions, can also be secreted whereupon they act as signaling molecules; and these intracrine enzymes act in the intracellular space either after internalization or retention in their cells of synthesis.[9–11] As is evident from Box 11.1,[6,9–22] the number of known intracrines is large. Thus intracrine action, although not widely appreciated, is not uncommon. Over time, the term intracrine has also been applied by others to steroid hormones which either directly or following intracellular modification act within the cells that synthesized them. While these mechanisms undoubtedly occur and while they are physiologically relevant, the principal focus of this chapter will be peptide intracrines because their role in hypertension has been studied in more detail. Indeed, one of the earliest studied intracrines was Ang II. In 1971, it was reported that the infusion of labeled Ang II into rats led to the detection of tracer in the nuclei and mitochondria of cardiac myocytes within seconds.[23] Although these early experiments could be challenged on methodological grounds, the basic finding has been reproduced over the years with ever more sophisticated imaging techniques.

Box 11.1 Intracrines

Insulin
Prolactin
Fibroblast growth factor (FGF) (1,2,3,10)
Midkine
Angiotensin
Angiogenin (RNase)
Vascular endothelial growth factor (VEGF)
Interferon (IFN)-β, γ
Interleukins
Nerve growth factor (NGF)
Platelet-derived growth factor (PDGF)
Parathyroid hormone-related protein (PTHrP)
Pleiotrophin
Proenkephalin
Homeoproteins
Insulin-like growth factor 1 (IGF-1)
Lactoferrin
Heregulin
Growth hormone
Somatostatin
Epidermal growth factor (EGF)
Tat
Thyrotropin-releasing hormone (TRH)
Luteinizing hormone-releasing hormone (LHRH)
Vasoactive intestinal polypeptide (VIP)
Defensins
Factor J
PLA2-I
Atrial natriuretic peptide (ANP)
Hepatoma-derived growth factor
Brain-derived neurotrophic factor
Gonadotropin
Chorionic gonadotropin
Pigmented epithelium-derived factor (a serpin)
Maspin (a serpin)
Schwannoma-derived growth factor
Leukemia inhibiting factor
Endogenous opioids (dynorphin)
Phosphoglucose isomerase/neuroleukin
Oxytocin
Macrophage colony-stimulating factor (CSF-1)
Hepatopoietin
Renin/prorenin (aspartyl-protease)
Leptin
Amphoterin (HMGB1)
PD-ECGF/thymidine phosphorylase
Transforming growth factor-α (TGF-α)
Insulin-like growth factor binding protein (IGFBP) 3, 5
Granzyme A, B
Hepatopoietin
ESkine/CCL 27
Thioredoxin
PAI-2 (a serpin)
Reelin
Sex hormone-binding globulin (SHBG)
Pancreatic bile salt-dependent lipase
Macrophage migration inhibitory factor
Urokinase
Endothelin
Ribosomal protein S 19
Trp-tRNA synthetase
Pituitary adenylate cyclase activating polypeptide
Neuropeptide Y
Erythropoietin
ACE (?)
Angiotensinogen
ACheR

References.[6,9–22]

THE INTRACRINE RENIN-ANGIOTENSIN SYSTEM (iRAS)

This chapter is, in part, intended to provide an overview and chronicle the published literature relating to intracellular Ang II and the AT_1 receptor (AT_1R), and the trafficking, function, and fate of intracellular components of the renin-angiotensin system (RAS). These will be presented in the venue of other peptide systems that are recognized to function as both archetypal endocrine and atypical intracellular hormone systems. These investigations are also tabulated according to specific study principles in Tables 11.1–11.4.[23–47] While this review is extensive it may not be comprehensive.

Table 11.1 Ang II associates with cellular nuclei (or other subcellular organelles) in experimental systems

Authors	*Cell type/tissue*	*Comments*
Robertson and Khairallah (1971)[23]	Labeled Ang II, injected into rat heart: associates with nuclei of smooth and cardiac muscle cells	
Goodfriend et al. (1972)[24]	Labeled Ang II binds to mitochondria from rat, rabbit and bovine (adrenals, heart, renal artery, brain)	
Sirett et al. (1977)[25]	Labeled Ang II binds to rat brain in a section-specific differential manner	90% of binding is in the crude microsomal fraction
Re et al. (1981)[26]	Rat liver and spleen nuclei	Ang II competes with labeled Ang II for nuclear binding; binding occurs through a specific receptor
Tang et al. (1992)[27]	Rat liver nuclei	Labeled Ang II binds to nuclei, binding is losartan-inhibited
Booz et al. (1992)[28]	Rat liver nuclei	Labeled Ang II binds specifically to nuclei, losartan inhibits binding, PD123177 does not
Haller et al. (1996)[29]	Rat aortic vascular smooth muscle cells	Nuclear fluorescein-labeled Ang II accumulates following Ang II cellular microinjection. Intracellular Ang II increases cytosolic and nuclear calcium

Overview: years 1970–1989

Studies suggesting that Ang II binding activity resides within intracellular organelles were reported as early as the 1970s. Robertson and Khairallah[23] found that labeled Ang II injected into the left ventricle of adult rats was preferentially localized in the nuclear zone of vascular and cardiac muscle cells, suggesting a potential nuclear function. They further showed the presence of labeled Ang II in or directly associated with mitochondria. These observations were, in part, corroborated by Goodfriend and colleagues,[24] who found Ang II binding activity to be high in mitochondrial fractions and intact mitochondria from bovine kidney and adrenal cortices.

In subsequent studies, our laboratory showed that isolated rat liver and spleen nuclei specifically bound ^{125}I-labeled Ang II with high affinity. In these studies, Ang II competed effectively for radiolabeled tracer, whereas Ang I did so less effectively and neurotensin not at all, suggesting that Ang II bound to a specific nuclear receptor. We further demonstrated ^{125}I-Ang II binding to solubilized rat liver chromatin fragments, the existence of a discrete Ang II-binding nucleoprotein particle by deoxynucleoprotein gel electrophoresis, and direct effects of nuclear angiotensin on transcription.[26,44,48,49] Ang treatment of nuclei led to enhanced solubilization of chromatin following micrococcal nuclease digestion, a finding consistent with enhanced gene transcription; Ang treatment also led to solubilization of its nuclear receptor. These findings strongly suggest a nuclear chromatin localization for at least some of the nuclear Ang receptors.

Consistent with these early studies and interpretations, Inagami and colleagues,[37] in the course of investigating a number of mouse and rat neuroblastoma cell lines, showed that at least three of these possessed renin, angiotensin converting enzyme (ACE), Ang I and Ang II, leading them to suggest that Ang II can be generated in an intracellular fashion.

Overview: years 1990–1999

Studies succeeding those of Inagami and colleagues[37] (see above) have confirmed the existence of intracellular Ang II in *normal* brain tissue. Erdmann and

Table 11.2 Endogenous Ang II, angiotensinogen and/or AT_1 receptor exist in native cells

Authors	*Cell type/tissue*	*Comments*
Erdmann et al. (1996)[30]	Rat cerebellum (also rat hepatocytes, rat adrenal glomerular cells)	Ang II immunoreactivity in nuclei of Purkinje, granule, basket, stellate cells. In endothelial and granule cells, Ang II clearly associated with euchromatin
Van Kats et al. (2001)[31]	Pig kidney and adrenals	Ang II synthesis occurs predominantly extracellularly and is followed by receptor-mediated endocytosis resulting in high intracellular levels of Ang II
Lu et al. (1998)[32]	Primary rat brain neurons	Ang II treatment induces nuclear targeting of the AT_1 receptor
Bkaily et al. (2003)[33]	Human vascular smooth muscle cells	Ang II induces internalization and nuclear transport of human AT_1R or human AT_1R-GFP in transfected cells
Jacques et al. (2003)[34]	Human endocardial endothelial cells	Native Ang II, AT_1R and AT_2R in these cells. Ang II throughout cell, cytosol > nucleus. AT_1R throughout cell, nucleus > cytoplasm. AT_2R only in nucleus
Licea et al. (2002)[35]	Rat kidney	AT_1R in nuclear and membrane fractions
Fu et al. (1998)[36]	Rat heart sections	Ang II receptors present in nuclei of cardiomyocytes
Okamura et al. (1981)[37]	Rat and mouse neuroblastoma cells	Immunoreactive Ang I and Ang II coexist with renin and ACE in juxtaglomerular cells, suggesting intracellular formation of angiotensins
Amedeo Modesti et al. (2002)[38]	Neonatal cardiac myocytes	Ang II present in granular cytoplasm
Mercure et al. (1998)[39]	Rat juxtaglomerular cells	Immunoreactive renin and Ang II in cells; renin suppression results in Ang II down-regulation suggesting that intracellular Ang II is generated from renin
Zhuo et al. (2002)[40]	Rat renal endosomes	Accumulation of Ang II in renal cortical endosomes
Thomas et al. (2003)[41]	Rat hypothalamus	Ang II and AT_1 receptor found within glia and neurons *in situ*
Vila-Porcile and Corvol (1998)[42]	Rat anterior pituitary	Angiotensinogen, prorenin and renin are colocalized in secretory granules, suggesting intracellular processing of angiotensinogen

colleagues,[30] using immunogold staining, found Ang II immunoreactivity to be prominent in cerebellar neurons including Purkinje, granule, basket, and stellate cells. The peptide was localized to nuclei and also to vesicle-like structures in cytoplasm. In some cell types such as endothelial and granule cells, the peptide was nearly exclusively present in the transcriptionally active euchromatin, leading the authors to suggest that Ang II directly regulates gene expression. Moreover, Vila-Porcile and Corvol,[42] also using immunogold labeling methods, found angiotensinogen (AGT), prorenin, and renin to be present in all the glandular cell types of

Table 11.3 Ang II associates with chromatin

Authors	*Cell type/tissue*	*Comments*
Re and Parab (1984)[43]	Rat liver nuclei	Ang II increases RNA synthesis
Re et al. (1984)[44]	Rat liver nuclei	Labeled Ang II binds chromatin, DNPP resolved by gel electrophoresis
Erdmann et al. (1996)[30]	Rat cerebellar cortex	Ang II immunoreactivity in Purkinje, granule, basket, stellant cells. In endothelial and granule cells, Ang II clearly associated with euchromatin
Eggena et al. (1993, 1996)[45,46]	Rat liver nuclei	Ang II increases angiotensinogen, renin, platelet-derived growth factor and *c-myc* transcription

Table 11.4 Characterization of the intracellular receptor

Authors	*Cell type/tissue*	*Comments*
Booz et al. (1992)[28]	Ang II binding sites on rat liver nuclei	Losartan inhibits binding, PD123177 does not. They suggested that nuclear envelopes have a G protein-coupled Ang II binding site, with properties different from the plasma membrane receptor
Tang et al. (1992)[27]	Ang II binding sites in rat liver	Partially characterized receptor: kinetics, size, pharmacokinetics. Similar to AT_1 receptor
Eggena et al. (1993, 1996)[45,46]	Ang II nuclear receptors exist in rat liver	Stimulate the production of renin, angiotensinogen, platelet-derived growth factor, *c-myc*
Jimenez et al. (1994)[47]	Ang II binding sites exist in rat liver	Ang II-receptor complexes identified, processing through the Golgi may be involved in the nuclear accumulation of Ang II

the rat anterior pituitary. The simultaneous detection of the substrate with the cleavage enzyme within the same granules led the authors to suggest intragranular processing of AGT and product secretion via the regulated secretory pathway.

This decade also coincided with further characterization of the intracellular receptor. Baker and colleagues[28] described the kinetics of Ang II binding (versus competitors) to rat liver nuclei and nuclear envelopes, and showed that inhibitors of AT_1R-Ang II binding (losartan) also inhibited Ang II–nuclear receptor interactions, suggesting that the nuclear receptor is of an AT_1-like nature. Dzau and colleagues,[27] in the same year, also characterized the Ang II rat liver nuclear receptor; their results suggested it to be AT_1-like (similar in size and losartan-inhibited) but distinct with respect to several physicochemical properties.

Jimenez and colleagues[47] further characterized Ang II receptors from rat liver nuclei using selective ligands for AT_1 and AT_2 subtypes in radioligand binding and isoelectric focusing assays. They found adult rat liver cells to possess only AT_1 receptors, although isoelectric focusing profiles revealed two Ang II–receptor complex peaks (pI=6.5 and 6.8) for plasma membrane and one peak (pI=6.8) for nuclear preparations. The authors suggest that this charge heterogeneity could account for the distinct physicochemical properties of nuclear versus plasma membrane receptors previously detected.[27] They also suggest that post-translational modifications could accompany receptor endocytosis and recycling and could account for the charge variability. They further showed that monensin, which disrupts Golgi trafficking, does inhibit nuclear accumulation of the labeled peptide, suggesting that Golgi bodies might be involved in Ang II nuclear accumulation.

Initial studies addressing the mechanism by which the receptor becomes associated with the nucleus were also performed late in this decade. In 1998, Raizada and colleagues[32] showed that Ang II-induced chronic neuromodulatory stimulation of rat primary neuronal cultures leads to nuclear sequestration of the AT_1 receptor, presumably involving the putative nuclear localization signal within the cytoplasmic tail of the receptor. Since other studies[27,47] suggest that the nuclear receptor is distinct from the plasma membrane receptor, it is possible that multiple receptors or multiple forms of the same receptor can reside in the nucleus depending on cell type and condition.

In studies that corroborate and extend our reports of the 1980s, Eggena and colleagues reported that Ang II treatment of rat liver nuclei induces specific transcriptional changes.[45,46] *c-myc*, platelet-derived growth factor (PDGF), renin and AGT mRNA levels were all found to increase (as determined by nuclear run-on assays), in a biphasic dose-dependent fashion, following Ang II exposure. The mechanics of Ang II–receptor stimulation of transcription were not apparent from these studies. No attempt was made to differentiate direct versus indirect effects upon transcription. Evidence also points to the rapid and direct stimulation of cellular Ca^{2+} uptake by vascular smooth muscle cells (VSMCs) injected with Ang II.[29] Haller and colleagues showed that microinjected fluorescein-labeled Ang II was rapidly distributed between the cytoplasm and nucleus and was accompanied by an increase in Ca^{2+} uptake, suggesting a direct effect of intracellular Ang II upon membrane-associated Ca^{2+} channels.[29] Moreover, De Mello and colleagues have shown that intracellular dialysis of either Ang II or renin into adult ventricular cardiac myocytes reduces junctional conductance. Ang II instillation is sensitive to co-dialysis of the AT_1 receptor blocker, losartan, while renin dialysis is sensitive to the ACE inhibitor, enaliprilat.[50–52] These results are consistent with the idea that (1) the reduction in junctional conductance (and thus electrical coupling) is the result of Ang action at an intracellular AT_1 receptor and (2) Ang II may be generated intracellularly in the presence of renin. As such the intracellular RAS may interfere with heart contractility and impulse propagation, contributing to heart failure. Further studies suggest that hypertension may increase intracellular myocyte accumulation of Ang II, which in turn may lead to oxidative damage and cardiac cell death.[53]

Collectively, these studies suggest that Ang II may be internalized or generated through an intracrine system and that it alters cellular properties both by modifying cytoplasmic pathways and by undergoing nuclear translocation, receptor binding, and transcriptional regulation of gene expression. Furthermore, the nuclear receptor is likely identical to, or distinct from but quite similar to, the plasma membrane AT_1 receptor.

Overview: years 2000–2004

The turn of the century coincided with a renewed interest in the intracellular RAS. Two reports from Canada corroborated and strengthened prior findings suggesting that extracellular Ang II treatment leads to intranuclear AT_1 receptor accumulation. Bkaily and co-investigators[33] showed that Ang II treatment of human primary aortic VSMCs induced internalization and nuclear translocation of the AT_1R as well as dose-dependent increases in nuclear and cytoplasmic calcium. In native as well as in normal human AT_1R or human AT_1R-GFP overexpressing VSMCs, Ang II induced internalization via clathrin-coated pits and nuclear translocation of the corresponding receptor. Furthermore, nuclear receptor accumulation appeared to stimulate *de novo* receptor production consistent with a pathologic positive feedback loop. Jacques and colleagues[34] showed the existence of Ang II, AT_1R and AT_2R in native human fetal endocardial endothelial cells. Ang II was found to be present in the nucleus and cytoplasm. They also showed that extracellular Ang II treatment induced a dose-dependent sustained increase in free cytosolic and nuclear calcium, suggesting signal transduction consequences.

Our laboratory, in the early 2000s, was possibly the first to report effects of intracellular Ang II–AT_1R interactions on cellular function and growth dynamics.[54] In order to investigate the effect of Ang II generation within cells, we mutated the rat AGT cDNA to remove the signal peptide-encoding region and ligated it into an expression plasmid to encode a non-secreted form of AGT.[54] Ang II produced from this construct is, in theory, generated through an intracrine mechanism. We investigated the effect of this plasmid, in the presence of various effectors, upon cellular proliferation. Rat hepatoma cells (H4-II-E-C3 cells, which produce renin and ACE mRNAs) were stably transfected with this experimental expression plasmid and mitotic indices were measured for stably transfected cell lines. Experimental clonal cell lines showed an average increase of $33 \pm 4.4\%$ ($p < 0.001$) in BrdU-labeled nuclei compared with control cell lines. The mitogenic effect was blocked by renin antisense phosphorothioate oligomers but not by candesartan. PDGF mRNA levels were found to be elevated 2.2-fold in transfected cell lines; addition of anti-PDGF antibodies to the culture medium partially blocked the mitogenic effect while anti-Ang II antibodies had no effect. Moreover, we showed that a GFP fusion of the experimental intracellular AGT product is retained intracellularly and is diffusely cytoplasmic.[55] These results suggest that the growth effect of the experimental plasmid is due, in part, to autocrine/paracrine stimulation by secreted PDGF following Ang II/Ang II receptor intracellular interactions. We also demonstrated that H4-II-E-C3 cells produce a recently identified alternative renin transcript, renin 1A, which lacks a signal sequence and is maintained intracellularly. Collectively, these studies of cultured cells suggest that some cell types may possess components of the RAS which permit intracellular processing of AGT to Ang II and that Ang II generated intracellularly may be mitogenic. Pending investigations in transgenic animals will allow us to further elucidate the mechanism, tissue specificity and prevalence of intracellular AGT processing as well as the function of Ang II generated in this fashion.

In more recent studies,[56] we reported that co-expression of ECFP/Ang II (Ang II fused to cyan fluorescent protein) and AT_1R/EYFP (AT_1 receptor fused to yellow fluorescent protein) enhances proliferation of COS-7 and CHO-K1 cells by 59% and 64%, respectively, compared with cells expressing the corresponding independent proteins ($p<0.001$ for both). The growth effect is independent of anti-Ang II antibodies, suggesting that it does not reflect Ang II secretion into the culture media; Ang II is also undetectable in the media. Expression of AT_1R/EYFP with ECFP/Ang II_C (control scrambled sequence Ang II fused to cyan fluorescent protein) has no effect upon cell proliferation. ECFP/Ang II also alters the cellular localization of AT_1R/EYFP. ECFP/Ang II is concentrated in the nucleus, but shows diffuse cytoplasmic fluorescence as well. Eighty-five percent of those cells expressing AT_1R/EYFP alone show plasma membrane-associated fluorescence. In contrast, in cells that express AT_1R/EYFP and ECFP/Ang II, both proteins accumulate in the nucleus and only 13% of the cells show visible plasma membrane-associated yellow fluorescence at 144 hours ($p<0.001$). Furthermore, co-expression of ECFP/Ang II with AT_1R/EYFP stimulates CREB activity in CHO-K1 and COS-7 cells. Exogenous Ang II similarly causes a redistribution of the AT_1R to the nucleus and significantly increases CREB activation in AT_1R/EYFP-stably transfected CHO-K1 and COS-cells. In conclusion, both intracellular and extracellular Ang II can result in AT_1R redistribution to the nucleus, enhanced CREB transcriptional activity, and augmented cellular proliferation.

In support and extension of our studies, Baker and colleagues have shown that intracellular Ang II generated from a plasmid vector introduced by mouse tail vein injection results in biventricular cardiac hypertrophy.[57] The expression vector was constructed by ligating the Ang II coding sequence between the α-MHC promoter and 3′-untranslated region of atrial natriuretic factor. Depending on the cell type and environment, intracellular Ang II expression can, therefore, lead to proliferation and/or hypertrophy.

It is important to note that, while we observed ligand-dependent AT_1R/EYFP nuclear transport in COS and CHO-K1 cells, O'Dowd and colleagues[58] showed agonist-independent transport of AT_1R-GFP in human embryonic kidney 293 cells. They observed constitutive nuclear localization of recombinant receptor in 70% of 293 cells and in an even higher proportion of D283 medulloblastoma cells. Ligand-dependent versus-independent receptor uptake may reflect cell type-specific differences and basal receptor turnover rates.

Is intracellular Ang II generated from intracellular AGT?

We have described above two experimental systems that we designed to generate intracellular Ang II. How might intracellular Ang II come to exist in nature? Obviously, intracellular Ang II exists following receptor: ligand internalization via receptor-mediated endocytosis and, in the classical pathway, is postulated to be degraded by lysosomal enzymes in a timely fashion. However, functional intracellular Ang II is probably not associated with lysosomes and, therefore, is likely functional in the endosomes, or following endosomal escape into the cytoplasm and/or nucleus. Alternatively, intracellular Ang II may be generated from intracellular AGT. Certainly these are not mutually exclusive possibilities and both may be valid. The notion that some cells can synthesize Ang intracellularly gained support from the observation that cultured rat juxtaglomerular cells, which do not express AGT, contain large amounts of Ang II in the same storage granules that contain renin. Administration of an AT_1 receptor blocker, however, does not diminish intracellular Ang II, implying that the Ang in juxtaglomerular cells is unlikely to have been internalized from the extracellular space.[39] The reasonable conclusion is that AGT is internalized into juxtaglomerular cells and is a substrate for intracellular formation of Ang II. Furthermore, limited evidence points to the existence of a cell surface receptor which could mediate AGT uptake. Competitive binding and displacement studies from the laboratory of Tewksbury and associates[59] suggest that placental cells have a specific receptor and can internalize AGT. This may be significant for hypertension in pre-eclamptic patients. Certainly, pre-eclampsia has been associated both with genetic polymorphisms and with up-regulation of members of the RAS.[60–63]

How might intracellular AGT be processed to intracellular Ang II? Peters and colleagues[64] have demonstrated that unglycosylated prorenin is taken up by adult cardiac myocytes (which have been documented to produce AGT mRNA and protein, see elsewhere for review[52]) and involved in generation of intracellular Ang II. In an inducible rat transgenic model that expresses the mouse Ren-2 product in a liver-specific fashion, plasma prorenin rises and contributes to hypertension and cardiac damage. Ren-2 prorenin lacks glycosylation sites and is not internalized via the mannose-6-phosphate receptor, yet the unglycosylated Ren-2 prorenin is internalized into cardiac myocytes and results in significantly enhanced steady-state levels of Ang II. Glycosylated prorenin is also taken up by cardiac myocytes but does not lead to increased intracellular Ang, suggesting that different pathways of internalization may affect activation properties or downstream availability to the substrate. Therefore, Ang I may be generated from AGT after prorenin internalization and activation. Subsequent generation of Ang II from Ang I likely involves ACE and/or chymase, both known to be expressed in the heart.

Another potential source of intracellular renin in rat is the alternative exon 1A renin.[65,66] This renin (renin 1A) generated by alternative splicing is expressed in a tissue-specific manner and lacks a detectable signal peptide. Therefore, it is predicted to be maintained intracellularly and could be available to cleave intracellular substrates in the adrenal gland, liver, and heart, among other organs. Corollaries of the alternate transcript exist in mouse and man.[67,68]

In the brain, AGT is expressed primarily in astrocytes[69] and influences blood pressure, salt intake, vasopressin release and sympathetic nerve activity. Despite the fact that AGT is synthesized primarily in astrocytes, Ang II accumulates to high levels intracellularly in several neuronal types. Pickel and associates,[70] using electron microscopic immunogold and immunocytochemistry, localized Ang II and the AT_1R to neurons of the area postrema and adjacent dorsomedial nucleus tractus solitarii of the rat sensory vagal complex, which has been implicated in central cardiovascular effects. In neurons of these areas, Ang II is often present in cytosolic granular deposits or granular deposits which appear to be fused with the nuclear membrane. AT_1R is often dispersed within the cytoplasm but also appears within the nucleus and even within the nucleolus. While it is not clear from these studies whether Ang II, or alternatively, AGT is internalized, the authors propose that intracellular Ang II is involved in intracrine effects in this region of the brain.

Clearly then, depending on the tissue or cell type and conditions, intracellular Ang II may be generated from AGT (either indigenous or internalized AGT) or internalized from the environment via receptor-mediated endocytosis.

INTRACRINE BIOLOGY

A review of the literature reveals that like angiotensin, many signaling peptides such as hormones and growth factors appear to act in the cellular interior either after internalization from the extracellular space or retention in the cells that synthesized them (Box 11.1).[1,3–8,11] Also, it appears that at least some transcription factors and some enzymes act as signaling molecules and therefore display both intracellular functionality and extracellular signaling capability. We introduced the term *intracrine* for the intracellular action of a peptide hormone after either retention in the cell that synthesized it or internalization from the extracellular space.[7,8] Because too little work has as yet been done on the intracellular actions of peptide hormone, we have functionally extended the definition to include cases in which binding to an intracellular organelle not related to secretion or degradation has been demonstrated; that is, binding to such an organelle is taken as presumptive evidence of action at that site. Moreover, if one isoform of a peptide acts as an extracellular signaling molecule and another appears to act within the cell, the peptide will be classified as an intracrine.

Defined in this way, intracrine function is displayed by a wide variety of peptide hormones, growth factors, enzymes (e.g. phosphoglucose isomerase, renin) and transcription factors/DNA binding proteins (e.g. *engrailed*, HMG B1), meaning that like hormones and growth factors, some enzymes and transcription factors demonstrate the capacity to act as intercellular signaling molecules.[6,11] We have proposed that intracrines act in ways other than simply refining hormone action at a target cell. For example, intracrines often form positive intracellular feedback loops (regulating either their own synthesis or that of components of their signaling cascades) within cells and also frequently interact with ribosomal RNA. This observation and others led to the suggestions (*'intracrine origin hypothesis'*) that peptide intracrines developed to coordinate trophic cellular events with ribosomal biology and that early in metazoan evolution, intracrines exited cells to signal at nearby cells, thereby coordinating tissue-wide differentiation.[5,6] In this, modern intracrine transcription factors act in a fashion reminiscent of certain plant transcription factors which traffic between cells through specialized pores termed plasmodesmata. A second hypothesis (*'intracrine memory hypothesis'*) suggests that the early intracrines up-regulated their own production, that of their signaling cascades or of other intracrines so as to produce a memory of the original trophic stimulus through the production of self-sustaining intracellular feedback loops. According to this view intracrines evolved to serve roles in cellular differentiation, memory of various sorts, and hormonal responsiveness.[3–6] We have, in addition, suggested that intracrine functionality plays an important role in neural tissues in the establishment and maintenance of neurological memory.[12]

Intracrine action occurs in the cardiovascular system and likely plays a role in vascular biology and pathobiology. For example, many intracrines are either angiogenic or anti-angiogenic and many of these intracrines traffic to nucleoli. Indeed, virtually every intracrine which is found in nucleoli is either angiogenic or anti-angiogenic, either directly or indirectly, through the regulation of another factor such as bFGF or vascular endothelial growth factor (VEGF), themselves intracrines.[5,6] For example, angiogenin is a weak RNase which is angiogenic only after internalization and trafficking to nucleus. Indeed, it appears that the nuclear translocation of endogenously synthesized angiogenin is required for endothelial cells to proliferate following exposure to the angiogenic factors fibroblast growth factor 1 (FGF1), FGF2, epidermal growth factor (EGF), and VEGF – which are also intracrines.[5,6,71] Another important intracrine in the cardiovascular system is parathyroid hormone-related protein (PTHrP). This protein is causative for certain forms of malignancy-associated hypercalcemia through its interaction with the parathyroid hormone receptor. It also can be synthesized in both secreted and retained (nuclear trafficking) isoforms. In this regard it is representative of many intracrines, which are often synthesized as multiple isoforms utilizing alternative transcription start sites, alternative splicing, alternative translational start sites, and apparently even internal ribosomal entry sites. In some cases externally applied PTHrP is internalized and traffics to the nucleus.[5,6] Thus this intracrine, like others, displays both modes of intracrine action. PTHrP in nucleus is proliferative for arterial smooth muscle cells, while surface receptor-bound PTHrP inhibits proliferation. Also the effects of PTHrP on growth of VSMCs are modulated by angiotensin, demonstrating the complexity of intracrine action in tissues.[5,6] Moreover, stretch induces transcriptional up-regulation of PTHrP in vascular smooth muscle and post-translation modulation of the protein's synthesis also occurs. This stretch-induced PTHrP up-regulation offsets stretch-related inhibition of cellular proliferation through an intracrine PTHrP action.[72] Thus, PTHrP likely supports the proliferative and remodeling actions of elevated pulse pressure on the vasculature and altered PTHrP regulation could have physiologically relevant effects on the vasculature response to hypertension.

It can be noted that (pro)renin is itself an intracrine. Evidence has been developed for the existence of three functional renin receptors, one of which generates intracellular second messengers and physiologic effects following (pro)renin binding. The other two receptors internalize renin – one of these may in part function as a clearance receptor, the other internalizes and activates non-glycosylated (pro)renin with the subsequent intracellular generation of Ang II.[11,64,73–75] This, along with the existence of non-secreted renin exon 1A indicates that (pro)renin could properly be deemed an enzyme intracrine.[65–68] Moreover, a recent report demonstrates that the introduction of a construct encoding the Ang II sequence induces hypertrophy in cardiac myocytes in the absence of Ang II secretion.[57] Thus it may well be that intracrine Ang II plays a role in the development of hypertrophy in the cardiovascular system. Finally, a recent preliminary report suggests that ACE may also function as an intracrine in that externally applied ACE can be internalized by VSMCs, traffic to nucleus and regulate the transcription of bradykinin B1 and B2 receptors.[13] If confirmed, this would indicate that ACE is an intracrine cardiovascular enzyme which is involved in a transcriptional regulatory loop with the receptors for one of its substrates.

The view of intracrine action described above has led to a variety of predictions. One was that the tumor suppressor protein p53 can function as an intracrine.[4–6] Recently developed evidence dealing with the activity of extracellular p53 fragments provides support for this hypothesis.[76] Similarly, the intracrine view suggested that the homeotranscription factor PDX-1, like other homeoproteins, could function as an intracrine.[5,6] The subsequent demonstration that the application of PDX-1 to pancreatic duct cells mimicked the intracellular action of endogenous PDX-1 to induce islet cell differentiation confirmed this suggestion.[77] Moreover, the recent demonstration of AGT trafficking to astrocyte cell nuclei is consistent with the earlier suggestion that AGT is an anti-angiogenic serpin intracrine.[5,6,11,78]

Also, it appears that intracrine action is closely associated with stem cell biology and development.[5,6,11] It is noteworthy that a complete RAS exists in the bone marrow and participates in hematopoetic stem cell development.[78] Indeed, some of the beneficial effects of angiotensin receptor blocker (ARB) therapy in hypercholesterolemic primates is associated with long-term effects on monocyte development such that monocyte homing to the injured vascular wall is suppressed for some time after withdrawal of the drug and after turnover of circulating monocytes.[79] This suggests an effect of ARBs on monocyte stem cell differentiation. Moreover, blockade of the RAS can reduce the growth of human glioblastoma and neuroblastoma cells, suggesting a role for autocrine, and likely intracrine, Ang action in some forms of neoplasm.[80,81] Thus, just as a variety of intracrine mechanisms are operative in the cardiovascular biology, cardiovascular intracrines likely participate in a wider biology outside the cardiovascular system.

These notions regarding an expanded view of intracrine action notwithstanding, our studies of intracellular Ang II, along with recent evidence indicating a direct effect of intracellular Ang II to induce hypertrophy in cardiac myocytes and the demonstration of likely intracrine actions of renin and AGT, strongly support the relevance of intracrine action in cardiovascular and other tissues. Intracrine action could well be important in fetal development (especially in the vasculature and kidney), atherosclerosis, vascular and cardiac hypertrophy, cardiac memory and arrhythmia, as well as other cardiovascular processes. Identifying such actions likely will open exciting new opportunities for therapy.

REFERENCES

1. Re RN. Tissue renin angiotensin systems. Med Clin North Am 2004; 88: 19–38.
2. Lifton RP, Wilson FH, Choate KA, Geller DS. Salt and blood pressure: new insight from human genetic studies. Cold Spring Harb Symp Quant Biol 2002; 67: 445–50.
3. Re R. The nature of intracrine peptide hormone action. Hypertension 1999; 34: 534–8.
4. Re RN. The origins of intracrine hormone action. Am J Med Sci 2002; 323: 43–8.
5. Re RN. Toward a theory of intracrine hormone action. Regul Pept 2002; 106: 1–6.
6. Re RN. The intracrine hypothesis and intracellular peptide hormone action. Bioessays 2003; 25: 401–9.
7. Re R, Bryan SE. Functional intracellular renin-angiotensin systems may exist in multiple tissues. Clin Exp Hypertens A 1984; 6: 1739–42.
8. Re RN. The cellular biology of angiotensin: paracrine, autocrine and intracrine actions in cardiovascular tissues. J Mol Cell Cardiol 1989; 21 (Suppl 5): 63–9.
9. Nijholt I, Farchi N, Kye M et al. Stress-induced alternative splicing of acetylcholinesterase results in enhanced fear memory and long-term potentiation. Mol Psychiatry 2004; 9: 174–83.
10. Grisaru D, Deutsch V, Shapira M et al. ARP, a peptide derived from the stress-associated acetylcholinesterase variant, has hematopoietic growth promoting activities. Mol Med 2001; 7: 93–105.
11. Re RN. Intracellular renin and the nature of intracrine enzymes. Hypertension 2003; 42: 117–22.
12. Re RN. A proposal regarding the biology of memory: participation of intracrine peptide networks. Med Hypotheses 2004; 63: 887–94.
13. Ignjacev IKE, Johns C, Vitseva O, Shenouda S, Gavras, I, Gavras H. Angiotensin-converting enzyme regulates bradykinin receptor gene expression. Am J Hypertens 2004; 17: 8A (abstract).
14. Sherrod M, Liu X, Zhang X, Sigmund CD. Nuclear localization of angiotensinogen in astrocytes. Am J Physiol Regul Integr Comp Physiol 2005; 288: R539–R546.
15. Hermine O, Beru N, Pech N, Goldwasser E. An autocrine role for erythropoietin in mouse hematopoietic cell differentiation. Blood 1991; 78: 2253–60.
16. Jacques D, Sader S, Perreault C et al. Presence of neuropeptide Y and the Y1 receptor in the plasma membrane and nuclear envelope of human endocardial endothelial cells: modulation of intracellular calcium. Can J Physiol Pharmacol 2003; 81: 288–300.
17. Tzima E, Reader JS, Irani-Tehrani M, Ewalt KL, Schwartz MA, Schimmel P. Biologically active fragment of a human tRNA synthetase inhibits fluid shear stress-activated responses of endothelial cells. Proc Natl Acad Sci U S A 2003; 100: 14903–7.
18. Martinis SA, Plateau P, Cavarelli J, Florentz C. Aminoacyl-tRNA synthetases: a family of expanding functions. Mittelwihr, France, October 10–15, 1999. Embo J 1999; 18: 4591–6.
19. Wakasugi K, Slike BM, Hood J et al. A human aminoacyl-tRNA synthetase as a regulator of angiogenesis. Proc Natl Acad Sci U S A 2002; 99: 173–7.
20. Wakasugi K, Slike BM, Hood J, Ewalt KL, Cheresh DA, Schimmel P. Induction of angiogenesis by a fragment of human tyrosyl-tRNA synthetase. J Biol Chem 2002; 277: 20124–6.
21. Li M, Funahashi H, Mbikay M, Shioda S, Arimura A. Pituitary adenylate cyclase activating polypeptide-mediated intracrine signaling in the testicular germ cells. Endocrine 2004; 23: 59–75.
22. Lindberg P, Baker MS, Kinnby B. The localization of the relaxed form of plasminogen activator inhibitor type 2 in human gingival tissues. Histochem Cell Biol 2001; 116: 447–5.
23. Robertson AL Jr, Khairallah PA. Angiotensin II: rapid localization in nuclei of smooth and cardiac muscle. Science 1971; 172: 1138–9.
24. Goodfriend TL GF, Knych E, Hollemans H, Allman D, Kent K, Cooper T. Clinical and Conceptual Uses of Angiotensin Receptors. New York: Springer-Verlag, 1972.
25. Sirett NE, McLean AS, Bray JJ et al. Distribution of angiotensin II receptors in rat brain. Brain Res 1977; 122: 299–312.
26. Re RN, MacPhee AA, Fallon JT. Specific nuclear binding of angiotensin II by rat liver and spleen nuclei. Clin Sci (Lond) 1981; 61 (Suppl 7): 245s–247s.
27. Tang SS, Rogg H, Schumacher R, Dzau VJ. Characterization of nuclear angiotensin-II-binding sites in rat liver and comparison with plasma membrane receptors. Endocrinology 1992; 131: 374–80.
28. Booz GW, Conrad KM, Hess AL, Singer HA, Baker KM. Angiotensin-II-binding sites on hepatocyte nuclei. Endocrinology 1992; 130: 3641–9.
29. Haller H, Lindschau C, Erdmann B, Quass P, Luft FC. Effects of intracellular angiotensin II in vascular smooth muscle cells. Circ Res 1996; 79: 765–72.
30. Erdmann B, Fuxe K, Ganten D. Subcellular localization of angiotensin II immunoreactivity in the rat cerebellar cortex. Hypertension 1996; 28: 818–24.

31. van Kats JP, van Meegen JR, Verdouw PD et al. Subcellular localization of angiotensin II in kidney and adrenal. J Hypertens 2001; 19: 583–89.
32. Lu D, Yang H, Shaw G, Raizada MK. Angiotensin II-induced nuclear targeting of the angiotensin type 1 (AT1) receptor in brain neurons. Endocrinology 1998; 139: 365–75.
33. Bkaily G, Sleiman S, Stephan J et al. Angiotensin II AT1 receptor internalization, translocation and de novo synthesis modulate cytosolic and nuclear calcium in human vascular smooth muscle cells. Can J Physiol Pharmacol 2003; 81: 274–87.
34. Jacques D, Abdel Malak NA, Sader S, Perreault C. Angiotensin II and its receptors in human endocardial endothelial cells: role in modulating intracellular calcium. Can J Physiol Pharmacol 2003; 81: 259–66.
35. Licea H, Walters MR, Navar LG. Renal nuclear angiotensin II receptors in normal and hypertensive rats. Acta Physiol Hung 2002; 89: 427–38.
36. Fu ML, Schulze W, Wallukat G et al. Immunohistochemical localization of angiotensin II receptors (AT1) in the heart with anti-peptide antibodies showing a positive chronotropic effect. Receptors Channels 1998; 6: 99–111.
37. Okamura T, Clemens DL, Inagami T. Renin, angiotensins, and angiotensin-converting enzyme in neuroblastoma cells: evidence for intracellular formation of angiotensins. Proc Natl Acad Sci U S A 1981; 78: 6940–3.
38. Amedeo Modesti P, Zecchi-Orlandini S, Vanni S et al. Release of preformed Ang II from myocytes mediates angiotensinogen and ET-1 gene overexpression in vivo via AT1 receptor. J Mol Cell Cardiol 2002; 34: 1491–500.
39. Mercure C, Ramla D, Garcia R, Thibault G, Deschepper CF, Reudelhuber TL. Evidence for intracellular generation of angiotensin II in rat juxtaglomerular cells. FEBS Lett 1998; 422: 395–9.
40. Zhuo JL, Imig JD, Hammond TG et al. Ang II accumulation in rat renal endosomes during Ang II-induced hypertension: role of AT(1) receptor. Hypertension 2002; 39(1): 116–21.
41. Thomas MA, Fleissner G, Hauptfleisch S et al. Subcellular identification of angiotensin I/II- and angiotensin II (AT1)-receptor-immunoreactivity in the central nervous system of rats. Brain Res 2003; 962: 92–104.
42. Vila-Porcile E, Corvol P. Angiotensinogen, prorenin, and renin are co-localized in the secretory granules of all glandular cells of the rat anterior pituitary: an immunoultrastructural study. J Histochem Cytochem 1998; 46: 301–11.
43. Re R, Parab M. Effect of angiotensin II on RNA synthesis by isolated nuclei. Life Sci 1984; 34: 647–51.
44. Re RN, Vizard DL, Brown J, Bryan SE. Angiotensin II receptors in chromatin fragments generated by micrococcal nuclease. Biochem Biophys Res Commun 1984; 119: 220–7.
45. Eggena P, Zhu JH, Sereevinyayut S et al. Hepatic angiotensin II nuclear receptors and transcription of growth-related factors. J Hypertens 1996; 14: 961–8.
46. Eggena P, Zhu JH, Clegg K, Barrett JD. Nuclear angiotensin receptors induce transcription of renin and angiotensinogen mRNA. Hypertension 1993; 22: 496–501.
47. Jimenez E, Vinson GP, Montiel M. Angiotensin II (AII)-binding sites in nuclei from rat liver: partial characterization of the mechanism of AII accumulation in nuclei. J Endocrinol 1994; 143: 449–53.
48. Re RN. Changes in nuclear initiation sites after the treatment of isolated nuclei with angiotensin II. Clin Sci 1982; 63: 191s–193s.
49. Re RN. Effect of angiotensin II on RNA synthesis by isolated nuclei. Life Sci 1984; 34: 647–51.
50. De Mello WC. Influence of intracellular renin on heart cell communication. Hypertension 1995; 25: 1172–7.
51. De Mello WC. Intracellular angiotensin II regulates the inward calcium current in cardiac myocytes. Hypertension 1998; 32: 976–82.
52. De Mello WC, Danser AH. Angiotensin II and the heart: on the intracrine renin-angiotensin system. Hypertension 2000; 35: 1183–8.
53. Frustaci A, Kajstura J, Chimenti C et al. Myocardial cell death in human diabetes. Circ Res 2000; 87: 1123–32.
54. Cook JL, Zhang Z, Re RN. In vitro evidence for an intracellular site of angiotensin action. Circ Res 2001; 89: 1138–46.
55. Cook JL, Giardina JF, Zhang Z, Re RN. Intracellular angiotensin II increases the long isoform of PDGF mRNA in rat hepatoma cells. J Mol Cell Cardiol 2002; 34: 1525–37.
56. Cook JL, Re R, Alam J, Hart M, Zhang Z. Intracellular angiotensin II fusion protein alters AT1 receptor fusion protein distribution and activates CREB. J Mol Cell Cardiol 2004; 36: 75–90.
57. Baker KM, Chernin MI, Schreiber T et al. Evidence of a novel intracrine mechanism in angiotensin II-induced cardiac hypertrophy. Regul Pept 2004; 120: 5–13.
58. Lee DK, Lanca AJ, Cheng R et al. Agonist-independent nuclear localization of the Apelin, angiotensin AT1, and bradykinin B2 receptors. J Biol Chem 2004; 279: 7901–8.
59. Tewksbury DA, Pan N, Kaiser SJ. Detection of a receptor for angiotensinogen on placental cells. Am J Hypertens 2003; 16: 59–62.
60. Choi H, Kang JY, Yoon HS et al. Association of angiotensin-converting enzyme and angiotensinogen gene polymorphisms with preeclampsia. J Korean Med Sci 2004; 19: 253–7.
61. Leung PS, Tsai SJ, Wallukat G, Leung TN, Lau TK. The upregulation of angiotensin II receptor AT(1) in human preeclamptic placenta. Mol Cell Endocrinol 2001; 184: 95–102.
62. Ito M, Itakura A, Ohno Y et al. Possible activation of the renin-angiotensin system in the feto-placental unit in preeclampsia. J Clin Endocrinol Metab 2002; 87: 1871–8.
63. Kim YJ, Park MH, Park HS, Lee KS, Ha EH, Pang MG. Associations of polymorphisms of the angiotensinogen M235 polymorphism and angiotensin-converting-enzyme intron 16 insertion/deletion polymorphism with preeclampsia in Korean women. Eur J Obstet Gynecol Reprod Biol 2004; 116: 48–53.
64. Peters J, Farrenkopf R, Clausmeyer S et al. Functional significance of prorenin internalization in the rat heart. Circ Res 2002; 90: 1135–41.
65. Clausmeyer S, Reinecke A, Farrenkopf R, Unger T, Peters J. Tissue-specific expression of a rat renin transcript lacking the coding sequence for the prefragment and its stimulation by myocardial infarction. Endocrinology 2000; 141: 2963–70.
66. Clausmeyer S, Sturzebecher R, Peters J. An alternative transcript of the rat renin gene can result in a truncated prorenin that is transported into adrenal mitochondria. Circ Res 1999; 84: 337–44.
67. Lee-Kirsch MA, Gaudet F, Cardoso MC, Lindpaintner K. Distinct renin isoforms generated by tissue-specific transcription initiation and alternative splicing. Circ Res 1999; 84: 240–6.
68. Sinn PL, Sigmund CD. Identification of three human renin mRNA isoforms from alternative tissue-specific transcriptional initiation. Physiol Genomics 2000; 3: 25–31.
69. Intebi AD, Flaxman MS, Ganong WF, Deschepper CF. Angiotensinogen production by rat astroglial cells in vitro and in vivo. Neuroscience 1990; 34: 545–54.
70. Huang J, Hara Y, Anrather J, Speth RC, Iadecola C, Pickel VM. Angiotensin II subtype 1A (AT1A) receptors in the rat sensory vagal complex: subcellular localization and association with endogenous angiotensin. Neuroscience 2003; 122: 21–36.
71. Kishimoto K, Liu S, Tsuji T, Olson KA, Hu GF. Endogenous angiogenin in endothelial cells is a general requirement for cell proliferation and angiogenesis. Oncogene 2005; 24: 445–56.

72. Schordan E, Welsch S, Rothhut S et al. Role of parathyroid hormone-related protein in the regulation of stretch-induced renal vascular smooth muscle cell proliferation. J Am Soc Nephrol 2004; 15: 3016–25.
73. Nguyen G, Delarue F, Burckle C, Bouzhir L, Giller T, Sraer JD. Pivotal role of the renin/prorenin receptor in angiotensin II production and cellular responses to renin. J Clin Invest 2002; 109: 1417–27.
74. Nguyen G, Delarue F, Berrou J, Rondeau E, Sraer JD. Specific receptor binding of renin on human mesangial cells in culture increases plasminogen activator inhibitor-1 antigen. Kidney Int 1996; 50: 1897–903.
75. Saris JJ, Derkx FH, Lamers JM, Saxena PR, Schalekamp MA, Danser AH. Cardiomyocytes bind and activate native human prorenin: role of soluble mannose 6-phosphate receptors. Hypertension 2001; 37: 710–15.
76. Mittelman JM, Gudkov AV. Generation of p53 suppressor peptide from the fragment of p53 protein. Somat Cell Mol Genet 1999; 25: 115–28.
77. Noguchi H, Kaneto H, Weir GC, Bonner-Weir S. PDX-1 protein containing its own antennapedia-like protein transduction domain can transduce pancreatic duct and islet cells. Diabetes 2003; 52: 1732–7.
78. Strawn WB, Richmond RS, Ann Tallant E, Gallagher PE, Ferrario CM. Renin-angiotensin system expression in rat bone marrow haematopoietic and stromal cells. Br J Haematol 2004; 126: 120–6.
79. Strawn WB, Chappell MC, Dean RH, Kivlighn S, Ferrario CM. Inhibition of early atherogenesis by losartan in monkeys with diet-induced hypercholesterolemia. Circulation 2000; 101: 1586–93.
80. Cook JL, Chen L, Bhandaru S, Bakris GL, Re RN. The use of antisense oligonucleotides to establish autocrine angiotensin growth effects in human neuroblastoma and mesangial cells. Antisense Res Dev 1992; 2: 199–210.
81. Juillerat-Jeanneret L, Celerier J, Chapuis Bernasconi C et al. Renin and angiotensinogen expression and functions in growth and apoptosis of human glioblastoma. Br J Cancer 2004; 90: 1059–68.

12

Nonmodulators and essential hypertension

Norman K Hollenberg and Gordon H Williams

INTRODUCTION

Everyone interested in the pathogenesis of essential hypertension believes that this does not represent a single process with a single pathogenesis. Indeed, over the past century and a half, advances in our understanding have had a characteristic sequence: a specific mechanism was identified in a subset of patients, which became a form of 'secondary hypertension'. Chronic renal failure recognized by Bright early in the nineteenth century remains the most common secondary cause. The last hundred years have seen the identification of Cushings syndrome, pheochromocytoma, primary aldosteronism, coarctation of the aorta, renovascular hypertension, and several monogenic forms of hypertension, e.g. glucocorticoid remedial hypertension (GRA), apparent mineralocorticoid excess syndrome, and Liddle's syndrome. Thus, essentially all of the identifiable causes to date are dominated by the kidney and the adrenal. Moreover, the logic has involved removing from a large group of patients with a similar phenotype – elevated blood pressure – subgroups of patients with an identifiable pathogenesis. It is appropo of nonmodulation that the first indication of an important renal and adrenal contribution was made by Bright and Addison in the same institution, Guys Hospital. This chapter will focus on one substantial subgroup involving perhaps 40% of patients with normal and high renin essential hypertension who show an abnormality involving the control of the kidney and the adrenal aldosterone release in response to shifts in sodium intake.[1] Again, a single institution was involved.

ANGIOTENSIN AND THE CONTROL OF ADRENAL ALDOSTERONE RELEASE AND RENAL PERFUSION

The relevant abnormalities were first recognized over 30 years ago.[2,3] In the case of the kidney, renal hemodynamic measurements identified a subset of patients with essential hypertension in whom renal perfusion did not change with changes in salt intake. In the case of adrenal aldosterone release, similar studies identified a patient subset in whom aldosterone release in response to shifts in salt intake was blunted.[3] The abnormality in control delineated is reflected in the absence of a normal shift in sensitivity (modulation) of their renal vascular and adrenal response to angiotensin II (Ang II) with changes in sodium intake.

When we first identified in normal humans the remarkable shift in sensitivity of the renal vasculature and adrenal aldosterone release in response to shifts in salt intake, we applied the term 'modulation' to that shift in sensitivity.[4] These studies were performed at a time when the influence of glucose and insulin concentration on tissue responsiveness to insulin were first being identified, and called modulation. We thought that we were probably studying the same phenomenon – as proved to be the case – and so we used the same term to describe the shifts in sensitivity. In the patients with the altered renal and adrenal response to salt intake, we identified the absence of the normal shift in sensitivity of the renal blood supply and adrenal to Ang II with changes in sodium intake.[1] Thus, we called then 'nonmodulators'.

The response of the adrenal and renal blood supply to Ang II is fixed at the level of least sensitivity in these patients. Restriction of salt intake normally enhances the adrenal response to Ang II and blunts the renovascular response. Conversely, a high-salt diet normally blunts adrenal responses to Ang II and enhances the renovascular response. In nonmodulators, the adrenal response is fixed at the level of characteristics of a high-salt diet in normal individuals, and the renal response is fixed at a level characteristic of low-salt intake. Renal blood flow does not display the normal change in response to shift in salt intake. Angotensin converting enzyme (ACE) inhibition corrected these abnormalities.[1]

ACE INHIBITION

The early studies evolved at a time when ACE inhibition first became available as a physiological tool and a therapeutic maneuver. The blunted renal plasma flow response to Ang II in these patients raised the intriguing possibility that these individuals suffered from excessive local intrarenal Ang II levels. If that were the case, one might anticipate a rise in renal perfusion in response to an ACE inhibitor in nonmodulators on a high-salt diet. That would indicate that the ACE inhibitor was more effective than a high-salt diet in influencing intrarenal Ang II formation in these patients. Indeed, a potentiated response to ACE inhibition had already been documented in some patients with essential hypertension.[5,6] ACE inhibition increased renal blood flow in nonmodulators substantially more than the minimal, appropriate response in normal subjects or essential hypertensives with intact modulation when the system was suppressed by a high-salt intake.[7]

Such an enhanced response does not necessarily reflect reversal of excessive Ang II formation. As an alternative the renal vasodilator response to ACE inhibition could reflect the local influence of prostaglandins or bradykinin. One would anticipate, however, if the latter was the explanation, that renal blood flow response to Ang II would be blunted further by ACE inhibition, as both prostaglandins and bradykinin reversed the renal vasoconstriction induced by Ang II. On the other hand, if the ACE inhibitor-induced increased renal perfusion reflected reduced Ang II formation, one would anticipate an enhanced renovascular response. Indeed, an enhanced renal blood flow response to Ang II was identified following ACE inhibition.[7]

INTRARENAL ANG II, RENAL SODIUM HANDLING, AND RENIN RELEASE

If there were extensive and inappropriate increases in tissue levels of Ang II in the kidney, one might anticipate an abnormality in renal sodium handling as one consequence. At about that time, Fujita, et al.[8] had identified a subset of patients with essential hypertension in whom blood pressure rose substantially on a shift from a low-salt to a high-salt diet. These individuals showed substantially more weight gain than normal subjects did on that shift, more positive sodium balance, and a striking sensitivity of blood pressure to salt intake. Our hypothesis was that these individuals represented nonmodulation. This proved to be the case.[9,10] Whether the acute natriuretic response to sodium load or the steady-state responses that develop over days when sodium intake has shifted from a low to a high level or a high to a low were assessed, the nonmodulators showed a blunting of the capacity to handle a salt load.[9,10] As might have been anticipated, treatment with an ACE inhibitor not only induced renal vasodilation, but also improved the capacity of the kidney to excrete sodium in response to an acute load – to a level seen in normal subjects.[9]

Similarly, one might anticipate that an excessive intrarenal Ang II level would influence renin release. Renin suppression by Ang II in subpressor doses failed to occur in about 50% of patients with essential hypertension.[11] This abnormality, as might be anticipated, if local Ang II was involved, was reversed by ACE inhibition.[12] The loss of Ang II mediated suppression of PRA occurs primarily in nonmodulators, as had been anticipated and is, indeed, reversed by ACE inhibition in that specific group of patients.[13]

As this array of functionally similar abnormalities occurred in the same patient,[14] it was difficult to avoid the conclusion that we had identified a syndrome that potentially had a common pathophysiological root. This syndrome is exceedingly common. In studies of over 400 patients documented before the mid-1990s, approximately 50% of patients with normal or high renin essential hypertension proved to be nonmodulators.[1] Thus, in addition to low renin hypertensives, this abnormality could account for nearly all of the salt-sensitive hypertension, estimated to have a frequency of 50–60% in the general hypertensive population.

FAMILY HISTORY AND GENES

A number of observations suggested that nonmodulation ought to be considered as a candidate intermediate phenotype for genetic studies. Perhaps most compelling was the extraordinarily strong positive family history of hypertension in nonmodulators.[10] In a study in which data were included only on the basis of primary ascertainment – either direct blood pressure measurement in family members or contact with their physicians – we found that 85% of nonmodulators had a positive family history for hypertension.[10] In contrast, the rest of the normal and the high renin essential hypertensives had a 25–30% positive family history. Moreover, the nonmodulating phenotype was observed in normotensive subjects in whom there was a positive family history for hypertension.[15] Beretta-Piccoli et al. confirmed and extended that observation by documenting that the aldosterone response to Ang II infusion in normotensive subjects with a positive family history for hypertension was significantly less than in those with a negative family history.[16] Van Hooft et al.

reported that basal renal plasma flow on a high-salt diet was lower in normotensive subjects with a positive family history of hypertension than in individuals with a negative family history despite a higher perfusion pressure.[17] Moreover, plasma aldosterone concentration was reduced significantly despite an identical or even somewhat higher plasma Ang II concentration. In Japanese subjects, Uneda et al.[18] documented that renal plasma flow response to ACE inhibition on a high-salt diet was influenced by a family history of hypertension. When hypertensive sibling pairs residing in Utah were tested for concordance of the renal plasma flow response to Ang II, a remarkable degree of concordance was observed.[19]

As the next step in the investigation, it was necessary to ascertain whether any of the features of nonmodulation showed a bimodal distribution in the community. Such a finding would suggest a discrete subgroup in whom genetic factors might be identified. In a study involving over 200 subjects and with maximum likelihood analysis employed to assess whether or not a bimodal[20] distribution was present, we identified four abnormalities that were clearly bimodal. The aldosterone secretory response to acute volume depletion, the plasma aldosterone response to Ang II infusion on a low-salt diet, the fall in plasma renin activity (PRA), which occurred in response to saline infusion, and the increase in renal perfusion with salt loading, all showed an unambiguous bimodal distribution. Thus, we were well positioned to conclude that nonmodulation is an intermediate phenotype and to pursue the genetic studies that were appropriate.

As a first step, genes governing the renin-angiotensin cascade offered an obvious target. In a study primarily reflecting the findings in normotensive subjects, we found that a single nucleotide polymorphism in the coding region of the angiotensinogen (AGT) gene was associated with a decreased renal blood flow response to Ang II, suggesting that this gene might be associated with nonmodulation.[21] This study was extended to include several hundred subjects with hypertension who showed the same association.[22] Moreover, the studies showed that in the same subjects, the polymorphism in the AGT locus was also associated with a decreased aldosterone response to Ang II.[22]

We then sought to ascertain whether other genes governing the renin-angiotensin system (RAS) might be involved and their interaction. In this study, the patient population had grown to 298 subjects with hypertension. Subjects were genotyped not only at the AGT locus, but also polymorphisms in the ACE, aldosterone synthase, renin, Ang II type 1 receptor, and adducing genes. As in earlier studies, the AGT locus was associated with nonmodulation. Although the ACE gene deletion polymorphism did not influence aldosterone responsiveness alone, the combination of the AGT and ACE gene polymorphisms had a larger influence than AGT alone – an example of genetic epistasis.[23] When the subjects were also required to possess an aldosterone synthase polymorphism, there was a further substantial reduction in aldosterone response to Ang II, one of the hallmarks of nonmodulation.

Overall, some 40% of subjects with normal or high renin essential hypertension show features of nonmodulation. Any individual gene in this complex polygenic model will account for only a few percent. Hence, it is crucial for us to search further. By the same logic that led us to examine the genes of the RAS in sequence, it is tempting to speculate on other genes that might be involved, given the fundamental contribution of different systems to responsiveness to Ang II.

There is, of course, an enormous array of potential targets. One very attractive candidate involves the largest group of receptors, the super family of seven-transmembrane receptors, as recently reviewed by Lefkowitz.[24] Several decades of research have identified a universal mechanism of receptor regulation via G protein-coupled receptor kinases and arrestins – originally discovered as a means of desensitizing G protein-mediated second-messenger generation. Today, it is clear that almost without exception seven-transmembrane receptors are regulated through these two pathways. That only a limited number of enzymes and only two forms of beta arrestin accomplish this emphasizes the remarkable ability of these proteins to interact with hundreds of different receptors. The key to their physiological specificity involves the fact that they interact only with the activated forms of the receptors. A systematic examination of these pathways should prove to be fruitful. This concept would account for the hitherto unexplained fact that nonmodulation, clearly specific for the angiotensin receptor, also shows up as variation in the physiology of a diverse host of hormones including insulin, atrial natriuretic peptide, and dopamine.[1] If one of the goals of science is to generate new hypotheses, nonmodulation clearly has the potential to lead to a broad range of studies.

REFERENCES

1. Hollenberg NK, Williams GH. Abnormal renal function, sodium-volume homeostasis and renin system behavior in normal-renin essential hypertension: the evolution of the nonmodulator concept. In: Laragh JH, Brenner BM (eds). Hypertension: Pathophysiology, Diagnosis, and Management, 2nd edn. New York: Raven Press, 1995, pp 1837–56.
2. Hollenberg NK, Merrill JP. Intrarenal perfusion in the young 'essential' hypertensive: a subpopulation resistant to sodium restriction. Trans Assoc Am Physicians 1970; 83: 93–101.

3. Williams GH, Rose LI, Dluhy RG et al. Abnormal responsiveness of the renin-aldosterone system to acute stimulation in patients with essential hypertension. Ann Intern Med 1970; 72: 317–26.
4. Hollenberg NK, Chenitz WR, Adams DF, Williams GH. Reciprocal influence of salt intake on adrenal glomerulosa and renal vascular responses to angiotensin II in normal man. J Clin Invest 1974; 54: 34–42.
5. Williams GH, Hollenberg NK. Accentuated vascular and endocrine responses to SQ 20881 in hypertension. N Engl J Med 1977; 297: 184–8.
6. Hollenberg NK, Meggs LG, Williams GH, Kiatz J, Garnic JD, Harrington DP. Sodium intake and renal responses to captopril in normal man and in essential hypertension. Kidney 1981; 20: 240–5.
7. Redgrave JE, Rabinowe SL, Hollenberg NK, Williams GH. Correction of abnormal renal blood flow response to angiotensin II by converting-enzyme inhibition in essential hypertensives. J Clin Invest 1985; 75: 1285–90.
8. Fujita T, Henry WL, Bartter FC, Lake CFR, Delea CS. Factors influencing blood pressure in salt-sensitive patients with hypertension. Am J Med 1980; 69: 334–4.
9. Rystedt LL, Williams GH, Hollenberg NK. The renal and endocrine response to saline infusion in essential hypertension. Hypertension 1986; 8: 217–22.
10. Hollenberg NK, Moore T, Shoback D, Redgrave J, Rabinowe S, Williams GH. Abnormal renal sodium handling in essential hypertension: relation to failure of renal and adrenal modulation of responses to Ang II. Am J Med 1986; 81: 412–18.
11. Williams GH, Hollenberg NK, Moore TJ et al. Failure of renin suppression by angiotensin II in hypertension. Circ Res 1978; 4: 46–52.
12. LeBoff MS, Dluhy RG, Hollenberg NK, Moore TJ, Koletsky RJ, Williams GH. Abnormal renin short feedback loop in essential hypertension is reversible with converting enzyme inhibition. J Clin Invest 1982; 70: 335–41.
13. Seely EW, Moore TJ, Rogacz S et al. Angiotensin-mediated renin suppression is altered in non-modulating hypertension. Hypertension 1989; 13: 31–7.
14. Williams GH, Tuck ML, Sullivan JM, Dluhy RG, Hollenberg NK. Parallel adrenal and renal abnormalities in the young patient with essential hypertension. Am J Med 1982; 72: 907–14.
15. Blackshear JL, Garnic D, Williams GH, Harrington DP, Hollenberg NK. Exaggerated renal vascular response to calcium entry blockade in first degree relatives of essential hypertensives: possible role of intrarenal Ang II. Hypertension 1987; 9: 384–9.
16. Beretta-Piccoli C, Pusterla C, Stadler P, Weidmann P. Blunted aldosterone responsiveness to Ang II in normotensive subjects with familial predisposition to essential hypertension. J Hypertens 1988; 61: 57–61.
17. Van Hooft IMS, Grobee DE, Derkx FHM, DeLeeuw PW, Schalekamp MA, Hofman A. Renal hemodynamics and the renin-angiotensin-aldosterone system in normotensive subjects with hypertensive and normotensive parents. N Engl J Med 1991; 324: 1305.
18. Uneda S, Fukishima S, Fujika Y, Tochikubo HO, Asahina S, Kaneko Y. Renal hemodynamics and renin-angiotensin system in adolescents genetically predisposed to essential hypertension. J Hypertens 1984; 263: 437–9.
19. Lifton RP, Hopkins PN, Williams RR, Hollenberg NK, Williams GH, Dluhy RG. Evidence for heritability of non-modulating essential hypertension. Hypertension 1989; 13: 884.
20. Williams GH, Dluhy RG, Lifton RP et al. Non-modulation as an intermediate phenotype in essential hypertension. Hypertension 1992; 20: 788–96.
21. Hopkins PN, Lifton RP, Hollenberg NK et al. Blunted renal vascular response to angiotensin I is associated with a common variant of the angiotensinogen gene and obesity. J Hypertens 1996; 14: 199–207.
22. Hopkins PN, Hunt SC, Jeunemaitre X et al. Angiotensin genotype effect on renal and adrenal responses to angiotensin II in essential hypertension. Circulation 2002; 105: 1921–7.
23. Kosachunhanun N, Hunt SC, Hopkins PN et al. Genetic determinants of nonmodulating hypertension. Hypertension 2003; 42: 901–8.
24. Lefkowitz RJ. Historical review: a brief history and personal retrospective of seven-transmembrane receptors. Trends Pharmacol Sci 2004; 25: 413–22.

13

Primary aldosteronism

Elise P Gomez-Sanchez and Celso E Gomez-Sanchez

INTRODUCTION

Aldosterone is the primary endogenous mineralocorticoid steroid. It is synthesized within the adrenal zona glomerulosa from cholesterol, the last step being the sequential 11β-hydroxylation of deoxycorticosterone by the enzyme aldosterone synthase to yield corticosterone, 18-hydroxylation to yield 18-hydroxycorticosterone followed by another hydroxylation leading to the formation of a diol which then spontaneously dehydrates to form aldosterone. The synthesis of aldosterone is primarily regulated by angiotensin II (Ang II) and potassium, and to a lesser extent by ACTH (adrenocorticotropic hormone) and sodium. Aldosterone acts through mineralocorticoid receptors (MRs) in transport epithelium, primarily that of the renal tubules, colon and salivary glands, to promote sodium and water reabsorption and potassium and proton excretion. Hyperaldosteronism results in hypertension, suppression of the renin-angiotensin system (RAS), hypokalemia, and metabolic alkalosis. In addition to modulating the vectorial transport of ions and water, aldosterone acts upon non-epithelial tissues, notably the cardiovascular and central nervous systems, where it has trophic effects in addition to altering ion transport and compartmentalization.[1–3] Because of the pathological cardiac, renal, and vascular remodeling associated with mineralocorticoid excess, it is crucial that conditions of excessive production of aldosterone be diagnosed and treated appropriately.

Primary aldosteronism (PA) is a group of disorders in which aldosterone production is inappropriately high and relatively autonomous of the RAS, potassium levels, and sodium intake. PA was first described by Jerome Conn in 1955 soon after aldosterone was isolated and described by Simpson and Tait.[4,5] It was considered relatively rare for the next 25 years because aldosterone was usually only measured in patients who presented with hypokalemia in addition to hypertension, even though Conn had described normokalemic primary aldosteronism in 1965.[6–8] PA is now known to be the most common form of secondary hypertension, affecting about 10% of the hypertensive population throughout the world[9] and up to 15% of the patients referred to hypertension clinics.[10,11] It is more common among patients with severe hypertension, being found in ~2% of patients with mild hypertension, 13% with severe hypertension,[12] and as high as 20% of patients with refractory hypertension.[13]

Hypokalemia was once considered a hallmark of PA along with hypertension, but normokalemic patients with PA are commonly identified with the increased use of the aldosterone/renin ratio (ARR) for screening for PA in unselected populations of normokalemic subjects diagnosed with essential hypertension.[9,11,14,15] However, the low incidence of hypokalemia[9,15] may be spurious. A potassium ≥ 3.6 mM was found in 69.1% of 152 patients with PA when the blood sample was obtained by the common procedure of using a tourniquet and clenching the fist; however, when the blood sample was obtained from the contralateral vein in the same patients without the fist clenching and tourniquet, only 10.5% of these patients had a potassium >3.6 mM.[16]

PA should be considered in hypertensive patients with spontaneous hypokalemia, hypokalemia due to low dose diuretics, refractory hypertension, family history of juvenile hypertension, family history of juvenile cerebrovascular events or adrenal incidentaloma.[10] While frequently severe or refractory, hypertension in PA may be mild or, rarely, malignant.[15] Hypertensive encephalopathy can occur with PA.[12,17–19] Compared to patients with pheochromocytoma, Cushing's syndrome, or essential hypertension, those with PA tend to have the highest office and 24-hour blood pressure values.[20] Nocturnal blood pressure decline is significantly attenuated in all forms of adrenal hypertension and returns to normal after specific treatment of the underlying disorder.[20]

Mineralocorticoid receptors are present in the heart, brain, and blood vessels, in addition to the kidney tubules and colon, and mediate proliferative and fibrotic disease in addition to blood pressure elevation when inappropriately activated. Reduction of blood pressure in the face of continued aldosterone excess does not prevent end organ damage.[2,3] Therefore, normalization of blood pressure is not the only goal in managing the patient with PA; the excessive production or action of aldosterone should be addressed. Mineralocorticoid excess in the presence of salt alters vascular function and promotes cardiac and vascular hypertrophy, remodeling and fibrosis independently of blood pressure elevation in experimental animals.[21,22] Structural alterations in subcutaneous small arteries seen in patients with PA are significant predictors of cardiovascular events.[23] Echocardiography with videodensitometric analysis of myocardial texture has been used to document cardiac hypertrophy due to increased collagen deposition. Ultrasonic integrated backscatter signal (IBS) in diastole correlates with the collagen content within the myocardium and is significantly increased in patients with PA compared to patients with essential hypertension matched for demographics, casual blood pressure, and known duration of hypertension.[24,25] Myocardial IBS increases with plasma aldosterone and immunoreactive endothelin.[25] Endothelin is an aldosterone secretagogue that may play an important role in pathological situations, particularly heart failure.[26]

Chronic aldosterone excess is associated with increased renal magnesium clearance despite normal plasma magnesium levels,[27] and PA is characterized by magnesium deficiency with decreased intralymphocyte ionized magnesium.[28] Magnesium deprivation of human fibroblasts in culture increases the expression of both collagen I and III mRNA genes, suggesting that chronic magnesium deficiency may be a mechanism for the myocardial remodeling associated with the combination of aldosterone and sodium excess.[22,28]

DIAGNOSIS OF PRIMARY ALDOSTERONISM (FIGURE 13.1)

The diagnosis of PA was originally established by the demonstration of a persistently suppressed plasma renin activity (PRA) upon stimulation of the RAS with the failure of salt loading to suppress aldosterone levels. The methods used to establish these criteria, however, are cumbersome and inimical to widespread screening. The recognition by Hiramatsu et al. that random measurements of plasma aldosterone and PRA expressed as a ratio reflected autonomy of aldosterone secretion led to the development of a rapid screening method used today.[29] The plasma aldosterone/PRA ratio is the ratio of plasma aldosterone concentration measured in ng/dl divided by the PRA in ng/ml/h. Notwithstanding problems with the lack of standardization, the ARR has become the screening test of choice for PA.[9] An ARR higher than 25 with plasma aldosterone concentrations >15 ng/dl suggests the diagnosis.[9,14,30] Its use led to a marked increase in the detection of PA in a retrospective evaluation of patients of different ethnicity in clinical centers on five different continents.[9] Ideally the patient is taken off medications for at least a week, but this is frequently difficult.[11] Although Ca^+ channel blockers, angiotensin converting enzyme (ACE) inhibitors, and AT_1 antagonists all decrease plasma aldosterone concentrations and increase PRA, the effect of Ca^+ channel blockers is less marked than agents that act directly upon the RAS. Nonetheless, the ARR is still fairly reliable as a screening test even if the patient is receiving antihypertensive therapy, except for beta blockers.[31,32] Measurement of the ARR after the administration of the ACE inhibitor captopril has been shown to improve the reliability of the screening.[33] Recently the use of a direct immunoassay to measure renin has become very popular because it is direct and much easier to do, and the results correlate well with the measurement of plasma renin activity.[34] The direct renin value is divided by 8 to approximate the PRA value.

Aldosterone secretion is variable. While regulated primarily by the RAS and Na^+ and K^+ levels, it does have a circadian rhythm and is acutely stimulated by ACTH. Plasma levels are therefore highly variable. Measurement of aldosterone metabolites in the urine gives an indication of its integrated production rate. The most commonly measured metabolite in the urine is the acid-labile aldosterone metabolite 18-oxo-glucuronide that corresponds to approximately 5–10% of the secreted aldosterone. However, about 45% of aldosterone is converted to 3α,5β-tetrahydroaldosterone in the liver and excreted in the urine. One of the first, and still perhaps best, integrated indexes of aldosterone production was that of 3α,5β-tetrahydroaldosterone.[35] The level of urinary tetrahydroaldosterone was found to be better than the ARR in the differentiation of PA from essential hypertension in a prospective study. The sensitivity and specificity of detection by

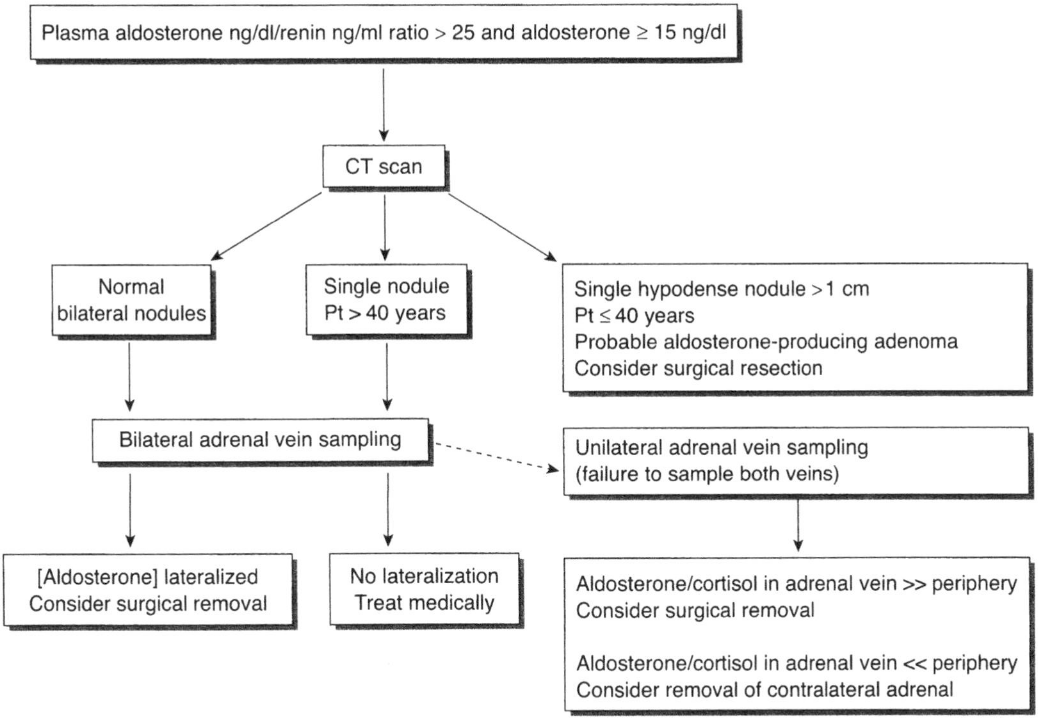

Figure 13.1 Diagnosis of primary aldosteronism

tetrahydroaldosterone levels were 96% and 95%, respectively.[16] Unfortunately 3α,5β-tetrahydroaldosterone is rarely measured because there are no commercial reagents for the assay at this time.

Once a screening test is positive, the diagnosis of PA must be confirmed by more definitive maneuvers. Three main techniques have been used. The most common is still the measurement of aldosterone in a 24-hour urine sample collected on the last day of a 4-day high-salt diet of 200 mmoles NaCl/day.[36] A urinary excretion of less than 12 μg/24 hour of aldosterone is considered normal. Suppression of plasma aldosterone with the infusion of 2 L of normal saline over 4 hours has also been used extensively, with a plasma aldosterone of >7.5 ng/dl or ≥5 ng/dl considered normal.[37–39] Others have advocated the administration of a high sodium diet and fludrocortisone 0.2 mg twice a day for 3 days with measurement of plasma aldosterone on the fourth day. A value of ≤5 ng/dl is considered normal.[11,14] Patients for whom there is a high degree of suspicion of PA, but who suppress below 7.5 ng/dl plasma aldosterone upon saline infusion may be diagnosed by the high sodium diet and fludrocortisone test.[40]

CLASSIFICATION OF PRIMARY ALDOSTERONISM

PA is classified by its diverse etiologies (Box 13.1). For the first two decades after PA was first described, Conn's syndrome, or aldosterone-producing adenoma, was the most commonly diagnosed cause of PA.[9,36,41] In a 1964 review of 10 years of experience, all patients with confirmed PA were found to have an adrenal adenoma.[42] Within a few years, however, patients were found that had PA without an adrenal tumor. This syndrome was called pseudoprimary aldosteronism or idiopathic hyperplasia.[43] The ability to identify milder forms of PA led to the realization that idiopathic adrenal hyperplasia, which is usually bilateral, occurs two to three times more commonly than aldosterone-producing adenoma.[9,10,36]

Box 13.1 Classification of primary aldosteronism

- Aldosterone-producing adenoma
  - Classic or ACTH-responsive
  - Angiotensin II-responsive
- Bilateral zona glomerulosa hyperplasia
  - Angiotensin II-responsive
  - Primary hyperplasia (ACTH-responsive)
- Unilateral hyperplasia
- Adrenal carcinoma
- Extra-adrenal aldosterone-producing tumors
- Familial hyperaldosteronism type I or glucocorticoid-responsive aldosteronism
- Familial hyperaldosteronism type II

Aldosterone-producing adenomas are further classified as classic, or ACTH-responsive, and Ang II-responsive. Idiopathic adrenal hyperplasia is subdivided into unilateral and bilateral zona glomerulosa hyperplasia which is usually Ang II responsive or, less commonly, ACTH-responsive (also called primary hyperplasia). Adrenal carcinoma and extra-adrenal aldosterone-producing tumors are rare causes of PA, as are inherited disorders, familial hyperaldosteronism type I, or glucocorticoid-responsive aldosteronism, and familial hyperaldosteronism type II.

Blood pressure levels vary widely among patients with PA and do not predict etiology. Determining the cause of PA is essential for appropriate treatment, which is surgical for aldosterone-producing adenoma and medical for idiopathic hyperaldosteronism. Multiple maneuvers have been employed to distinguish between patients having an aldosterone-producing adenoma and idiopathic hyperaldosteronism. Aldosterone secretion in idiopathic hyperaldosteronism tends to be very sensitive to Ang II stimulation, while in aldosterone-producing adenoma production it is more commonly independent of the RAS. One of the earliest tests, and one that is still used, is based upon this difference.[44] Changes in aldosterone secretion in response to an elevation in Ang II induced by a postural change from supine to standing are measured. Plasma aldosterone and PRA levels are compared in blood samples drawn upon waking in the morning before the patient sits up, then after 4 hours of ambulation. Patients with an adrenal adenoma usually experience a decrease in aldosterone after the upright posture, reflecting the circadian decrease in ACTH and independence from the RAS. Aldosterone in patients with idiopathic hyperaldosteronism increased after standing due to extreme sensitivity to even minor changes in Ang II produced by the change in posture.[44] Sensitivity to Ang II was then confirmed using Ang II infusions.[45] This test is still used in conjunction with imaging using computed tomography (CT) scans or magnetic resonance imaging (MRI) to more accurately differentiate between the two types of PA.[46,47] However, subsequent studies have demonstrated heterogeneity among the response of aldosterone-producing adrenal adenomas to ACTH and Ang II. Some tumors, up to 40%, are not sensitive to ACTH, but are sensitive to Ang II.[48] Aldosterone secretion in these patients behaves similarly to those with idiopathic hyperaldosteronism. Some patients with idiopathic hyperplasia are not responsive to Ang II, but are responsive to ACTH, the incidence of which is unknown.[49] Elevated concentrations of the intermediate metabolites 18 hydroxycorticosterone, 18 hydroxy-cortisol and 18 oxo-cortisol suggest an aldosterone-producing adrenal adenoma or glucocorticoid-suppressible aldosteronism, while lower levels suggest idiopathic hyperaldosteronism.[50,51] However, the diagnostic usefulness of these tests remains to be confirmed.[10]

Bilateral adrenal vein sampling is the preferred predictive test for unilateral disease amenable to surgical treatment.[11,52,53] Blood samples from each adrenal vein and the inferior vena cava or another peripheral vein are taken for aldosterone and cortisol measurements. Results are expressed as plasma aldosterone/cortisol ratio to verify the position of the catheter in the adrenal vein and to correct for dilutional effects of sampling. If the aldosterone/cortisol ratio on one side is greater than four to five times that of the other, removal of the adrenal on that side is indicated.[15]

While adrenal vein sampling is still considered the best test to differentiate between adenoma and hyperplasia, there have been rare patients described who clearly had unilateral aldosterone production upon adrenal vein catheterization, yet the histopathology of the removed gland demonstrated adrenal zona glomerulosa hyperplasia with no tumor[54] or multiple 'microadenomas'.[55]

Bilateral adrenal vein sampling is a difficult procedure because the right adrenal vein is small; the success rate depends on the proficiency of the angiographer.[11,52,53] In cases where cannulation of one of the adrenal veins fails, a ratio of aldosterone to cortisol in the sampled side that is less than the ratio in peripheral plasma sample strongly suggests a contralateral adenoma.[47] However, this interpretation has been established in retrospective studies of overtly hypokalemic PA and may not be as useful in the prospective evaluation of patients.[11,15,36,56,57]

Adrenal CT scan, with an estimated sensitivity of 50%, is more sensitive than nuclear magnetic resonance (NMR) imaging in distinguishing between aldosterone-producing adenoma and idiopathic hyperaldosteronism. Adrenal adenomas tend to have more lipid-rich cells, producing less pre-contrast on CT.[58] When a solitary unilateral macroadenoma (> 1 cm) and normal contralateral morphology are found on CT in a patient less than 40 years old with PA, unilateral adrenalectomy is a reasonable therapeutic option; however, there are occasional patients with idiopathic hyperaldosteronism with unilateral nodules that are large enough to be confused with an aldosterone-producing adenoma. Because the majority of aldosterone-producing adenomas do not exceed 1 cm in diameter, however, CT scan cannot distinguish with adequate accuracy between idiopathic hyperaldosteronism and aldosterone-producing adenoma in most cases and CT-negative microadenomas are not uncommon.[36]

In a prospective study at the Mayo Clinic between September 1990 and October 2003, 203 patients with PA were studied by adrenal vein catheterization and CT scanning. Of 194 patients in whom both adrenal veins were catheterized, 110 patients (57%) had unilateral aldosterone secretion. Of the 143 who also had adrenal CT, 58 appeared to have normal adrenals by CT scan, yet 24 of these (41%) had unilateral hypersecretion of aldosterone. Only 51% of the 47 patients with a unilateral micronodule (≤10 mm) visualized by CT also had lateralization of aldosterone secretion; in 7 of these the unilateral aldosterone hypersecretion was from the contralateral adrenal that had no nodule on the CT scan. Of 32 with unilateral macronodule (>10 mm) apparent on CT, 21 had unilateral aldosterone hypersecretion, one of these being from the contralateral adrenal. Unilateral aldosterone secretion was found in 16 of 33 patients with bilateral micronodules, and 2 of 6 with bilateral macronodules visualized by CT. In this study CT findings were misleading in almost half the patients and would have incorrectly excluded 22% patients as candidates for adrenalectomy, while 25% might have had unnecessary or inappropriate adrenalectomy.[53] The fallibility of CT scans in diagnosing aldosterone-producing adenomas has been reported by others.[52] Adrenal vein sampling is the only method to distinguish between unilateral and bilateral adrenal aldosterone hypersecretion because nonfunctional adrenal incidentalomas are not uncommon. Notwithstanding, if the patient with PA is under 40 years old and a single adenoma is found on CT, removal of the gland is recommended.[53]

Adrenocortical scintigraphy with radiolabeled 131-I-cholesterol analogs, performed after dexamethasone suppression, can be done without the discontinuation of antihypertensive medications and has the advantage of correlating function with anatomic abnormalities.[59] Scintigraphy can augment CT and MRI results when bilateral adrenal vein sampling is not possible; however, the sensitivity of scintigraphy with radiolabeled 131-I-cholesterol analogs cannot distinguish nodules < 1.5 cm in diameter, so is not very helpful in most cases.

As previously discussed, hypersecretion of aldosterone from a unilateral lesion suppresses aldosterone production by the contralateral gland. Accordingly, in those patients in which adrenal vein sampling was possible in only one vein, an adrenal vein aldosterone/cortisol ratio less than that of peripheral blood was shown to correctly diagnose an aldosterone-producing adenoma in the contralateral gland. Finding that the aldosterone/cortisol ratio was elevated in a single adrenal vein effluent compared with the peripheral sample in patients positive by the postural test predicted an aldosterone-producing tumor on the sampled side.[47] However, these patients had PA with overt hypokalemia; this interpretation has not been very reliable when applied to less severe cases of primary aldosteronism.[36,53]

GENETIC FORMS OF HYPERALDOSTERONISM

The cause of idiopathic hyperaldosteronism is uncertain, but insight may be gained by studying the molecular mechanisms of the control of aldosterone secretion, starting with genetic causes of hyperaldosteronism. Of the inherited forms of PA, only glucocorticoid-remediable aldosteronism is well understood at this time. The CYP11B2 gene coding for the aldosterone synthase enzyme and the CYP11B1 gene coding for the 11β-hydroxylase that produces cortisol by 11β-hydroxylation of the 17-hydroxysteroid, deoxycortisol within the zona fasciculata, are highly homologous and lie in tandem on chromosome 8 in the human.[60] The first variety of familial PA recognized was glucocorticoid-suppressible (remediable) aldosteronism, or familial hyperaldosteronism type I (FH-I), caused by a cross-over recombination between the CYP11B2 and CYP11B1 genes. The resulting gene has the 5′ sequences comprising the coding and regulatory sequences of the 11β-hydroxylase gene and 3′ sequences including most of the coding sequences of the aldosterone synthase gene.[56,61] This hybrid gene is regulated by ACTH and expressed in the zona fasciculata-reticularis,[62] but produces aldosterone. The phenotype of those with the FH-I mutation is highly variable, from little or no pathology to severe childhood-onset hypertension leading to early cerebrovascular events.[63,64]

A second form of inherited PA, FH-II, has also been described that is probably more common than FH-I.[56] This familial variety of PA is neither glucocorticoid-remediable nor associated with the 'hybrid gene' mutation. In some families, linkage was found to a locus mapped to chromosome 7p22.[56,65]

The associations between CYP11B2 polymorphisms and hypertension and cardiac hypertrophy have been sought by several laboratories with variable results. Several polymorphisms of the CYP11B2 gene have been implicated in left ventricular mass or volume, including C344T, G5937C, A4550C and a gene conversion in intron2 (Int2C).[66–68] C344T, a polymorphism in the CYP11B2 promoter region coding for the steroidogenic factor-1 binding site, has been found to be associated with an increase in essential hypertension and cardiac hypertrophy in several predominantly Caucasian populations,[69–73] but not by others in similar cohorts.[74,75] The C344T polymorphism has been associated with an increased aldosterone/renin ratio in hypertensive patients, particularly when combined with the Int2C variant, suggesting that altered production of aldosterone may be mediating the increased blood pressure in these patients.[69,70,76] The C344T CYP11B2 gene polymorphism is also associated with an elevation in plasma 11-deoxycortisol, the substrate for cortisol production by 11β-hydroxylase, in both normotensive and hypertensive people.[71] Production of 11-deoxycortisol was shown to be elevated in essential and low renin hypertension over 25 years ago.[77,78] It is postulated that this increase in the substrate for 11β-hydroxylase, the gene product of CYP11B1, may be caused by a linkage disequilibrium between the C344T polymorphism, the CYP11B2 gene, and variants in the nearby CYP11B1 gene rendering the 11β-hydroxylase less efficient.[14,70,73,79,80]

TREATMENT

The treatment of choice for an aldosterone-producing adenoma is unilateral adrenalectomy. Removal of the offending adrenal in patients with aldosterone-producing adenoma results in normal potassium homeostasis and improvement in hypertension in all patients; 30–60% are cured of their hypertension.[57] Currently laparoscopic adrenalectomy is the preferred surgical approach because it is associated with less morbidity and shorter hospital stays.[36,81] Risk factors for persistent hypertension include advanced age, lack of response to spironolactone, and hypertension upon discharge from hospital.[82] A significant proportion of patients with lateralization of aldosterone production and assumed to have an adenoma are found upon pathological examination of the resected adrenal to have unilateral zona glomerulosa hyperplasia.[83] Removal of the affected adrenal usually results in a cure or marked improvement of the hypertension, but patients retain a deficient suppression of plasma aldosterone when given salt and fludrocortisone.[84] This suggests that many cases of PA with unilateral hypersecretion represent cases of adrenal hyperplasia with 'hot' unilateral nodules that overexpress the enzymes of aldosterone production. This would be a situation analogous to that of hyperthyroidism produced by multinodular goiter with a hot nodule.

The mineralocorticoid receptor antagonist spironolactone has been the drug of choice to treat primary aldosteronism for more than three decades. The starting dose of spironolactone is 25–50 mg twice daily with food, increasing it weekly as necessary to a maximum of 200 mg twice daily. Many patients respond to low doses of spironolactone.[18,85] In addition to binding the mineralocorticoid receptors, spironolactone is also an antagonist of the androgen receptor and, to a lesser extent, an agonist of the progesterone receptor. At higher doses spironolactone frequently causes painful gynecomastia and erectile dysfunction or menstrual irregularity.[57] Eplerenone is a recently FDA-approved mineralocorticoid receptor antagonist that has significantly less binding affinity for the androgen and progesterone receptors compared with spironolactone and a lower incidence of side effects.[36,86] Effective pharmacological treatment made possible by the advent of mineralocorticoid receptor antagonists with fewer side effects may decrease the number of patients seeking surgical treatment. Among the multiple effects mediated by aldosterone through the mineralocorticoid receptor is the increased movement of sodium ions through the epithelial sodium channel leading indirectly to potassium loss in the urine. Amiloride, an epithelial sodium channel antagonist, can be used for its potassium-sparing properties in patients who are intolerant of spironolactone. Amiloride dosing may be started at 5 mg twice daily and increased up to 15 mg twice daily. Amiloride is not a very effective antihypertensive or diuretic, so hydrochlorothiazide may also be required.

CONCLUSION

PA is an important cause of hypertension that is associated with significant cardiovascular pathology in addition to and independent of the elevation of blood pressure. It is therefore imperative that in addition to normalizing the blood pressure, levels of aldosterone be normalized or its effects be antagonized. When lowering of the aldosterone levels cannot be achieved, an inhibitor of the mineralocorticoid receptor should be used alone, or in addition to other antihypertensive agents. To select the most effective therapy, surgical or medical, one must distinguish between idiopathic hyperaldosteronism and aldosterone-producing adenomas as the cause of the PA.

REFERENCES

1. Gomez-Sanchez EP. Central hypertensive effects of aldosterone. Front Neuroendocrinol 1997; 18: 440–62.
2. Gomez-Sanchez CE, Gomez-Sanchez EP. Role of central mineralocorticoid receptors in cardiovascular disease. Curr Hypertens Rep 2001; 3: 263–9.
3. Gomez-Sanchez EP. Brain mineralocorticoid receptors: orchestrators of hypertension and end-organ disease. Curr Opin Nephrol Hypertens 2004; 13: 191–6.
4. Conn JW. Primary aldosteronism, a new clinical syndrome. J Lab Clin Med 1955; 45: 3–7.
5. Simpson SA, Tait JF, Wettstein A, Neher R, Van Euw J, Reichstein T. Isolierung eines neuen kristallisierten hormons aus nebennieren mit besonders hoher wirksamkeit auf den mineralostoffwechsel. Experientia 1953; 9: 333–5.
6. Conn JW, Cohen EL, Rovner DR, Nesbit RM. Normokalemic primary aldosteronism. A detectable cause of curable 'essential' hypertension. JAMA 1965; 193: 200–6.
7. Berglund G, Andersson O, Wilhelmsen L. Prevalence of primary and secondary hypertension: studies in a random population sample. Br Med J 1976; 2: 554–6.
8. Fishman LM, Kuchel O, Liddle GW, Michelakis AM, Gordon RD, Chick WT. Incidence of primary aldosteronism uncomplicated 'essential' hypertension. A prospective study with elevated aldosterone secretion and suppressed plasma renin activity used as diagnostic criteria. JAMA 1968; 205: 497–502.
9. Mulatero P, Stowasser M, Loh KC et al. Increased diagnosis of primary aldosteronism, including surgically correctable forms, in centers from five continents. J Clin Endocrinol Metab 2004; 89: 1045–50.
10. Veglio F, Morello F, Rabbia F, Leotta G, Mulatero P. Recent advances in diagnosis and treatment of primary aldosteronism. Minerva Med 2003; 94: 259–65.
11. Stowasser M, Gordon RD, Gunasekera TG et al. High rate of detection of primary aldosteronism, including surgically treatable forms, after 'non-selective' screening of hypertensive patients. J Hypertens 2003; 21: 2149–57.
12. Mosso L, Carvajal C, Gonzalez A et al. Primary aldosteronism and hypertensive disease. Hypertension 2003; 42: 161–5.
13. Calhoun DA, Nishizaka MK, Zaman MA, Thakkar RB, Weissmann P. Hyperaldosteronism among black and white subjects with resistant hypertension. Hypertension 2002; 40: 892–6.
14. Fardella CE, Mosso L, Gomez-Sanchez CE et al. Primary hyperaldosteronism in essential hypertensives: prevalence, biochemical profile and molecular biology. J Clin Endocrinol Metab 2000; 85: 1863–7.
15. Stowasser M, Gordon RD. Primary aldosteronism. Best Pract Res Clin Endocrinol Metab 2003; 17: 591–605.
16. Abdelhamid S, Blomer R, Hommel G et al. Urinary tetrahydroaldosterone as a screening method for primary aldosteronism: a comparative study. Am J Hypertens 2003; 16: 522–30.
17. Calhoun DA, Nishizaka MK, Zaman MA, Harding SM. Aldosterone excretion among subjects with resistant hypertension and symptoms of sleep apnea. Chest 2004; 125: 112–7.
18. Nishizaka MK, Zaman MA, Calhoun DA. Efficacy of low-dose spironolactone in subjects with resistant hypertension. Am J Hypertens 2003; 16: 925–30.
19. Bortolotto LA, Cesena FH, Jatene FB, Silva HB. Malignant hypertension and hypertensive encephalopathy in primary aldosteronism caused by adrenal adenoma. Arq Bras Cardiol 2003; 81: 97–100, 93–6.
20. Zelinka T, Strauch B, Pecen L, Widimsky J Jr. Diurnal blood pressure variation in pheochromocytoma, primary aldosteronism and Cushing's syndrome. J Hum Hypertens 2004; 18: 107–11.
21. Berecek KH, Bohr DF. Whole body vascular reactivity during the development of deoxycorticosterone acetate hypertension in the pig. Circ Res 1978; 42: 764–71.
22. Weber KT. Aldosteronism revisited: perspectives on less well-recognized actions of aldosterone. J Lab Clin Med 2003; 142: 71–82.
23. Rizzoni D, Muiesan M, Porteri E et al. Relations between cardiac and vascular structure in patients with primary and secondary hypertension. J Am Coll Cardiol 1998; 32: 985–992.
24. Rossi GP, Di Bello V, Ganzaroli C et al. Excess aldosterone is associated with alterations of myocardial texture in primary aldosteronism. Hypertension 2002; 40: 23–7.
25. Kozakova M, Buralli S, Palombo C et al. Myocardial ultrasonic backscatter in hypertension: relation to aldosterone and endothelin. Hypertension 2003; 41: 230–6.
26. Rossi GP, Cavallin M, Nussdorfer GG, Pessina AC. The endothelin-aldosterone axis and cardiovascular diseases. J Cardiovasc Pharmacol 2001; 38: S49–S52.
27. Horton R, Biglieri EG. Effect of aldosterone on the metabolism of aldosterone. J Clin Endocrinol Metab 1962; 22: 1187–92.
28. Delva P, Lechi A. Intralymphocyte magnesium decrease in patients with primary aldosteronism. Possible links with cardiac remodelling. Magnes Res 2003; 16: 206–9.
29. Hiramatsu K, Yamada T, Yukimura Y et al. A screening test to identify aldosterone-producing adenoma by measuring plasma renin activity. Results in hypertensive patients. Arch Intern Med 1981; 141: 1589–93.
30. Lim PO, MacDonald TM. Primary aldosteronism, diagnosed by the aldosterone to renin ratio, is a common cause of hypertension. Clin Endocrinol (Oxf) 2003; 59: 427–30.
31. Mulatero P, Rabbia F, Milan A et al. Drug effects on aldosterone/plasma renin activity ratio in primary aldosteronism. Hypertension 2002; 40: 897–902.
32. Tanabe A, Naruse M, Takagi S, Tsuchiya K, Imaki T, Takano K. Variability in the renin/aldosterone profile under random and standardized sampling conditions in primary aldosteronism. J Clin Endocrinol Metab 2003; 88: 2489–94.
33. Castro OL, Yu X, Kem DC. Diagnostic value of the post-captopril test in primary aldosteronism. Hypertension 2002; 39: 935–8.
34. Unger N, Lopez Schmidt I, Pitt C et al. Comparison of active renin concentration and plasma renin activity for the diagnosis of primary hyperaldosteronism in patients with an adrenal mass. Eur J Endocrinol 2004; 150: 517–23.
35. Ulick S, Laragh JH, Lieberman S. The isolation of urinary metabolite of aldosterone and its use to measure the rate of secretion of aldosterone by the adrenal cortex of man. Trans Assoc Am Physicians 1958; 71: 225–35.
36. Young WF Jr. Minireview: primary aldosteronism – changing concepts in diagnosis and treatment. Endocrinology 2003; 144: 2208–13.
37. Kem DC, Weinberger MH, Mayes DM, Nugent CA. Saline suppression of plasma aldosterone in hypertension. Arch Intern Med 1971; 128: 380–6.

38. Streeten DHP, Tomycz N, Anderson GH. Reliability of screening methods for the diagnosis of primary aldosteronism. Am J Med 1979; 67: 403–13.
39. Weinberger MH, Grim CE, Hollifield JW et al. Primary aldosteronism. Diagnosis, localization and treatment. Ann Intern Med 1979; 90: 386–95.
40. Holland O, Brown H, Kuhnert L, Fairchild C, Risk M, Gomez-Sanchez CE. Further evaluation of saline infusion for the diagnosis of primary aldosteronism. Hypertension 1984; 6: 717–23.
41. Young WF Jr. Primary aldosteronism: management issues. Ann N Y Acad Sci 2002; 970: 61–76.
42. Conn JW, Knopf RF, Nesbit RM. Clinical characteristics of primary aldosteronism from an analysis of 145 cases. Am J Surg 1964; 107: 159–72.
43. Baer L, Sommers SC, Krakoff LR, Newton MA, Laragh JH. Pseudo-primary aldosteronism. An entity distinct from true primary aldosteronism. Circ Res 1970; 27: 203–20.
44. Ganguly A, Melada GA, Luetscher JA, Dowdy AJ. Control of plasma aldosterone in primary aldosteronism: distinction between adenoma and hyperplasia. J Clin Endocrinol Metab 1973; 37: 765–75.
45. Wisgerhof M, Brown RD, Hogan MJ, Carpenter PC, Edis AJ. The plasma aldosterone response to angiotensin II infusion in aldosterone-producing adenoma and idiopathic hyperaldosteronism. J Clin Endocrinol Metab 1981; 52: 195–8.
46. Phillips JL, Walther MM, Pezzullo JC et al. Predictive value of preoperative tests in discriminating bilateral adrenal hyperplasia from an aldosterone producing adrenal adenoma. J Clin Endocrinol Metab 2000; 85: 4526–33.
47. Espiner EA, Ross DG, Yandle TG, Richards AM, Hunt PJ. Predicting surgically remedial primary aldosteronism: role of adrenal scanning, posture testing, and adrenal vein sampling. J Clin Endocrinol Metab 2003; 88: 3637–44.
48. Tunny TJ, Klemm SA, Stowasser M, Gordon RD. Angiotensin-responsive aldosterone-producing adenomas: postoperative disappearance of aldosterone response to angiotensin. Clin Exp Pharmacol Physiol 1993; 20: 306–9.
49. Irony I, Kater CE, Biglieri EG, Shackleton CH. Correctable subsets of primary aldosteronism. Primary adrenal hyperplasia and renin responsive adenoma. Am J Hypertens 1990; 3: 576–82.
50. Gomez-Sanchez CE, Montgomery M, Ganguly A et al. Elevated urinary excretion of 18-oxocortisol in glucocorticoid suppressible aldosteronism. J Clin Endocrinol Metab 1984; 59: 1022–4.
51. Gomez-Sanchez CE, Gill JJR, Ganguly A, Gordon RD. Glucocorticoid-suppressible aldosteronism: a disorder of the adrenal transitional zone. J Clin Endocrinol Metab 1988; 67: 444–8.
52. Magill SB, Raff H, Shaker JL et al. Comparison of adrenal vein sampling and computed tomography in the differentiation of primary aldosteronism. J Clin Endocrinol Metab 2001; 86: 1066–71.
53. Young WF, Stanson AW, Thompson GB, Grant CS, Farley DR, van Heerden JA. Role for adrenal venous sampling in primary aldosteronism. Surgery 2004; 136: 1227–35.
54. Ganguly A, Zager PG, Luetscher JA. Primary aldosteronism due to unilateral adrenal hyperplasia. J Clin Endocrinol Metab 1980; 51: 1190–4.
55. Omura M, Sasano H, Fujiwara T, Yamaguchi K, Nishikawa T. Unique cases of unilateral hyperaldosteronemia due to multiple adrenocortical micronodules, which can only be detected by selective adrenal venous sampling. Metabolism 2002; 51: 350–5.
56. Stowasser M, Gordon RD. Primary aldosteronism: from genesis to genetics. Trends Endocrinol Metab 2003; 14: 310–17.
57. Young WF Jr. Primary aldosteronism – treatment options. Growth Horm IGF Res 2003; 13 (Suppl A): S102–S108.
58. Yamada T, Ishibashi T, Saito H et al. Adrenal adenomas: relationship between histologic lipid-rich cells and CT attenuation number. Eur J Radiol 2003; 48: 198–202.
59. Nocaudie-Calzada M, Huglo D, Lambert M et al. Efficacy of iodine-131 6beta-methyl-iodo-19-norcholesterol scintigraphy and computed tomography in patients with primary aldosteronism. Eur J Nuclear Med 1999; 26: 1326–32.
60. Taymans S, Pack S, Pak E, Torpy D, Zhuang Z, Stratakis C. Human CYP11B2 (aldosterone synthase) maps to chromosome 8q24.3. J Clin Endocrinol Metab 1998; 83: 1033–6.
61. Lifton RP, Dluhy RG, Powers M et al. A chimaeric 11β-hydroxylase/aldosterone synthase gene causes glucocorticoid-remediable aldosteronism and human hypertension. Nature 1992; 355: 262–5.
62. Pascoe L, Jeunemaitre X, Lebrethon MC et al. Glucocorticoid suppressible hyperaldosteronism and adrenal tumors occurring in a single French pedigree. J Clin Invest 1995; 96: 2236–46.
63. Mulatero P, di Cella SM, Williams TA et al. Glucocorticoid remediable aldosteronism: low morbidity and mortality in a four-generation Italian pedigree. J Clin Endocrinol Metab 2002; 87: 3187–91.
64. Litchfield WR, Anderson BF, Weiss RJ, Lifton RP, Dluhy RG. Intracranial aneurysm and hemorrhagic stroke in glucocorticoid-remediable aldosteronism. Hypertension 1998; 31: 445–50.
65. Lafferty AR, Torpy DJ, Stowasser M et al. A novel genetic locus for low renin hypertension: familial hyperaldosteronism type II maps to chromosome 7 (7p22). J Med Genet 2000; 37: 831–5.
66. Kupari M, Hautanen A, Lankinen L, Koskinen P, Virolainen J, Nikkila H. Associations between human aldosterone synthase (CYP11B2) gene polymorphisms and left ventricular size, mass, and function. Circulation 1998; 97: 569–75.
67. White PC, Hautanen A, Kupari M. Aldosterone synthase (cyp11b2) polymorphisms and cardiovascular function. J Steroid Biochem Mol Biol 1999; 69: 409–12.
68. Mayosi BM, Keavney B, Watkins H, Farrall M. Measured haplotype analysis of the aldosterone synthase gene and heart size. Eur J Hum Genet 2003; 11: 395–401.
69. Davies E, Holloway CD, Ingram MC et al. Aldosterone excretion rate and blood pressure in essential hypertension are related to polymorphic differences in the aldosterone synthase gene CYP11B2. Hypertension 1999; 33: 703–7.
70. Lim PO, MacDonald TM, Holloway C et al. Variation at the aldosterone synthase (CYP11B2) locus contributes to hypertension in subjects with a raised aldosterone-to-renin ratio. J Clin Endocrinol Metab 2002; 87: 4398–402.
71. Keavney B, Mayosi B, Gaukrodger N et al. Genetic variation at the locus encompassing 11-beta hydroxylase and aldosterone synthase accounts for heritability in cortisol precursor (11-deoxycortisol) urinary metabolite excretion. J Clin Endocrinol Metab 2005; 90: 1072–7.
72. Stella P, Bigatti G, Tizzoni L et al. Association between aldosterone synthase (CYP11B2) polymorphism and left ventricular mass in human essential hypertension. J Am Coll Cardiol 2004; 43: 265–70.
73. Ganapathipillai S, Laval G, Hoffmann IS et al. CYP11B2-CYP11B1 haplotypes associated with decreased 11 beta-hydroxylase activity. J Clin Endocrinol Metab 2005; 90: 1220–5.
74. Schunkert H, Hengstenberg C, Holmer SR et al. Lack of association between a polymorphism of the aldosterone synthase gene and left ventricular structure. Circulation 1999; 99: 2255–60.
75. Ortlepp JR, Breithardt O, Ohme F, Hanrath P, Hoffmann R. Lack of association among five genetic polymorphisms of the renin-angiotensin system and cardiac hypertrophy in patients with aortic stenosis. Am Heart J 2001; 141: 671–6.

76. Connell JM, Kenyon CJ, Ingram M et al. Corticosteroids in essential hypertension: multiple candidate loci and phenotypic variation. Clin Exp Pharmacol Physiol 1996; 23: 369–74.
77. Honda M, Nowaczynski W, Guthrie GP Jr et al. Response of several adrenal steroids to ACTH stimulation in essential hypertension. J Clin Endocrinol Metab 1977; 44: 264–72.
78. de Simone G, Tommaselli AP, Rossi R et al. Partial deficiency of adrenal 11-hydroxylase: a possible cause of primary hypertension. Hypertension 1985; 7: 204–10.
79. White PC, Slutsker L. Haplotype analysis of CYP11B2. Endocr Res 1995; 21: 437–42.
80. Davies E, Holloway CD, Ingram MC et al. An influence of variation in the aldosterone synthase gene (CYP11B2) on corticosteroid responses to ACTH in normal human subjects. Clin Endocrinol (Oxf) 2001; 54: 813–17.
81. Harris DA, Au-Yong I, Basnyat PS, Sadler GP, Wheeler MH. Review of surgical management of aldosterone secreting tumours of the adrenal cortex. Eur J Surg Oncol 2003; 29: 467–74.
82. Wheeler MH, Harris DA. Diagnosis and management of primary aldosteronism. World J Surg 2003; 27: 627–31.
83. Neville AM, O'Hare MJ. The Human Adrenal Cortex, Pathology and Biology. An Integrated Approach. Heidelberg: Springer-Verlag, 1982.
84. Rutherford JC, Taylor WL, Stowasser M, Gordon RD. Success of surgery for primary aldosteronism judged by residual autonomous aldosterone production. World J Surg 1998; 22: 1243–5.
85. Lim PO, Young WF, MacDonald TM. A review of the medical treatment of primary aldosteronism. J Hypertens 2001; 19: 353–61.
86. de Gasparo M, Joss U, Ramjoue HP et al. Three new epoxy-spirolactone derivatives: characterization in vivo and in vitro. J Pharmacol Exp Ther 1987; 240: 650–6.

14

Mineralocorticoid hypertension

Nathaniel Winer

INTRODUCTION

Mineralocorticoids raise blood pressure by increasing salt reabsorption via renal cortical tubular epithelial sodium channels (ENaC), which are highly regulated by the renin-angiotensin system (RAS). Primary aldosteronism, the most striking example of mineralocorticoid excess, is discussed in Chapter 13. Other forms of mineralocorticoid hypertension may be attributed to excessive adrenal mineralocorticoid secretion, an inability to metabolize cortisol to its inactive metabolite, cortisone, or mutations that alter the function of either the glucocorticoid or mineralocorticoid receptor (Box 14.1).

Box 14.1 Disorders associated with mineralocorticoid hypertension

Excessive mineralocorticoid hormone secretion
- Primary aldosteronism
- Glucocorticoid-remediable aldosteronism
- Congenital adrenal hyperplasia
  - 11β-hydroxylase deficiency
  - 17α-hydroxylase deficiency

Conditions affecting cortisol metabolism
- Syndrome of apparent mineralocorticoid excess
- Chronic licorice ingestion
- Carbenoxolone treatment
- Ectopic ACTH syndrome

Glucocorticoid or mineralocorticoid receptor mutations
- Glucocorticoid receptor resistance
- Pregnancy-exacerbated hypertension
- Liddle syndrome

EXCESSIVE MINERALOCORTICOID HORMONE SECRETION

Glucocorticoid-remediable aldosteronism

Glucocorticoid-remediable aldosteronism (GRA), also known as dexamethasone-suppressible hyperaldosteronism and familial hyperaldosteronism type I, was first described in 1966 in a father and son with hypertension, hypokalemia, increased aldosterone secretion, and suppressed plasma renin activity (PRA).[1] Reversal of these manifestations with glucocorticoid treatment suggested that adrenocorticotropic hormone (ACTH) was regulating aldosterone secretion in these patients.[1] Subsequently, GRA has been reported worldwide, most frequently in North America among families of Celtic ancestry, but not in black people.

Pathophysiology

In GRA aldosterone secretion is regulated by ACTH, rather than angiotensin II (Ang II) and potassium, the principal secretogogues of aldosterone under normal conditions. Consequently, aldosterone levels are unaffected by changes in sodium balance, but instead parallel the diurnal variation of ACTH and cortisol. The resultant chronic mineralocorticoid excess can be countered by the administration of glucocorticoids to suppress ACTH. In addition, the zona fasciculata produces the hybrid compounds, 18-oxocortisol and 18-hydroxy cortisol, which have characteristics of both aldosterone and cortisol and may have sodium-retaining properties (Figure 14.1).

Clinical features

GRA may present as moderate or severe hypertension, often in early childhood or adolescence.[2] Blood

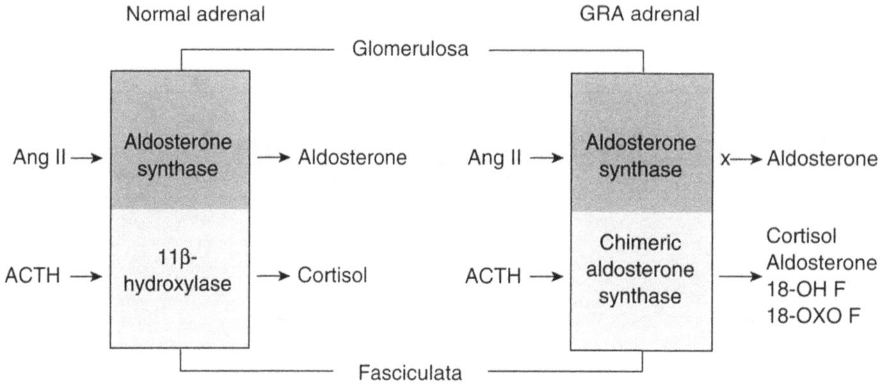

Figure 14.1 Mechanism underlying glucocorticoid-remediable aldosteronism. Unequal crossing over of two closely related genes results in a chimeric gene that combines the regulatory sequences of the 11β-hydroxylase gene with the coding sequences of the aldosterone synthase gene. The encoded gene product, which is located ectopically in the adrenal fasciculata, expresses aldosterone synthase enzymatic activity. Because aldosterone secretion is regulated by ACTH rather than angiotensin II (Ang II), maintenance of normal cortisol levels results in constitutive aldosterone secretion, leading to salt and water retention and hypertension. In addition the hybrid aldosterone synthase produces 18-hydroxy cortisol (18-OH F) and 18-oxocortisol (18-OXO F), which may have mineralocorticoid properties

pressure control is frequently resistant to conventional antihypertensive agents, such as angiotensin converting enzyme (ACE) inhibitors and β-blockers. In affected relatives blood pressure may range from normal to severely elevated. An analysis of families with GRA has shown an increased prevalence of cerebral aneurysms, leading to fatal cerebral hemorrhage.[2] Screening for aneurysms with magnetic resonance angiography (MRA) at 5-year intervals beginning at puberty has been advocated for patients with GRA.[3] Although hypokalemia was believed to be a hallmark of GRA, most patients are normokalemic, possibly because both a blunted aldosterone secretory response to K^+ and a greater nocturnal decline in aldosterone secretion reduce kaliuresis, compared with other forms of primary aldosteronism.[4]

Genetics

GRA is inherited as an autosomal dominant disorder without gender preference.[5] GRA arises from unequal crossing over of the genes for 11β-hydroxylase (CYP11B1) and aldosterone synthase (CYP11B2). Located on chromosome 8, these genes, which share a high degree of nucleotide homology, produce a chimeric gene that fuses the 5′ regulatory sequence of CYP11B1 with the 3′ coding sequence of CYP11B2, conferring aldosterone synthase enzymatic activity and responsiveness to ACTH on the gene product.[6] At least eight independent mutations with five different cross-over sites have been identified.[6] Although the sites of fusion from different pedigrees vary, encoded amino acids upstream of exon 5 are essential for aldosterone synthase activity.[5]

Diagnosis

GRA should be considered in children and adolescents with hypertension or in patients who are resistant to conventional antihypertensive medications. A family history of early hemorrhagic stroke should also raise suspicion for GRA. Serum K^+ levels are generally normal unless diuretic therapy has been prescribed. Often plasma renin activity (PRA) is suppressed and serum aldosterone is inappropriately elevated relative to sodium intake, since aldosterone is responsive to ACTH rather than the RAS. While 24-hour urine collections for 18-oxygenated steroids are sensitive and specific for the diagnosis of GRA, assays for these compounds are not widely available. Plasma aldosterone levels <4 ng/dL after administration of dexamethasone 0.5 mg every 6 hours over 2–4 days are also highly specific and sensitive for the diagnosis of GRA,[7] but the testing is inconvenient. Genetic screening has a specificity and sensitivity of 100% and requires only a blood specimen for evaluation of leucocyte DNA. The chimeric gene can be detected by the Southern blot technique[8] or by the more rapid long-PCR method.[9,10]

Treatment

The diagnosis of GRA allows targeted monotherapy with glucocorticoids and aldosterone antagonists, in conjunction with dietary sodium restriction. Prednisone or hydrocortisone are effective in suppressing the hypothalamic-pituitary axis and controlling blood pressure. The smallest possible dose should be used, particularly in children, to avoid stunting linear growth and hypoaldosteronism, as manifested by salt wasting, hypotension, and hyperkalemia. In adult patients blood pressure may be controlled by spironolactone alone (100–400 mg/day) or in combination with hydrochlorothiazide or furosemide. In men who develop gynecomastia or erectile dysfunction or women who complain of menstrual irregularity, eplerenone, an aldosterone antagonist with reduced affinity for androgen and progesterone receptors, may be substituted. Alternative therapeutic agents are amiloride and triamterene, both of which inhibit epithelial Na^+ channels in the distal tubule. Dihydropyridine calcium channel blockers, such as extended-release nifedipine and amlodipine, may be used, but are considered second-line drugs.[7]

Congenital adrenal hyperplasia (CAH)

Among the family of inborn errors of steroidogenesis only 11β-hydroxylase (CYP11B1) deficiency and 17α-hydroxylase/17,20-lyase deficiency (CYP17) are associated with hypertension. 11β-Hydroxylase deficiency ranks second to impaired 21-hydroxylation as the most common cause of CAH in the US and Western Europe, accounting for 5–8% of cases.[11] Among Israeli Jews of Moroccan ancestry the incidence of CYP11B1 deficiency may be as high as 1 in 5000 live births.[12]

Pathophysiology

11β-Hydroxylase deficiency reduces the conversion of 11-deoxycorticosterone to corticosterone and 11-deoxycortisol to cortisol, leading to increased production of ACTH and accumulation of 11-deoxy-precursors and adrenal androgens. Clinical manifestations of the disorder result from the mineralocorticoid effects of 11-deoxycorticosterone and the virilizing effects of the androgens (Figure 14.2).

Genetics

11β-Hydroxylase deficiency is an autosomal recessive disorder that results from mutations of the CYP11B1 gene located on chromosome 8q21-q22. Loss of enzyme activity is a consequence of missense, nonsense, or frameshift mutations of the CYP11B gene.[13]

Clinical manifestations

Hypertension occurs in about two-thirds of patients, usually early in life. Although 11-deoxycorticosterone is thought to cause hypertension, the correlation between serum 11-deoxycorticosterone and blood pressure is weak.[14] Among neonates females may have ambiguous genitalia and males may have penile enlargement. Androgen effects may be variable in time of onset with some patients showing signs of androgen excess only during adolescence.[14] Laboratory findings include hypokalemia, low plasma renin activity, and increased serum concentrations of 11-deoxycorticosterone, 11-deoxycortisol, and adrenal androgens, including dehydroepiandrosterone (DHEA), dehydroepiandrosterone sulfate (DHEA sulfate), androstenedione, and testosterone. Aldosterone levels are usually low because of suppression of the RAS by deoxycorticosterone.

Treatment

The goal of therapy is to reduce serum 11-deoxycorticosterone and androgens. Hydrocortisone in doses of 10–25 mg/m^2 will generally reduce blood pressure and suppress hyperandrogenism without growth retardation, delay in sexual maturation, or development of manifestations of Cushing's syndrome.

17α-Hydroxylase/17,20-lyase deficiency (CYP17) is an unusual cause of CAH, representing about 1% of cases in the US, but is more common among Brazilians of Spanish or Portuguese origin.[15] Both 17α-hydroxylase and 17,20-lyase enzymes are encoded by a single gene, located on chromosome 10, region q24–q25.[16,17] Approximately 30 mutations have been described to date.[18]

Pathophysiology

Patients present with low renin hypertension, hypokalemia and metabolic alkalosis because reduced cortisol synthesis leads to enhanced ACTH secretion and accumulation of corticosterone and deoxycorticosterone. Reduced 17α-hydroxylase/17,20-lyase enzymatic activity results in decreased production of C19 sex steroids in the adrenals and gonads[19] (Figure 14.2). As a consequence of testosterone deficiency affected females have normal genitalia at birth but absent secondary sexual characteristics in adolescence, while affected males may have female genitalia at birth.[19]

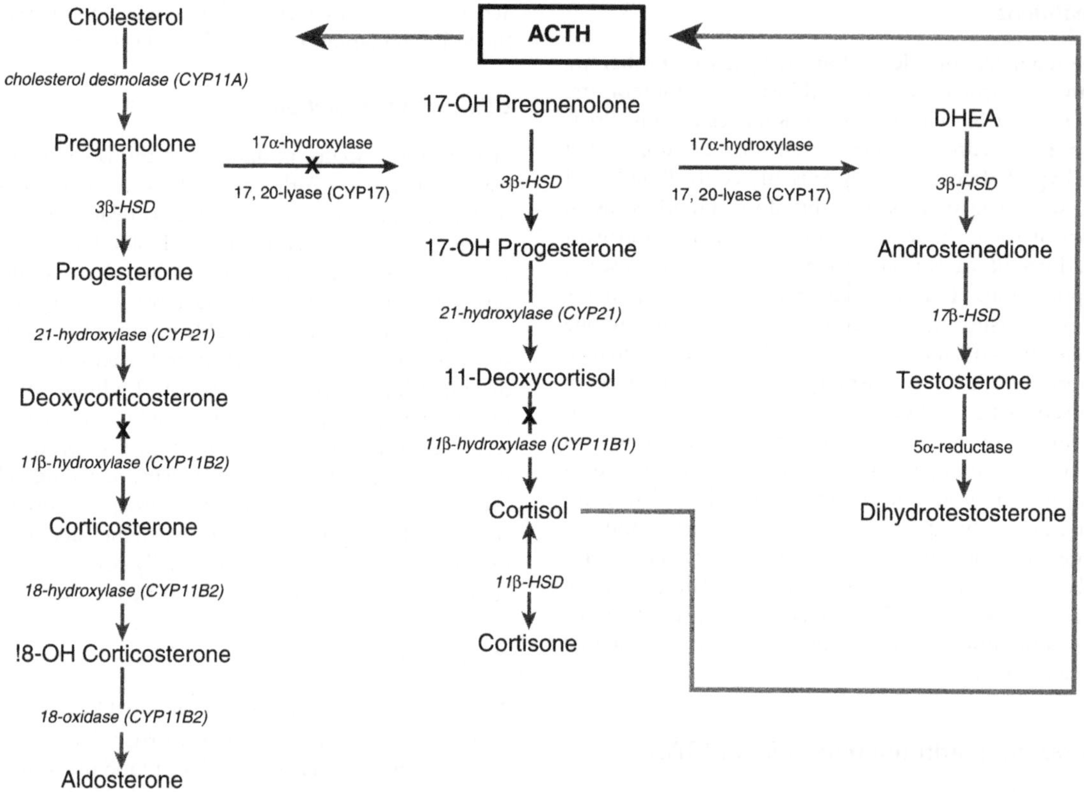

Figure 14.2 Biosynthetic pathways for mineralocorticoids, glucocorticoids, and androgens. Deficiency of 11β-hydroxylase activity (blue X) results in upstream accumulation of deoxycorticosterone and testosterone and dihydrotestosterone, leading to hypertension and virilization and/or ambiguous genitalia, respectively. Loss of 17α-hydroxylase/17,20-lyase activity (red X) is associated with hypertension because of high deoxycorticosterone levels, while diminished estrogen levels lead to absence of sexual development in adolescent females and testosterone deficiency results in external female genitalia in males. Enzyme activities mediated by specific P450 cytochromes are designated as 'CYP'. CYP11B2 (aldosterone synthase) and CYP17 have multiple enzymatic activities. 'HSD' designates hydroxysteroid dehydrogenase

Diagnosis

The diagnosis can be established by elevated levels of corticosterone and deoxycorticosterone and their metabolites, reduced circulating concentrations of cortisol and gonadal steroids, and elevated gonadotropins. Hypokalemia and suppressed renin may reduce aldosterone concentrations.

Treatment

The goals of therapy are to treat hypertension by reducing deoxycorticosterone levels with corticosteroid therapy and to correct androgen deficiency, if needed.

CONDITIONS AFFECTING CORTISOL METABOLISM

Syndrome of apparent mineralocorticoid excess

In 1979, Ulick et al.[20] described children with 'apparent mineralocorticoid excess' (AME), who presented with hypertension, hypokalemic alkalosis, and suppressed renin, but very low or undetectable aldosterone levels. Steroid patterns in these patients were characterized by an increased ratio of cortisol to cortisone, reflected by high urinary levels of 5β- and 5α-tetrahydrocortisol (5β-THF and 5α-THF) and very low or absent tetrahydrocortisone (THE). Although the half-life of cortisol

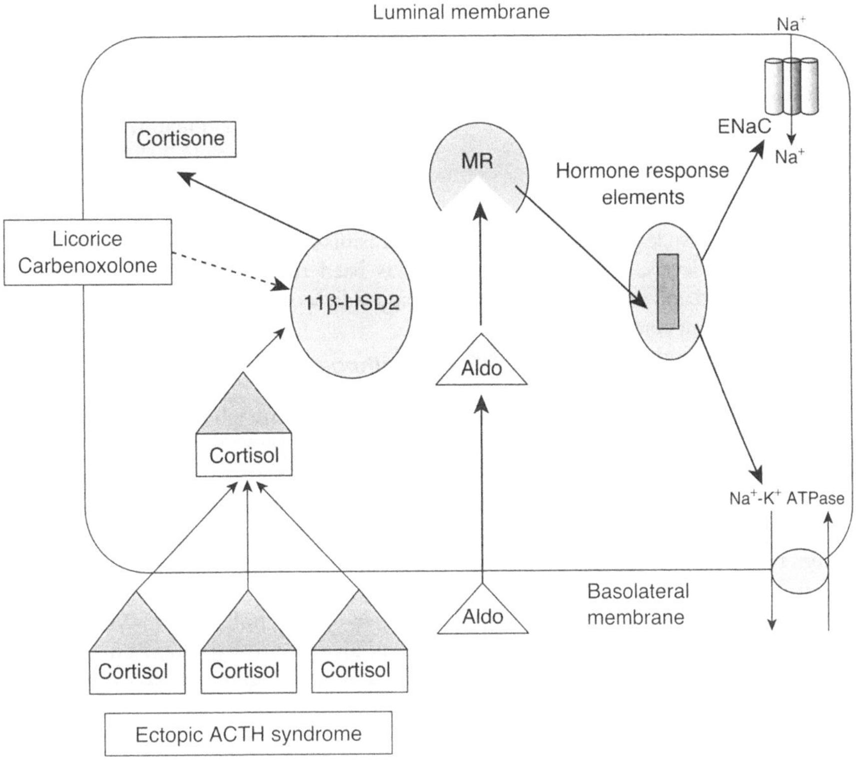

Figure 14.3 Role of 11β-HSD2 in protecting the mineralocorticoid receptor (MR). MR binds aldosterone (Aldo) and cortisol with equal affinity. Since plasma cortisol concentrations are 100-fold greater than those of aldosterone 11β-HSD2 protects MR from cortisol activation by converting cortisol to its inactive metabolite, cortisone. In the syndrome of apparent mineralocorticoid excess mutations in the gene encoding 11β-HSD2 lead to loss of enzymatic activity, increased cortisol binding to MR, hypertension and hypokalemia. High levels of plasma cortisol in ectopic ACTH syndrome may overwhelm the capacity of 11β-HSD2 to metabolize cortisol, producing a mineralocorticoid excess state. Similar findings may result from the ingestion of licorice or carbenoxolone, which competitively inhibit 11β-HSD2. The aldosterone- or cortisol-MR complex binds to DNA hormone response elements, increasing transcription of target genes, such as the luminal ENaC or basolateral sodium-potassium (Na^+-K^+) ATPase, causing sodium reabsorption and potassium excretion. (Adapted from Quinkler et al. Mol Cell Endocrinol 2004; 217: 143–9.[22])

was prolonged, circulating cortisol levels were normal because of the negative feedback effect of cortisol on ACTH secretion. The significance of these findings became apparent with the cloning of the mineralocorticoid receptor (MR),[21] which led to the unexpected observation that cortisol and aldosterone were nearly equipotent in activating MRs in vitro. Since serum cortisol concentrations are at least 100-fold greater than those of aldosterone, MR is protected from activation by conversion of hormonally active cortisol to biologically inactive cortisone by 11β-hydroxysteroid dehydrogenase type 2 (11β-HSD2). This enzyme, which co-localizes with MR, is found mainly in mineralocorticoid target tissues, including kidney, colon, and salivary glands.

Pathophysiology

Deficiency of 11β-HSD2 in AME permits cortisol to activate renal tubular MRs, leading to increased ENaC activity and hypertension (Figure 14.3). Nearly 100 cases of AME in about 60 kindreds and more than 30 different mutations in 11β-HSD2 have been reported.[22] Most patients with AME are homozygous for 11β-HSD2 mutations resulting in complete or partial loss of enzyme activity. Such patients present early in life with low birth weight, failure to thrive, short stature, severe and often life-threatening hypertension, and hypokalemia, which may cause rhabdomyolysis and nephrogenic diabetes insipidus. Renal cysts and nephrocalcinosis may lead to renal insufficiency. In contrast, patients presenting in late adolescence or early adulthood (type II AME) have mutations associated with greater enzymatic activity and milder abnormalities of blood pressure, serum potassium, and cortisol metabolite excretion.[22]

Related conditions

Chronic licorice ingestion may also lead to hypertension, and low renin and aldosterone levels, since the metabolites of licorice (glycerrhizic acid and its hydrolytic product, glycerrhetinic acid) are potent competitive inhibitors of 11β-HSD2.[23] Similarly, the anti-peptic ulcer agent, carbenoxolone, a synthetic licorice derivative, may cause hypertension, hypokalemia, and suppressed aldosterone and renin, since its metabolites (glycerrhizic and glycerrhetinic acids) inhibit 11β-HSD2, as well.[24] In ectopic ACTH syndrome and in some cases of pituitary-dependent Cushing's syndrome markedly elevated levels of cortisol may exceed the metabolizing capacity of renal 11β-HSD2, leading to hypertension.

Diagnosis

The diagnosis of AME should be suspected in patients from tribal societies in which the prevalence of consanguinity is high and the likelihood of homozygosity is increased. Initial evaluation should consist of determination of plasma renin activity (PRA) and serum aldosterone, both of which are suppressed in AME. Measurement of urinary cortisol/cortisone metabolites should follow, and the diagnosis should be confirmed by genetic testing.[25]

Treatment

Patients with life-threatening hypokalemia and hypertension often respond to dexamethasone therapy if cortisol is adequately suppressed; however, in about 40% of cases additional medication may be required to control blood pressure. Triamterene and/or amiloride have also been effective. Thiazide diuretics are indicated if hypercalciuria and/or nephrocalcinosis are present. Renal transplant has been reported to be curative in a single patient.[26]

GLUCOCORTICOID RECEPTOR MUTATIONS

Glucocorticoid resistance is a rare familial or sporadic disorder of partial end-organ insensitivity to physiological glucocorticoid concentrations.[27] The glucocorticoid receptor (GR), a 94-kDa intracellular protein, is a member of the superfamily of steroid/thyroid/retinoic acid receptor proteins that act as ligand-dependent transcription factors. Mutations in the human glucocorticoid receptor-alpha (hGRα) gene, mostly within the ligand-binding domain, may impair the ability of the receptor to transduce the glucocorticoid signal and lead to variations in the clinical phenotype of affected subjects and in the autosomal dominant or recessive transmission of the disorder. To date the condition has been reported in more than 10 kindreds and in sporadic cases.[28]

Pathogenesis

Because mutant glucocorticoid receptors impair glucorticoid action compensatory increases in ACTH secretion raise levels of cortisol and steroids with mineralocorticoid or androgenic activity.[29–31] Patients may be asymptomatic or may present with manifestations of mineralocorticoid excess and/or severe hyperandrogenism, but without clinical evidence of adrenal hyper- or hypofunction. Mineralocorticoid excess may give rise to hypertension and hypokalemic alkalosis, whereas androgen excess may lead to precocious puberty, acne, hirsutism, male and female infertility, sexual ambiguity at birth, male-pattern hair loss, menstrual irregularities, adrenal rests in the testes, and oligospermia. Many subjects may be asymptomatic, presenting with only biochemical changes.[29,30]

Treatment

Administration of high doses of mineralocorticoid-sparing synthetic glucocorticoids, such as dexamethasone (1–3 mg/day), activate the mutated and/or wild-type GR, and suppress the endogenous secretion of ACTH.[29] Appropriate treatment is particularly important in cases of severe impairment of GR function, because an ACTH-secreting adenoma might ensue from chronic corticotroph stimulation.[31]

Progesterone-induced hypertension

Geller et al.[32] have described a mutation in the mineralocorticoid receptor that leads to early-onset hypertension which is exacerbated during pregnancy, increasing the risk of pre-eclampsia and maternal and perinatal mortality. The mutant receptor contains a leucine for serine substitution at codon 810 (MR_{L810}) in its hormone-binding domain that increases the constitutive MR activity and the receptor specificity for progesterone and other steroids. First detected in a 15-year-old boy with severe hypertension and suppressed renin and aldosterone levels, MR_{L810}

was found in 11 family members who developed hypertension prior to age 20, whereas 12 normotensive relatives expressed the wild-type receptor (MR_{WT}). Two MR_{L810} carriers suffered marked exacerbation of hypertension during pregnancy, accompanied by suppressed levels of aldosterone and renin.[32]

Pathophysiology

In monkey kidney cells aldosterone activated MR_{WT} and MR_{L810} equally. In contrast, progesterone and spironolactone, which, unlike aldosterone, lack a 21-hydroxy group and normally antagonize MR_{WT}, activated MR_{L810}, but not MR_{WT}. Steroids with 17-keto groups, such as estrogen and testosterone, activated neither receptor. Biochemical and structural studies suggested that the MR_{L810} mutation leads to a gain of function resulting from a van der Waals interaction between helices 5 and 3 in the hormone-binding domain of the progesterone receptor in place of the interaction of the steroid 21-hydroxyl group. Ligand binding may result in conformational changes, such as the bending of helix 3, that may be important for receptor activation. The 100-fold rise of progesterone during gestation[33] may explain the development of severe hypertension in pregnant women with the MR_{L810} mutation in the absence of pre-eclampsia. Further investigation will be required to determine the role of progesterone in pregnancy-related hypertension, a condition that affects 6% of pregnancies.[34] Since progesterone levels in men are normally low, hypertension in affected males may arise from constitutive receptor activation sufficient to raise blood pressure or from normal levels of 17-hydroxyprogesterone, an agonist of MR_{L810}, which circulates in levels similar to those of aldosterone.

Treatment

Spironolactone is contraindicated in the treatment of hypertensive carriers of the mutant receptor, since the aldosterone antagonist is a potent activator of MR_{L810}. Female carriers of the MR_{L810} mutation should avoid pregnancy.

Liddle syndrome

In 1963 Liddle et al. described a family with early-onset hypertension, hypokalemia, and suppressed PRA, suggesting primary aldosteronism; however, aldosterone levels were low, and triamterene (an inhibitor of ENaC) corrected the hypertension and hypokalemia, whereas spironolactone was ineffective. The authors speculated that in these patients increased renal tubular sodium transport led to a state simulating mineralocorticoid excess.[35] Sixteen years later the woman who was the index case in this family underwent renal transplantation with normalization of the renin/aldosterone abnormality, confirming the likelihood of an intrinsic renal tubular abnormality as the cause of the syndrome.[36]

Pathophysiology

Liddle syndrome is characterized by early-onset volume-expanded hypertension, hypokalemic alkalosis, suppressed PRA, and low aldosterone levels. Inappropriate renal sodium retention results from constitutive activation of the amiloride-sensitive ENaC in terminal nephron segments. The ENaC complex is composed of three homologous subunits, each with two membrane-spanning domains with amino- and carboxy (C)-terminal domains located in the cytoplasm. Normally the interaction of Nedd4-1 and Nedd4-2 proteins with the amino acid sequence of the ENaC C-terminal cytoplasmic tail leads to endocytosis through clathrin-coated pits.[37] Ubiquitin ligase domains of the Nedd proteins tag C-terminal proline-tyrosine motifs (PPPXY) for destruction by proteosomes, leading to ENaC degradation.[38] In Liddle syndrome mutations that delete cytoplasmic β or δ subunits of C-termini[39] prevent targeted destruction of these motifs, leading to prolonged half-life and increased numbers of channels on the cell surface.[40] Enhanced EnaC activity results in increased sodium reabsorption and hypertension (Figure 14.4).[41]

Diagnosis

The finding of low renin in a child should raise suspicion of a monogenic cause of hypertension, such as Liddle syndrome, especially in the context of a strong family history of hypertension accompanied by target organ damage. Although suppressed aldosterone and renin levels are characteristic of Liddle syndrome, patients may not be overtly hypokalemic.

Treatment

Either triamterene or amiloride, both of which block EnaC, may control blood pressure in patients with Liddle syndrome, while spironolactone is ineffective.[41] The antihypertensive action of these agents can be enhanced by dietary sodium restriction. Thiazide diuretics may worsen renal K^+ wasting in patients who have hypokalemia or fail to reduce their sodium intake. If blood pressure is not adequately controlled with triamterene or amiloride, conventional antihypertensive agents, including ACE inhibitors, angiotensin receptor blockers, calcium channel antagonists or beta blockers,

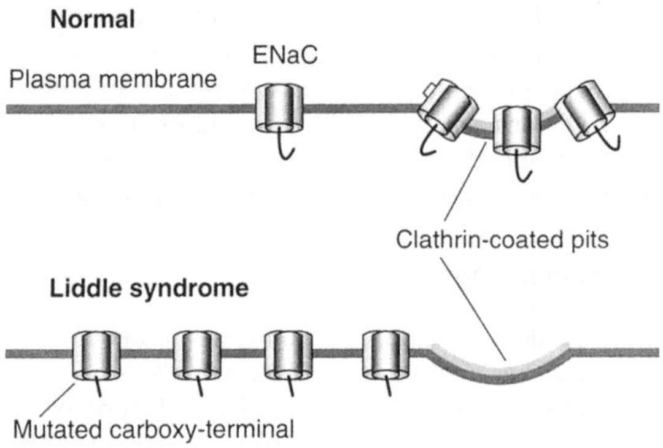

Figure 14.4 Mechanism of Liddle syndrome. ENaC is composed of homologous α, β, and γ subunits that facilitate entry of Na^+ from the lumen into the cells of the cortical collecting duct under tight control by aldosterone. In Liddle syndrome mutations in the genes of either of the β or γ carboxy-terminal tails prevent the interaction between PY motifs (xPPxY, where P = proline, Y = tyrosine, x = any polar amino acid) and the WW domain-containing proteins, Nedd4-1 and Nedd4-2. These proteins contain ubiquitin ligase domains that label ENaC for destruction, leading to inhibition of endocytosis via clathrin-coated pits,[37] reduced clearance, and prolonged half-life of mutant channels on the cell surface of the plasma membrane. The increased number of EnaC results in enhanced salt reabsorption and hypertension. (Adapted from Lifton et al[41] with permission from Elsevier)

may be added to reduce potential cardiovascular and cerebrovascular risk.

REFERENCES

1. Sutherland DJ, Ruse JL, Laidlaw JC. Increased aldosterone secretion and low plasma renin activity relieved by dexamethasone. Can Med Assoc J 1966; 95: 1109–19.
2. Dluhy RG, Anderson B, Harlin B et al. Glucocorticoid-remediable aldosteronism is associated with severe hypertension in early childhood. J Pediatr 2001; 138: 715–20.
3. Litchfield WR, Anderson BF, Weiss RJ et al. Intracranial aneurysm and hemorrhagic stroke in glucocorticoid-remediable aldosteronism. Hypertension 1998; 31: 445–50.
4. Litchfield WR, Coolidge C, Silva P et al. Impaired potassium-stimulated aldosterone production: a possible explanation for normokalemic glucocorticoid-remediable aldosteronism. J Clin Endocrinol Metab 1997; 82: 1507–10.
5. Dluhy RG, Lifton RP. Glucocorticoid-remediable aldosteronism. J Clin Endocrinol Metab 1999; 84: 4341–4.
6. Lifton RP, Dluhy RG, Powers M et al. A chimaeric 11 beta-hydroxylase/aldosterone synthase gene causes glucocorticoid-remediable aldosteronism and human hypertension. Nature 1992; 355: 262–5.
7. Litchfield WR, New MI, Coolidge C et al. Evaluation of the dexamethasone suppression test for the diagnosis of glucocorticoid-remediable aldosteronism. J Clin Endocrinol Metab 1997; 82: 3570–3.
8. Lifton RP, Dluhy RG, Powers M et al. Hereditary hypertension caused by chimaeric gene duplications and ectopic expression of aldosterone synthase. Nat Genet 1992; 2: 66–74.
9. Stowasser M, Gartside MG, Gordon RD. A PCR-based method of screening individuals of all ages, from neonates to the elderly, for familial hyperaldosteronism type I. Aust N Z J Med 1997; 27: 685–90.
10. MacConnachie AA, Kelly KF, McNamara A et al. Rapid diagnosis and identification of cross-over sites in patients with glucocorticoid remediable aldosteronism. J Clin Endocrinol Metab 1998; 83: 4328–31.
11. White PC, Curnow KM, Pascoe L. Disorders of steroid 11 beta-hydroxylase isozymes. Endocr Rev 1994; 15: 421–38.
12. Rosler A, Leiberman E, Cohen T. High frequency of congenital adrenal hyperplasia (classic 11 beta-hydroxylase deficiency) among Jews from Morocco. Am J Med Genet 1992; 42: 827–34.
13. Curnow KM, Slutsker L, Vitek J et al. Mutations in the CYP11B1 gene causing congenital adrenal hyperplasia and hypertension cluster in exons 6, 7, and 8. Proc Natl Acad Sci U S A 1993; 90: 4552–6.
14. Zachmann M, Tassinari D, Prader A. Clinical and biochemical variability of congenital adrenal hyperplasia due to 11 beta-hydroxylase deficiency. A study of 25 patients. J Clin Endocrinol Metab 1983; 56: 222–9.
15. Costa-Santos M, Kater CE, Dias EP et al. Two intronic mutations cause 17-hydroxylase deficiency by disrupting splice acceptor sites: direct demonstration of aberrant splicing and absent enzyme activity by expression of the entire CYP17 gene in HEK-293 cells. J Clin Endocrinol Metab 2004; 89: 43–8.
16. Matteson K, Picado-Leonard J, Chung B et al. Assignment of the gene for adrenal P450c17 (steroid 17alpha-hydroxylase/17,20 lyase) to human chromosome 10. J Clin Endocrinol Metab 1986; 63: 789–91.
17. Sparkes R, Klisak I, Miller W. Regional mapping of genes encoding human steroidogenic enzymes: P450scc to 15q23-q24, adrenodoxin to 11q22; adrenodoxin reductase to 17q24–q25; and P450c17 to 10q24–q25. DNA Cell Biol 1991; 10: 359–65.
18. New MI. Inborn errors of adrenal steroidogenesis. Mol Cell Endocrinol 2003; 211: 75–83.
19. Zachmann M, Vollmin W, Hamilton W et al. Steroid 17,20-desmolase deficiency: a new cause of male pseudohermaphroditism. Clin Endocrinol 1972; 1: 369–85.
20. Ulick S, Levine LS, Gunczler P et al. A syndrome of apparent mineralocorticoid excess associated with defects in the peripheral metabolism of cortisol. J Clin Endocrinol Metab 1979; 49: 757–64.
21. Arriza JL, Weinberger C, Cerelli G et al. Cloning of human mineralocorticoid receptor complementary DNA: structural and functional kinship with the glucocorticoid receptor. Science 1987; 237: 268–75.
22. Quinkler M, Bappal B, Draper N et al. Molecular basis for the apparent mineralocorticoid excess syndrome in the Oman population. Mol Cell Endocrinol 2004; 217: 143–9.
23. Stewart PM, Wallace AM, Valentino R et al. Mineralocorticoid activity of liquorice: 11-beta-hydroxysteroid dehydrogenase deficiency comes of age. Lancet 1987; 2: 821–4.
24. Stewart PM, Wallace AM, Atherden SM et al. Mineralocorticoid activity of carbenoxolone: contrasting effects of carbenoxolone and liquorice on 11 beta-hydroxysteroid dehydrogenase activity in man. Clin Sci 1990; 78: 49–54.

25. Quinkler M, Stewart PM. Hypertension and the cortisol-cortisone shuttle. J Clin Endocrinol Metab 2003; 88: 2384–92.
26. Palermo M, Cossu M, Shackleton CH. Cure of apparent mineralocorticoid excess by kidney transplantation. N Engl J Med 1998; 339: 1787–8.
27. Charmandari E, Kino T, Souvatzoglou E et al. Natural glucocorticoid receptor mutants causing generalized glucocorticoid resistance: molecular genotype, genetic transmission, and clinical phenotype. J Clin Endocrinol Metab 2004; 89: 1939–49.
28. Chrousos GP, Detera-Wadleigh SD, Karl M. Syndromes of glucocorticoid resistance. Ann Intern Med 1993; 119: 1113–24.
29. Kino T, Vottero A, Charmandari E et al. Familial/sporadic glucocorticoid resistance syndrome and hypertension. Ann N Y Acad Sci 2002; 970: 101–11.
30. Mendonca BB, Leite MV, de Castro M et al. Female pseudohermaphroditism caused by a novel homozygous missense mutation of the GR gene. J Clin Endocrinol Metab 2002; 87: 1805–9.
31. Karl M, Lamberts SW, Koper JW et al. Cushing's disease preceded by generalized glucocorticoid resistance: clinical consequences of a novel, dominant negative glucocorticoid receptor mutation. Proc Assoc Am Physicians 1996; 108: 296–307.
32. Geller DS, Farhi A, Pinkerton N et al. Activating mineralocorticoid receptor mutation in hypertension exacerbated by pregnancy. Science 2000; 289: 119–23.
33. Dunn JF, Nisula BC, Rodbard D. Transport of steroid hormones: binding of 21 endogenous steroids to both testosterone-binding globulin and corticosteroid-binding globulin in human plasma. J Clin Endocrinol Metab 1981; 53: 58–68.
34. August P, Lindheimer MD. Pathophysiology, diagnosis, and management. In: Laragh JH, Brenner BM (eds). Hypertension. New York: Raven, 1995, pp 2407–26.
35. Liddle GW, Bledsoe T, Coppage WS Jr. A familial renal disorder simulating primary aldosteronism but with negligible aldosterone secretion. Trans Assoc Am Physicians 1963; 76: 199–213.
36. Botero-Velez M, Curtis JJ, Warnock DG. Brief report: Liddle's syndrome revisited – a disorder of sodium reabsorption in the distal tubule. N Engl J Med 1994; 330: 178–81.
37. Shimkets RA, Lifton RP, Canessa CM. The activity of the epithelial sodium channel is regulated by clathrin-mediated endocytosis. J Biol Chem 1997; 272: 25537–41.
38. Warnock DG. Liddle syndrome. An autosomal dominant form of human hypertension. Kidney Int 1998; 53: 18–24.
39. Snyder PM, Price MP, McDonald FJ et al. Mechanism by which Liddle's syndrome mutations increase activity of a human epithelial Na^+ channel. Cell 1995; 83: 969–78.
40. Kamynina E, Debonneville C, Bens M et al. A novel mouse Nedd4 protein suppresses the activity of the epithelial Na+ channel. FASEB J 2001; 15: 204–14.
41. Lifton RP, Gharavi AG, Geller DS. Molecular mechanisms of human hypertension. Cell 2001; 104: 545–56.

15

Pathophysiologic effects of aldosterone in cardiovascular tissues

Ricardo Rocha and Gordon H Williams

INTRODUCTION

Over the last 40 years, numerous clinical and experimental studies have demonstrated that blockade of the renin-angiotensin-aldosterone system (RAAS) with either angiotensin converting enzyme (ACE) inhibitors or angiotensin (Ang) II receptor antagonists provides significant cardiovascular protection. More recently, a growing body of evidence has indicated that pharmacological antagonism of aldosterone, the third component of this neurohormonal axis, also provides significant incremental benefit against the deleterious consequences of abnormal activation of this system on cardiovascular tissues. In the present chapter, we examine the most relevant clinical and experimental evidence around the pathophysiologic role for aldosterone in the development of cardiovascular disease. Specifically, we discuss the relative roles of the classic epithelial effects versus the novel nonepithelial effects of this steroid that lead to the development of hypertension and related complications such as renal disease and congestive heart failure.

NOVEL CONCEPTS OF ALDOSTERONE BIOLOGY

Epithelial versus nonepithelial aldosterone effects

The classic aldosterone receptor (type I corticoid receptor or mineralocorticoid receptor, MR) forms part of the steroid/thyroid/retinoid/orphan receptor family of nuclear transactivating factors.[1] When unbound, these receptors remain in an inactive but ligand-friendly conformation associated with a multiprotein complex of chaperones.[2] Upon binding aldosterone, the receptor undergoes a conformational change in which specific helices of the ligand binding domain, primarily helices 12, 3, and 5, are repositioned to form a pocket where transcriptional activators can bind. Importantly, Zhang and co-workers have recently shown that an interaction between helix 3 and helix 5 seems to play a critical role on the sensitivity and or specificity of the MR, as well as probably other steroid receptors.[3] In addition, Hultman and collaborators documented that an intact helix 12 is indispensable for corticoid activation of the MR and that depending on the ligand bound, the conformational changes may differ so that different sets of coactivators and corepressors will interact with the ligand–receptor complex.[4] In addition, they have identified two key residues (K785 and E962) in the MR ligand binding domain, the site for binding and activation of MR by corticoids, that are critical for the differential nuclear effects of the MR upon activation by mineralocorticoids, glucocorticoids or the MR antagonist eplerenone. Upon modification of the conformation of the aldosterone–MR complex, receptor chaperones are released and the receptor/hormone complex is translocated into the nucleus. The complex then binds to hormone response elements on DNA interacting with transcription–initiation complexes and other transcription factors to modulate gene expression.

In the kidney, MRs are located in epithelial cells of the distal nephron, primarily in principal cells. Although the affinity of the MR for aldosterone binding is higher than for the GR (Kd approximately 10^{-9} and 3×10^{-8} M, respectively),[5] the MR can bind with similar affinity other corticoids such as cortisol or corticosterone. However, glucocorticoid binding to the

MR is limited in aldosterone target cells by the enzyme 11β-hydroxysteroid dehydrogenase type 2 (11β-HSD2), which converts cortisol (in humans) or corticosterone (in rats) to inactive metabolites,[6] whereas it has no effect on the metabolism of aldosterone. This allows for the access of aldosterone to the MR in target tissues despite a much higher circulating concentration of glucocorticoids. Activation of MR by aldosterone in epithelial cells induces the rapid expression of serum and glucocorticoid inducible kinase (sgk)-1 which, when phosphorylated, modulates the trafficking of ion transporter such as the epithelial sodium channel.[7] This initiates a cascade of events, which leads to potent stimulation of Na^+ transport and, secondarily, activation of K^+ secretion and Cl^- reabsorption. Importantly, under normal conditions, this increase is transient and a rapid return to sodium balance occurs, even in the presence of continued stimulation of the tubular epithelium by aldosterone, the mechanisms for which are not yet well understood.[8]

Growing evidence supports the presence and activity of aldosterone receptors in nonepithelial tissues. Aldosterone receptors have been identified in the heart,[9] brain,[10] and blood vessels.[11] Activation of these receptors can elicit important biological responses. In vitro stimulation of cultured neonatal rat cardiac myocytes with aldosterone, but not with dexamethasone, has an anabolic effect as assessed by increased leucine incorporation into proteins.[12] This effect was significantly increased by the presence of increased glucose in the media and involved activation of the protein kinase C pathway. More recently, aldosterone has been shown to inhibit the sarcolemmal Na^+/K^+ pump[13] through mechanisms that involve the isoform –ε of protein kinase C.[14] Using the isolated perfused rat heart, Moreau et al. have shown that aldosterone can decrease coronary blood flow and increase aortic flow and cardiac output.[15] Finally, Vassort and co-workers have shown that aldosterone can up-regulate calcium transport into cardiomyocytes.[16] Nonepithelial effects of aldosterone have also been demonstrated in the brain. Administration of small doses of aldosterone into the cerebral ventricles in rats induced hypertension, whereas the same doses administered systemically had no effect.[17] Likewise, intracerebroventricular infusion of low doses of the aldosterone receptor antagonist RU 28318 prevented the development of hypertension in aldosterone/salt hypertensive rats,[18] an intervention that did not prevent the pathologic effects of aldosterone in the heart.[19] Thus, multiple lines of evidence indicate that aldosterone can activate its nonepithelial receptors. The physiological or pathophysiological significance of these effects remains to be clarified, as do the mechanisms by which they are regulated.

Rapid nongenomic effects of aldosterone

The above-mentioned nonepithelial actions of aldosterone were typically slow to develop, consistent with aldosterone-induced activation of gene transcription. However, rapid effects of aldosterone in cardiovascular tissues have also been reported. In cultured vascular smooth muscle cells, aldosterone induced a prompt (< 1 minute) increase in intracellular Ca^{2+} concentration.[20] This increase was dependent on activation of phospholipase C and protein kinase C and was elicited by subnanomolar concentrations of aldosterone, which are in the physiologic range. Interestingly, the rapid effects of aldosterone on intracellular Ca^{2+} concentration were not inhibited by spironolactone. In addition, aldosterone has been shown to induce rapid Na^+ influx in vascular smooth muscle cells,[21] apparently via activation of the Na^+/H^+exchange.[22] The effects of aldosterone on Na^+ influx were observed within 5 minutes, were mimicked by fludrocortisone and deoxycorticosterone (but not by glucocorticoids), and were inhibited by RU 28318[22] but not by canrenone or spironolactone.[21,22] However, Alzamora et al. showed that although cortisol is without effect on Na/H exchange in vascular smooth muscle cells (VSMC), when 11β-HSD2 activity is blocked by carbenoxolone, cortisol shows agonist effects indistinguishable from aldosterone.[22] The existence of a novel membrane receptor for aldosterone has been proposed to mediate these rapid effects. However, although membrane receptors for steroids have been recently cloned,[23] a specific membrane receptor for aldosterone has yet to be identified. Moreover, the fact that nongenomic rapid effects of aldosterone can be blocked by the classic aldosterone antagonist RU 28318,[22] suggests that the cytosolic aldosterone receptor may also be responsible for these rapid effects, either directly by interaction with intracellular signaling pathways or through one of the chaperones released upon aldosterone binding to the receptor, as suggested previously.[24,25]

ROLE OF ALDOSTERONE IN CARDIOVASCULAR END ORGAN DAMAGE

Experimental evidence

Since the 1940s, the model of mineralocorticoid hypertension has been used in animals to mimic the multiple deleterious changes that occur in target tissues of hypertensive vascular disease. Indeed, Hans Selye was the first to document that administration of deoxycorticosterone acetate, and sodium chloride to chicken[26] and later to rats[27] induced the development of severe hypertension with accompanying vascular lesions in the brain, heart, kidney, pancreas, and mesenteric arteries. These lesions are almost identical to those observed in other hypertensive models that display an abnormal activation of the RAAS, such as Ang II/salt hypertensive rats,[28,29] L-NAME/Ang II hypertensive rats[30] or stroke-prone spontaneously hypertensive rats (SHRSP)[31] and are greatly dependent on the presence of an elevated dietary salt environment. In studies to determine the contribution of aldosterone to vascular lesion development in several of these models, we and others have found that administration of aldosterone antagonists or adrenalectomy markedly reduced the incidence of stroke,[33] coronary vascular lesions and fibrosis,[29,30,34] and attenuated the development of proteinuria, renal microvascular lesions, and glomerulopathy.[30,32,33,35,36] These vascular protective effects of aldosterone antagonism were achieved despite minor or no reductions in blood pressure, which suggested that the effects of aldosterone on target organ damage are not solely dependent on elevations in arterial pressure.

We have also recently demonstrated that the vascular structural damage induced by aldosterone in the heart and in the kidney is accompanied by the expression of a vascular inflammatory phenotype, which may be the triggering mechanism for the perivascular leukocyte accumulation typically observed in the coronary arteries of mineralocorticoid/salt hypertensive rats.[34,36] Whether aldosterone causes this injury solely by its effects on epithelial tissues or whether activation of nonepithelial receptors also participates, remains to be elucidated.

Clinical evidence

For more than 40 years, the aldosterone receptor antagonist, spironolactone, has been available for the treatment of hypertension, hyperaldosteronism, and edematous states, primarily in patients with uncompensated heart failure. However, it has only been during the last decade that aldosterone has emerged as a major risk factor for cardiovascular disease. This is despite early evidence from the original work by Jerome Conn in which he described 145 cases of primary aldosteronism (PA) secondary to an aldosterone-producing adenoma.[37] Every patient demonstrated hypertension. More importantly, cardiomegaly was documented in 41% of the patients, retinopathy in 50%, and proteinuria in 85%. More recently, Nishimura and collaborators have investigated the incidence of cardiovascular complications in a population of patients with PA secondary to an aldosterone-producing adenoma.[38] These investigators identified cardiovascular complications in 34% of the patients: stroke was demonstrated in 16% and proteinuria in 24%. In addition 78% of the patients in which left ventricular mass index was evaluated had evidence of left ventricular hypertrophy (LVH). Finally, Milliez and co-workers reported results from an evaluation of 124 consecutive patients with the diagnosis of PA in comparison to 465 patients with essential hypertension randomly matched for age, gender, and systolic and diastolic blood pressure. A history of stroke was documented in 12.9% of patients with PA and 3.4% of patients with essential hypertension whereas nonfatal myocardial infarction was diagnosed in 4.0% of patients with PA and in 0.6% of patients with essential hypertension. Interestingly, atrial fibrillation was diagnosed in 7.3% of the patients with PA and in 0.6% of patients with essential hypertension.[39] The above reports are particularly relevant as recent reports have documented that the prevalence of PA in patients with hypertension seems to be much higher than previously believed and can be as high as 20%.[40]

Despite the documented evidence of cardiovascular complications in patients with aldosterone excess, for many years it was assumed that the cardiovascular damage observed in these patients was simply the result of elevated blood pressure. However, recent clinical studies have shown that aldosterone may have deleterious effects on cardiovascular tissues that are largely independent of elevations in blood pressure. In a recent study, Pitt and co-workers studied the effects of the selective aldosterone blocker, eplerenone, on LV mass in patients with essential hypertension.[41] A total of 202 subjects with echocardiographic evidence of LVH were randomized in a double-blind fashion to receive therapy with eplerenone 200 mg daily, or enalapril 40 mg daily or a combination of eplerenone 200 mg and enalapril 10 mg daily for a period of 9 months. In an attempt to achieve comparable blood pressure reductions in the three groups, patients were allowed to receive hydrochlorothiazide and/or amlodipine treatment as add-on medications if necessary after 8 weeks of randomization. Change in left ventricular mass as assessed by magnetic resonance imaging (MRI) was the primary end-point. All treatments reduced systolic blood pressure and diastolic blood pressure from baseline to a similar degree, although the combination of enalapril and eplerenone produced slightly higher blood pressure reductions compared with eplerenone alone. Eplerenone significantly reduced left ventricular mass from baseline (−14.5 ± 3.36 g; $n = 50$) similarly to enalapril (−19.7 ± 3.20 g; $n = 54$; $p = 0.258$). Combined treatment with eplerenone/enalapril (−27.2 ± 3.39 g; $n = 49$) was more effective than eplerenone alone in reducing left ventricular mass ($p = 0.007$). In a similar study examining the potential beneficial effects of aldosterone blockade on renal disease, hypertensive diabetic patients with proteinuria were randomized into the same treatment arms as stated for the LVH study above.[42] Protein excretion was assessed before and after 6 months of therapy, with a significant 45% reduction in protein excretion with eplerenone, 63% with enalapril, and 74% with combination therapy ($p < 0.001$). Combination therapy was significantly more effective than monotherapy. These differences in proteinuria reductions occurred despite the fact that there were no significant differences in blood pressure reduction between the three arms. The effect of lower doses of eplerenone on microalbuminuria was examined more recently in a study in which diabetic subjects were started on enalapril 20 mg/day 1 month before being randomized into placebo, 50 mg of eplerenone or 100 mg of eplerenone groups.[43] Both 50 and 100 mg of eplerenone produced similar 45–50% reduction in proteinuria, compared with only 11% in patients receiving enalapril alone. Thus, blockade of the MR with eplerenone or reduction in Ang II formation are similarly effective in reducing the degree of LVH and level of proteinuria, two surrogate markers for cardiovascular/renal damage. Importantly, the combination of these two strategies produces the maximum end organ protection, although the doses at which these agents should be used to achieve an optimal risk benefit balance remain to be determined.

The Randomized Aldactone Evaluation Study (RALES) represented the most important piece of evidence that aldosterone receptor antagonism may offer significant cardiovascular protection that translates into marked reductions in morbidity and mortality in patients with advanced cardiovascular disease, namely congestive heart.[44] In that study, over 1600 patients with a history of severe heart failure (NYHA class IV within the 6 months prior to entry into the study) and treatment with standard therapy including an ACE inhibitor, beta blocker, diuretic, and digoxin were randomized to spironolactone 25–50 mg/day or placebo. The primary end-point was all-cause mortality. Patients entered into the study had to have evidence of systolic left ventricular dysfunction (SLVD) with a left ventricular ejection fraction (LVEF) ≤35%. The study was stopped prematurely at a mean follow-up of 2 years when it was found that patients randomized to spironolactone had a significant 30% reduction in total mortality as well as a 35% reduction in the incidence of hospitalization for heart failure. Aldosterone blockade has also been shown to be beneficial in patients following an acute myocardial infarction. Indeed, the study EPHESUS[45] randomized over 6600 patients with an acute myocardial infarction and clinical signs of heart failure or SLVD (LVEF ≤40%) to usual care plus eplerenone 25 mg/day titrated upto 50 mg/day at 1 month or placebo. Over 85% of patients were on an ACE inhibitor or an angiotensin receptor blocker (ARB) and 75% on a beta blocker. At a mean follow-up of 16 months, patients randomized to eplerenone had a significant 15% reduction in total mortality and a 13% reduction in the co-primary end-point of cardiovascular mortality/cardiovascular hospitalization. The major cause of cardiovascular death in EPHESUS was sudden cardiac death, which was significantly reduced by 21%. Interestingly, in a retrospective analysis of those patients with an LVEF ≤30% at baseline there was a 33% reduction in sudden cardiac death. Both in RALES and EPHESUS there was an increase in the incidence of serious hyperkalemia ($K \geq 6.0$ meq/l). However, the risk was relatively small and no patients in RALES or EPHESUS randomized to an aldosterone blockade had a death attributable to hyperkalemia.

CONCLUSION

Accumulating evidence suggests that the classic characterization of aldosterone as an epithelial-acting, electrolyte-regulator hormone should be carefully re-evaluated. It is now clear that in addition to its epithelial effects, aldosterone has major functions in nonepithelial tissues that, under certain conditions, may lead to cardiovascular injury, renal disease, and stroke. Thus, aldosterone should be considered as a critical independent risk factor for end organ damage in cardiovascular disease.

REFERENCES

1. Mangelsdorf DJ, Thummel C, Beato M et al. The nuclear receptor superfamily: the second decade. Cell 1995; 83: 835–9.
2. Pratt WB. The role of heat shock proteins in regulating the function, folding and trafficking of the glucocorticoid receptor. J Biol Chem 1993; 268: 21455–8.
3. Zhang J, Simisky J, Tsai FTF, Geller DS. A critical role of helix 3-helix 5 interaction in steroid hormone receptor function. Proc Natl Acad Sci U S A 2005; 102: 2707–12.
4. Hultman M, Krasnoperova NV, Li S et al. The ligand-dependent interaction of mineralocorticoid receptor with coactivator and corepressor peptides suggests multiple activation mechanisms. Mol Endocrinol 2005; 19: 1460–73.

5. Funder JW. Mineralocorticoid receptors and hypertension. J Steroid Biochem Mol Biol 1995; 53: 53–5.
6. Funder JW. 11 beta-Hydroxysteroid dehydrogenase: new answers, new questions. Eur J Endocrinol 1996; 134: 267–8.
7. Bhargava A, Wang J, Pearce D. Regulation of epithelial ion transport by aldosterone through changes in gene expression. Mol Cell Endocrinol 2004; 217: 189–96.
8. Granger JP, Kassab S, Novak J et al. Role of nitric oxide in modulating renal function and arterial pressure during chronic aldosterone excess. Am J Physiol 1999; 276: R197–R202.
9. Lombes M, Alfaidy N, Eugene E et al. Prerequisite for cardiac aldosterone action: mineralocorticoid receptor and 11 β-hydroxysteroid dehydrogenase in the human heart. Circulation 1995; 92: 175–82.
10. Roland BL, Krozowski ZS, Funder JW. Glucocorticoid receptor, mineralocorticoid receptors, 11 beta-hydroxysteroid dehydrogenase-1 and -2 expression in rat brain and kidney: in situ studies. Mol Cell Endocrinol 1995; 111: R1–R7.
11. Takeda Y, Miyamori I, Inaba S et al. Vascular aldosterone in genetically hypertensive rats. Hypertension 1997; 29: 45–8.
12. Sato A, Funder JW. High glucose stimulates aldosterone-induced hypertrophy via type I mineralocorticoid receptors in neonatal rat cardiomyocytes. Endocrinology 1996; 137: 4145–53.
13. Mihailidou AS, Bundgaard H, Mardini M et al. Hyperaldosteronemia in rabbits inhibits the cardiac sarcolemmal Na(+)-K(+) pump. Circ Res 2000; 86: 37–42.
14. Mihailidou AS, Mardini M, Raison M et al. Protein kinase C-ε regulates cardiac Na+–K+ pump function in hyperaldosteronemia. Circulation 2000; 102: 135 (abstract).
15. Moreau D, Chardigny JM, Rochette L. Effects of aldosterone and spironolactone on the isolated perfused rat heart. Pharmacology 1996; 53: 28–36.
16. Benitah JP, Vassort G. Aldosterone upregulates Ca(2+) current in adult rat cardiomyocytes. Circ Res 1999; 85: 1139–45.
17. Gómez-Sánchez EP, Venkataraman MT, Thwaites D et al. ICV infusion of corticosterone antagonizes ICV-aldosterone hypertension. Am J Physiol 1990; 258: E649–E653.
18. Gómez-Sánchez EP, Fort CM, Gómez-Sánchez CE. Intracerebroventricular infusion of RU 28318 blocks aldosterone-salt hypertension. Am J Physiol 1990; 258: E482–E484.
19. Young M, Head G, Funder JW. Determinants of cardiac fibrosis in experimental hypermineralocorticoid states. Am J Physiol 1995; 269: E657–E662.
20. Wehling M, Neylon CB, Fullerton M et al. Nongenomic effects of aldosterone on intracellular Ca2+ in vascular smooth muscle cells. Circ Res 1995; 76: 973–9.
21. Christ M, Douwes K, Eisen C et al. Rapid effects of aldosterone on sodium transport in vascular smooth muscle cells. Hypertension 1995; 25: 117–23.
22. Alzamora R, Michea L, Marusic ET. Role of 11beta-hydroxysteroid dehydrogenase in nongenomic aldosterone effects in human arteries. Hypertension 2000; 35: 1099–104.
23. Gerdes D, Wehling M, Leube B et al. Cloning and tissue expression of two putative steroid membrane receptors. Biol Chem 1998; 379: 907–11.
24. Someren JS, Faber LE, Klein JD et al. Heat shock proteins 70 and 90 increase calcineurin activity in vitro through calmodulin-dependent and independent mechanisms. Biochem Biophys Res Commun 1999; 260: 619–25.
25. Stier CT Jr, Chander PN, Zuckerman A et al. Non-epithelial effects of aldosterone. Curr Opin Endocrinol Diabetes 1998; 5: 211–16.
26. Selye H, Hall CE, Rowley EM. Malignant hypertension produced by treatment with deoxycorticosterone acetate and sodium chloride. Can Med Assoc J 1943; 49: 88–92.
27. Selye H. The general adaptation syndrome and the diseases of adaptation. J Clin Endocrinol. 1946; 6: 117–230.
28. Mistry M, Muirhead EE, Yamaguchi Y et al. Renal function in rats with angiotensin II-salt-induced hypertension: effect of thromboxane synthesis inhibition and receptor blockade. J Hypertens 1990; 8: 77–83.
29. Rocha R, Martin-Berger CL, Yang P, Scherrer R, Delyani JA, McMahon EG. Selective aldosterone blockade prevents angiotensin II/salt-induced vascular inflammation in the rat heart. Endocrinology 2002; 143: 4828–36.
30. Rocha R, Stier CT, Kifor I et al. Aldosterone: a mediator of myocardial necrosis and renal arteriopathy. Endocrinology 2000; 141: 3871–8.
31. Stier CT Jr, Chander PN, Gutstein WH et al. Therapeutic benefit of captopril in salt-loaded stroke-prone spontaneously hypertensive rats is independent of hypotensive effect. Am J Hypertens 1991; 4: 680–7.
32. Martinez DV, Rocha R, Matsumura M et al. Cardiac damage prevention by eplerenone: comparison with low sodium diet or potassium loading. Hypertension 2002; 39 (2 Pt 2): 614–18.
33. Rocha R, Chander PN, Khanna K et al. Mineralocorticoid blockade reduces vascular injury in stroke-prone hypertensive rats. Hypertension 1998; 31: 451–8.
34. Rocha R, Rudolph AE, Frierdich GE et al. Aldosterone induces a vascular inflammatory phenotype in the rat heart. Am J Physiol Heart Circ Physiol 2002; 283: H1802–H1810.
35. Chander PN, Rocha R, Ranaudo J, Singh G, Zuckerman A, Stier CT Jr. Aldosterone plays a pivotal role in the pathogenesis of thrombotic microangiopathy in SHRSP. J Am Soc Nephrol 2003; 14: 1990–7.
36. Blasi ER, Rocha R, Rudolph AE, Blomme EA, Polly ML, McMahon EG. Aldosterone/salt induces renal inflammation and fibrosis in hypertensive rats. Kidney Int 2003; 63: 1791–800.
37. Conn JW, Knopf RF, Nesbit RM. Clinical characteristics of primary aldosteronism from an analysis of 145 cases. Am J Surg 1964; 107: 159–72.
38. Nishimura M, Uzu T, Fuji T et al. Cardiovascular complications in patients with primary aldosteronism. Am J Kidney Dis 1999; 33: 261–6.
39. Milliez P, Girerd X, Plouin PF, Blacher J, Safar ME, Mourad JJ. Evidence for an increased rate of cardiovascular events in patients with primary aldosteronism. J Am Coll Cardiol 2005; 45: 1243–8.
40. Mulatero P, Stowasser M, Loh KC et al. Increased diagnosis of primary aldosteronism, including surgically correctable forms, in centers from five continents. J Clin Endocrinol Metab 2004; 89: 1045–50.
41. Pitt B, Reichek N, Willenbrock R et al. Effects of eplerenone, enalapril, and eplerenone/enalapril in patients with essential hypertension and left ventricular hypertrophy: the 4E-left ventricular hypertrophy study. Circulation 2003; 108: 1831–8.
42. Epstein M, Buckalew V, Martinez F et al. Antiproteinuric efficacy of eplerenone, enalapril, and eplerenone/enalapril combination in diabetic hypertensives with microalbuminuria. Am J Hypertens 2002; 15: 24A.
43. Epstein M, Williams GH, Lewin AJ et al. Characterization of the antiproteinuric effect of eplerenone in patients with type 2 diabetes mellitus. American Society of Hypertension Meeting, 2003: Abstract P-181a.
44. Pitt B, Zannad F, Remme WJ et al. The effect of spironolactone on morbidity and mortality in patients with severe heart failure. Randomized Aldactone Evaluation Study Investigators. N Engl J Med 1999; 341: 709–17.
45. Pitt B, Remme W, Zannad F et al. Eplerenone Post-Acute Myocardial Infarction Heart Failure Efficacy and Survival Study Investigators. Eplerenone, a selective aldosterone blocker, in patients with left ventricular dysfunction after myocardial infarction. N Engl J Med 2003; 348: 1309–21.

PART II

16

Endothelins: molecular mechanisms in hypertension and cardiovascular diseases

Gian Paolo Rossi and Achille Cesare Pessina

INTRODUCTION

The isolation and chemical identification by Masashi Yanagisawa in Professor Masaki's laboratory of a peptide, named endothelin (ET), was first reported in *Nature* in March 1988.[1] This discovery was triggered by that of an endothelium-derived contracting factor in the mid-1980s.[2,3] The seminal paper, which described the sequence of the peptide and the cDNA, the putative biosynthetic pathway and the vasoconstrictor activity of ET, aroused much interest in the scientific community and a *deluge* of studies that have enormously improved the understanding of the mechanisms of cardiovascular diseases, as summarized in this chapter. More importantly, the discovery of ET has led in less than 15 years to the development of a novel effective strategy for the treatment of pulmonary hypertension.

ISOFORMS AND FUNCTION

The peptide, later defined endothelin (ET)-1, at first sight differed from all other known peptides. However, it was soon discovered that it has a striking similarity to sarafotoxin peptides present in the venom of snakes of the *Atractaspis* family. It also became evident that ET-1 was the prototype of a larger family of structurally similar isopeptides including ET-1, ET-2, and ET-3, which have remarkable differences in tissue distribution[4] and are encoded by genes that have been mapped on chromosomes 6, 1, and 20, for ET-1, ET-2, and ET-3, respectively. The most widely studied isopeptide is ET-1 and therefore we shall refer mostly to this isoform, unless otherwise specified.

BIOSYNTHESIS AND REGULATION

ET-1 is a 21-amino acid residue peptide predominantly made by endothelial cells (ECs) from which it is released abluminally toward the vascular smooth muscle cells (SMCs), where it acts in a paracrine fashion.[5] Other cells involved in cardiovascular disease, such as smooth muscle cells,[6] leukocytes, macrophages, cardiomyocytes, and mesangial cells, can also produce ET-1 under disease conditions.[7]

Transcription of the preproET-1 gene is regulated through binding sites for nuclear factor-1, GATA-2, AP-1,[8–10] the phorbol ester-sensitive *c-fos* and *c-jun* complexes,[11] and acute phase reactant regulatory elements.[12] The translation of preproET mRNA results in the formation of a 212-amino acid preproET peptide, which undergoes a further intracellular processing as described below.

ET-FORMING ENZYMES

Once formed, the preproET-1 is cleaved by a furin convertase, to the 38-amino acid inactive precursor big(pro)ET-1_{1-38}. This is followed by a cleavage of the Trp_{21}-Val_{22} bond by a specific ET-converting enzyme-1 (ECE-1), or by ECE-2. ECE-3 selectively converts big ET-1 into ET-3. ECEs belong to the metalloprotease family,[13–16] share functional and structural similarity with neutral endopeptidases, and are partially inhibited by phosphoramidon. They are localized in ECs, and SMCs,[6] cardiomyocytes, and macrophages. The ECE-1 gene is widely expressed in human tissues,[17] and has been finely mapped on chromosome 1p36.[18] It exists in different isoforms termed *a, b, c,* and *d*, whose functional differences are still poorly explored.[13,14,16,19,20] ECE-1 expression is regulated through protein kinase C-dependent mechanisms, ET_B-receptors,[21] the transcription factor ets-1, and cytokines.

ECE-independent pathways also contribute substantively to ET-1 production since in ECE-1 knockout mice the tissue levels of ET-1 are reduced by only about 30%.[22] Indeed, chymase, a major angiotensin (Ang) II-forming enzyme in the human cardiovascular system,[23,24] can generate $ET\text{-}1_{1\text{-}21}$.[25] It also cleaves big ET-1 at the Tyr_{31}-Gly_{32} bond, resulting in the formation of $ET\text{-}1_{1\text{-}31}$, which acts as a selective ET_A receptor agonist.[39]

In addition, two novel $ET\text{-}1_{1\text{-}21}$-forming enzymes, a non-ECE metalloprotease and a vascular smooth muscle cell chymase have been cloned.

FACTORS REGULATING ET SYNTHESIS

ET synthesis is regulated by physicochemical factors, such as pulsatile stretch,[26] shear stress,[27] hypoxia, and pH,[28] as illustrated in Figure 16.1.[7] Exercise upregulates myocardial ET-1 expression, thus suggesting that ET-1 intervenes in the functional cardiac adaptation to exercise.[29] ET-1 biosynthesis is stimulated by cardiovascular risk factors such as elevated levels of oxidized LDL cholesterol[30] and glucose,[31] estrogen deficiency,[32] obesity,[33] cocaine use, aging, and procoagulant mediators such as thrombin.[34] Furthermore, vasoconstrictors like norepinephrine and Ang II,[35–37] growth factors,[38,40,41] cytokines,[42,43] and adhesion molecules also stimulate ET production. Inhibitors of ET-1 synthesis include nitric oxide (NO),[34] prostacyclin,[44] atrial natriuretic peptides (ANPs),[45] homocysteine,[46] and estrogens,[10] and alcohol-free extracts of red wine.[47]

ET RECEPTOR CLASSIFICATION AND FUNCTION

The biologic effects of ET (Table 16.1) are mediated in mammals by two different G_i protein-coupled, 7-transmembrane domain receptors, termed ET_A,[48,49] and ET_B,[50,51] which are encoded by different genes and characterized by distinct tissue distribution and pharmacological properties. In the vasculature, ET_A receptors are found in SMCs,[52] whereas ET_B receptors are localized on ECs and, to some extent, in SMCs, and macrophages.[53] The affinity of ET_A receptors for ET-1 and ET-2 is >100-fold higher than for ET-3, whereas ET_B receptors bind ET isopeptides with a similar affinity. A cross-talk between ET_A and ET_B receptors has been described,[54,55] but its functional relevance remains unclear. Transactivation of the epidermal growth factor (EGF) receptor can also mediate at least two of the major actions of ET-1 in the vascular tissue, e.g. contractility and fibrogenesis,[56] indicating a cross-talk of ET-1 with other peptide systems.[24]

The binding of ET-1 to ET_A receptors activates phospholipase C, which leads to an accumulation of inositol trisphosphate (IP_3) and intracellular Ca and thereby to long-lasting vasoconstriction.[1,57] The activation of ET_A receptors by ET-1 or $ET\text{-}1_{1\text{-}31}$ also induces cell proliferation in different tissues,[58,59] including the adrenal cortex, which express chymase and therefore can synthesize $ET\text{-}1_{1\text{-}31}$.[39] By contrast, the activation of endothelial ET_B subtype mediates the release of endothelial-derived relaxing factors (EDRFs), like NO, adrenomedullin and prostacyclin,[60,61] prevents apoptosis, and inhibits ECE-1 expression in ECs.[21] ET_B receptors also mediate the pulmonary clearance of circulating ET-1, the reuptake of ET-1 by ECs and the release of aldosterone.[62] However, under disease conditions ET_B receptors can also be expressed in vascular SMCs and mediate vasoconstriction.[63,64]

ET-1-MEDIATED MECHANISMS OF CARDIOVASCULAR DISEASES

Fifteen years of research have convincingly shown that ET-1 is much more than an extremely potent vasoconstrictor and displays its multiple actions by deeply interacting with other peptide systems. ET-1 is endowed with mitogenic effects,[58,65] stimulates the production of cytokines[66,67] and growth factors such as vascular EGF,[41] basic fibroblast growth factor-2,[68] and epiregulin.[69] It also promotes the formation of reactive oxygen species (ROS),[70,71] induces deposition of extracellular matrix proteins,[72] and enhances collagen I gene activity.[55] ET-1 promotes expression of fibronectin and potentiates the effects of transforming growth factor-β[73] and platelet-derived growth factor.[74] Of note, ET-1 interacts with the blood cells stimulating neutrophil adhesion, and platelet aggregation, and is a chemotactic factor for macrophages. ET-1 promotes cell cycle progression in an autocrine fashion.[75–77] Finally, the mature ET-1 peptide stimulates synthesis and secretion of hormones and autacoids, such as aldosterone, arginine-vasopressin, NO, adrenomedullin, and prostacyclin.[78]

Effect of ET-1 on ROS

NADH/NADPH oxidases (NAD(P)Hox) are the most important source of ROS, which include plausible

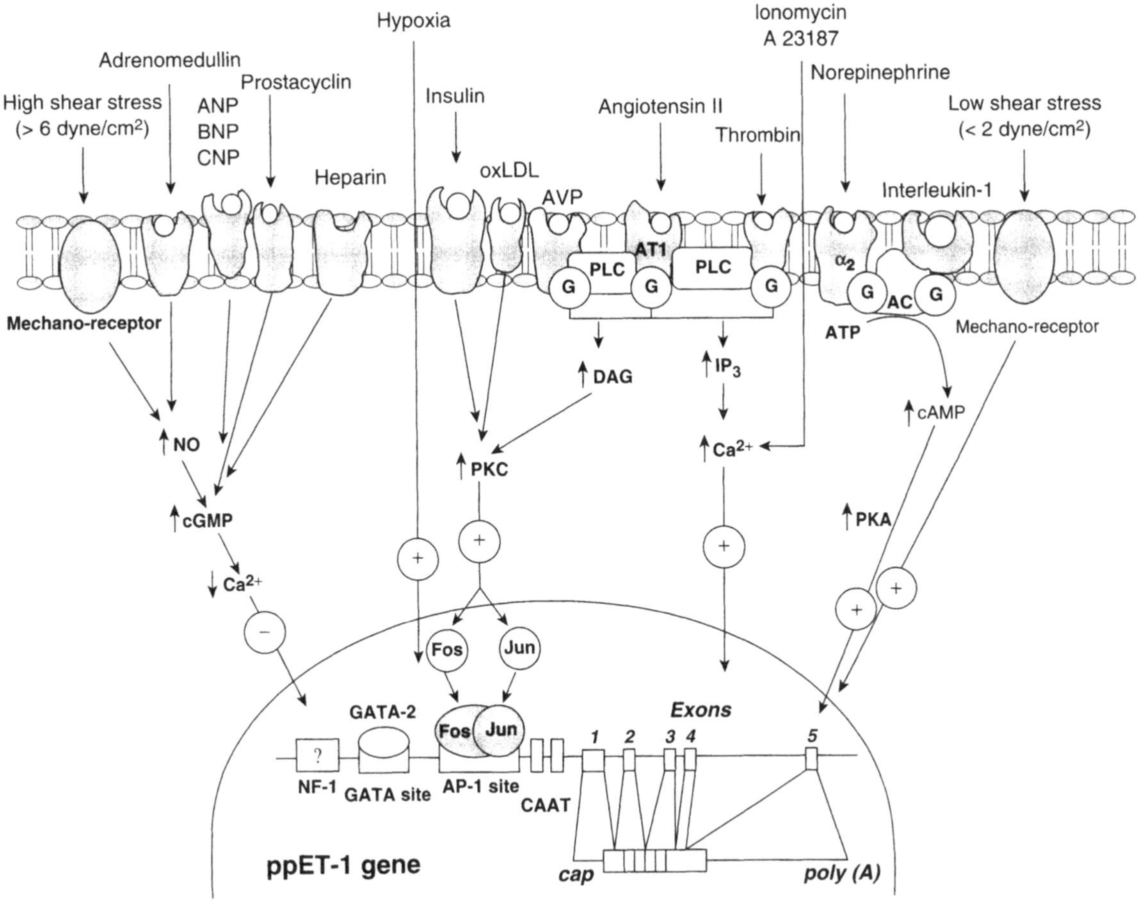

Figure 16.1 The cartoon summarizes the factors affecting ET-1 synthesis and related intracellular signaling pathways. Those acting via activation of the phospholipase C (PLC)-protein kinase C (PKC) pathway, such as insulin, LDL (low-density lipoprotein), oxidized LDL (oxLDL) AVP (arginine vasopressin), angiotensin II, and thrombin, enhance ET-1 production by binding of the AP-1 complex, consisting of a heterodimer *Fos-Jun*, to the specific motif in the ppET-1 promoter. Natriuretic peptides, PGI_2, and heparin blunt ppET-1 gene transcription by increasing cGMP, whereas adrenomedullin acts by increasing nitric oxide (NO) production. Norepinephrine and IL-1 increase ET-1 synthesis by increasing cAMP and PKA. Shear stress affects, in a bidirectional way, ppET-1 expression. Exons and consensus sequences in the promoter are schematically depicted in the nucleus

candidate molecules for atherogenesis, and cardiovascular events, in neutrophils, ECs, vascular SMCs, adventitial fibroblasts,[79] and monocyte-macrophages infiltrating the atherosclerotic plaques. In the vasculature they generate superoxide anion ($O_2^{\cdot -}$), which can oxidatively modify LDL,[79,80] scavenge NO,[81–83] and activate the family of nuclear transcription factor (NF)κB (see later). In a low-renin model of hypertension, where the ET-1 system is up-regulated,[84] activation of NAD(P)Hox with ensuing enhanced ROS generation occurs.[70,71] Furthermore, ET-1 induces VCAM-1 expression,[85] and mediates the NAD(P)Hox activation induced by vasopressin, which is also up-regulated in this model of hypertension.[86] Thus, enhanced ROS generation represents one important molecular mechanism of the detrimental cardiovascular effects of ET-1.

Effect of ET-1 on NF-κB

The binding of the homo- and heterodimers p50/p65 or p50/p65 NF-κB complexes to specific DNA binding κB motifs in the promoter of genes coding for adhesins (VCAM-1, ICAM-1, E-selectin) and inflammatory cytokines (IL-6 and IL-8), triggers the expression of these proatherogenic and proinflammatory molecules, which can also activate matrix metalloproteases (MMPs). Therefore, NF-κB activation is instrumental

Table 16.1 Main biological effects of ET-1 and receptor subtype involved (ET_A and ET_B)

ET_A	ET_B
Vasoconstriction	Release of NO (nitric oxide), prostacyclin, adrenomedullin,
Cell growth	ET-1 clearance
Stimulation of synthesis of cytokines and growth factors: VEGF (vascular endothelial growth factor) and bFGF (basic fibroblast growth factor-2)	Inhibition of ECE-1
Deposition of extracellular matrix (increased synthesis of structural proteins and fibronectin)	Endothelial reuptake of ET-1
Increase of TGF-β (transforming growth factor-β) and PDGF (platelet-derived growth factor) effects	Migration and proliferation of endothelial cells
Neutrophil adhesion	Release of aldosterone
Platelet adhesion	
Macrophage chemotaxis	

for the induction and progression of atherosclerosis, as well as for the transition from a stable to an unstable atherosclerotic plaque. Under conditions of normal NO bioactivity ET-1 can blunt the activity of the family of NF-κB via ET_B-mediated NO release (Figure 16.2). By contrast, under conditions of blunted NO bioactivity, ET-1 activates NF-κB via ET_A receptors and through phosphorylation and enhanced degradation of the inhibitory subunit I-κB.[87] The ensuing instability of the inactive complex consisting of I-κB and NF-κB monomers leads to active dimeric p50/p65 or p50/p65 complexes and to their translocation in the nucleus with induction of adhesin and cytokine genes transcription. Thus, these mechanisms likely mediate some effects of ET-1 that are relevant for hypertension and atherogenesis.

Effect of ET-1 on cardiovascular remodeling and fibrosis

Remodeling of the small resistance arteries plays a crucial role in maintaining high blood pressure levels, contributing to cardiovascular damage and complications. With pharmacological or molecular inhibition of ET-1 it was shown that the peptide contributes to vascular hypertrophy, and that local expression of ET-1 increases in vascular and renal tissue in most,[36,88–90] although not all, forms of experimental hypertension.[91,92] For instance, in the mouse renin Ren2 transgenic rats (TGRen2) that overexpress renin in cardiovascular tissues and develop severe hypertension and early cardiovascular damage and fibrosis, blockade of ET_A and ET_B receptor does prevent vascular and cardiac hypertrophy and fibrosis even without lowering blood pressure.[93] Thus, an increase in blood pressure *per se* may not be sufficient to activate the ET system, as indicated also by findings in rats transgenic for the human ET-1 gene that exhibit vascular hypertrophy, renal interstitial fibrosis, and glomerulosclerosis but lack hypertension.[94] Accordingly, the ET-1 system plays a role in inducing cardiovascular damage even in the models of hypertension where it does not play a major role in raising blood pressure.

Blockade of the ET system and therapeutic targets

Theoretically the inhibition of ECE can inhibit the production of ET-1 and its effects, but the ECE-independent pathways of ET-1 formation would likely limit the effectiveness of this strategy. Blunting of ET-1 production can also be attained indirectly through renin-angiotensin system (RAS) inhibitors,[95,96] or statins,[97] and therefore might contribute to the beneficial effect of these therapies.

Peptides and nonpeptide ET receptor blockers are available as research tools, some are in clinical development[98] and one, bosentan, has been approved for clinical use (see later). Given the opposing actions of the ET_A and ET_B receptors and the fact that the tissue expression of both receptor subtypes can change dramatically in disease conditions, the therapeutic applications must be

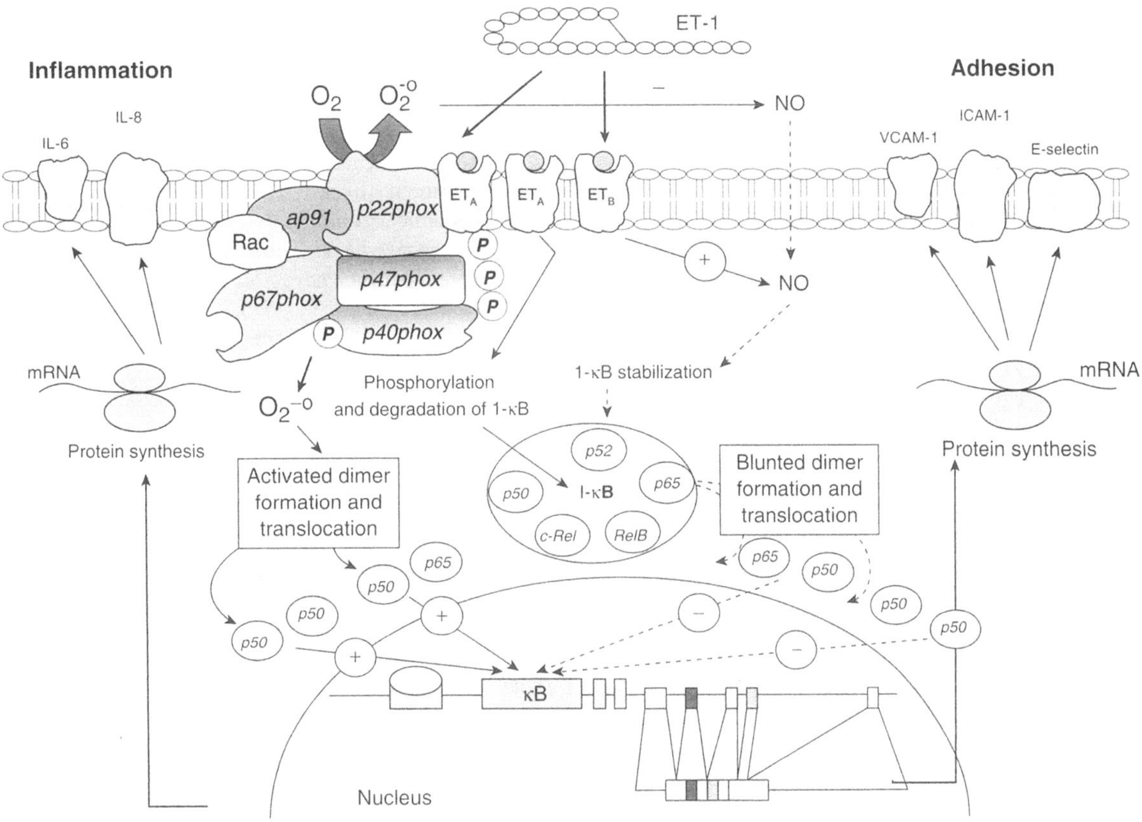

Figure 16.2 Effects of ET-1 on NF-κB and NAD(P)H oxidase activity. ET-1 can enhance the activity of NAD(P)H oxidase via ET_A receptor and thus increase production of superoxide O_2^{-o}, which scavenges nitric oxide (NO). Under conditions of blunted NO bioactivity ET-1 enhances activation of NF-κB that, by binding to specific DNA binding κB motifs in the promoters of genes coding for adhesins (VCAM-1, ICAM-1, E-selectin) and inflammatory cytokines (IL-6 and IL-8), can trigger the expression of these proatherogenic and proinflammatory molecules. NF-κB activation can also result from phosphorylation and degradation of I-κB that, in turn, lead to a reduced stability of the inactive complex, consisting of transcription factors p50, p52, p65, c-Rel, RelB, plus the inhibitory factor I-κB. Thus, increased availability of the active complex, constituted by dimeric complex p50/p65 or p50/p65, may derive. Dashed lines indicate the NO-mediated pathway, leading to blunting dimer formation and translocation and, therefore, to reduced levels of NF-κB active complex + and – signs indicate stimulation and inhibition, respectively

carefully assessed in each indication. ET antagonists can block either ET_A or ET_B receptors or both, but blockade of the ET_B receptors impairs the pulmonary clearance of ET-1 and reduces NO-mediated vasodilatation.[99] Furthermore, ET_B receptor deficiency is associated with hypertension in mice and ET_B blockade increases systemic vascular resistance in humans.[100] Thus, since ET_B-mediated NO-induced vasodilation is mostly beneficial, selective ET_B receptor antagonists have not been exploited for therapeutic use. However, in most experimental and clinical studies, combined ET_A and ET_B receptor antagonists improved cardiovascular function and structure, suggesting that ET_A receptor blockade is obligatory for the therapeutic effects, regardless of concomitant ET_B receptor blockade.

ET-1 AND CARDIOVASCULAR DISEASES

Since ET-1 synthesis can be triggered by several factors that can be involved in arterial hypertension and atherosclerosis and since picomolar concentrations of ET-1 induce a sustained and dose-dependent vasoconstriction, the peptide has been implicated in the pathogenesis of conditions that feature excess vasoconstriction and cell proliferation (Box 16.1).

Arterial hypertension and renal disease

The role of ET-1 differs markedly across the experimental models of hypertension.[24,84,101] In Ang II-induced and in salt-sensitive hypertension, as in deoxycorticosterone acetate–salt-treated and in Dahl rats, the ET-1 system is up-regulated and chronic ET receptor blockade lowers blood pressure. By contrast, in spontaneously hypertensive rats and in transgenic TGRen2 rats this does not occur.[102] The different role played by ET-1 in experimental models is mirrored in human hypertension. In the rare patients with ET-1-producing hemangioendothelioma, both hypertension and the raised ET-1 levels were cured by tumorectomy and recurred with tumor recurrence,[103] thus underlying the crucial pathophysiologic role of the peptide. At variance, in primary (essential) hypertension the evidence supporting the involvement of ET-1 is far more controversial. Most clinical studies, except those in black populations, showed that ET-1 levels were low in hypertensive subjects and that the ET-1 plasma levels in hypertensive patients were not increased compared to normotensive subjects. However, ET-1 plasma levels estimate only roughly the activation of the system, because of the abluminal ET-1 secretion.[5] Additionally, in most studies the statistical power was inadequate to provide conclusive data.[104] Furthermore, given the pathophysiological diversity of essential hypertension the contention that ET-1 is consistently enhanced in this condition can be a naive one. Nonetheless, data on ET receptor blockade in hypertensive patients showed a consistent picture. In patients with mild to moderate hypertension, bosentan showed an antihypertensive efficacy similar to the angiotensin converting enzyme (ACE) inhibitor enalapril.[105] Combined ET_A/ET_B receptor blockade with TAK 044 induced an enhanced vasodilatory response in essential hypertensive patients compared with normal subjects, thereby suggesting an enhanced vasoconstriction to endogenous ET-1.[106] A similar significant fall of blood pressure was also documented in hypertensive patients with primary and secondary aldosteronism, e.g. contrasting degree of activation of the RAS after infusion of low doses of the ET_A receptor antagonist BQ-123, alone or combined with the ET_B receptor antagonist BQ-788.[107] Thus, available data collectively suggest that ET-1 contributes to maintaining elevated blood pressure level in a wide range of hypertensive patients. Studies in L-N^G-nitroarginine methyl ester hypertension also suggest that ET-1 is linked to the dysfunction of the L-arginine/NO pathway,[108] because ET_A-selective but not combined ET blockade[109] improves endothelial function, independent of blood pressure.[99]

Box 16.1 Cardiovascular diseases with increased ET-1 levels

- Atherosclerosis
- Acute myocardial ischemia
- Pulmonary hypertension
- Systemic arterial hypertension
- Congestive heart failure
- Renal insufficiency
- Scleroderma
- Hemangioendothelioma
- Conn's syndrome

ET-1 promotes vasoconstriction and cell growth in the vasculature and in the kidney, mainly via ET_A receptors. Accordingly, in experimental models, chronic ET receptor blockade inhibits vascular injury, reduces hypertension-associated and other forms of renal and vascular injury,[110–116] and also prolongs survival.[117] However, the concomitant blockade of ET_B receptors can abolish the beneficial effects of an ET_A-selective antagonist on vascular structure.

Hyperaldosteronism

Consistent animal data showed that the ET-1 system is up-regulated in models of hypertension with increased mineralocorticoid activity.[71,102,118] Chronic ET-1 infusion induces zona glomerulosa cell hyperplasia and an increase of the steroidogenic machinery.[119] Furthermore, in vitro ET-1 exerts a secretagogue effect on aldosterone which is mediated via ET_B receptors.[120] In keeping with the animal data it was found that preproET-1 gene, ECE-1, and both ET_A and ET_B receptor genes are expressed in the human adrenocortical zona glomerulosa and in aldosteronoma tissue and that plasma ET-1 levels are elevated in patients with primary aldosteronism.[62]

Thus, local and systemic activation of the ET-1 system can play a relevant role in the pathophysiology of primary and secondary aldosteronism, as well as in inducing its cardiovascular consequences including vascular remodeling and cardiac hypertrophy and fibrosis.

Atherosclerosis and coronary artery disease

Increased ET levels in plasma and tissue along with endothelial dysfunction were found in hypercholesterolemia.[121] Furthermore, the most atherogenic oxidized low-density lipoproteins (LDLs) up-regulate ET-1 gene expression in ECs[30] (Figure 16.1) and enhance vascular SMC proliferation via ET_A receptors.[121] In turn, ET-1 stimulates the synthesis of growth factors and adhesins that are implicated in atherogenesis, as previously mentioned. ET-1 also increases neutrophil and platelet adhesion, thereby promoting plaque growth and coronary thrombosis.[122] In experimental hypercholesterolemia, ET_A receptor blockade reduced macrophage infiltration in fatty streaks,[123] and combined ET_A/ET_B receptor blockade improved the impaired endothelium-dependent vasodilatation.[124]

ET-1 also contributes to myocardial infarction in atherosclerotic mice[125] and in apolipoprotein E-deficient mice, long-term ET_A blockade reduces the extent of atherosclerosis, corrects endothelial dysfunction and prevents increased vascular ET-1, even without affecting blood pressure or plasma cholesterol.[126]

In patients with angina pectoris but normal angiograms and in those with coronary artery disease[127] and acute myocardial infarction,[128] ET-1 plasma levels are increased. In human atherosclerotic lesions, the expression of ET-1 and ECE is enhanced.[6,129,130] A functional role for tissue ET-1 in coronary artery disease is suggested by the observation that the extent of immunoreactive staining for ET-1 in atheromatous lesions is related to angina class[129] and the plasma levels of ET-1 correlate with number of coronary artery diseased vessels.[131] In line with these findings, combined ET receptor blockade causes vasodilation, at least in certain patients with coronary atherosclerosis.[132] ET-1 also plays a role in determining the severity of stroke and its sequelae, because ET receptor blockade reduces ischemic brain injury and vasospasm.[133]

Data on ET_A receptors in atherosclerosis are more controversial, since they appear to be down-regulated in humans, and increased in atherosclerotic mice.[126] ET-1 can also be involved in restenosis that is a major limitation of balloon angioplasty.[134]

Heart allograft and transplant-associated vasculopathy

Kidney, heart, and lung transplantation is associated with raised circulating ET-1 levels, probably because the ET system is activated in the transplanted organ.[135,136] Accelerated arteriosclerosis of coronary vessels of transplanted heart can contribute to worsening the outcome of heart transplant recipients. Compelling evidence indicates that immunologic mechanisms leading to chronic nonspecific inflammatory changes and EC activation (induced by cytokines released by infiltrating mononuclear cells and lymphocytes) can be major underlying mechanisms. Enhanced local synthesis of ET-1, with ensuing ROS production, NF-κB activation and stimulation of adhesins and proinflammatory cytokine expression, contributes to SMC proliferation. A causal role of ET-1 up-regulation in the accelerated arteriosclerosis of heart transplant is also supported by the effectiveness of treatment with bosentan in preventing the development of arteriolar narrowing of transplanted heart, at least in rats.[137]

Congestive heart failure and left ventricular dysfunction

ET-1 has emerged as an important player in congestive heart failure (CHF). The ET-1 plasma levels are increased in experimental animals and in patients with CHF and predict survival. The ECE-1, the preproET-1 and ET_A receptor genes are up-regulated in CHF in rodents and humans[138–140] and contribute to impaired ventricular function. The synthesis of ET-1 can take place in cardiomyocytes in CHF, possibly as a result of Ang II- and catecholamine-induced preproET-1 gene expression.[141,142] The growth-promoting effects of ET-1 on cardiomyocytes[35,44,143,144] may facilitate the development of hypertrophy during hypoxia, which is important in chronic ischemia. In addition, ET-1-mediated cardiac hypertrophy is enhanced by the RAS,[44,145] which is also up-regulated in CHF.

It is likely, however, that ET-1 plays a dual role: prolonged exercise in rats up-regulates myocardial ET-1 expression[29] and ET-1 maintains cardiac function in early stages of CHF.[138] In animal models of CHF, prolonged ET blockade improves hemodynamics, reduces ventricular dilatation, and prolongs survival.[140,146–148] Beneficial hemodynamic and clinical effects occur with ET receptor blockade, both with selective and nonselective ET antagonists, but concomitant ET_B blockade markedly increases circulating ET-1 levels and may abrogate the beneficial effects of ET_A receptor blockade on hemodynamics and renal function in heart failure.[149,150] On the other hand, increased ET_B-mediated systemic vasoconstriction can occur in CHF patients;[151] thus, whether selective ET_A or nonselective ET blockade should be favored in CHF remains unclear.

The first hemodynamic studies of ET-1 receptor blockade in humans have been promising,[152,153] but clinical trials thereafter failed to prove the clinical efficacy of either nonselective (bosentan and tezosentan) or ET_A-selective (darusentan) receptor ET-1 antagonists in patients with acute and chronic CHF.[154–158] Thus, in contrast to expectations, to date there is no evidence for clinical efficacy for ET-1 receptor antagonists in patients with CHF. Issues concerning timing for starting treatment, drug dosages, concomitant therapies and selection of the patients, as well as the fact that ET blockade can interfere with scar formation in injured myocardium, might explain these negative results.

Pulmonary hypertension

The vasculature of the lung is a site of intense NO and ET-1 production and clearance, which can be altered in lung disease and pulmonary hypertension.[159] An imbalance between NO and ET-1 synthesis is a hallmark of both primary and secondary pulmonary hypertension.[159,160] In primary pulmonary hypertension the expression of eNOS and the bioavailability of NO is decreased in the pulmonary vasculature[161] and this can play a causal role. Conversely, ET-1 expression is enhanced in pulmonary hypertension.[159] Furthermore, the ET_A receptor is highly expressed in both conduit and resistance arteries of the lung, which can explain why they are so exquisitely sensitive to the vasoconstrictor effect of ET-1. ET-1 was also shown to exert a clear-cut proliferative effect on pulmonary artery SMCs via ET_A receptors.[162] In addition, the transcription of the ppET-1 gene can be turned on by hypoxia and both an activation of the ET-1 system and a beneficial effect of ET-1 receptor antagonists on the course of pulmonary hypertension have been documented.[156,163] Thus, compelling evidence indicates a pathogenic role for ET-1 in raising pulmonary artery pressure and causing adverse structural changes in the vasculature. A first pilot study[164] in a few patients with primary and scleroderma-induced pulmonary hypertension showed impressive hemodynamic improvement. A larger multicenter study thereafter conclusively demonstrated an impressive amelioration of the clinical course of this serious disease.[161] Based on these findings, and despite its effects on liver enzymes, bosentan has been approved in both the US and Europe for the treatment of pulmonary hypertension in patients in NYHA class III/IV. An open label 2-year follow-up study of patients on bosentan indicated a doubling of the survival as compared with the survival rate expected on the basis of the NHI equation (M. Clozel, personal communication).

CONCLUSIONS

The ET system is involved in cardiovascular control and disease progression. In most conditions associated with generation of ROS and blunted NO bioactivity, such as hypertension, atherosclerosis, and heart failure, the ET-1 system is up-regulated. The diversity of the underlying mechanisms and their complex interplay with variation of genes involved in EC function and regulation likely account for the different individual susceptibility to cardiovascular disease. ET receptor blockade offers a possibility of restoring the imbalance between NO and ET-1 and has been shown to have therapeutic potential in hypertension, atherosclerosis, heart failure, pulmonary disease, and renal damage. Controlled clinical studies will determine whether these new drugs, which promise to be powerful tools in cardiovascular medicine, have the potential to reduce morbidity and mortality.

REFERENCES

1. Yanagisawa M, Kurihara H, Kimura S et al. A novel potent vasoconstrictor peptide produced by vascular endothelial cells. Nature 1988; 332: 411–15.
2. Hickey KA, Rubanyi G, Paul RJ, Highsmith RF. Characterization of a coronary vasoconstrictor produced by cultured endothelial cells. Am J Physiol 1985; 248: C550–C556.
3. O'Brien RF, McMurtry IF. Endothelial cells in culture produce a vasoconstrictor substance. J Cell Physiol 1987; 132: 263–70.
4. Masaki T, Yanagisawa M, Goto K. Physiology and pharmacology of endothelins. Med Res Rev 1992; 12: 391–421.
5. Wagner OF, Christ G, Wojta J et al. Polar secretion of endothelin-1 by cultured endothelial cells. J Biol Chem 1992; 267: 16066–8.
6. Rossi GP, Colonna S, Pavan E et al. Endothelin-1 and its mRNA in the wall layers of human arteries ex vivo. Circulation 1999; 99: 1147–55.
7. Rubanyi GM, Polokoff MA. Endothelins: molecular biology, biochemistry, pharmacology, physiology, and pathophysiology. Pharmacol Rev 1994; 46: 325–415.
8. Benatti L, Fabbrini MS, Patrono C. Regulation of endothelin-1 biosynthesis. Ann N Y Acad Sci 1994; 714: 109–21.
9. Dorfman DM, Wilson DB, Bruns GA, Orkin SH. Human transcription factor GATA-2. Evidence for regulation of preproendothelin-1 gene expression in endothelial cells. J Biol Chem 1992; 267: 1279–85.
10. Morey AK, Razandi M, Pedram A, Hu RM, Prins BA, Levin ER. Oestrogen and progesterone inhibit the stimulated production of endothelin-1. Biochem J 1998; 330: 1097–105.
11. Lee ME, Bloch KD, Clifford JA, Quertermous T. Functional analysis of the endothelin-1 gene promoter. Evidence for an endothelial cell-specific cis-acting sequence. J Biol Chem 1990; 265: 10446–50.
12. Inoue A, Yanagisawa M, Takuwa Y, Mitsui Y, Kobayashi M, Masaki T. The human preproendothelin-1 gene. Complete nucleotide sequence and regulation of expression. J Biol Chem 1989; 264: 14954–9.
13. Xu D, Emoto N, Giaid A, Slaughter C, Kaw S, deWit D, Yanagisawa M. ECE-1: a membrane-bound metalloprotease that catalyzes the proteolytic activation of big endothelin-1. Cell 1994; 78: 473–85.
14. Valdenaire O, Rohrbacher E, Mattei MG. Organization of the gene encoding the human endothelin converting enzyme (ECE-1). J Biol Chem 1995; 270: 29794–8.
15. Emoto N, Yanagisawa M. Endothelin-converting enzyme-2 is a membrane-bound, phosphoramidon-sensitive metalloprotease with acidic pH optimum. J Biol Chem 1995; 270: 15262–8.

16. Schweizer A, Valdenaire O, Nelbock P et al. Human endothelin-converting enzyme (ECE-1): three isoforms with distinct subcellular localizations. Biochem J 1997; 328: 871–7.
17. Rossi GP, Albertin G, Franchin E et al. Expression of the endothelin-converting enzyme gene in human tissues. Biochem Biophys Res Commun 1995; 211: 249–53.
18. Albertin G, Rossi GP, Majone F et al. Fine mapping of the human ECE gene by fluorescent in situ hybridization and radiation hybrids. Biochem Biophys Res Commun 1996; 221: 682–7.
19. Schmidt M, Kröger B, Jacob E et al. Molecular characterization of human and bovine endothelin converting enzyme (ECE-1). FEBS Lett 1994; 356: 238–43.
20. Valdenaire O, Lepailleur-Enouf D, Egidy G et al. A fourth isoform of endothelin-converting enzyme (ECE-1) is generated from an additional promoter molecular cloning and characterization. Eur J Biochem 1999; 264: 341–9.
21. Naomi S, Iwaoka T, Disashi T et al. Endothelin-1 inhibits endothelin-converting enzyme-1 expression in cultured rat pulmonary endothelial cells. Circulation 1998; 97: 234–6.
22. Yanagisawa H, Yanagisawa M, Kapur RP et al. Dual genetic pathways of endothelin-mediated intercellular signaling revealed by targeted disruption of endothelin converting enzyme-1 gene. Development 1998; 125: 825–36.
23. Urata H, Kinoshita A, Misono KS, Bumpus FM, Husain A. Identification of a highly specific chymase as the major angiotensin II-forming enzyme in the human heart. J Biol Chem 1990; 265: 22348–57.
24. Rossi GP, Sacchetto A, Cesari M, Pessina AC. Interactions between endothelin-1 and the renin-angiotensin-aldosterone system. Cardiovasc Res 1999; 43: 300–7.
25. Wypij DM, Nichols JS, Novak PJ, Stacy DL, Berman J, Wiseman JS. Role of mast cell chymase in the extracellular processing of big-endothelin-1 to endothelin-1 in the perfused rat lung. Biochem Pharmacol 1992; 43: 845–53.
26. Macarthur H, Warner TD, Wood EG, Corder R, Vane JR. Endothelin-1 release from endothelial cells in culture is elevated both acutely and chronically by short periods of mechanical stretch. Biochem Biophys Res Commun 1994; 200: 395–400.
27. Malek A, Izumo S. Physiological fluid shear stress causes downregulation of endothelin-1 mRNA in bovine aortic endothelium. Am J Physiol 1992; 263: C389–C396.
28. Wesson DE, Simoni J, Green DF. Reduced extracellular pH increases endothelin-1 secretion by human renal microvascular endothelial cells. J Clin Invest 1998; 101: 578–83.
29. Maeda S, Miyauchi T, Sakai S et al. Prolonged exercise causes an increase in endothelin-1 production in the heart in rats. Am J Physiol 1998; 275: H2105–H2112.
30. Boulanger CM, Tanner FC, Bea ML, Hahn AW, Werner A, Luscher TF. Oxidized low density lipoproteins induce mRNA expression and release of endothelin from human and porcine endothelium. Circ Res 1992; 70: 1191–7.
31. Yamauchi T, Ohnaka K, Takayanagi R, Umeda F, Nawata H. Enhanced secretion of endothelin-1 by elevated glucose levels from cultured bovine aortic endothelial cells. FEBS Lett 1990; 267: 16–18.
32. Akishita M, Ouchi Y, Miyoshi H et al. Estrogen inhibits endothelin-1 production and c-fos gene expression in rat aorta. Atherosclerosis 1996; 125: 27–38.
33. Barton M, Carmona R, Morawietz H et al. Obesity is associated with tissue-specific activation of renal angiotensin-converting enzyme in vivo: evidence for a regulatory role of endothelin. Hypertension 2000; 35: 329–36.
34. Boulanger C, Luscher TF. Release of endothelin from the porcine aorta. Inhibition by endothelium-derived nitric oxide. J Clin Invest 1990; 85: 587–90.
35. Ito H, Hirata Y, Adachi S et al. Endothelin-1 is an autocrine/paracrine factor in the mechanism of angiotensin II-induced hypertrophy in cultured rat cardiomyocytes. J Clin Invest 1993; 92: 398–403.
36. Barton M, Shaw S, d'Uscio LV, Moreau P, Luscher TF. Angiotensin II increases vascular and renal endothelin-1 and functional endothelin converting enzyme activity in vivo: role of ETA receptors for endothelin regulation. Biochem Biophys Res Commun 1997; 238: 861–5.
37. Imai T, Hirata Y, Emori T, Yanagisawa M, Masaki T, Marumo F. Induction of endothelin-1 gene by angiotensin and vasopressin in endothelial cells. Hypertension 1992; 19: 753–7.
38. Hahn AW, Resink TJ, Scott Burden T, Powell J, Dohi Y, Buhler FR. Stimulation of endothelin mRNA and secretion in rat vascular smooth muscle cells: a novel autocrine function. Cell Regul 1990; 1: 649–59.
39. Rossi GP, Andreis PG, Colonna S et al. Endothelin-1[1-31]: a novel autocrine-paracrine regulator of human adrenal cortex secretion and growth. J Clin Endocrinol Metab 2002; 87: 322–8.
40. Boulanger CM, Luscher TF. Hirudin and nitrates inhibit the thrombin-induced release of endothelin from the intact porcine aorta. Circ Res 1991; 68: 1768–72.
41. Matsuura A, Yamochi W, Hirata K, Kawashima S, Yokoyama M. Stimulatory interaction between vascular endothelial growth factor and endothelin-1 on each gene expression. Hypertension 1998; 32: 89–95.
42. Bodin P, Milner P, Marshall J, Burnstock G. Cytokines suppress the shear stress-stimulated release of vasoactive peptides from human endothelial cells. Peptides 1995; 16: 1433–8.
43. Corder R, Carrier M, Khan N, Klemm P, Vane JR. Cytokine regulation of endothelin-1 release from bovine aortic endothelial cells. J Cardiovasc Pharmacol 1995; 26 (Suppl 3): S56–S58.
44. Stewart DJ, Cernacek P, Mohamed F, Blais D, Cianflone K, Monge JC. Role of cyclic nucleotides in the regulation of endothelin-1 production by human endothelial cells. Am J Physiol 1994; 266: H944–H951.
45. Fujisaki H, Ito H, Hirata Y et al. Natriuretic peptides inhibit angiotensin II-induced proliferation of rat cardiac fibroblasts by blocking endothelin-1 gene expression. J Clin Invest 1995; 96: 1059–65.
46. Drunat S, Moatti N, Demuth K. Homocysteine decreases endothelin-1 expression by interfering with the AP-1 signaling pathway. Free Radic Biol Med 2002; 33: 659–68.
47. Corder R, Douthwaite JA, Lees DM et al. Endothelin-1 synthesis reduced by red wine. Nature 2001; 414: 863–4.
48. Arai H, Hori S, Aramori I, Ohkubo H, Nakanishi S. Cloning and expression of a cDNA encoding an endothelin receptor. Nature 1990; 348: 730–2.
49. Lin HY, Kaji EH, Winkel GK, Ives HE, Lodish HF. Cloning and functional expression of a vascular smooth muscle endothelin 1 receptor. Proc Natl Acad Sci U S A 1991; 88: 3185–9.
50. Sakurai T, Yanagisawa M, Takuwa Y et al. Cloning of a cDNA encoding a non-isopeptide-selective subtype of the endothelin receptor. Nature 1990; 348: 732–5.
51. Sakamoto A, Yanagisawa M, Sakurai T, Takuwa Y, Yanagisawa H, Masaki T. Cloning and functional expression of human cDNA for the ETB endothelin receptor. Biochem Biophys Res Commun 1991; 178: 656–63.
52. White DG, Cannon TR, Garratt H, Mundin JW, Sumner MJ, Watts IS. Endothelin ETA and ETB receptors mediate vascular smooth-muscle contraction. J Cardiovasc Pharmacol 1993; 22 (Suppl 8): S144–S148.
53. Bacon CR, Cary NR, Davenport AP. Endothelin peptide and receptors in human atherosclerotic coronary artery and aorta. Circ Res 1996; 79: 794–801.

54. Simonson MS, Herman WH. Protein kinase C and protein tyrosine kinase activity contribute to mitogenic signaling by endothelin-1. Cross-talk between G protein-coupled receptors and pp60c-src. J Biol Chem 1993; 268: 9347–57.
55. Ozaki S, Ohwaki K, Ihara M, Ishikawa K, Yano M. Coexpression studies with endothelin receptor subtypes indicate the existence of intracellular cross-talk between ET(A) and ET(B) receptors. J Biochem (Tokyo) 1997; 121: 440–7.
56. Flamant M, Tharaux PL, Placier S et al. Epidermal growth factor receptor trans-activation mediates the tonic and fibrogenic effects of endothelin in the aortic wall of transgenic mice. FASEB J 2003; 17: 327–9.
57. Pollock DM, Keith TL, Highsmith RF. Endothelin receptors and calcium signaling. FASEB J 1995; 9: 1196–204.
58. Alberts GF, Peifley KA, Johns A, Kleha JF, Winkles JA. Constitutive endothelin-1 overexpression promotes smooth muscle cell proliferation via an external autocrine loop. J Biol Chem 1994; 269: 10112–18.
59. Ohlstein EH, Arleth A, Bryan H, Elliott JD, Sung CP. The selective endothelin ETA receptor antagonist BQ123 antagonizes endothelin-1-mediated mitogenesis. Eur J Pharmacol 1992; 225: 347–50.
60. Warner TD, Mitchell JA, de Nucci G, Vane JR. Endothelin-1 and endothelin-3 release EDRF from isolated perfused arterial vessels of the rat and rabbit. J Cardiovasc Pharmacol 1989; 13 (Suppl 5): S85–S88.
61. Hirata Y, Emori T, Eguchi S et al. Endothelin receptor subtype B mediates synthesis of nitric oxide by cultured bovine endothelial cells. J Clin Invest 1993; 91: 1367–73.
62. Rossi G, Albertin G, Belloni A et al. Gene expression, localization, and characterization of endothelin A and B receptors in the human adrenal cortex. J Clin Invest 1994; 94: 1226–34.
63. Dagassan PH, Breu V, Clozel M et al. Up-regulation of endothelin-B receptors in atherosclerotic human coronary arteries. J Cardiovasc Pharmacol 1996; 27: 147–53.
64. Teerlink JR, Breu V, Sprecher U, Clozel M, Clozel JP. Potent vasoconstriction mediated by endothelin ETB receptors in canine coronary arteries. Circ Res 1994; 74: 105–14.
65. Komuro I, Kurihara H, Sugiyama T, Yoshizumi M, Takaku F, Yazaki Y. Endothelin stimulates c-fos and c-myc expression and proliferation of vascular smooth muscle cells [published erratum appears in FEBS Lett 1989; 244: 509]. FEBS Lett 1988; 238: 249–52.
66. Agui T, Xin X, Cai Y, Sakai T, Matsumoto K. Stimulation of interleukin-6 production by endothelin in rat bone marrow-derived stromal cells. Blood 1994; 84: 2531–8.
67. Hofman FM, Chen P, Jeyaseelan R, Incardona F, Fisher M, Zidovetzki R. Endothelin-1 induces production of the neutrophil chemotactic factor interleukin-8 by human brain-derived endothelial cells. Blood 1998; 92: 3064–72.
68. Peifley KA, Winkles JA. Angiotensin II and endothelin-1 increase fibroblast growth factor-2 mRNA expression in vascular smooth muscle cells. Biochem Biophys Res Commun 1998; 242: 202–8.
69. Taylor S, Cheng X, Pawlowski JE, Wallace AR, Ferrer P, Molloy CJ. Epiregulin is a potent vascular smooth muscle cell-derived mitogen induced by angiotensin II, endothelin-1, and thrombin. Proc Natl Acad Sci U S A 1999; 96: 1633–8.
70. Li L, Watts SW, Banes AK, Galligan JJ, Fink GD, Chen AF. NADPH oxidase-derived superoxide augments endothelin-1-induced venoconstriction in mineralocorticoid hypertension. Hypertension 2003; 42: 316–21.
71. Li L, Fink GD, Watts SW et al. Endothelin-1 increases vascular superoxide via endothelin(A)-NADPH oxidase pathway in low-renin hypertension. Circulation 2003; 107: 1053–8.
72. Guidry C, Hook M. Endothelins produced by endothelial cells promote collagen gel contraction by fibroblasts. J Cell Biol 1991; 115: 873–80.
73. Weissberg PL, Witchell C, Davenport AP, Hesketh TR, Metcalfe JC. The endothelin peptides ET-1, ET-2, ET-3 and sarafotoxin S6b are co-mitogenic with platelet-derived growth factor for vascular smooth muscle cells. Atherosclerosis 1990; 85: 257–62.
74. Yang Z, Krasnici N, Luscher TF. Endothelin-1 potentiates human smooth muscle cell growth to PDGF: effects of ETA and ETB receptor blockade. Circulation 1999; 100: 5–8.
75. Jahan H, Kobayashi S, Nishimura J, Kanaide H. Endothelin-1 and angiotensin II act as progression but not competence growth factors in vascular smooth muscle cells. Eur J Pharmacol 1996; 295: 261–9.
76. Pedram A, Razandi M, Hu RM, Levin ER. Astrocyte Progression from G1 to S phase of the cell cycle depends upon multiple protein interaction. J Biol Chem 1998; 273: 13966–72.
77. Suzuki E, Nagata D, Kakoki M et al. Molecular mechanisms of endothelin-1-induced cell-cycle progression: involvement of extracellular signal-regulated kinase, protein kinase C, and phosphatidylinositol 3-kinase at distinct points. Circ Res 1999; 84: 611–19.
78. Nussdorfer GG, Rossi GP, Malendowicz LK, Mazzocchi G. Autocrine-paracrine endothelin system in the physiology and pathology of steroid-secreting tissues. Pharmacol Rev 1999; 51: 403–38.
79. Griendling KK, Sorescu D, Ushio-Fukai M. NAD(P)H oxidase: role in cardiovascular biology and disease. Circ Res 2000; 86: 494–501.
80. Cahilly C, Ballantyne CM, Lim DS, Gotto A, Marian AJ. A variant of p22(phox), involved in generation of reactive oxygen species in the vessel wall, is associated with progression of coronary atherosclerosis. Circ Res 2000; 86: 391–5.
81. Mohazzab KM, Kaminski PM, Wolin MS. NADH oxidoreductase is a major source of superoxide anion in bovine coronary artery endothelium. Am J Physiol 1994; 266: H2568–H2572.
82. Howard AB, Alexander RW, Nerem RM, Griendling KK, Taylor WR. Cyclic strain induces an oxidative stress in endothelial cells. Am J Physiol Cell Physiol 1997; 272: C421–C427.
83. De Keulenaer GW, Chappell DC, Ishizaka N, Nerem RM, Alexander RW, Griendling KK. Oscillatory and steady laminar shear stress differentially affect human endothelial redox state: role of a superoxide-producing NADH oxidase. Circ Res 1998; 82: 1094–101.
84. Schiffrin EL. Endothelin: role in experimental hypertension. J Cardiovasc Pharmacol 2000; 35: S33–S35.
85. Li L, Chu Y, Fink GD, Engelhardt JF, Heistad DD, Chen AF. Endothelin-1 stimulates arterial VCAM-1 expression via NADPH oxidase-derived superoxide in mineralocorticoid hypertension. Hypertension 2003; 42: 997–1003.
86. Li L, Galligan JJ, Fink GD, Chen AF. Vasopressin induces vascular superoxide via endothelin-1 in mineralocorticoid hypertension. Hypertension 2003; 41: 663–8.
87. Ishizuka T, Takamizawa-Matsumoto M, Suzuki K, Kurita A. Endothelin-1 enhances vascular cell adhesion molecule-1 expression in tumor necrosis factor alpha-stimulated vascular endothelial cells. Eur J Pharmacol 1999; 369: 237–45.
88. Li JS, Lariviere R, Schiffrin EL. Effect of a nonselective endothelin antagonist on vascular remodeling in deoxycorticosterone acetate-salt hypertensive rats. Evidence for a role of endothelin in vascular hypertrophy. Hypertension 1994; 24: 183–8.
89. Moreau P, d'Uscio LV, Shaw S, Takase H, Barton M, Luscher TF. Angiotensin II increases tissue endothelin and induces vascular hypertrophy: reversal by ETA-receptor antagonist. Circulation 1997; 96: 1593–7.

90. Barton M, d'Uscio LV, Shaw S, Meyer P, Moreau P, Luscher TF. ET(A) receptor blockade prevents increased tissue endothelin-1, vascular hypertrophy, and endothelial dysfunction in salt-sensitive hypertension. Hypertension 1998; 31: 499–504.
91. Li JS, Schiffrin EL. Effect of chronic treatment of adult spontaneously hypertensive rats with an endothelin receptor antagonist. Hypertension 1995; 25 (Pt 1): 495–500.
92. Li JS, Knafo L, Turgeon A, Garcia R, Schiffrin EL. Effect of endothelin antagonism on blood pressure and vascular structure in renovascular hypertensive rats. Am J Physiol 1996; 271: H88–H93.
93. Seccia TM, Belloni AS, Kreutz R et al. Cardiac fibrosis occurs early and involves endothelin and AT-1 receptors in hypertension due to endogenous angiotensin II. J Am Coll Cardiol 2003; 41: 666–73.
94. Hocher B, Thone-Reineke C, Rohmeiss P et al. Endothelin-1 transgenic mice develop glomerulosclerosis, interstitial fibrosis, and renal cysts but not hypertension. J Clin Invest 1997; 99: 1380–9.
95. Clavell AL, Mattingly MT, Stevens TL et al. Angiotensin converting enzyme inhibition modulates endogenous endothelin in chronic canine thoracic inferior vena caval constriction. J Clin Invest 1996; 97: 1286–92.
96. d'Uscio LV, Shaw S, Barton M, Luscher TF. Losartan but not verapamil inhibits angiotensin II-induced tissue endothelin-1 increase. Role of blood pressure and endothelial function. Hypertension 1998; 31: 1305–10.
97. Hernandez-Perera O, Perez-Sala D, Navarro-Antolin J et al. Effects of the 3-hydroxy-3-methylglutaryl-CoA reductase inhibitors, atorvastatin and simvastatin, on the expression of endothelin-1 and endothelial nitric oxide synthase in vascular endothelial cells. J Clin Invest 1998; 101: 2711–19.
98. Luscher TF, Barton M. Endothelins and endothelin receptor antagonists: therapeutic considerations for a novel class of cardiovascular drugs. Circulation 2000; 102: 2434–40.
99. Verhaar MC, Strachan FE, Newby DE et al. Endothelin-A receptor antagonist-mediated vasodilatation is attenuated by inhibition of nitric oxide synthesis and by endothelin-B receptor blockade. Circulation 1998; 97: 752–6.
100. Strachan FE, Spratt JC, Wilkinson IB, Webb DJ. Systemic blockade of the ETB receptor increases peripheral vascular resistance in healthy volunteers in vivo. Hypertension 1999; 33: 581–5.
101. Schiffrin EL. Role of endothelin-1 in hypertension and vascular disease. Am J Hypertens 2001; 14: 83S–89S.
102. Rossi GP, Sacchetto A, Rizzoni D et al. Blockade of angiotensin II type 1 receptor and not of endothelin receptor prevents hypertension and cardiovascular disease in transgenic TGR(mRen2)27 rats via adrenocortical steroid-independent mechanisms. Arterioscl Thromb Vasc Biol 2000; 20: 949–56.
103. Yokokawa K, Tahara H, Kohno M et al. Hypertension associated with endothelin-secreting malignant hemangioendothelioma. Ann Intern Med 1991; 114: 213–15.
104. Rossi GP, Seccia TM, Albertin G, Pessina AC. Measurement of endothelin: clinical and research use. Ann Clin Biochem 2000; 37: 608–26.
105. Krum H, Viskoper RJ, Lacourciere Y, Budde M, Charlon V. The effect of an endothelin-receptor antagonist, bosentan, on blood pressure in patients with essential hypertension. Bosentan Hypertension Investigators. N Engl J Med 1998; 338: 784–90.
106. Taddei S, Virdis A, Ghiadoni L, Sudano I, Notari M, Salvetti A. Vasoconstriction to endogenous endothelin-1 is increased in the peripheral circulation of patients with essential hypertension. Circulation 1999; 100: 1680–3.
107. Rossi GP, Ganzaroli C, Cesari M et al. Endothelin receptor blockade lowers plasma aldosterone levels via different mechanisms in primary aldosteronism and high-to-normal renin hypertension. Cardiovasc Res 2003; 57: 277–83.
108. Panza JA, Casino PR, Badar DM, Quyyumi AA. Effect of increased availability of endothelium-derived nitric oxide precursor on endothelium-dependent vascular relaxation in normal subjects and in patients with essential hypertension. Circulation 1993; 87: 1475–81.
109. Moreau P, Takase H, Kung CF, Shaw S, Luscher TF. Blood pressure and vascular effects of endothelin blockade in chronic nitric oxide-deficient hypertension. Hypertension 1997; 29: 763–9.
110. Benigni A, Zoja C, Corna D et al. A specific endothelin subtype A receptor antagonist protects against injury in renal disease progression. Kidney Int 1993; 44: 440–4.
111. Forbes JM, Leaker B, Hewitson TD, Becker GJ, Jones CL. Macrophage and myofibroblast involvement in ischemic acute renal failure is attenuated by endothelin receptor antagonists. Kidney Int 1999; 55: 198–208.
112. Moreau P, d'Uscio LV, Shaw S, Takase H, Barton M, Luscher TF. Angiotensin II increases tissue endothelin and induces vascular hypertrophy: reversal by ET(A)-receptor antagonist. Circulation 1997; 96: 1593–7.
113. Benigni A, Zola C, Corna D et al. Blocking both type A and B endothelin receptors in the kidney attenuates renal injury and prolongs survival in rats with remnant kidney. Am J Kidney Dis 1996; 27: 416–23.
114. Verhagen AM, Rabelink TJ, Braam B et al. Endothelin A receptor blockade alleviates hypertension and renal lesions associated with chronic nitric oxide synthase inhibition. J Am Soc Nephrol 1998; 9: 755–62.
115. Kassab S, Miller MT, Novak J, Reckelhoff J, Clower B, Granger JP. Endothelin-A receptor antagonism attenuates the hypertension and renal injury in Dahl salt-sensitive rats. Hypertension 1998; 31: 397–402.
116. Barton M, Vos I, Shaw S et al. Dysfunctional renal nitric oxide synthase as a determinant of salt-sensitive hypertension: mechanisms of renal artery endothelial dysfunction and role of endothelin for vascular hypertrophy and glomerulosclerosis. J Am Soc Nephrol 2000; 11: 835–45.
117. Orth SR, Esslinger JP, Amann K, Schwarz U, Raschack M, Ritz E. Nephroprotection of an ETA-receptor blocker (LU 135252) in salt-loaded uninephrectomized stroke-prone spontaneously hypertensive rats. Hypertension 1998; 31: 995–1001.
118. Deng LY, Day R, Schiffrin EL. Localization of sites of enhanced expression of endothelin-1 in the kidney of DOCA-salt hypertensive rats. J Am Soc Nephrol 1996; 7: 1158–64.
119. Mazzocchi G, Rebuffat P, Meneghelli V, Malendowicz LK, Kasprzak A, Nussdorfer GG. Effects of prolonged infusion with endothelin-1 on the function and morphology of rat adrenal cortex. Peptides 1990; 11: 767–72.
120. Belloni A, Rossi GP, Andreis PG et al. Endothelin adrenocortical secretagogue effect is mediated by the B receptor in rats. Hypertension 1996; 27: 1153–9.
121. Lerman A, Holmes DR Jr, Bell MR et al. Endothelin in coronary endothelial dysfunction and early atherosclerosis in humans. Circulation 1995; 92: 2426–31.
122. Lopez Farre A, Riesco A, Espinosa G et al. Effect of endothelin-1 on neutrophil adhesion to endothelial cells and perfused heart. Circulation 1993; 88: 1166–71.
123. Kowala MC, Rose PM, Stein PD et al. Selective blockade of the endothelin subtype A receptor decreases early atherosclerosis in hamsters fed cholesterol. Am J Pathol 1995; 146: 819–26.

124. Best PJM, McKenna CJ, Hasdai D, Holmes DR Jr, Lerman A. Chronic endothelin receptor antagonism preserves coronary endothelial function in experimental hypercholesterolemia. Circulation 1999; 99: 1747–52.
125. Caligiuri G, Levy B, Pernow J, Thoren P, Hansson GK. Myocardial infarction mediated by endothelin receptor signaling in hypercholesterolemic mice. Proc Natl Acad Sci U S A 1999; 96: 6920–4.
126. Barton M, Haudenschild CC, d'Uscio LV, Shaw S, Munter K, Luscher TF. Endothelin ETA receptor blockade restores NO-mediated endothelial function and inhibits atherosclerosis in apolipoprotein E-deficient mice. Proc Natl Acad Sci U S A 1998; 95: 14367–72.
127. Lerman A, Edwards BS, Hallett JW, Heublein DM, Sandberg SM, Burnett JC. Circulating and tissue endothelin immunoreactivity in advanced atherosclerosis. N Engl J Med 1991; 325: 997–1001.
128. Stewart DJ, Kubac G, Costello KB, Cernacek P. Increased plasma endothelin-1 in the early hours of acute myocardial infarction. J Am Coll Cardiol 1991; 18: 38–43.
129. Zeiher AM, Goebel H, Schachinger V, Ihling C. Tissue endothelin-1 immunoreactivity in the active coronary atherosclerotic plaque. A clue to the mechanism of increased vasoreactivity of the culprit lesion in unstable angina. Circulation 1995; 91: 941–7.
130. Ihling C, Szombathy T, Bohrmann B, Brockhaus M, Schaefer HE, Loeffler BM. Coexpression of endothelin-converting enzyme-1 and endothelin-1 in different stages of human atherosclerosis. Circulation 2001; 104: 864–9.
131. Salomone OA, Elliott PM, Calvino R, Holt D, Kaski JC. Plasma immunoreactive endothelin concentration correlates with severity of coronary artery disease in patients with stable angina pectoris and normal ventricular function. J Am Coll Cardiol 1996; 28: 14–19.
132. Wenzel RR, Fleisch M, Shaw S et al. Hemodynamic and coronary effects of the endothelin antagonist bosentan in patients with coronary artery disease. Circulation 1998; 98: 2235–40.
133. Blezer ELA, Nicolay K, Goldschmeding R et al. Early-onset but not late-onset endothelin-A-receptor blockade can modulate hypertension, cerebral edema, and proteinuria in stroke-prone hypertensive rats. Hypertension 1999; 33: 137–44.
134. Kirchengast M, Munter K. Endothelin and restenosis. Cardiovasc Res 1998; 39: 550–5.
135. Giaid A, Saleh D, Yanagisawa M, Forbes RD. Endothelin-1 immunoreactivity and mRNA in the transplanted human heart. Transplantation 1995; 59: 1308–13.
136. Ravalli S, Szabolcs M, Albala A, Michler RE, Cannon PJ. Increased immunoreactive endothelin-1 in human transplant coronary artery disease. Circulation 1996; 94: 2096–102.
137. Okada K, Nishida Y, Murakami H et al. Role of endogenous endothelin in the development of graft arteriosclerosis in rat cardiac allografts: antiproliferative effects of bosentan, a nonselective endothelin receptor antagonist. Circulation 1998; 97: 2346–51.
138. Sakai S, Miyauchi T, Sakurai T et al. Endogenous endothelin-1 participates in the maintenance of cardiac function in rats with congestive heart failure: marked increase in endothelin-1 production in the failing heart. Circulation 1996; 93: 1214–22.
139. Krum H, Itescu S. Spontaneous endothelin production by circulating mononuclear cells from patients with chronic heart failure but not from normal subjects. Clin Exp Pharmacol Physiol 1994; 21: 311–13.
140. Sakai S, Miyauchi T, Kobayashi M, Yamaguchi I, Goto K, Sugishita Y. Inhibition of myocardial endothelin pathway improves long-term survival in heart failure. Nature 1996; 384: 353–5.
141. Iwanaga Y, Kihara Y, Hasegawa K et al. Cardiac endothelin-1 plays a critical role in the functional deterioration of left ventricles during the transition from compensatory hypertrophy to congestive heart failure in salt-sensitive hypertensive rats. Circulation 1998; 98: 2065–73.
142. Ruetten H, Thiemermann C. Endothelin-1 stimulates the biosynthesis of tumour necrosis factor in macrophages: ET-receptors, signal transduction and inhibition by dexamethasone. J Physiol Pharmacol 1997; 48: 675–88.
143. Ponicke K, Heinroth HI, Becker K, Brodde OE. Trophic effect of angiotensin II in neonatal rat cardiomyocytes: role of endothelin-1 and non-myocyte cells. Br J Pharmacol 1997; 121: 118–24.
144. Inada T, Fujiwara H, Hasegawa K et al. Upregulated expression of cardiac endothelin-1 participates in myocardial cell growth in Bio14.6 Syrian cardiomyopathic hamsters. J Am Coll Cardiol 1999; 33: 565–71.
145. Gray MO, Long CS, Kalinyak JE, Li HT, Karliner JS. Angiotensin II stimulates cardiac myocyte hypertrophy via paracrine release of TGF-beta 1 and endothelin-1 from fibroblasts. Cardiovasc Res 1998; 40: 352–63.
146. Borgeson DD, Grantham JA, Williamson EE et al. Chronic oral endothelin type A receptor antagonism in experimental heart failure. Hypertension 1998; 31: 766–70.
147. Moe GW, Albernaz A, Naik GO, Kirchengast M, Stewart DJ. Beneficial effects of long-term selective endothelin type A receptor blockade in canine experimental heart failure. Cardiovasc Res 1998; 39: 571–9.
148. Zolk O, Quattek J, Sitzler G et al. Expression of endothelin-1, endothelin-converting enzyme, and endothelin receptors in chronic heart failure. Circulation 1999; 99: 2118–23.
149. Love MP, Haynes WG, Gray GA, Webb DJ, McMurray JJ. Vasodilator effects of endothelin-converting enzyme inhibition and endothelin ETA receptor blockade in chronic heart failure patients treated with ACE inhibitors. Circulation 1996; 94: 2131–7.
150. Wada A, Tsutamoto T, Fukai D et al. Comparison of the effects of selective endothelin ETA and ETB receptor antagonists in congestive heart failure. J Am Coll Cardiol 1997; 30: 1385–92.
151. Cowburn PJ, Cleland JG, McArthur JD et al. Endothelin B receptors are functionally important in mediating vasoconstriction in the systemic circulation in patients with left ventricular systolic dysfunction. J Am Coll Cardiol 1999; 33: 932–8.
152. Kiowski W, Sutsch G, Hunziker P et al. Evidence for endothelin-1-mediated vasoconstriction in severe chronic heart failure. Lancet 1995; 346: 732–6.
153. Sutsch G, Kiowski W, Yan XW et al. Short-term oral endothelin-receptor antagonist therapy in conventionally treated patients with symptomatic severe chronic heart failure. Circulation 1998; 98: 2262–8.
154. Kaluski E, Kobrin I, Zimlichman R et al. RITZ-5: randomized intravenous TeZosentan (an endothelin-A/B antagonist) for the treatment of pulmonary edema: a prospective, multicenter, double-blind, placebo-controlled study. J Am Coll Cardiol 2003; 41: 204–10.
155. O'Connor CM, Gattis WA, Adams KF Jr, Shah MR, Frey A, Gheorghiade M. Tezosentan in patients with acute heart failure and acute coronary syndromes: design of the fourth Randomized Intravenous Tezosentan Study (RITZ-4). Am Heart J 2003; 145: S58–S59.
156. Rich S, McLaughlin VV. Endothelin receptor blockers in cardiovascular disease. Circulation 2003; 108: 2184–90.
157. Louis AA, Manousos IR, Coletta AP, Clark AL, Cleland JG. Clinical trials update: The Heart Protection Study, IONA, CARISA, ENRICHD, ACUTE, ALIVE, MADIT II and

REMATCH. Impact of Nicorandil on Angina. Combination Assessment of Ranolazine In Stable Angina. Enhancing Recovery In Coronary Heart Disease patients. Assessment of Cardioversion Using Transoesophageal Echocardiography. AzimiLide post-Infarct surVival Evaluation. Randomised Evaluation of Mechanical Assistance for Treatment of Chronic Heart failure. Eur J Heart Fail 2002; 4: 111–16.

158. Luscher TF, Enseleit F, Pacher R et al. Hemodynamic and neurohumoral effects of selective endothelin A (ET(A)) receptor blockade in chronic heart failure: the Heart Failure ET(A) Receptor Blockade Trial (HEAT). Circulation 2002; 106: 2666–72.
159. Dupuis J, Cernacek P, Tardif JC et al. Reduced pulmonary clearance of endothelin-1 in pulmonary hypertension. Am Heart J 1998; 135: 614–20.
160. Giaid A, Michel RP, Stewart DJ, Sheppard M, Corrin B, Hamid Q. Expression of endothelin-1 in lungs of patients with cryptogenic fibrosing alveolitis. Lancet 1993; 341: 1550–4.
161. Rubin LJ, Badesch DB, Barst RJ et al. Bosentan therapy for pulmonary arterial hypertension. N Engl J Med 2002; 346: 896–903.
162. Zamora MA, Dempsey EC, Walchak SJ, Stelzner TJ. BQ123, an ETA receptor antagonist, inhibits endothelin-1-mediated proliferation of human pulmonary artery smooth muscle cells. Am J Respir Cell Mol Biol 1993; 9: 429–33.
163. Chen YF, Oparil S. Endothelin and pulmonary hypertension. J Cardiovasc Pharmacol 2000; 35: 49–54.
164. Williamson DJ, Wallman LL, Jones R et al. Hemodynamic effects of Bosentan, an endothelin receptor antagonist, in patients with pulmonary hypertension. Circulation 2000; 102: 411–18.

17

Role of vascular endothelin in hypertension

Ernesto L Schiffrin

THE ENDOTHELIN SYSTEM

The existence of a potent vasoconstrictor peptide secreted by endothelial cells was initially demonstrated in 1985,[1] but it was Yanagisawa et al.[2] who isolated and cloned the 21-amino acid peptide endothelin (ET) shortly afterwards. Several ETs have since been discovered, called ET-1, ET-2, and ET-3, as well as bigger 31-amino acid peptides. ET-1 is the most abundant ET produced in blood vessels and the one this chapter is concerned with, whereas ET-3 is mainly a neuropeptide. ET-1 is released normally by endothelial cells toward underlying smooth muscle,[3] upon which it exerts its vasoconstrictor effects.

Furin and other enzymes act on proETs to generate 38–39-amino acid peptides (big ETs). These are then converted into the mature 21-amino acid ETs by endothelin converting enzymes (ECE-1 and ECE-2). ECE-1 is found in endothelial cells. There are four differentially spliced isoforms of ECE-1 encoded by a single gene (ECE-1a, ECE-1b, ECE-1c, and ECE-1d) resulting from the presence of four alternative promoters.[4] The four isoforms of ECE-1 only differ by their N-terminal amino acid, responsible for their cellular localization. ECE-1a, -c, and -d are located extracellularly, whereas ECE-1b is an intracellular enzyme.[4] ECE-1b heterodimerizes with other ECE-1 isoforms and exerts a regulatory role on their activity.[5] ECE-2 is present on the surface of smooth muscle cells and converts big ET-1 to ET-1 in the vicinity of ET receptors. This may protect ET-1 from degradation. Other ET-generating enzymes include chymase and neutral endopeptidase.[6]

Regulators of ET generation in blood vessels include shear stress[7] and nitric oxide (NO), which reduce ET-1 production by the endothelium, and epinephrine, thrombin, angiotensin II (Ang II), vasopressin, cytokines, insulin, growth factors (TGF-β1) and hypoxia, which stimulate ET-1 generation. NO production is enhanced by increased shear stress and may mediate its effect to inhibit ET-1 generation.[8] Leptin stimulates ET-1 generation by endothelial cells.[9] This may be one of the mechanisms linking ET-1 and obesity, and that contributes to vascular damage in the metabolic syndrome and type 2 diabetes mellitus. Peroxisome proliferator-activated receptors (PPARs) exert anti-inflammatory and anti-growth properties[10–12] on blood vessels. PPARα activators (lipid-lowering fibrates) and γ agonists (insulin-sensitizing thiazolidinediones or glitazones) inhibit in vivo ET-1 production and prevent progression of blood pressure elevation and vascular damage in Ang II-induced[10–12] and deoxycorticosterone acetate (DOCA)-salt rats,[13] hypertensive models in which the ET system is activated.[14]

PHARMACOLOGICAL EFFECTS OF ET-1 ON BLOOD VESSELS

ET-1 acts on two subtypes of ET receptors: ET_A and ET_B. In the vascular wall, ET_A and ET_B receptors are present on smooth muscle cells, whereas endothelial cells only possess ET_B receptors. ET_A and ET_B receptors on vascular smooth muscle cells have vasoconstrictor and growth promoting effects. They are present in systemic arteries and veins,[15] and pulmonary vessels.[16–18] In all vessels, ET_A receptors predominate over ET_B. ET_B receptors on endothelial cells stimulate the generation of NO and prostacyclin and thus are vasodilatory. In some vascular beds such as coronary arteries there are few endothelial vasodilator ET_B receptors[19] and thus at these sites ET-1 acts mainly as a vasoconstrictor, whereas in other vascular beds it may be predominantly a vasodilator.[20,21] Whether the physiological role of ETs is vasoconstrictor or vasodilator remains unclear, but under pathophysiological conditions when large amounts of ET-1 are produced by endothelial or smooth muscle cells, its effects appear to be mainly vasoconstrictor, mitogenic, growth promoting, stimulatory of cell migration and inflammation (see below).

EFFECTS OF PREPROET-1 OR ET RECEPTOR GENE DELETION

ETs play important roles in development, as demonstrated by naturally occurring mutations or experimental deletion of ET peptide or receptor genes. Deletion of the ET-1 or the ET_A receptor gene in mice results in slight blood pressure elevation. Elevation of blood pressure in this gene knockout model is a consequence of abnormal craniofacial development that impairs respiration, leading to hypoxia.[22,23] There is also abnormal conduit artery development. The phenotype mimics the Pierre Robin syndrome in humans.

ET-3 is the preferred ligand of ET_B receptors and plays a role in the migration of neural crest cells during development. Mutations or gene inactivation of ET_B receptors induce aganglionic megacolon and pigmentary abnormalities.[24] Many instances of hereditary and sporadic human aganglionic megacolon (Hirschsprung's disease) are associated with mutations of the ET_B receptor gene. Heterozygous ET_B receptor knockout mice have slightly elevated blood pressure, which supports the idea mentioned above that ET_B receptors physiologically exert a vasodilator effect.[20,21]

MECHANISM OF ACTION OF ETs

When ET-1 stimulates ET receptors, phospholipase C is activated, inositol trisphosphate is generated and calcium release occurs, followed by activation of the calcium-calmodulin pathway, production of diacylglycerol and stimulation of protein kinase C, all contributing to trigger vascular smooth muscle cell constriction.[25] As well, as with other peptides that activate G protein-coupled receptors, the ras-raf-mitogen-activated kinase (MAPK) cascade is also stimulated to induce growth. In small arteries, ET-1 induced an initial effect that was completely dependent on calcium influx and inhibited by herbimycin A.[26] A second phase was only 50% calcium-dependent, insensitive to herbimycin A, but 50% inhibited by the non-selective tyrosine kinase inhibitor genistein. p38MAPK activity returned to basal by 30 minutes. A p38MAPK inhibitor, SB203580, which inhibited norepinephrine-induced contraction, had little effect on endothelin-induced vasoconstriction, indicating that p38MAPK is not activated by ET-1 in small arteries.

The role of reactive oxygen species (ROS) has been increasingly appreciated as an intracellular signal transduction mechanism involved in either transactivation of growth factor receptors or activation of the MAPK cascade.[27] ET-1 generation in blood vessels of DOCA-salt rats[14] is accompanied by enhanced production of superoxide.[28,29] Superoxide is derived from different sources, that include reduced nicotinamide adenine dinucleotide phosphate (NAD(P)H) oxidase, xanthine oxidase, mitochondria, and uncoupled NO synthase (the latter resulting from low concentrations of tetrahydrobiopterin, derived from folic acid). In human smooth muscle cells ET-1 stimulates superoxide generation mainly from mitochondrial sources, in contrast to angiotensin, that stimulates generation of ROS mostly from NAD(P)H oxidase.[30] In rat vessels, xanthine oxidase and mitochondria also appear to be important sources (E Viel and EL Schiffrin, 2005, unpublished observations), whereas in mice, NA(D)PH oxidase seems to be the main source of superoxide after ET-1 stimulation.[31] Increased ROS generation contributes to the decreased bioavailability of NO and the endothelial dysfunction found in DOCA-salt rats.[13] On the other hand, ROS are potent stimulators of ET-1 synthesis by endothelial cells.[32]

The mechanisms whereby ET-1 induces vascular remodeling have been investigated in organoid culture of small arteries.[33] ET-1 induced vasoconstriction and eutrophic remodeling (in contrast to in vivo models cited below in which hypertrophic remodeling was induced by ET-1). This response was enhanced by an antibody directed to β_3-integrin. Inward eutrophic remodeling was the result of sustained contraction, which may involve collagen reorganization through β_3-integrins. The same group showed that stimulation with ET-1 induced significant increase in *c-fos* mRNA which could not be blocked by inhibitors of MAP kinases, conventional protein kinase C, nor tyrosine kinases, but was inhibited by staurosporine and the calcium chelator BAPTA, suggesting a role for intracellular calcium in ET-1-induced vascular remodeling.[34]

ET_A and ET_B receptors may have countervailing or cooperative effects in different cells. ET_A receptors induce cell growth and apoptosis through NFκB activation.[35] ET_B receptors may have apoptotic effects on cells.[36] The overall effect of ET-1, however, appears to be anti-apoptotic and a survival effect that is associated with a reduction of the activation of the caspase-3 pathway.[36,37]

PATHOPHYSIOLOGY OF THE ENDOTHELIN SYSTEM

The endothelin system plays a pathophysiological role in hypertension, atherosclerosis, coronary artery disease, heart failure, subarachnoid hemorrhage and cerebral vasospasm, diabetes, primary pulmonary hypertension (the only approved indication for ET antagonists), pulmonary fibrosis, scleroderma, renal failure, hepatorenal syndrome, glaucoma, prostate cancer and its metastasis, etc. Of these, the present review will only briefly address the role of endothelin in experimental and clinical hypertension.

ET-1-induced vascular, cardiac and renal effects in experimental hypertension

ET-1 induces vasoconstriction and growth, and accordingly, when production of ET-1 is enhanced in experimental hypertension, it contributes to the remodeling of large and small arteries.[38,39] This is found primarily in salt-dependent models of experimental hypertension such as DOCA-salt hypertension or Dahl salt-sensitive rats, and in models with severe hypertension. In contrast, there appears to be little role of ETs in spontaneously hypertensive rats (SHR).[14,40] However, in stroke-prone SHR the endothelin system is activated and does play a role, particularly if rats are loaded with salt,[41] or if they are treated with the NO synthase inhibitor L-NAME.[42] In the models in which the endothelin system is activated, such as salt-loaded and low-renin models, hypertrophic remodeling of resistance arteries with increased cross-sectional area is found, rather than the 'eutrophic' remodeling without true vascular hypertrophy more often found in essential hypertension and in SHR. Hypertrophic remodeling in these hypertensive models regresses after treatment with ET antagonists.[38]

To unambiguously demonstrate the direct effects of ETs on the vasculature, we generated a genetically engineered mouse that transgenically expresses human preproET-1 restricted to the endothelium using the endothelium-specific promoter Tie-2.[31] ET-1 overexpression in the endothelium resulted in small artery hypertrophic remodeling and endothelial dysfunction despite the fact that blood pressure was not elevated, underlining the ability of ET-1 to induce blood pressure-independent vascular effects.

Similarly to what is found in the DOCA-salt hypertensive rat,[38,39] systolic blood pressure, plasma ET, systemic oxidative stress, and vascular NADPH activity are increased in association with small artery hypertrophic remodeling in aldosterone-infused rats.[43] Laser confocal microscopy showed increased vascular collagen, fibronectin, and intercellular adhesion molecule (ICAM-1). All these changes were decreased by ET_A receptor antagonism, whereas hydralazine lowered blood pressure and reduced vascular NADPH activity but did not affect the other changes.

ET-1 contributes to renal and cardiac target organ damage in hypertension. ET-1 production is increased by salt loading, which by activation of renal ET_B receptors inhibits sodium reabsorption.[44] Ang II infusion combined with high salt increased renal ET-1.[45] Whereas in Ang II-infused mice the dual ET_A/ET_B receptor blocker bosentan partially prevented activation of the procollagen gene,[46] in transgenic rats overexpressing the ren2 gene (TGR(mRen2)27) that have renin-dependent hypertension, treatment between 10 and 30 weeks of age with the selective ET_A receptor blocker darusentan or the ET_A/ET_B receptor antagonist LU420627[47] neither lowered blood pressure nor reduced mortality. Proteinuria and glomerulosclerosis, tubulointerstitial damage and renal osteopontin mRNA expression were unchanged in ET receptor blocker-treated rats. ET-1 thus does not appear to play a role in renal damage in renin-dependent hypertension. However, rats overexpressing human angiotensinogen and human renin, which develop malignant hypertension, exhibited reduced renal and myocardial damage after treatment with bosentan,[48,49] in agreement with evidence that the endothelin system may mediate part of Ang II actions on the vasculature in Ang II-infused rats.[50] Whether ET-1 does or does not mediate actions of Ang II is still controversial. We have pointed out in a recent editorial that Ang II-infused models may be a special situation where high Ang II levels are achieved in a steady-state condition in the circulation, and that the rat overexpressing human angiotensinogen and human renin may be an exception because of the severity of BP elevation.[51] ET-1 may be thus activated in both models by different mechanisms and erroneously suggest an effect of Ang II, which does not occur in other conditions with renin-dependent hypertension such as 2-kidney 1 clip Goldblatt hypertension.[52]

In salt-loaded SHR-SP, in which the endothelin system is activated,[41] increased expression of ET-1 was associated with enhanced generation of transforming growth factor (TGF)-β1, basic fibroblast growth factor (bFGF), procollagen I expression and matrix metalloproteinase (MMP)-2 activity.[53] These were reduced by a selective ET_A antagonist, indicating that involvement of ET-1 in renal fibrosis is mediated by triggering an inflammatory response and stimulation of growth factors.

ET_A blockade prevented enhanced TGF-β1 expression and collagen deposition in the hearts of DOCA-salt hypertensive rats.[54] Expression of inflammatory mediators (NFκB and adhesion molecules) and activation of the anti-apoptotic molecule X inhibitor of apoptosis peptide (xIAP) was modulated by ET_A receptors.[55] Inhibition of NFkB prevented anti-apoptotic and hypertrophic actions of ET-1.[56] ET-1 induced cardiac hypertrophy through stimulation of reactive oxygen species generated by NAD(P)H oxidase, and via activation of MAPK.[57] Of the components of the renin-angiotensin-aldosterone system, aldosterone appears to contribute to cardiac and vascular damage via stimulation of the production of ET-1. ET_A antagonism prevented vascular remodeling and cardiac and vascular fibrosis in aldosterone-infused rats,[43,58,59] suggesting that ET-1, whose expression is enhanced in aldosterone-infused rats, mediates in part the effects of aldosterone on the heart and blood vessels. The potential implication of ET-1 stimulated by Ang II has already been discussed above.

ET-1 and essential hypertension

Circulating levels of immunoreactive ET in plasma are normal in primary human hypertension,[60] except in hypertensive African Americans, in whom plasma ET is elevated.[61] The latter result is interesting in that African Americans appear to have a form of volume expanded hypertension, which is that associated with activation of the endothelin system in experimental models. Multiple stepwise regression analysis demonstrated in a recent study that age, creatinine, and smoking were significantly correlated to plasma ET in 1492 subjects, but there was no correlation with blood pressure.[62] It was suggested that high ET is related to subclinical renal dysfunction and smoking rather than hypertension. Vascular levels of immunoreactive ET are increased in patients with stage 2 of the JNC 7 classification, compared with normotensive subjects or patients with stage 1 hypertension,[63] which agrees with plasma levels of ET being an unreliable index of tissue production of the peptide. A predominant role of ET_A receptors in the regulation of vascular tone by endogenous ET-1 has been suggested in essential hypertensive patients, since ET_A receptor antagonists caused greater vasodilatation in the forearm compared with normotensive individuals.[64] Impaired vasodilation in hypertensive patients was improved by the ET_A antagonist BQ-123. The ET_B antagonist BQ-788 constricted forearm resistance arteries in normotensive subjects,[61] indicating that ET_B receptors have a vasodilator role in normotensive subjects. In contrast, BQ-788 dilated the forearm in hypertensive subjects.[65] African American hypertensive subjects may have increased smooth muscle vasoconstrictor ET_B receptors.[66,67] Forearm blood flow response to BQ-123 in normotensives was similar in white and black subjects, whereas in hypertensive patients ET_A receptor blockade had a significantly greater vasodilator effect in black subjects than in white subjects.[68] ET-1 induced significant vasoconstriction equally in white and black patients. These data suggest that in hypertensive black patients there is increased ET_A-mediated vascular tone that may contribute to hypertension.

Ang II has been implicated in induction of expression of ET-1 in experimental models. The controversy[51] surrounding this mechanism has been described above. In humans intravenous infusion of Ang II increased blood pressure and renal vascular resistance and accordingly decreased renal plasma flow and glomerular filtration rate, but none of these changes were altered by the ET_A receptor antagonist BQ-123.[69] This indicates that the pressor responses to Ang II cannot be mediated by ET-1, as discussed earlier.[51] Other investigators observed less blood pressure rise or decrement in renal blood flow and glomerular filtration with Ang II plus an ET_A receptor antagonist than with Ang II alone,[70] which leaves the question unresolved.

It has been proposed that ET-1 at concentrations of 10^{-11} mol/L may potentiate other vasoconstrictors (e.g. phenylephrine or serotonin),[71] a mechanism which may be accentuated in hypertensive patients.[72] There is evidence that this mechanism is under the influence of the *EDN1 K198N* polymorphism in the coding region of the preproET-1 gene,[73] and could lead to enhanced vascular tone in hypertensive patients.

In patients with essential hypertension, primary aldosteronism or renovascular hypertension, ultrasound backscatter signal analysis arising from tissue heterogeneity in the myocardium correlated with plasma aldosterone and immunoreactive ET, which suggested that aldosterone and ET-1 induce myocardial fibrosis in human hypertension,[74] as occurs in experimental animal models.[54,55,58]

Clinical trials of ET antagonists in human hypertension have been carried out with both the combined ET_A/ET_B antagonist bosentan and the ET_A antagonist darusentan. Bosentan lowered diastolic blood pressure in patients with mild-to-moderate essential hypertension, similarly to the angiotensin converting enzyme (ACE) inhibitor enalapril.[75] Darusentan also reduced systolic blood pressure.[76] Whereas bosentan induced liver enzyme elevation, darusentan did not. However, ET receptor antagonists have not yet been incorporated in the therapeutic arsenal for the treatment of essential hypertension and target organ damage associated with high blood pressure because of side effects.

GENETICS OF THE ENDOTHELIN SYSTEM

There is a polymorphism (*EDN1 K198N*) in the coding region of the preproET-1 gene associated with increased vasoreactivity that may contribute to blood pressure elevation in hypertensive patients[69] and has also been associated with hypertension in overweight individuals.[77] *ECE1 C-388A* is a polymorphism present in the 5'-regulatory region of the ECE-1b gene that results in a binding site for the transcription factor E2F-2,[78] and induces increased promoter activity. This polymorphism was present in untreated hypertensive German women in whom the A allele had co-dominant effect on daytime and night-time systolic and diastolic BP.[78] In 1198 subjects (698 women) from a French epidemiological study (Étude du Vieillissement Artériel or EVA) the association of blood pressure and the polymorphism was present in women but not in men.[79] Females homozygous for the A allele had significantly higher systolic, diastolic and mean blood pressure levels. Thus, there may be a recessive effect of this variant in this French population. The A allele may raise expression of ECE-1b, with increased generation of ET-1. The *EDN1 K198N* polymorphism of the preproET-1 gene was not associated with blood pressure values in either men or women in this study, but interacted with the *ECE1 C-338A* variant to influence systolic and mean blood pressure levels in women.[75] Although the *EDN1* variant did not correlate with blood pressure, the effect of the *ECE1 C-338A* variant on blood pressure was found only in homozygous *EDN1* KK women. Why the ECE-1b effect was observed only in females remains unclear. The association may be related to interactions between ET and sex hormones, and stimulation of ET by androgens could explain the absence of effect in males.

CONCLUSION

ET-1 promotes cardiovascular inflammation, hypertrophy, and fibrosis in the vasculature, the heart, and the kidney. ET receptor antagonists may prevent complications of hypertension, atherosclerosis, and diabetes, and make it possible to obtain blood pressure-independent effects on cardiovascular pathology. These effects may contribute to the therapeutic potential of ET antagonism in hypertension, heart failure, atherosclerosis, chronic renal failure, and diabetes.

ACKNOWLEDGMENTS

The work of the author was supported by grant 37917 and a Group Grant to the Multidisciplinary Research Group on Hypertension, both from the Canadian Institutes of Health Research.

REFERENCES

1. Hickey KA, Rubanyi G, Paul RJ, Highsmith RF. Characterization of a coronary vasoconstrictor produced by cultured endothelial cells. Am J Physiol 1985; 248: C550–C556.
2. Yanagisawa M, Kurihara H, Kimura S et al. A novel potent vasoconstrictor peptide produced by vascular endothelial cells. Nature 1988; 332: 411–15.
3. Wagner OF, Christ G, Wojta J et al. Polar secretion of endothelin-1 by cultured endothelial cells. J Biol Chem 1992; 267: 16066–8.
4. Valdenaire O, Lepailleur-Enouf D, Egidy G et al. A fourth isoform of endothelin-converting enzyme (ECE-1) is generated from an additional promoter molecular cloning and characterization. Eur J Biochem 1999; 264: 341–9.
5. Muller L, Barret A, Etienne E et al. Heterodimerization of endothelin-converting enzyme-1 isoforms regulates the subcellular distribution of this metalloprotease. J Biol Chem 2003; 278: 545–55.
6. D'Orléans-Juste P, Plante M, Honoré JC, Carrier E, Labonté J. Synthesis and degradation of endothelin-1. Can J Physiol Pharmacol 2003; 81: 503–10.
7. Malek A, Izumo S. Physiological fluid shear stress causes downregulation of endothelin-1 mRNA in bovine aortic endothelium. Am J Physiol 1992; 263: C389–C396.
8. Boulanger C, Luscher TF. Release of endothelin from the porcine aorta. Inhibition by endothelium-derived nitric oxide. J Clin Invest 1990; 85: 587–90.
9. Quehenberger P, Exner M, Sunder-Plassmann R et al. Leptin induces endothelin-1 in endothelial cells in vitro. Circ Res 2002; 90: 711–18.
10. Diep QN, El Mabrouk M, Cohn JS et al. Structure, endothelial function, cell growth, and inflammation in blood vessels of angiotensin II-infused rats. Role of peroxisome proliferator-activated receptor-γ. Circulation 2002; 105: 2296–302.
11. Diep QN, Amiri F, Touyz RM, Cohn JS, Endemann D, Schiffrin EL. PPARα activator effects on Ang II-induced vascular oxidative stress and inflammation. Hypertension 2002; 40: 866–71.
12. Schiffrin EL. Peroxisome proliferator-activated receptors and cardiovascular remodeling. Am J Physiol Heart Circ Physiol 2005; 288: H1037–H1043.
13. Iglarz M, Touyz RM, Amiri F, Lavoie M-F, Diep QN, Schiffrin EL. Effect of peroxisome proliferator-activated receptor-α and -γ activators on vascular remodeling in endothelin-dependent hypertension. Arterioscl Thromb Vasc Biol 2003; 23: 45–51.
14. Larivière R, Thibault G, Schiffrin EL. Increased endothelin-1 content in blood vessels of deoxycorticosterone acetate-salt hypertensive but not in spontaneously hypertensive rats. Hypertension 1993; 21: 294–300.
15. Moreland S, McMullen DM, Delaney CL, Lee VG, Hunt JT. Venous smooth muscle contains vasoconstrictor ET_B-like receptors. Biochem Biophys Res Commun 1992; 184: 100–6.
16. Russell FD, Davenport AP. Characterization of endothelin receptors in the human pulmonary vasculature using bosentan, SB209670, and 97-139. J Cardiovasc Pharmacol 1995; 26: S346–S347.
17. Sato K, Oka M, Hasunuma K, Ohnishi M, Kira S. Effects of separate and combined ET_A and ET_B blockade on ET-1-induced constriction in perfused rat lungs. Am J Physiol 1995; 269: L668–L672.
18. Davie N, Haleen SJ, Upton PD et al. ET(A) and ET(B)-receptors modulate the proliferation of human pulmonary artery smooth muscle cells. Am J Respir Crit Care Med 2002; 165: 398–405.

19. Bacon CR, Davenport AP. Endothelin receptors in human coronary artery and aorta. Br J Pharmacol 1996; 117: 986–92.
20. Verhaar MC, Strachan FE, Newby DE et al. Endothelin-A receptor antagonist-mediated vasodilatation is attenuated by inhibition of nitric oxide synthesis and by endothelin-B receptor blockade. Circulation 1998; 97: 752–6.
21. Goddard J, Johnston NR, Hand MF et al. Endothelin-A receptor antagonism reduces blood pressure and increases renal blood flow in hypertensive patients with chronic renal failure: a comparison of selective and combined endothelin receptor blockade. Circulation 2004; 109: 1186–93.
22. Kurihara Y, Kurihara H, Suzuki H et al. Elevated blood pressure and craniofacial abnormalities in mice deficient in endothelin-1. Nature 1994; 368: 703–10.
23. Clouthier DE, Hosoda K, Richardson JA et al. Cranial and cardiac neural crest defects in endothelin-A receptor-deficient mice. Development 1998; 125: 813–24.
24. Hosoda K, Hammer RE, Richardson JA et al. Targeted and natural (piebald-lethal) mutations of endothelin-B receptor gene produce megacolon associated with spotted coat color in mice. Cell 1994; 79: 1267–76.
25. Touyz RM, Schiffrin EL. Reactive oxygen species in vascular biology: implications in hypertension. Histochem Cell Biol 2004; 122: 339–52.
26. Schiffrin EL, Touyz RM. Vascular biology of endothelin. J Cardiovasc Pharmacol 1998; 32: S2–S13.
27. Ohanian J, Cunliffe P, Ceppi E et al. Activation of p38 mitogen-activated protein kinases by endothelin and noradrenaline in small arteries, regulation by calcium influx and tyrosine kinases, and their role in contraction. Arterioscler Thromb Vasc Biol 2001; 21: 1921–7.
28. Li LX, Fink GD, Watts SW et al. Endothelin-1 increases vascular superoxide via endothelinA-NADPH oxidase pathway in low-renin hypertension. Circulation 2003; 107: 1053–8.
29. Callera GE, Touyz RM, Teixeira SA et al. ET_A receptor blockade decreases vascular superoxide generation in DOCA-salt hypertension. Hypertension 2003; 42: 811–17.
30. Touyz RM, Yao G, Viel E, Amiri F, Schiffrin EL. Angiotensin II and endothelin-1 regulate MAP kinases through different redox-dependent mechanisms in human vascular smooth muscle cells. J Hypertens 2004; 22: 1141–9.
31. Amiri F, Virdis A, Fritsch Neves M et al. Endothelium-restricted overexpression of human endothelin-1 causes vascular remodeling and endothelial dysfunction. Circulation 2004; 110: 2233–40.
32. Kahler J, Mendel S, Weckmuller J et al. Oxidative stress increases synthesis of big endothelin-1 by activation of the endothelin-1 promoter. J Mol Cell Cardiol 2000; 32: 1429–37.
33. Bakker ENTP, Buus CL, VanBavel E et al. Activation of resistance arteries with endothelin-1: from vasoconstriction to functional adaptation and remodeling. J Vasc Res 2004; 41: 174–82.
34. Buus CL, Kristensen HB, Bakker ENTP et al. Force-independent expression of c-fos mRNA by endothelin-1 in rat intact small mesenteric arteries. Acta Physiol Scand 2004; 181: 1–11.
35. Mangelus M, Galron R, Naor Z, Sokolovsky M. Involvement of nuclear factor-kappaB in endothelin-A-receptor-induced proliferation and inhibition of apoptosis. Cell Mol Neurobiol 2001; 21: 657–74.
36. Shichiri M, Kato H, Marumo F, Hirata Y. Endothelin-1 as an autocrine/paracrine apoptosis survival factor for endothelial cells. Hypertension 1997; 30: 1198–203.
37. Diep QN, Intengan HD, Schiffrin EL. Endothelin-1 attenuates omega3 fatty acid-induced apoptosis by inhibition of caspase 3. Hypertension 2000; 35: 287–91.
38. Li JS, Larivière R, Schiffrin EL. Effect of a nonselective endothelin antagonist on vascular remodeling in deoxycorticosterone acetate-salt hypertensive rats. Evidence for a role of endothelin in vascular hypertrophy. Hypertension 1994; 24: 183–8.
39. Schiffrin EL. Endothelin: potential role in hypertension and vascular hypertrophy. Hypertension 1995; 25: 1135–43.
40. Li JS, Schiffrin EL. Effect of chronic treatment of adult spontaneously hypertensive rats with an endothelin receptor antagonist. Hypertension 1995; 25 (Pt 1): 495–500.
41. Touyz RM, Turgeon A, Schiffrin EL. Endothelin-A-receptor blockade improves renal function and doubles the lifespan of stroke-prone spontaneously hypertensive rats. J Cardiovasc Pharmacol 2000; 36 (Suppl 1): S300–S304.
42. Li JS, Deng LY, Grove K, Deschepper CF, Schiffrin EL. Comparison of effect of endothelin antagonism and angiotensin-converting enzyme inhibition on blood pressure and vascular structure in spontaneously hypertensive rats treated with N^{ω}-nitro-L-arginine methyl ester. Correlation with topography of vascular endothelin-1 gene expression. Hypertension 1996; 28: 188–95.
43. Pu Q, Neves MF, Virdis A, Touyz RM, Schiffrin EL. Endothelin antagonism on aldosterone-induced oxidative stress and vascular remodeling. Hypertension 2003; 42: 49–55.
44. Plato CF, Pollock DM, Garvin JL. Endothelin inhibits thick ascending limb chloride flux via ET(B) receptor-mediated NO release. Am J Physiol 2000; 279: F326–F333.
45. Sasser JM, Pollock JS, Pollock DM. Renal endothelin in chronic angiotensin II hypertension. Am J Physiol 2002; 283: R243–R248.
46. Fakhouri F, Placier S, Ardaillou R, Dussaule JC, Chatziantoniou C. Angiotensin II activates collagen type I gene in the renal cortex and aorta of transgenic mice through interaction with endothelin and TGF-beta. J Am Soc Nephrol 2001; 12: 2701–10.
47. Rothermund L, Kossmehl P, Neumayer H-H, Paul M, Kreutz R. Renal damage is not improved by blockade of endothelin receptors in primary renin-dependent hypertension. J Hypertens 2003; 21: 2389–97.
48. Muller DN, Mervaala EM, Schmidt F et al. Effect of bosentan on NF-kappaB, inflammation, and tissue factor in angiotensin II-induced end-organ damage. Hypertension 2000; 36: 282–90.
49. Muller DN, Mullally A, Dechend R et al. Endothelin-converting enzyme inhibition ameliorates angiotensin II-induced cardiac damage. Hypertension 2002; 40: 840–6.
50. Rajagopalan S, Laursen JB, Borthayre A et al. Role for endothelin-1 in angiotensin II-mediated hypertension. Hypertension 1997; 30: 29–34.
51. Schiffrin EL. The angiotensin-endothelin relationship: does it play a role in cardiovascular and renal pathophysiology? Editorial commentary. J Hypertens 2003; 21: 2245–7.
52. Li JS, Knafo L, Turgeon A, Garcia R, Schiffrin EL. Effect of endothelin antagonism on blood pressure and vascular structure in renovascular hypertensive rats. Am J Physiol 1996; 40: H88–H93.
53. Tostes RC, Touyz RM, He G, Ammarguellat F, Schiffrin EL. Endothelin A receptor blockade decreases expression of growth factors and collagen and improves matrix metalloproteinase-2 activity in kidneys from stroke-prone spontaneously hypertensive rats. J Cardiovasc Pharmacol 2002; 39: 892–900.
54. Ammarguellat F, Larouche I, Schiffrin EL. Myocardial fibrosis in DOCA-salt hypertensive rats: effect of endothelin ET(A) receptor antagonism. Circulation 2001; 103: 319–24.
55. Ammarguellat FZ, Gannon PO, Amiri F, Schiffrin EL. Fibrosis, matrix metalloproteinases, and inflammation in the heart of DOCA-salt hypertensive rats: role of ET(A) receptors. Hypertension 2002; 39: 679–84.
56. Hirotani S, Otsu K, Nishida K et al. Involvement of nuclear factor-kappaB and apoptosis signal-regulating kinase 1 in

G-protein-coupled receptor agonist-induced cardiomyocyte hypertrophy. Circulation 2002; 105: 509–15.
57. Tanaka K, Honda M, Takabatake T. Redox regulation of MAPK pathways and cardiac hypertrophy in adult rat cardiac myocyte. J Am Coll Cardiol 2001; 37: 676–85.
58. Park JB, Schiffrin EL. Cardiac and vascular fibrosis and hypertrophy in aldosterone-infused rats: role of endothelin-1. Am J Hypertens 2002; 15: 164–9.
59. Park JB, Schiffrin EL. ET(A) receptor antagonist prevents blood pressure elevation and vascular remodeling in aldosterone-infused rats. Hypertension 2001; 37: 1444–9.
60. Schiffrin EL, Thibault G. Plasma endothelin in human essential hypertension. Am J Hypertens 1991; 4: 303–8.
61. Ergul S, Parish DC, Puett D et al. Racial differences in plasma endothelin-1 concentrations in individuals with essential hypertension. Hypertension 1996; 28: 652–5.
62. Hirai Y, Adachi H, Fujiura Y, Hiratsuka A, Enomoto M, Imaizumi T. Plasma endothelin-1 level is related to renal function and smoking status but not to blood pressure: an epidemiological study. J Hypertens 2004; 22: 713–18.
63. Schiffrin EL, Deng LY, Sventek P, Day R. Enhanced expression of endothelin-1 gene in resistance arteries in severe human essential hypertension. J Hypertens 1997; 15: 57–63.
64. Cardillo C, Kilcoyne CM, Waclawiw M, Cannon RO 3rd, Panza JA. Role of endothelin in the increased vascular tone of patients with essential hypertension. Hypertension 1999; 33: 753–8.
65. Cardillo C, Campia U, Kilcoyne CM, Bryant MB, Panza JA. Improved endothelium-dependent vasodilation after blockade of endothelin receptors in patients with essential hypertension. Circulation 2002; 105: 452–6.
66. Ergul A, Tackett RL, Puett D. Distribution of endothelin receptors in saphenous veins of African Americans: implications of racial differences. J Cardiovasc Pharmacol 1999; 34: 327–32.
67. Grubbs AL, Anstadt MP, Ergul A. Saphenous vein endothelin system expression and activity in African American patients. Arterioscler Thromb Vasc Biol 2002; 22: 1122–7.
68. Campia U, Cardillo C, Panza JA. Ethnic differences in the vasoconstrictor activity of endogenous endothelin-1 in hypertensive patients. Circulation 2004; 109: 3191–5.
69. Bayerle-Eder M, Langenberger H, Pleiner J et al. Endothelin ET_A receptor-subtype specific antagonism does not mitigate the acute systemic or renal effects of exogenous angiotensin II in humans. Eur J Clin Invest 2002; 32: 230–5.
70. Montanari A, Biggi A, Carra N et al. Endothelin-A receptors mediate renal hemodynamic effects of exogenous angiotensin II in humans. Hypertension 2003; 42: 825–30.
71. Yang ZH, Richard V, von Segesser L et al. Threshold concentrations of endothelin-1 potentiate contractions to norepinephrine and serotonin in human arteries. A new mechanism of vasospasm? Circulation 1990; 2: 188–95.
72. Haynes WG, Hand MF, Johnstone HA, Padfield PL, Webb DJ. Direct and sympathetically mediated venoconstriction in essential hypertension. Enhanced responses to endothelin-1. J Clin Invest 1994; 94: 1359–64.
73. Iglarz M, Benessiano J, Philip I et al. Preproendothelin-1 gene polymorphism is related to a change in vascular reactivity in the human mammary artery in vitro. Hypertension 2002; 39: 209–13.
74. Kozàkovà M, Buralli S, Palombo C et al. Myocardial ultrasonic backscatter in hypertension – relation to aldosterone and endothelin. Hypertension 2003; 41: 230–6.
75. Krum H, Viskoper RJ, Lacourcière Y, Budde M, Charlon V. The effect of an endothelin-receptor antagonist, bosentan, on blood pressure in patients with essential hypertension. Bosentan Hypertension Investigators. N Engl J Med 1998; 338: 784–90.
76. Nakov R, Pfarr E, Eberle S. Darusentan: an effective endothelin A receptor antagonist for treatment of hypertension. Am J Hypertens 2002; 15: 583–9.
77. Tiret L, Poirier O, Hallet V et al. The Lys198Asn polymorphism in the endothelin-1 gene is associated with blood pressure in overweight people. Hypertension 1999; 33: 1169–74.
78. Funke-Kaiser H, Reichenberger F, Köpke K et al. Differential binding of transcription factor E2F-2 to the endothelin-converting enzyme-1b promoter affects blood pressure regulation. Hum Mol Genet 2003; 12: 423–33.
79. Funalot B, Courbon D, Brousseau T et al. Genes encoding endothelin-converting enzyme-1 and endothelin-1 interact to influence blood pressure in women: the EVA study. J Hypertens 2004; 22: 739–43.

18

Molecular effects of vasopressin, thyroid hormones, parathyroid hormone, and growth hormone on blood pressure

Alan Sacerdote, Surender Arora, Karolina Weiss, Tri Tran, Marina Goikhberg, Samy I McFarlane

INTRODUCTION

The goal of this chapter is to explore the known molecular pathogenesis of hypertension in states of vasopressin excess, hyperparathyroidism, hyper- and hypothyroidism, and acromegaly. We will present the current evidence and understanding of the molecular mechanisms of hypertension in various endocrine disorders. Mechanistic insights into blood pressure regulation as it relates to vasopressin, parathyroid, thyroid, and growth hormone actions are presented.

VASOPRESSIN

Vasopressin or arginine-vasopressin (AVP) is a neurohypophysial hormone produced by the magnocellular neurons in the supraoptic (SON) and paraventricular (PVN) nuclei of the hypothalamus. It is stored in the posterior pituitary and is released in response to decrease in blood volume and increase in serum osmolality. Baroreceptors located in the carotid artery aortic arch and left atrium sense falls in blood pressure (BP) and directly stimulate the SON and PVN nuclei. Osmoreceptors located in the hypothalamus sense small changes in osmolality, resulting in either an increase or decrease in AVP secretion from neurons in the stalk or posterior pituitary. The physiological effects of AVP include osmoregulation mediated by antidiuretic action (V2 receptor) and acute regulation of BP through vasoconstriction (V1 receptor). These specific receptors belong to a seven-membrane-spanning receptor family and signal through G protein, resulting in the formation of distinct second messengers.[1] At least three AVP receptor subtypes[1] have been identified (Table 18.1).

Table 18.1 Arginine vasopressin (AVP) receptor subtypes, location, and functions

Receptor	*Location*	*Action*
V1A	Vascular smooth muscle cell Hepatocytes Platelets Mesangial cells	• Contraction, proliferation and hypertrophy of cells • Vascular resistance control • Platelet aggregation • Hepatocyte glycogenolysis
V1B	Anterior pituitary	ACTH release
V2	Distal tubules of kidney	Free water absorption Vasodilatation

AVP is one of the most powerful vasoconstricting agents in vitro[2] and its vasoconstrictive effect is even more potent than angiotensin II (Ang II).[1] However, it is also capable of producing vasodilatation through its action on V2 receptors and the vasodilatory effects are more clearly demonstrated following V1 receptor antagonist administration.[3] Based on its biological effects on vascular resistance (V1) and water excretion (V2), AVP plays an important role in the maintenance of BP in several conditions with true or relative hypovolemia, including dehydration, upright posture, hemorrhage, adrenal insufficiency, and heart failure, and during surgery.[4] AVP is also implicated in the pathogenesis of arterial hypertension via its mitogenic and vasoconstrictive properties.[5] Indeed, AVP has been demonstrated to play a central role in the genesis and maintenance of several models of experimental hypertension, based on measurements of plasma and urinary AVP levels and responses to peptide and nonpeptide AVP receptor antagonists.[6]

In one study,[7] attenuation of genetic hypertension in young spontaneously hypertensive rats (SHR) was demonstrated after short-term administration of nonpeptide V1 receptor antagonist. Similarly, others[8] demonstrated that Brattleboro rats with hereditary AVP deficiency failed to develop hypertension with deoxycorticosterone (DOCA)-salt unless supplemented with AVP. Many other workers have reported similar results in experimental models of hypertension such as the DOCA-salt model, thereby suggesting a primary pathogenic role of AVP.[9,10] Although the exact mechanism involved in the pathogenesis of this experimental hypertension is not clearly understood, the vasoconstrictor and renal actions of AVP may play a significant role, in addition to possible increase in sympathetic outflow.[11] One investigative group[12] reported an increase in plasma AVP levels during the early phase of mineralocorticoid-induced hypertension in seven normotensive young volunteers treated with fludrocortisone 0.8 mg/day for 1 week. The blood pressure increased from 117/67 to 121/76 mm Hg ($p<0.05$) within 1 week while plasma AVP (0.45 ± 0.1 pg/ml) increased within 3 days (0.68 ± 0.5 pg/ml) and rose further to 1.53 ± 0.27 pg/ml after 1 week. The plasma osmolality remained unaltered during the study. However, the changes in plasma AVP were not correlated with alteration in BP. The authors concluded that AVP could contribute to increase in BP during mineralocorticoid treatment. The role of AVP in human hypertension has been examined in a series of studies. Many workers have reported an increase in plasma AVP levels in hypertensive patients,[13–15] with AVP levels correlating with severity of hypertension,[16] thereby suggesting a role of AVP in pathogenesis of hypertension. However, a positive correlation between BP and AVP levels has not been consistently reported. This could be explained on the basis of increase in vascular reactivity and sensitivity to AVP. Although slight increase in pressor sensitivity to AVP has been reported by some workers, this is not sufficient to explain the increase in BP in most studies.[17]

Sex and racial differences in the role of AVP in blood pressure control have been reported.[14,18] One group[14] reported significant sex differences in endocrine predictors of hypertension, with increased AVP levels in hypertensive men as compared with hypertensive women. Others[18] have reported important racial differences in the role of AVP in hypertension, with higher basal AVP levels and low renin activity in African American hypertensive subjects compared with Caucasians. The administration of selective AVP receptor antagonist lowered mean arterial pressure in African American subjects but not in Caucasians. Moreover, AVP receptor blockade further reduced the arterial pressure after clonidine pretreatment in African Americans but not in Caucasian subjects. This study illustrated that pressor function of AVP is probably more important in low-renin hypertension as seen in African Americans and after sympathetic suppression. This has also been demonstrated in another study;[19] patients with accelerated or malignant hypertension had a small fall in BP after treatment with V1 receptor antagonist alone, but after pretreatment with a sympatholytic agent (clonidine), the V1 receptor antagonist produced a significant fall in diastolic BP. The same group also reported a significant orthostatic diastolic BP fall in diabetic hypertensive patients after V1 receptor antagonist, without any alteration in supine BP, thereby suggesting an important role for AVP in sustaining BP in the upright posture when the baroreflex system is altered. Similarly, AVP may also play a predominant role in the presence of decreased activity of the sympathetic system and suppression of the renin-angiotensin system (RAS). A greater BP reduction in upright BP in the elderly (altered baroreflex function) and black patients (suppressed RAS) than in young and white patients has been reported.[20]

Another report[21] demonstrated equivalent reduction in systemic vascular resistance in normal and quadriplegic subjects after incremental infusions of AVP following V1 receptor blockade. However, mean arterial pressure was reduced only in quadriplegic subjects but not in normal subjects and was attributed to a difference in the magnitude of increase in cardiac output, which was twofold greater in normal than in quadriplegic subjects. This study again suggests an important role for AVP in maintaining BP in subjects with impaired baroreflex function with deficient sympathetic efferent responses. Furthermore, significant reduction in plasma AVP levels was reported after captopril treatment, thereby suggesting that RAS influences the release of AVP. However, the interaction between AVP and RAS is complex and is not completely understood.[22]

Overall, AVP has multiple and diverse actions on the cardiovascular system, including direct vasoconstriction, antidiuresis, vasodilatation of renal vasculature, and modulation of baroreflex control. AVP acts in concert with the sympathetic nervous system and RAS as an integrated neurohormonal system in the control of BP.[5] It plays an important role in vascular homeostasis mediated by its vasoconstrictive action whenever volume is depleted such as in dehydration, hemorrhage, adrenal insufficiency, and orthostasis.[5] Although AVP is a very potent vasoconstrictor, its pressor function is partly offset by its sensitizing influence on baroreflexes[23] and is usually not apparent unless the other two systems have been impaired. Therefore, the pressor role is most visible in patients with autonomic insufficiency, as seen in diabetics and elderly individuals.

To summarize, the relationship between AVP and hypertension is complex and not completely understood. Although AVP plays an important role in the pathogenesis of hypertension in experimental models, its role in the development and maintenance of human essential hypertension is not clear. Present evidence indicates that it may be an important back-up pressor system in hypovolemic states, impaired baroreflex mechanisms, and autonomic insufficiency, as well as in the presence of low-renin states. It may also be an important factor in the pathogenesis of mineralocorticoid-induced hypertension.

PARATHYROID HORMONE

Hypertension is a common co-morbidity in patients with primary hyperparathyroidism, with a reported prevalence of up to 30% in this patient population.[24] Whether hyperparathyroidism causes the hypertension is questionable and the pathogenetic mechanisms of hypertension in these patients is largely unknown. In a study of 124 patients with hyperparathyroidism, 73% of these were hypertensive as compared with controls matched for, age, race, sex, and days in the hospital admitted for conditions of comparable surgical magnitude.[25] The systolic and diastolic BP was significantly higher in hyperparathyroid patients ($143 \pm 26.8/89 \pm 13.6$ mm Hg) compared with the controls ($130 \pm 19.8/81.1 \pm 10.8$ mm Hg). There was a significant difference in the mean postoperative decrease in BP between the two groups. However, there was no linear correlation between the serum calcium and BP in the hyperparathyroid patients either pre- or postoperatively. The investigators concluded that hyperparathyroidism is associated with hypertension and is probably caused by parathyroid hormone (PTH) rather than indirectly by hypercalcemia, although they did not specifically correlate PTH with BP.[25]

One investigative group evaluated the pressor response to graded infusion of Ang II and norepinephrine (NE) in 7 normotensive hyperparathyroid patients before and after surgical cure, 10 patients with idiopathic hypertension and 10 normal controls.[26] The pressor dose was defined as the dose of Ang II or NE needed to increase diastolic BP by 20 mm Hg. The pressor doses of Ang II and NE were significantly lower in normotensive hyperparathyroid patients than in normal controls, and were similar to the pressor dose in idiopathic hypertensive patients. The pressor dose 2–6 months after surgical cure of hyperparathyroidism remained unchanged from the preoperative values. The authors concluded that hyperparathyroidism can disrupt the normal responsiveness to pressor agents, even in the absence of clinical hypertension.

A significant inverse relationship has been noted between mean arterial pressure and 51Cr-labeled ethylene-diaminetetra-acetate (EDTA) clearance in patients with hyperparathyroidism both before and after parathyroidectomy, but not in patients with essential hypertension, thereby suggesting a possible role of renal dysfunction in the causation of hypertension in hyperparathyroidism.[27] These authors reported no significant change in BP or glomerular filtration rate as measured by 51Cr-EDTA after parathyroidectomy in these patients. The plasma renin activity (PRA) and plasma aldosterone levels did not differ between normotensive and hypertensive patients with primary hyperparathyroidism and were unchanged after surgery.

To elucidate the mechanisms involved in calcium-mediated BP control, an investigative group[28] studied cardiovascular pressor responsiveness to NE and Ang II before and during acute mild hypercalcemia induced by intravenous calcium infusion and after short-term calcium inhibition with nifedipine in 20 normal and 5 borderline hypertensive patients. They reported significant increase in systolic BP, plasma NE and epinephrine concentrations ($p < 0.05$) in normal subjects during acute rise in serum calcium by 3.1 mg/dl but not following an increase of 1 mg/dl. However, in the borderline hypertensive group, elevation of serum calcium levels by 1 mg/dl was associated with a slight increase in systolic BP ($p < 0.05$) and plasma catecholamines. In both groups, pressor responsiveness to infused NE and Ang II, and plasma renin and Ang II levels were unchanged during mild to moderate hypercalcemia. Nifedipine given for 2 weeks reduced BP significantly ($p < 0.05$) in the borderline hypertensive subjects only and NE pressor response in both groups ($p < 0.05$) without any significant effect on plasma catecholamines, renin or Ang II levels.

In another study,[29] PRA, plasma aldosterone levels and pressor response to NE were compared among 10 hypertensive and 10 normotensive hyperparathyroid patients and in 10 controls. The authors reported significantly high PRA, plasma aldosterone levels, and pressor response to NE in the hypertensive group as compared with the other two groups. After parathyroidectomy, the PRA and aldosterone levels normalized in 8 of 10 hypertensive patients with normal pressor response to NE. The authors hypothesized a direct effect of PTH on renin secretion that could contribute to pathogenesis of hypertension and abnormal vascular reactivity in hyperparathyroid patients. If such an effect of PTH on renin secretion is confirmed, it would also partially explain the hypertension seen in conditions of secondary hyperparathyroidism, i.e. chronic renal failure.

A higher plasma cortisol level and PRA in patients with primary hyperparathyroidism before surgery as compared with after parathyroidectomy has been reported.[30] There was no significant difference in plasma aldosterone and catecholamine levels from the preoperative values.

An inverse relationship between serum phosphate levels and BP has been reported in hypertensive patients with hyperparathyroidism as compared with normotensive hyperparathyroid subjects.[31] The mean serum phosphate level in hypertensive patients was significantly lower (2.20 ± 0.06 mg/dl) than that in normotensive patients (2.69 ± 0.09 mg/dl, $p < 0.02$).

It has been reported that PTH can increase adrenocorticotropin hormone (ACTH) and AVP release.[32] Others have demonstrated a direct effect of PTH on dispersed adrenal cortex cells to stimulate aldosterone and cortisol production with complete inhibition of this effect with a PTH receptor inhibitor.[33] They further showed that the presence of an ACTH receptor inhibitor failed to attenuate the response to PTH, thereby suggesting that ACTH does not mediate the stimulation of aldosterone and cortisol release. They also reported that specific inhibitors of adenylate cyclase and phospholipase C, which are second messengers of PTH signaling pathways, together could abolish the PTH stimulation of cortisol and aldosterone. Therefore, it is possible that cortisol and aldosterone could contribute to the pathogenesis of hypertension seen in patients with primary hyperparathyroidism.

To summarize, despite a higher incidence of hypertension seen in hyperparathyroid patients and some reversal to normotensive state after parathyroid surgery, the association between hyperparathyroidism and hypertension remains unclear. Suggested mechanisms of hypertension in patients with hyperparathyroidism include stimulation of the RAS and increased PRA. However, high plasma aldosterone levels in this patient population have not been consistently demonstrated. Although there is some evidence that high serum calcium may be associated with abnormal pressor responsiveness, linear correlation between serum calcium and BP has not been reported. Instead, the degree of BP elevation in this population correlates more with serum phosphate levels. Thus, the association between primary hyperparathyroidism and hypertension remains unclear and a causal relationship cannot be established on the basis of present evidence.

THYROID HORMONE

Hypothyroidism

Hypothyroidism is frequently associated with hypertension, usually diastolic, and has been identified as a cause of hypertension in 3% of patients with high BP.[34,35] The reported prevalence of hypertension in hypothyroid patients is estimated to be increased threefold and occurs in up to 50% of the patients.[35,36]

A significantly increased diastolic BP was observed in 16 patients in a group of 40 patients rendered hypothyroid by radioiodine treatment for thyrotoxicosis. Restoration of euthyroidism with thyroxine treatment significantly reduced the systolic and diastolic BP in these patients. However, while achievement of euthyroidism is associated with normalization of BP in many patients, replacement therapy is not always successful in reversing the hypertensive state.[34]

The pathogenesis of sustained hypertension in the setting of hypothyroidism is not completely understood. Investigators reported direct vasodilator effects of T3, and to a lesser extent T4, on the rat skeletal muscle resistance arteries.[37] Similarly, other investigations[38] have demonstrated that T3 induced relaxation of the aortic endothelial and vascular smooth muscle cells in primary cultures, thereby suggesting increase in vascular resistance in the hypothyroid state.

An investigative group[39] studied the peripheral and central pressure waveforms noninvasively in 12 untreated hypothyroid patients and 12 age-, sex-, and BMI-matched controls. They reported increased augmentation of central aortic pressure and central arterial stiffness, with reversal of these abnormalities after adequate thyroid replacement therapy. Another group[34] studied the elastic properties of the aorta before and after thyroid hormone replacement therapy in patients with hypothyroidism and high BP. The study group consisted of 30 patients with hypothyroidism and hypertension, 15 patients with hypothyroidism and normal BP, 15 patients with hypertension with normal thyroid functions, and 30 healthy age- and sex-matched controls with normal thyroid function. The aortic stiffness index was significantly increased in all the three study groups as compared with the control group. Complete normalization of BP, both systolic and diastolic, was seen in 15 of 30 patients with hypothyroidism and hypertension after levothyroxine therapy compared with the remaining 15 patients who showed only a small decrease in BP with thyroxine replacement. The aortic stiffness index was significantly increased in the latter group ($p<0.01$), both before and after treatment, compared with the former and decreased significantly after treatment with felodipine.

Collectively, these data indicate that impairment of aortic elastic properties may also contribute to sustained hypertension in hypothyroid patients and may be partially reversible with thyroid replacement therapy. Furthermore, in hypothyroid patients, there is an impairment of flow-mediated endothelium-dependent vasodilation that could – in part – explain the high blood pressure in these patients.[40]

Although the exact mechanism for increase in systemic vascular resistance and increased vascular stiffness in hypothyroidism is not clear, the following factors may be crucial to the pathogenesis:

1. Altered responsiveness to sympathetic stimulation with increased activity in vascular smooth muscles.
2. Modulation of adrenergic receptors with decrease in number of and response to β-adrenergic receptors with corresponding increase in α-adrenergic responses.
3. Decreased flow-mediated endothelium-dependent vasodilation.

Hyperthyroidism

Hyperthyroidism is associated with systolic hypertension in nearly one-third of patients, especially in the elderly. This contrasts with predominantly diastolic hypertension in hypothyroidism. Circulating blood volume, and hence preload, is increased in hyperthyroidism, possibly related to up-regulation of erythropoietin secretion and activation of the RAS[41] with resultant increase in sodium absorption. Relaxation of arterial smooth muscle by T4 causes decrease in systemic vascular resistance by 50–60%.[37,38] Increased preload and low systemic vascular resistance (SVR) together contribute to increased stroke volume of the heart which, in combination with T4-induced increase in heart rate, result in a two to threefold increase in cardiac output and systolic hypertension.[42] The fall in SVR causes a decrease in diastolic pressure and explains the low mean arterial pressure and rare occurrence of diastolic hypertension in hyperthyroidism.[36] The establishment of the euthyroid state leads to a complete reversal of these changes.

The RAS may play a significant role in the pathogenesis of hypertension associated with hyperthyroidism. In a preclinical study, an investigative group[43] demonstrated elevation of mean arterial pressure in rats treated with T4 alone as compared with rats treated with both T4 and captopril. The authors concluded that increase in blood pressure caused by T4 is likely mediated by the RAS and blockade of the RAS with captopril prevented the increase in BP in the captopril group.

To summarize: hypothyroidism is known to be associated with increase in total peripheral vascular resistance and arterial wall thickness. These, in combination with hypothyroidism-induced endothelial dysfunction, may contribute to the development of diastolic hypertension in hypothyroid patients that may be partially reversible after adequate thyroid hormone replacement. In contrast, hyperthyroidism is associated with predominantly systolic hypertension contributed by low systemic vascular resistance and increase in preload mediated by increased sodium absorption, possibly through activation of the RAS. As with hypothyroidism, these changes are also usually reversible with achievement of the euthyroid state.

Growth hormone and IGF-1

Hypertension is a common problem in acromegaly. In various published series, the prevalence of hypertension in patients with acromegaly has been reported as 18–60%.[44] In general, hypertension in acromegaly is reported to be mild and readily controlled.[45] Factors influencing the prevalence of hypertension in acromegaly are similar to those in the general population and include:[45]

1. Age: prevalence of hypertension increases with increasing age.
2. Gender: borderline hypertension is equally common in both sexes but stable, sustained hypertension is more common in women.
3. Ethnicity: hypertension is significantly more prevalent in black acromegalic patients than in patients of other ethnicity.
4. Obesity: hypertensive acromegalics tend to have higher weight than normotensive patients.
5. Genetic factors: positive correlation between IGF-1 level and BP has been reported in patients with a family history of hypertension, suggesting that genetic factors may influence the expression of IGF-1 on the vasculature.
6. Increased insulin resistance associated with direct actions of GH.
7. Other factors: presence of concomitant central hypothyroidism, sleep apnea syndrome (≥50% of acromegalics) and hyperparathyroidism (MEN-1).

Most, but not all, growth hormone (GH) actions are mediated through stimulation of the production and release of other peptide hormones known as insulin-like growth factors (IGFs). The most important among these growth factors is IGF-1, which is structurally similar to pro-insulin and exerts a number of insulin-like effects.

In hypertensive patients with acromegaly, a correlation between the GH level and BP has not been established. However, the IGF-1 level is positively correlated with BP in acromegalic patients with a family history of hypertension.[46] The apparent lack of correlation between GH level and blood pressure may be explained by episodic secretion of GH, making levels in a given patient highly variable over the course of a few minutes, while IGF-1 levels are more stable, reflecting the integrated effect of GH. It is likely that pooled GH level measured from frequently sampled GH specimens might correlate with BP in this population.

The pathogenesis of hypertension in acromegaly appears to be multifactorial, although the precise mechanism is not clear. Factors likely to be contributing to pathogenesis of hypertension in acromegaly include those discussed below.[47]

Expansion of plasma volume

There is evidence that exchangeable sodium (Na_e), total body sodium, extracellular water, and plasma volume are all increased in acromegaly.[48] The sodium retaining effect of GH, as measured by Na_e, is positively correlated with both BP and log GH level in untreated acromegalics. It has been suggested that both GH and IGF-1 increase tubular sodium and water absorption. Receptors for GH and the IGF are expressed in the kidneys and direct activation of distal tubular sodium channels by IGF-1 has been suggested. A positive correlation between IGF-1 and erythrocyte sodium transport has been demonstrated,[49] with an increased intracellular sodium content which normalized after successful pituitary surgery.

Insulin resistance and hyperinsulinemia

Most acromegalic patients are insulin-resistant, whether they have normal or abnormal glucose tolerance.[50] In this population, BP increases with rise of their insulin levels, while the insulin response to an oral glucose load is greater in hypertensive than in normotensive acromegalics. Hypersecretion of GH is central to the pathogenesis of this resistance. GH acts by inhibiting the phosphorylation of the insulin receptor (IR) and the signaling molecule, insulin receptor substrate-1 (IRS-1)[50,51] (Figure 18.1). This results in reduced peripheral glucose uptake and diminished suppression of hepatic gluconeogenesis in response to insulin.[51] Compensatory hyperinsulinemia leads to overexpression of other insulin actions for which there is no resistance, such as a vasoconstrictor rather than a normal vasodilator response to acetylcholine via insulin stimulation of the mitogen-activated phosphorylation (MAP) kinase pathway. Another proposed mechanism of GH-mediated insulin resistance is by mobilization of free fatty acids, which inhibit insulin-stimulated glucose oxidation by acting as an alternative energy source. The hypertension-promoting actions of insulin are mediated via binding to the IGF-1 receptor. Together, insulin and IGF-1 stimulate vascular smooth muscle growth via the MAP kinase cascade.[50,51] Other MAP kinase-mediated insulin actions include endothelial inflammation and media-intima cellular proliferation, which may also contribute to pathogenesis of hypertension.[51] Insulin resistance associated with GH excess is largely ameliorated by the GH receptor antagonist, pegvisomant, independent of weight loss,[52] supporting the evidence for the direct action of GH in inducing insulin resistance.[50,51] This effect of pegvisomant does not, however, rule out an IGF-1 effect. A summary of our current understanding of the interplay of GH excess and insulin excess in the pathogenesis of acromegalic hypertension is presented in Figure 18.2.

Direct pressor effects of GH and/or IGF-1

The IGF-1 gene is expressed in both endothelial and vascular smooth muscle cells and IGF-1 is an important mitogen for both these cell types.[53] Proliferation of vascular smooth muscle and endothelial dysfunction mediated by IGF may be contributory to hypertension seen in acromegaly. Studies in IGF-1 knockout animals have shown that IGF-1 causes structural changes in the arterial wall, such as an increase in thickness and collagen content and possibly contributes to increased intimal-medial thickness of carotid arteries in acromegaly.[53]

Reduced secretion of atrial natriuretic peptide (ANP)

GH may attenuate the secretion of ANP, resulting in increased sodium reabsorption.[54,55] A summary of our current state of knowledge regarding atrial natriuretic factor (ANF) in the pathogenesis of acromegalic hypertension is presented in Figure 18.3.[54,55]

Sympathetic nervous system hyperactivity

Studies on the activity and role of the sympathoadrenal system in acromegaly are few and conflicting. Although the addition of IGF-1 has been shown to increase catecholamine biosynthesis in vitro, IGF

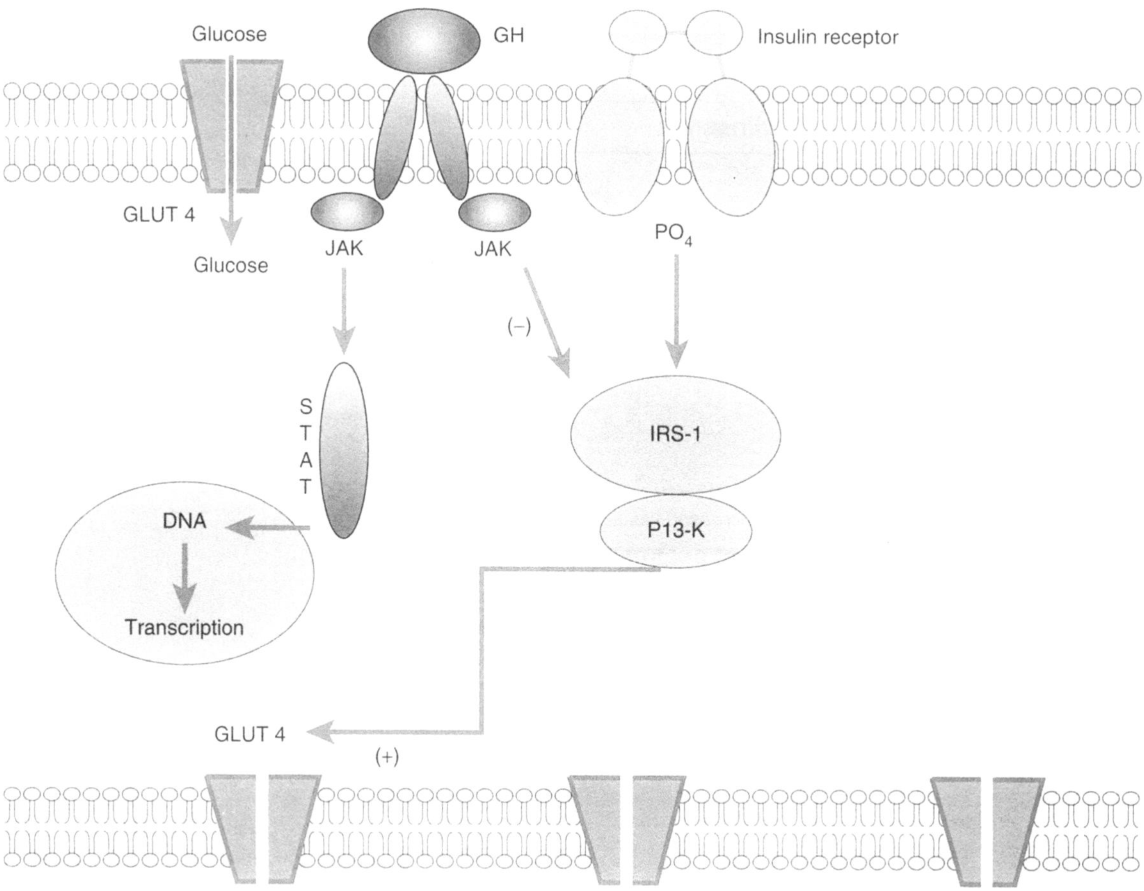

Figure 18.1 Effect of growth hormone (GH) on insulin signaling pathway. GH inhibition of the phosphorylation of insulin receptor substrate 1 (IRS-1) is mediated via Janus kinase (JAK). (Data taken from Rose and Clemmons. Growth Horm IGF Res 2002; 12: 418–24.[51])

infusion failed to increase circulating catecholamine levels in normal volunteers.[56] Acromegaly is associated with flattening of 24-hour profile for both norepinephrine and BP, instead of the normal circadian BP fluctuation.[57,58] Sleep apnea has been reported in 60–75% of acromegalics and increases catecholamine release during apneic/hypopneic episodes, which may contribute to both the insulin resistance and the hypertension in the acromegalic patients.[59–61]

Overexpression of the renin-angiotensin-aldosterone system (RAAS)

Stimulation of the RAAS in the pathogenesis of hypertension in acromegalic patients has been postulated;[62,63] however, no relationship between plasma aldosterone concentration and blood pressure could be detected.[62] GH receptors have been identified in the zona glomerulosa of the adrenal cortex,[63] pointing to the possibility of a direct GH effect on aldosterone synthesis.

Cardiac hyperkinesis

Increased peripheral blood flow in acromegaly reportedly results in cardiac hyperkinesis over the short term, which may contribute to the development of hypertension as acromegaly becomes long-standing.[64]

To summarize, the prevalence of hypertension is increased in acromegaly and has a multifactorial etiology, including hereditary factors, sodium and water

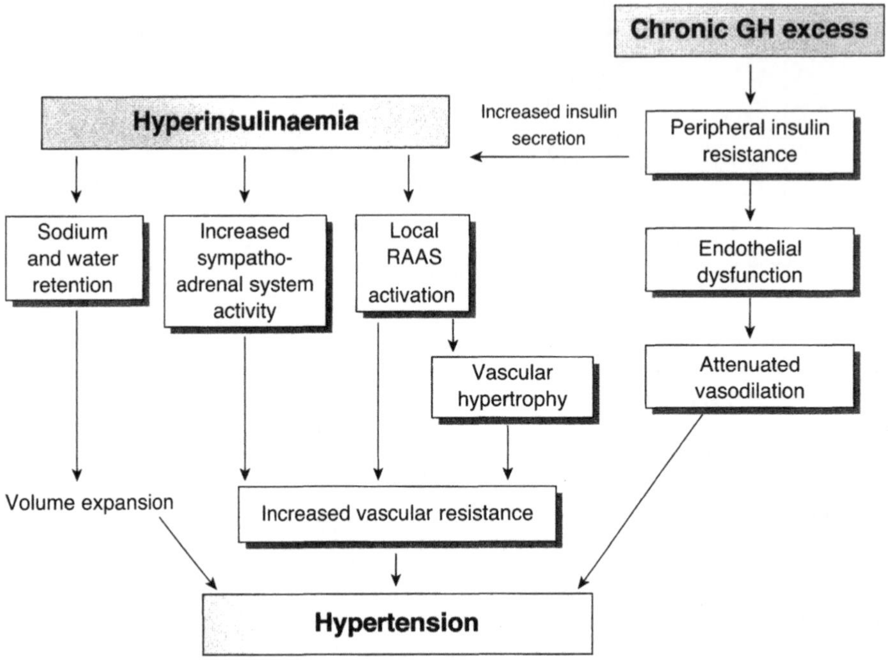

Figure 18.2 Role of insulin resistance and hyperinsulinemia in the development of hypertension in the acromegaly/renin-angiotensin-aldosterone system (RAAS)

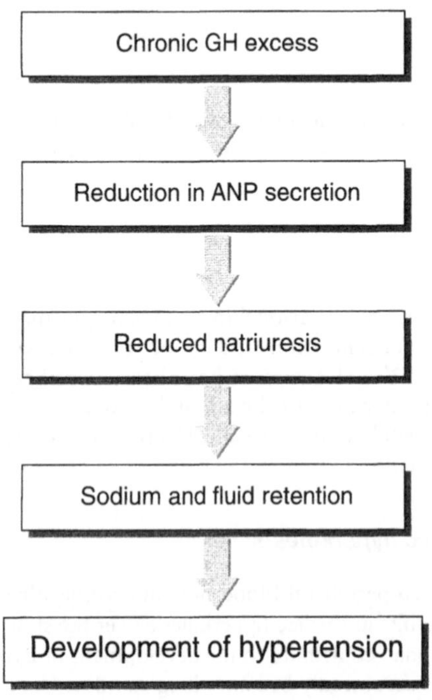

Figure 18.3 Role of atrial natriuretic factor (ANP) secretion in the development of hypertension in acromegaly

retention with increased plasma volume, effects of GH and IGF-1 on insulin sensitivity, RAAS activity, vascular and sympathetic tone, and sleep apnea.

CONCLUSIONS

In this chapter we have presented an overview of the complex subject of the molecular pathophysiology of hypertension in several endocrine disorders. The existence of multiple mechanisms and complementary as well as opposing pathways in these disorders makes it challenging to gain a unified comprehension of how hypertension develops in these patients. It is hoped that the information presented will be useful to basic and clinical investigators as well as to clinicians caring for these patients.

REFERENCES

1. Tahara A, Tomura Y, Wada KI et al. Pharmacological profile of YM087, a novel potent non peptide vasopressin V1A and V2 receptor antagonist, in vitro and in vivo. J Pharmacol Exp Ther 1997; 282: 301–8.
2. Altura BM, Altura BT. Vascular smooth muscle and neurohypophyseal hormones. Fed Proc 1977; 36: 1853–60.

3. Huch KM, Runyun KR, Wall BM et al. Hemodynamic response to vasopressin during V1 receptor antagonism in baroreflex-deficient subjects. Am J Physiol 1995; 268: R156–R163.
4. Share L. Role of vasopressin in cardiovascular regulation. Physiol Rev 1988; 68: 1248–84.
5. Johnston CI. Vasopressin in circulatory control and hypertension. J Hypertens 1985; 3: 557–69.
6. Thibonnier M, Kilani A, Rahman M et al. Effects of the nonpeptide V1 vasopressin receptor antagonist SR49059 in hypertensive patients. Hypertension 1999; 34: 1293–300.
7. Burrell LM, Phillips PA, Risvanis J et al. Attenuation of genetic hypertension after short-term vasopressin V1A receptor antagonism. Hypertension 1995; 26: 828–34.
8. Berecek KH, Murray RD, Gross F et al. Vasopressin and vascular reactivity in the development of DOCA hypertension in rats with hereditary diabetes insipidus. Hypertension 1982; 4: 3–12.
9. Bayorh MA, Ogbolu EC, Williams E et al. Possible mechanisms of salt-induced hypertension in Dahl salt-sensitive rats. Physiol Behav 1998; 65: 563–8.
10. Crofton JT, Ota M, Share L et al. Role of vasopressin, the renin-angiotensin system and sex in Dahl salt-sensitive hypertension. J Hypertens 1993; 11: 1031–8.
11. Tachikawa K, Yokoi H, Nagasaki H et al. Altered cardiovascular regulation in arginine vasopressin-overexpressing transgenic rat. Am J Physiol Endocrinol Metab 2003; 285: E1161–E1166.
12. Haller H, Bahr V, Bock A et al. Vasopressin is increased in mineralocorticoid-induced blood pressure increase in man. J Hypertens Suppl 1987; 5: S111–S113.
13. Padfield PL, Brown JJ, Lever AF et al. Blood pressure in acute and chronic vasopressin excess. N Engl J Med 1981; 304: 1067–70.
14. Cowley AW Jr, Skelton MM, Velasquez MT et al. Sex differences in the endocrine predictors of essential hypertension. Vasopressin versus renin. Hypertension 1985; 7: I151–60.
15. Zhang X, Hense HW, Riegger GA et al. Association of arginine vasopressin and arterial blood pressure in a population-based sample. J Hypertens 1999; 17: 319–24.
16. Johnston CI. Vasopressin in circulatory control and hypertension. J Hypertens 1985; 3: 557–69.
17. Morton JJ, Padfield PL. Vasopressin and hypertension in man. J Cardiovasc Pharmacol 1986; 8: S101–S106.
18. Bakris G, Bursztyn M, Gavras I et al. Role of vasopressin in essential hypertension: racial differences. J Hypertens 1997; 15: 545–50.
19. Ribeiro A. Sequential elimination of pressor mechanism in severe hypertension in humans. Hypertension 1986; 8: I-169–73.
20. De Paula RB, Plavnik FL, Rodrigues CI et al. Age and race determine vasopressin participation in upright blood pressure control in essential hypertension. Ann N Y Acad Sci 1993; 689: 534–6.
21. Cooke CR, Wall BM, Huch KM et al. Cardiovascular effects of vasopressin following V(1) receptor blockade compared to effects of nitroglycerin. Am J Physiol Regul Integr Comp Physiol 2001; 281: R887–R893.
22. Santucci A, Leonetti Luparini R et al. Relationship between vasopressin and the renin-angiotensin-aldosterone system in essential hypertension: effect of converting enzyme inhibitor on plasma vasopressin. J Hypertens Suppl 1985; 3: S133–S134.
23. Aylward PE, Floras JS, Leimbach WN Jr et al. Effects of vasopressin on the circulation and its baroreflex control in healthy men. Circulation 1986; 73: 1145–54.
24. Broulik PD, Horky K, Pacovsky V. Blood pressure in patients with primary hyperparathyroidism before and after parathyroidectomy. Exp Clin Endocrinol 1985; 86: 346–52.
25. Nainby-Luxmore JC, Langford HG, Nelson NC et al. A case-comparison study of hypertension and hyperparathyroidism. J Clin Endocrinol Metab 1982; 55: 303–6.
26. Rodriguez-Portales JA, Fardella C. Primary hyperparathyroidism and hypertension: persistently abnormal pressor sensitivity in normotensive patients after surgical cure. J Endocrinol Invest 1994; 17: 307–11.
27. Salahudeen AK, Thomas TH, Sellars L et al. Hypertension and renal dysfunction in primary hyperparathyroidism: effect of parathyroidectomy. Clin Sci (Lond) 1989; 76: 289–96.
28. Bianchetti MG, Beretta-Piccoli C, Weidmann P et al. Calcium and blood pressure regulation in normal and hypertensive subjects. Hypertension 1983; 5: II57–65.
29. Gennari C, Nami R, Gonnelli S. Hypertension and primary hyperparathyroidism: the role of adrenergic and renin-angiotensin-aldosterone systems. Miner Electrolyte Metab 1995; 21: 77–81.
30. Richards AM, Espiner EA, Nicholls MG et al. Hormone, calcium and blood pressure relationships in primary hyperparathyroidism. J Hypertens 1988; 6: 747–52.
31. Daniels J, Goodman AD. Hypertension and hyperparathyroidism. Inverse relation of serum phosphate level and blood pressure. Am J Med 1983; 75: 17–23.
32. Nussdorfer GG, Bahcelioglu M, Neri G et al. Secretin, glucagon, gastric inhibitory polypeptide, parathyroid hormone, and related peptides in the regulation of the hypothalamus-pituitary-adrenal axis. Peptides 2000; 21: 309–24.
33. Mazzocchi G, Aragona F, Malendowicz LK et al. PTH and PTH-related peptide enhance steroid secretion from human adrenocortical cells. Am J Physiol Endocrinol Metab 2001; 280: E209–13.
34. Dernellis J, Panaretou M. Effects of thyroid replacement therapy on arterial blood pressure in patients with hypertension and hypothyroidism. Am Heart J 2002; 143: 718–24.
35. Streeten DH, Anderson GH Jr, Howland T et al. Effects of thyroid function on blood pressure. Recognition of hypothyroid hypertension. Hypertension 1988; 11: 78–83.
36. Saito I, Saruta T. Hypertension in thyroid disorders. Endocrinol Metab Clin North Am 1994; 23: 379–86.
37. Park KW, Dai HB, Ojamaa K et al. The direct vasomotor effect of thyroid hormones on rat skeletal muscle resistance arteries. Anesth Analg 1997; 85: 734–8.
38. Ojamaa K, Klemperer JD, Klein I. Acute effects of thyroid hormone on vascular smooth muscle. Thyroid 1996; 6: 505–12.
39. Obuobie K, Smith J, Evans LM et al. Increased central arterial stiffness in hypothyroidism. J Clin Endocrinol Metab 2002; 87: 4662–6.
40. Lekakis J, Papamichael C, Alevizaki M et al. Flow-mediated, endothelium-dependent vasodilation is impaired in subjects with hypothyroidism, borderline hypothyroidism, and high-normal serum thyrotropin (TSH) values. Thyroid 1997; 7: 411–14.
41. Resnick LM, Laragh JH. Plasma renin activity in syndromes of thyroid hormone excess and deficiency. Life Sci 1982; 30: 585–6.
42. Fadel BM, Ellahham S, Ringel MD et al. Hyperthyroid heart disease. Clin Cardiol 2000; 23: 402–8.
43. Garcia del Rio C, Moreno MR, Osuna A et al. Role of the renin-angiotensinogen system in the development of thyroxine-induced hypertension. Eur J Endocrinol 1997; 136: 656–60.
44. Bondanelli M, Ambrosio MR, Degli Uberti EC. Pathogenesis and prevalence of hypertension in acromegaly. Pituitary 2001; 4: 239–49.
45. Ezzat S, Forster MJ, Berchtold P et al. Acromegaly. Clinical and biochemical features in 500 patients. Medicine 1994; 73: 233–40.
46. Ohtsuka H, Komiya I, Aizawa T et al. Hypertension in acromegaly: hereditary hypertensive factor produces hypertension by enhancing IGF-I production. Endocr J 1995; 42: 781–7.
47. Ritchie CM, Sheridan B, Fraser R et al. Studies on the pathogenesis of hypertension in Cushing's disease and acromegaly. Q J Med 1990; 76: 855–67.

48. Davies DL, Beastall GH, Connell JM et al. Body composition, blood pressure and the renin-angiotensin system in acromegaly before and after treatment. J Hypertens Suppl 1985; 3 (Suppl): S413–S415.
49. Herlitz H, Jonsson O, Bengtsson BA. Relationship between plasma growth hormone concentration and cellular sodium transport in acromegaly. Acta Endocrinol (Copenh) 1992; 127: 38–43.
50. Jorgensen JO, Krag M, Jessen N et al. Growth hormone and glucose homeostasis. Horm Res 2004; 62 (Suppl 3): 51–5.
51. Rose DR, Clemmons DR. Growth hormone receptor antagonist improves insulin resistance in acromegaly. Growth Horm IGF Res 2002; 12: 418–24.
52. Chen Y, Capron L, Magnusson JO et al. Insulin-like growth factor-1 stimulates vascular smooth muscle cell proliferation in rat aorta in vivo. Growth Horm IGF Res 1998; 8: 299–303.
53. Dirsch VM, Wolf E, Wanke R, Schulz R, Hermanns W, Vollmar AM. Effect of chronic GH overproduction on cardiac ANP expression and circulating ANP levels. Mol Cell Endocrinol 1998; 144: 109–18.
54. Moller J, Jorgensen JO, Moller N, Hansen KW, Pedersen EB, Christiansen JS. Expansion of extracellular volume and suppression of atrial natriuretic peptide after growth hormone administration in normal man. J Clin Endocrinol Metab 1991; 72: 768–72.
55. Dahmer MK, Hart PM, Perlman RL. Studies on the effect of insulin-like growth factor-I on catecholamine secretion from chromaffin cells. J Neurochem 1990; 54: 931–6.
56. Terzolo M, Matrella C, Boccuzzi A et al. Twenty-four hour profile of blood pressure in patients with acromegaly. Correlation with demographic, clinical and hormonal features. J Endocrinol Invest 1999; 22: 48–54.
57. Fallo F, Barzon L, Boscaro M, Casiglia E, Sonino N. Effect of octreotide on 24-h blood pressure profile in acromegaly. Am J Hypertens 1998; 11: 591–6.
58. Blanco Perez JJ, Blanco-Ramos MA, Zamarron Sanz C, Souto Fernandez A, Mato Mato A, Lamela Lopez J. [Acromegaly and sleep apnea.] Arch Bronconeumol 2004; 40: 355–9 (in Spanish).
59. Bottini P, Tantucci C. Sleep apnea syndrome in endocrine diseases. Respiration 2003; 70: 320–7.
60. Weiss V, Sonka K, Pretl M et al. Prevalence of the sleep apnea syndrome in acromegaly population. J Endocrinol Invest 2000; 23: 515–19.
61. Zdrojewicz Z. [The renin-angiotensin-aldosterone (RAA) system in endocrine diseases.] Wiad Lek 1990; 43: 679–84 (in Polish).
62. Kraatz C, Benker G, Weber F, Ludecke D, Hirche H, Reinwein D. Acromegaly and hypertension: prevalence and relationship to the renin-angiotensin-aldosterone system. Klin Wochenschr 1990; 68: 583–7.
63. Lin CJ, Mendonca BB, Lucon AM, Guazzelli IC, Nicolau W, Villares SM. Growth hormone receptor messenger ribonucleic acid in normal and pathologic human adrenocortical tissues – an analysis by quantitative polymerase chain reaction technique. J Clin Endocrinol Metab 1997; 82: 2671–6.
64. Theusen L, Christensen SE, Weeke J et al. A hyperkinetic heart in uncomplicated active acromegaly. Explanation of hypertension in acromegalic patients? Acta Med Scand 1988; 223: 337–43.

19

Vasopressin receptors: molecular mechanisms in hypertension and cardiovascular diseases

Marc Thibonnier

INTRODUCTION

The antidiuretic hormone arginine vasopressin (AVP) is a nonapeptide released from the posterior pituitary gland in response to a small (1%) increase of plasma osmolality and/or larger decreases of arterial blood pressure and cardiopulmonary blood volume. AVP regulates free water reabsorption, body fluid osmolality, blood volume, blood pressure, cell contraction, cell proliferation, and ACTH secretion via the stimulation of specific G protein-coupled receptors (GPCRs) currently classified into V1 vascular, V2 renal, and V3 pituitary subtypes having distinct pharmacological profiles and intracellular second messengers.[1]

This chapter reviews the involvement of AVP receptors in the molecular mechanisms underlying arterial hypertension and cardiovascular diseases as well as the potential therapeutic benefits expected from the use of peptide and nonpeptide AVP analogs. Research work in this field has been facilitated by the cloning and expression of AVP receptor subtypes in various species, site-directed mutagenesis experiments, immunofluorescence, immunoprecipitation, 3-dimensional modeling of wild-type and mutated AVP receptors, and administration of peptide and nonpeptide AVP analogs.[2]

AVP RECEPTORS AND EXPERIMENTAL MODELS OF ARTERIAL HYPERTENSION

Although AVP is a potent vasoactive hormone that plays a significant role in blood pressure maintenance after rapid hemorrhage, its vasoconstrictive effect does not translate into a sustained elevation of blood pressure under normal conditions because of resetting of the cardiac baroreflex to a lower pressure.[3] This action, which is mediated by V1 receptors in the area postrema of the brain, causes a leftward shift of the heart rate-arterial pressure baroreflex curve. This event explains why for a given blood pressure elevation, AVP produces more bradycardia than other vasoconstrictors. Furthermore, AVP stimulates nitric oxide (NO) release from the renal medulla, which may buffer blood pressure elevation.[4] Intra-brachial artery administration of AVP in healthy subjects produces a dose-dependent biphasic change in blood flow with a modest vasoconstriction at lower doses (3–30 pmol/min) and a substantial vasodilation at higher doses (>100 pmol/min).[5] NO release was a major contributor to AVP-induced vasodilation in these conditions.

Nevertheless, AVP has been implicated in the pathogenesis of some experimental models of animal hypertension. For instance, in the model of mineralocorticoid-induced hypertension in the rat, AVP may be involved in the blood pressure elevation and remodeling of resistance arteries. Chronic treatment with a AVP V1 receptor antagonist lowers blood pressure in this experimental model of hypertension.[6] Furthermore, in this deoxycorticosterone acetate (DOCA)-salt hypertension model, AVP up-regulates vascular preproendothelin-1 (ET-1) gene expression.[7] Increased arterial ET-1 levels result in increased superoxide anion (O_2^-) production and vascular growth, events that are reduced in the presence of a selective AVP V1 receptor antagonist.[8] This up-regulation of ET-1 gene expression is absent in AVP-deficient Brattleboro rats treated with DOCA-salt, which did not develop vascular structure alteration and wall component stiffness.[9]

Previous studies have shown that AVP may be a contributor in the pathogenesis of hypertension in the spontaneously hypertensive rat (SHR), presumably through the V1 receptor, as blocking of this receptor subtype with a specific V1 receptor antagonist delays the development of hypertension in SHR.[10] Young SHRs have an increased renal vascular reactivity to AVP with enhanced release of intracellular calcium when compared with age-matched Wistar-Kyoto (WKY) rats.[11] Vagnes et al. found an increased expression of the V1 receptor in young SHRs.[12] However, in 40-week-old SHRs, the vascular response to AVP became equal to that of age-matched WKY rats.[13] This age-dependent alteration of AVP V1 receptors in preglomerular vessels from SHRs was examined by real-time PCR and ligand binding studies.[14] These studies showed an increase of the V1 receptor protein and mRNA levels from 5- and 10-week-old SHR rats when compared with 20- and 70-week-old SHRs. Another group of investigators have found that the expression of V2 receptors is increased in the renal medulla of young SHRs and suggested that the increased density of renal AVP receptors plays a role in the pathophysiology of hypertension in these animals.[15] Furthermore, in SHR animals mineralocorticoid treatment up-regulates the paraventricular hypothalamic nucleic V1 receptors, which contributes to the blood pressure elevation of these animals.[16]

AVP RECEPTORS AND HUMAN ARTERIAL HYPERTENSION

Limited studies have assessed the blood pressure response of human subjects to the V1 receptor peptide antagonist d(CH2)5Tyr(Me)AVP. In well hydrated and resting normal subjects, this peptide V1 receptor antagonist did not alter blood pressure.[17] In patients with mild uncomplicated essential hypertension, d(CH2)5Tyr(Me)AVP did not alter blood pressure unless AVP release was stimulated through various maneuvers such as cigarette smoking or a sauna.[18] In patients with severe salt-induced hypertension and end-stage renal disease, d(CH2)5Tyr(Me)AVP produced a 9–12 mm Hg fall of supine systolic blood pressure.[19] In patients with 'accelerated' or malignant hypertension who were pretreated with the sympatholytic agent clonidine, d(CH2)5Tyr(Me)AVP treatment led to a diastolic blood pressure reduction up to 18 mm Hg.[20] In a small series of 27 essential hypertensive patients, a 0.5 mg intravenous bolus of d(CH2)5Tyr(Me)AVP induced a blood pressure reduction that was greater in the elderly and black patients than in the young and white patients (−15 mm Hg vs −7 to −8 mm Hg, respectively).[21]

We assessed the clinical and pharmacological profile of the orally active V1 vascular AVP receptor nonpeptide antagonist SR49059 during the osmotic stimulation of AVP release in hypertensive patients.[22] In a double-blind cross-over versus placebo study, 24 untreated stage I or II essential hypertensive patients (12 Caucasians and 12 African Americans) received a single 300 mg oral dose of SR49059 2 hours prior to stimulation of AVP secretion by a 5% hypertonic saline infusion. Hemodynamic, humoral and hormonal parameters were monitored for up to 28 hours after drug administration.

SR49059 did not alter blood pressure or heart rate before the saline infusion and did not reduce the blood pressure increment induced by the hypertonic saline infusion. However, the blood pressure peak at the end of the hypertonic saline infusion was slightly lower in the presence of SR49059 ($p=0.04$). Heart rate was significantly faster between 4 and 6 hours after SR49059 administration ($p=0.02$). The rise of plasma sodium and osmolality triggered by the saline infusion was not modified by SR49059, but AVP release was slightly greater in the presence of SR49059 ($p<0.0003$). AVP-induced aggregation of blood platelets in vitro was significantly reduced by SR49059, with a peak effect 2 hours after drug administration that coincided with the SR49059 peak plasma concentration. Plasma renin activity and aldosterone before and after the saline infusion were not modified by SR49059. Urine volume and osmolality were not altered by SR49059 administration. SR49059 effects were similar in the two ethnic groups as well as in salt-sensitive versus salt-resistant patients. Thus, in a situation of AVP osmotic release and volume expansion in hypertensive patients, a single oral dose of the V1 vascular AVP receptor nonpeptide antagonist SR49059 able to block AVP-induced platelet aggregation exerts a transient vasodilating effect which is not associated with a sustained blood pressure reduction. SR49059 is a pure V1 vascular receptor antagonist devoid of V2 renal receptor actions. As of today, no published study has reported the effects of chronic treatment with an orally active AVP receptor antagonist on the blood pressure of hypertensive patients.

AVP RECEPTOR VARIANTS AND ARTERIAL HYPERTENSION

Polymorphism of AVP V1 receptors

We have reported the structure and functional expression of the human V1 receptor cDNA and described the genomic characteristics, tissue expression, chromosomal localization, and regional mapping of the human V1 receptor gene, AVPR1A.[23] To test whether the V1 receptor is a marker for human essential hypertension, we sequenced the human AVPR1A gene and its 5′ upstream region and found several DNA microsatellite motifs.[24] One $(GT)_{14}$-$(GA)_{13}$-$(A)_8$ microsatellite is located 2983 bp downstream of the transcription start site, within a 2.2 kbp intron interrupting the coding sequence of the receptor. Three other microsatellites are present in the 5′ flanking DNA of the AVPR1A gene: a $(GT)_{25}$ dinucleotide repeat, a complex $(CT)_4$-TT-$(CT)_8$-$(GT)_{24}$ motif, and a $(GATA)_{14}$ tetranucleotide repeat located, respectively, 3956 bp, 3625 bp and 553 bp upstream of the transcription start site. Analysis of these polymorphisms in 79 hypertensive and 86 normotensive subjects for the $(GT)_{14}$-$(GA)_{13}$-$(A)_8$ and the $(GT)_{25}$ motifs revealed a high percentage of heterozygosity but no difference in allele frequencies between the two groups. A linkage study using the affected sib pair method and the $(GT)_{25}$ repeat in 446 hypertensive sib pairs from 282 French Caucasian pedigrees showed no excess of allele sharing at the AVPR1A locus. No linkage was found in the subgroups of patients with early-onset hypertension (diagnosis before age 40) or severe hypertension (diastolic blood pressure ≥100 mm Hg or requirement for two or more medications). These findings suggest that molecular variants of the V1 receptor gene are not involved in unselected forms of essential hypertension. Although the analysis of more than 400 hypertensive sib pairs should have prevented the generation of false negative results, one cannot exclude rare mutations affecting either the promoter or the coding sequence of the AVPR1A gene that could affect blood pressure. Furthermore, testing linkage with a highly polymorphic marker can lead to false negative results if different alleles share a same common susceptibility variant. Finally, the absence of linkage could be due to either a modest increase in the relative risk of the disease, or if variants of the human V1 vascular AVP receptor gene have a detectable phenotypic effect but are too rare to be detectable in a large common population of hypertensive subjects. In this regard, it could be of interest to analyze an intermediate phenotype such as salt sensitivity that may be more directly influenced by changes in the vasopressinergic system. Several large-scale studies of candidate genes in human arterial hypertension are currently in progress and should provide a more definitive answer about the role of AVPR1A gene polymorphism in cardiovascular diseases.

In their quest to identify genes whose expression results in hypertension, Kotchen et al. studied more than 200 hypertensive, hyperlipidemic black sib pairs.[25] Various anthropometric and phenotypic markers were assessed. Heritability was estimated on the basis of sib-sib correlations and with an association model. Among various hemodynamic, hormonal, and renal parameters, significant heritability was observed for plasma AVP levels measured after saline infusion. The identification of specific genetic determinants of hypertension in black subjects is currently in progress. Further studies will be required to define the role of the vasopressin system in the genetic component of human arterial hypertension. However, in a meta-analysis of genome-wide linkage scans for hypertension in four large multicenter networks of patient groups of various racial background ($n > 6000$ patients), no genomic region showed uniformly large effects of blood pressure.[26] This suggests that no blood pressure/hypertension gene with a large effect is present across diverse ethnic groups.

AVP RECEPTORS AND CONGESTIVE HEART FAILURE

In congestive heart failure (CHF), several neurohormonal systems (sympathetic nervous system, renin-angiotensin-aldosterone system – RAAS, endothelin, cytokines, and AVP) are simulated to maintain arterial pressure and circulatory homeostasis.[27] However, excessive activation of these systems may lead to increased cardiac preload via water and sodium retention, peripheral vasoconstriction, reduced renal blood flow and cardiac remodeling. This situation fuels a vicious cycle, worsening CHF, that could be interrupted by specific blockers of these systems.

AVP circulating levels are often elevated during the progression and/or exacerbation of CHF in response to various non-osmotic stimuli including low arterial pressure and diminished effective arterial volume.[28] This increased release of AVP is aimed at maintaining systemic perfusion in low output states and may occur even in the presence of low plasma osmolality and hyponatremia. The increase of AVP, as well as the increase of catecholamines, is inversely correlated with the prognosis of CHF. In infants and children with CHF related to left ventricular dysfunction or pulmonary overcirculation attributable to large left-to-right shunts, plasma AVP levels were increased and correlated with New York Heart Association (NYHA) functional class.[29]

The abnormal proliferation of cardiac fibroblasts plays an important role in the pathophysiology of left ventricular hypertrophy (LVH). Plasma AVP levels have been shown to be higher in hypertensive patients with LVH than in patients without LVH. Furthermore,

AVP increases the rate of protein synthesis in rat heart and cardiomyocytes, thus raising the possibility that AVP induces the proliferation of cardiac fibroblasts.[30] Indeed, in cardiac fibroblasts of neonatal Sprague-Dawley rats, AVP increased DNA synthesis and the number of cells. The cell number, cell cycle S-stage percentage, and phosphatidyl inositol levels induced by AVP were decreased by the selective V1 receptor antagonist $d(CH_2)_5Tyr(Me)Arg$ vasopressin. These findings suggest that AVP may promote the proliferation of cardiac fibroblasts via stimulation of V1 receptors. In the Studies of Left Ventricular Dysfunction (SOLVD) population (ejection fraction 35% or less), patients with asymptomatic left ventricular dysfunction had higher AVP levels (mean median plasma AVP = 2.2 pg/ml) than control patients (mean median plasma AVP = 1.8 pg/ml), whereas patients with symptomatic mild-to-moderate CHF had even higher AVP levels (mean median plasma AVP = 3.0 pg/ml).[31] Sustained AVP release may worsen CHF via its V1 receptor-mediated vasoconstrictor effect and its V2 receptor-mediated water retention effect. Furthermore, activation of V1 receptors in the myocardium can lead to hypertrophy and stimulation of V_3 receptors may lead to ACTH-mediated aldosterone secretion and subsequent sodium reabsorption. In the Survival and Ventricular Enlargement (SAVE) population of post-myocardial infarction patients with left ventricular dysfunction, AVP levels 1 month after the infarction were independently associated with long-term cardiovascular outcomes, including heart failure, recurrent myocardial infarction, and death.[32]

Accordingly, blockade of AVP receptors may prove beneficial in the treatment of CHF.[33] In several studies of acute and chronic models of heat failure in animals, selective blockade of V1 receptors and/or V2 receptors produced hemodynamic and volume status improvement as previously reported in several species (rat, pig, and dog).[34]

In a pig model of CHF induced by rapid pacing for 3 weeks, administration of the nonpeptide V1 receptor antagonist SR49059 ((2S)1-[(2R3S)-5-chloro-3-(2-chloro-phenyl)-1-(3,4-dimethoxy benzene-sulfonyl)-3-hydroxy-2,3-dihydro-1H-indole-2-carbonyl]-pyrrolidine-2-carboxamide) (60 mg/kg b.i.d.) reduced left ventricular end-diastolic dimension and peak wall stress, two indexes of left ventricular loading conditions.[35] Plasma norepinephrine and angiotensin II were reduced on treatment. When V1 receptor blockade was combined with selective blockade of the angiotensin 1 receptor by irbesartan (30 mg/kg b.i.d.), then left ventricular fractional shortening was increased and myocyte contractile function was improved.

In a rat model of post-infarction-induced CHF with left ventricular remodeling, impaired systolic function, increased cardiac and lung weight, animals were treated for 6 months with the nonpeptide V2 receptor antagonist OPC-31260 (5-dimethylamino-1-[4-(2-methylbenzoylamino) benzoyl]-2,3,4,5-tetrahydro-1H-benzazepine hydrochloride) at a dose of 10 mg/kg/day orally.[36] Chronic V2 receptor blockade increased urine volume and decreased urine osmolality with no natriuretic effect. Baseline plasma sodium and AVP were not altered in this model of CHF. Plasma AVP increased on OPC-31260 treatment, whereas the renin-angiotensin system was not activated. V2 receptor blockade did not modify cardiac remodeling, cardiac function, or survival. This study suggested that blockade of V2 receptors may represent an alternative to standard diuretic therapy in the management of water retention observed in CHF.

In the anesthetized dog, intravenous infusion of AVP (up to 4 mU/kg/min) dose-dependently decreases cardiac contractility and cardiac output while increasing left ventricular end-diastolic pressure and total peripheral resistance – typical manifestations of CHF.[37] Intravenous bolus injection (0.1 mg/kg) of the dual V1 and V2 receptor nonpeptide antagonist conivaptan (YM087, 4′-[(2-methyl-1,4,5,6-tetrahydroimidazo [4,5-*d*][1]benzoazepine-6-carbonyl]-2-phenylbenzanilide monohydrochloride) rapidly attenuated the AVP-induced hemodynamic alterations. In a dog model of CHF induced by rapid right ventricular pacing for 2–3 weeks, intravenous administration of conivaptan (0.1 mg/kg) significantly increased left ventricular pressure and cardiac output while decreasing left ventricular end-diastolic pressure and total peripheral resistance.[38] Conivaptan also increased urine flow and reduced urine osmolality. These results indicate that a mixed V1/V2 receptor nonpeptide antagonist produces hemodynamic improvement and marked aquaresis in dogs with CHF.

In a rat model of CHF induced by left coronary artery ligation, oral administration of conivaptan (3.0 mg/kg) attenuated the changes in left ventricular end-diastolic pressure, lung and right ventricular weight induced by heart failure while reducing blood pressure.[39] In the same model of rat CHF, oral administration of conivaptan (1 mg/kg/day for 4 weeks) decreased urine osmolality while urine volume and plasma AVP increased.[34] Conivaptan did not alter left ventricular mass but significantly reduced right ventricular mass. Combination treatment with the angiotensin converting enzyme (ACE) inhibitor captopril (50 mg/kg/day) lowered blood pressure and plasma natriuretic peptide, caused further increase in aquaresis, and reduced both left and right ventricular mass as well as pulmonary congestion and body weight. These results suggest that a dual AVP receptor antagonist may be a useful addition to ACE inhibitor treatment in the management of vasoconstriction and fluid retention present in CHF.

Consequently, randomized clinical trials were designed to assess the efficacy and safety of AVP receptor antagonists in patients with CHF. VPA-985 (5-fluoro-2-methyl-N-[4-(5H-pyrrolo[2,1-c][1,4]benzodiazepin-10(11H)-yl carbonyl)-3-chlorophenyl]benzamide) is a specific and selective nonpeptide V2 renal receptor antagonist which has been shown to be a potent aquaretic compound in rats and dogs.[40] In a multicenter randomized placebo-controlled trial assessing the efficacy and safety of VPA-985, 44 hospitalized patients with stable hyponatremia <130 mmol/L for 3 consecutive days were randomized to receive per os either placebo or 25 mg, 125 mg or 250 mg of VPA-985 twice daily for 7 days.[41] All patients were maintained on the usual doses of medications, including diuretics and 1.5 liter fluid intake. Six patients had CHF (5 in relation to ischemic heart disease and 1 to idiopathic dilated cardiomyopathy), 33 had cirrhosis of the liver and 5 had a syndrome of inappropriate secretion of AVP. Serum sodium measurements were repeated after every daily dose and the next dose withheld for excessive serum sodium rise. Fluid intake was adjusted according to previous daily urinary outputs. Throughout the study, all patients were maintained on their usual dose of diuretic(s). Thirty-two patients completed the study. VPA-985 produced a significant dose-related aquaretic response compared with placebo with significant dose-related increase in free water clearance, serum sodium and serum osmolality, without significant changes in orthostatic blood pressure and serum creatinine. There was no change in urinary sodium excretion. Plasma AVP increased significantly at the end of the study for both the VPA-985 125 and 250 mg dose groups. Thirst score was significantly increased in the 250 mg group. No patient on placebo had their medication withheld because of an increase in serum sodium by >8 mmol/L. At variance, one patient in the 25 mg group, one patient in the 125 mg group, and five patients in the 250 mg group had to have VPA-985 withheld because of an increase in serum sodium by>8 mmol/L. In conclusion, this study demonstrated the beneficial effect of VPA-985 in improving renal water handling was maintained with continued administration for 7 days in patients with hyponatremia. The higher dose of 250 mg b.i.d. was associated with dehydration as reflected by increased thirst and serum sodium concentration, requiring frequent dose withdrawals. Consequently, administration of high doses of VPA-985 would require careful monitoring of hydration state and should not be administered to patients without appropriate access to fluids.

Tolvaptan (OPC-41061, (±)-7-chloro-5-hydroxy-1-[2-methyl-4-(2-methylbenzoylamino) benzoyl]-2,3,4,5-tetrahydro-1H-1-benzazepine) is a specific and selective nonpeptide V2 renal receptor antagonist which has been shown to be a potent aquaretic compound in rats and dogs.[42] Tovalptan is orally available and has a half-life of 6–8 hours. In a double-blind study, the effects of three doses of tolvaptan (30, 45 or 60 mg) and placebo were tested in 254 patients with CHF (mostly NYHA class II and class III) who were kept on their standard treatment including loop diuretics, ACE inhibitors, digoxin, beta-blockers, hydralazine, and nitrates.[43] Patients were not fluid restricted. Study medications were administered daily for 25 days in an outpatient setting; 87% of patients completed the study. At day 1 a decrease in body weight of -0.79 ± 0.99, -0.96 ± 0.93, -0.84 ± 0.02 kg was observed in the 30, 45, and 60 mg tolvaptan groups, respectively, whereas weight increased by 0.32 ± 0.46 kg in the placebo group ($p<0.001$). The decrease in body weight was similar in all tolvaptan-treated patients irrespective of left ventricular ejection fraction (LVEF). An increase in urine volume was observed with tolvaptan when compared with placebo (3.9 ± 0.6, 4.2 ± 0.9, 4.6 ± 0.4 vs 2.3 ± 0.2 l/24 hours at day 1 for 30, 45, 60 mg tolvaptan groups and placebo, respectively. Tolvaptan-treated patients had decreases in urine osmolality from baseline throughout the study. Patients treated with tolvapatan had small increases (<4 mEq/l) from baseline in serum sodium concentrations. A decrease in edema and a normalization of serum sodium in patients with hyponatremia were observed in the tolvaptan groups but not in the placebo group. No significant changes in heart rate, blood pressure, serum potassium or renal function were observed. A trend toward an increase in plasma AVP concentrations was noted at the end of the treatment period in the tolvaptan-treated patients. This study demonstrated that a decrease in body weight, normalization of serum sodium in patients with hyponatremia, and amelioration of edema can be achieved in patients with CHF with mild signs of congestion on chronic diuretic therapy in response to the V2 receptor antagonist tolvaptan.

The short- and intermediate-term effects of tolvaptan were also studied in patients hospitalized with acute exacerbation of CHF. The Acute and Chronic Therapeutic Impact of a Vasopressin Antagonist in Congestive Heart Failure (ACTIV in CHF) trial was a prospective, randomized, double-blind, placebo-controlled, parallel group trial that studied three doses of tolvaptan (30, 60, and 90 mg) given orally once a day to patients hospitalized for worsening heart failure.[44] Daily therapy was given during hospitalization for 10 days. The patients remaining in the hospital after 10 days were considered as treatment failures and the drug was discontinued. The other patients continued to receive tolvaptan for 7 weeks of outpatient therapy. The primary end-point for the inpatient phase was the change in body weight at 24 hours after the first dose of tolvaptan. The primary end-point for the 7-week outpatient phase was the clinical worsening of CHF. Three hundred and nineteen patients with LVEF of <40% from 45 centers in the USA and Argentina were enrolled into the study. There was a significant reduction of body weight at 24 hours after randomization in all tolvaptan groups versus placebo (−1.80, −2.10 and −2.05 vs −0.60 kg, $p < 0.008$). The weight reduction with tolvaptan was not associated with alterations in heart rate, blood pressure, serum potassium, and renal function. There was no difference in worsening heart failure at 60 days between the tolvaptan and placebo groups. In *post hoc* analysis, 60-day mortality was lower in tolvaptan-treated patients with renal dysfunction or severe systemic congestion. The results of this well designed and well controlled trial suggest that AVP receptor antagonists may complement the symptomatic treatment of CHF. Outcome studies are in progress to test the hypothesis that aquaretics may influence cardiovascular morbidity and mortality in patients with CHF.

Conivaptan (YM087 (4′-[(2-methyl-1,4,5,6-tetrahydroimidazo[4,5-d][1]benzazepin-6-yl)-carbonyl]-2-phenylbenzanilide monochloride)) is a nonpeptide AVP antagonist which has a high affinity for both V1 receptor and V2 receptor.[45] In a group of six healthy volunteers, a single oral dose of 60 mg conivaptan and a single intravenous dose of 50 mg conivaptan produced a significant sevenfold increase in urine flow rate and a fall in urine osmolality from 600 to <100 mosm/L, with a peak effect 2 hours after drug administration.[46] Simultaneously, plasma osmolality and plasma AVP levels increased significantly. The aquaretic effect of these single doses lasted at least 6 hours. When administered intravenously, conivaptan inhibited AVP-induced skin vasoconstriction via blockade of the V1 receptors. However, antagonism of the V1 receptors was less marked than blockade of the V2 receptors. No significant change in blood pressure or heart rate was found in these single-dose studies. One hundred and forty-two patients with symptomatic heart failure (NYHA class III and IV) were randomized to double-blind administration of single intravenous doses (10, 20 or 40 mg) of the dual V1/V2 receptor nonpeptide antagonist conivaptan or placebo.[47] Mean age was 60 years, 75% were men and about 60% were Caucasians. Most of the patients were in NYHA class III and average LVEF ranged from 21% to 26% across groups. Ischemic heart disease was the most frequent etiology, followed by idiopathic/dilated cardiomyopathy and hypertension. All patients were on loop diuretics ± spironolactone, half were on beta-blockers, and about 80% were on digoxin. Compared with placebo, conivaptan at 20 and 40 mg significantly reduced pulmonary capillary wedge pressure (−2.6 ± 0.7, −5.4 ± 0.7, and −4.6 ± 0.7 mm Hg for placebo and 20 and 40 mg groups, respectively, $p < 0.05$) and right arterial pressure (−2.0 ± 0.4, −3.7 ± 0.4, and −3.5 ± 0.4 mm Hg for placebo and 20 and 40 mg groups, respectively, $p < 0.05$) during the 3–6-hour interval after intravenous administration. Conivaptan significantly increased urine output in a dose-dependent fashion (−11 ± 17, 68 ± 17, 152 ± 19, and 176 ± 18 ml/hour for placebo and 10, 20 and 40 mg groups, respectively, $p < 0.001$) during the first 4 hours after the dose. Urine osmolality was significantly reduced by all doses of conivaptan relative to placebo. Serum osmolality, serum sodium and potassium levels were not statistically different between the various subgroups. Changes in cardiac index, systemic and pulmonary vascular resistance, blood pressure, and heart rate did not differ significantly between conivaptan and placebo groups. Acute conivaptan treatment was well tolerated and there were fewer adverse events reported on conivaptan than on placebo. The most commonly reported adverse event was headache, occurring in 7.9% of the placebo patients and 5.8% of the conivaptan patients. The pharmacokinetic profile of conivaptan was best described by a two-compartment model with a terminal half-life of 7.8 hours (range from 5 to 12 hours). The results of this adequate and well-designed placebo-controlled study demonstrate that short-term blockade of AVP receptors with the dual antagonist conivaptan improved the hemodynamic profile while increasing the urine output of patients with advanced CHF. Systemic blood pressure, heart rate, and serum electrolytes were not affected. The absence of significant correlation between conivaptan pharmacodynamic effects and baseline AVP or serum sodium levels suggests that the benefits of this kind of treatment are not limited to patients with hyponatremia and elevated circulating AVP levels.

In view of these encouraging results, additional randomized clinical trials are being executed to assess the efficacy and safety profile of conivaptan in patients with CHF. For instance, the ADVANCE (A Dose evaluation of a Vasopressin ANtagonist in CHF patients undergoing Exercise) trial is a multicenter, double-blind, placebo-controlled, randomized trial investigating the effects of conivaptan on functional capacity in patients with CHF. The primary end-point is the change in the exercise time to reach 70% of peak oxygen consumption during an incremental exercise test using a modified Naughton exercise protocol. Secondary end-points include changes in peak oxygen consumption and other exercise parameters as well as quality of life parameters. The study includes several unique features to lessen potential methodological errors of exercise testing in heart failure, including a core laboratory to evaluate exercise tests, a computer program to determine the exercise end-points, and validation of each site before patient enrollment. Three hundred and forty-five patients with class II to IV CHF and LVEF $\geq$35% will be randomized to placebo or three conivaptan doses (10, 20 or 40 mg daily doses) for 12 weeks of chronic oral treatment. Changes in both functional capacity during treadmill exercise and the symptoms of heart failure will be assessed. The time to reach 70% of peak VO_2 is the primary efficacy end-point; secondary end-points include change in submaximal VO_2 at 70% of peak work load, change in exercise time to peak work load, change in heart rate$\times$systolic blood pressure at peak exercise, and change in peak VO_2. The results of this study will provide valuable information about the use of AVP receptor antagonists for CHF treatment and also about the value of exercise testing and gas exchange determination for the evaluation of new drug therapies in CHF.

Another approach to treat CHF via modulation of AVP receptors rests on the hypothesis that expression of recombinant V2 receptors in the myocardium could result in a positive inotropic effect via the activation of the Gs/adenylyl cyclase system by elevated circulating levels of AVP. Laugwitz et al. constructed a recombinant adenovirus encoding the human V2 receptor (Ad-V2R) and infected rat ventricular cardiomyocytes and H9c2 cardiomyoblasts.[48] A virus concentration-dependent expression of the transgene was obtained and led to a marked increase in cAMP formation in recombinant V2 receptor expressing cardiomyocytes after exposure to AVP. Enhancement of AVP-induced contraction amplitude was blocked by the V2 receptor antagonist SR121463A. Gene transfer of AdV2R in rat and rabbit myocardium led to a significant increase of AVP binding and a significant increase in contraction amplitude after exposure to AVP or the V2 receptor-specific agonist dDAVP.[49] Local fractional shortening was documented by echocardiography after administration of dDAVP. Simultaneous measurement of global contractility (dP/dtmax) confirmed a positive inotropic effect of dDAVP on left ventricular function in the Ad-V2R-injected animals. These experiments suggested that the heterologous expression of cAMP-stimulating receptors in the myocardium could lead to novel strategies in the treatment of CHF by bypassing desensitized beta-adrenergic receptor-signaling cascade.

AVP AND SEPTIC SHOCK

In the United States, about 700 000 cases of sepsis occur each year and 210 000 are fatal. Sepsis is associated with a cytokine-mediated induction of NO synthesis that decreases systemic vascular resistance.[50] Sites of major vasodilation in sepsis include the splanchnic territory, the muscles, and the skin, vascular beds that contain high density of V1 receptors. During the initial phase of septic shock, plasma AVP concentration increases dramatically to the 200–300 pg/ml range. Subsequently, the neurohypophysial stores of AVP are depleted within an hour and plasma AVP concentrations fall to the 30 pg/ml range.[51] Several studies have shown that AVP plasma levels are inappropriately low in vasodilatory shock, most likely because of impaired baroreflex-mediated secretion.[52] This deficiency in AVP presumably contributes to the hypotension of vasodilatory shock. As a matter of fact, the administration of AVP in patients with sepsis-related vasodilatory shock may help maintain blood pressure despite the relative ineffectiveness of other vasopressor hormones such as norepinephrine and angiotensin.[53] Administration of exogenous AVP can raise blood pressure by 25–50 mm Hg, in relation to a large increase in systemic vascular resistances. Furthermore, AVP constricts the glomerular efferent arterioles and therefore can increase renal filtration pressure and glomerular filtration rate. A prospective randomized controlled study was performed to evaluate differences in hemodynamic response and organ functions in 48 patients with advanced vasodilatory shock receiving either a combined infusion of AVP and norepinephrine (NE) or NE alone.[54] Patients receiving AVP (4 U/h) had significantly lower heart rate, NE requirements, and incidence of new onset tachyarrhythmias than patients receiving NE only. Mean arterial pressure, cardiac index, stroke volume index, and left ventricular stroke work index were significantly higher in AVP patients. Gastrointestinal perfusion was better preserved in AVP-treated patients. This study concluded that the combined infusion of AVP and NE is superior to the infusion of NE alone in the treatment of cardiocirculatory failure in catecholamine-resistant vasodilatory shock.

CONCLUSIONS

Over the last decade, the vasoactive properties of AVP have been confirmed in various animal models and in human subjects. However, there is still no evidence that chronic treatment with an AVP receptor antagonist may be beneficial in human arterial hypertension. On the other hand, nonpeptide AVP receptor antagonists can provide symptomatic improvement in patients with advanced CHF. Such compounds are nearing regulatory approval and outcome studies are in progress to assess their impact on cardiovascular outcomes and quality of life. Administration of AVP has been shown to be beneficial in septic shock with systemic vasodilation.

ACKNOWLEDGMENTS

This work was supported by the National Institutes of Health (grant HL39757). We would like to thank Mrs Irene Bayous for her skilled assistance.

REFERENCES

1. Thibonnier M, Conarty DM, Preston JA, Wilkins PL, Berti-Mattera LN, Mattera R. Molecular pharmacology of human vasopressin receptors. Adv Exp Med Biol 1998; 449: 251–76.
2. Thibonnier M, Coles P, Thibonnier A, Shoham M. The basic and clinical pharmacology of nonpeptide vasopressin receptor antagonists. Annu Rev Pharmacol Toxicol 2001; 41: 175–202.
3. Cowley AW Jr. Vasopressin in cardiovascular regulation. In: Guyton AC, Hall JE (eds). International review of physiology. Baltimore, MD: University Park Press, 1982, pp 189–242.
4. Mori T, Dickhout JG, Cowley AW Jr. Vasopressin increases intracellular NO concentration via Ca2+ signaling in inner medullary collecting duct. Hypertension 2002; 39: 465–9.
5. Affolter JT, McKee SP, Helmy A, Jones CR, Newby DE, Webb DJ. Intra-arterial vasopressin in the human forearm: pharmacodynamics and the role of nitric oxide. Clin Pharmacol Ther 2003; 74: 9–16.
6. Burrell LM, Phillips PA, Stephenson JM, Risvanis J, Rolls KA, Johnston CI. Blood pressure lowering effect of an orally active vasopressin V1 receptor antagonist in mineralocorticoid hypertension in the rat. Hypertension 1994; 23: 737–43.
7. Intengan HD, Park JB, Schiffrin EL. Blood pressure and small arteries in DOCA-salt-treated genetically AVP-deficient rats: role of endothelin. Hypertension 1999; 34: 907–13.
8. Intengan HD, He G, Schiffrin EL. Effect of vasopressin antagonism on structure and mechanics of small arteries and vascular expression of endothelin-1 in deoxycorticosterone acetate-salt hypertensive rats. Hypertension 1998; 32: 770–7.
9. Li L, Galligan JJ, Fink GD, Chen AF. Vasopressin induces vascular superoxide via endothelin-1 in mineralocorticoid hypertension. Hypertension 2003; 41 (3 Pt 2): 663–8.
10. Burrell LM, Phillips PA, Risvanis J, Aldred KL, Hutchins AM, Johnston CI. Attenuation of genetic hypertension after short-term vasopressin V1a receptor antagonism. Hypertension 1995; 26: 828–34.
11. Iversen BM, Arendshorst WJ. Exaggerated calcium signaling in preglomerular arteriolar smooth muscle cells of genetically hyertensive rats. Am J Physiol 1999; 276: F260–F270.
12. Vagnes B, Feng JJ, Iversen BM, Arendshorst WJ. Upregulation of V1 receptors in renal resistance vessels of rats developing genetic hypertension. Am J Physiol Renal Physiol 2000; 278: F940–F948.
13. Christiansen RE, Roald AB, Gjerstad C, Tensatd O, Iversen BM. Renal hemodynamics in young and old spontaneously hypertensive rats during intrarenal infusion of arginine vasopressin. Kidney Blood Press Res 2001; 24: 176–84.
14. Vagnes BO, Hansen FH, Christiansen RE, Gjerstad C, Iversen BM. Age-dependent regulation of vasopressin V1a receptors in preglomerular vessels from the spontaneously hypertensive rat. Am J Physiol Renal Physiol 2004; 286: F997–F1003.
15. Tahara A, Tsukada J, Tomura Y et al. Alterations of renal vasopressin V1a and V2 receptors in spontaneously hypertensive rats. Pharmacology 2002; 67: 106–12.
16. Pietranera L, Saravia F, Roig P, Lima A, De Nicola AF. Mineralocorticoid treatment upregulates the hypothalamic vasopressinergic system of spontaneously hypertensive rats. Neuroendocrinology 2004; 80: 100–10.
17. Bussien JP, Waeber B, Nussberger J et al. Does vasopressin sustain blood pressure of normally hydrated healthy volunteers? Am J Physiol 1984; 246: H143–H147.
18. Waeber B, Nussberger J, Hofbauer KG, Nicod P, Brunner HR. Clinical studies with a vascular vasopressin antagonist. J Cardiovasc Pharmacol 1986; 8 (Suppl 7): S111–S116.
19. Papadoliopoulou-Diamandopoulou N, Papagalanis N, Gavras I, Gavras H. Vasopressin in end-stage renal disease: relationship to salt, catecholamines and renin activity. Clin Exp Theory Practice 1987; A9: 1197–208.
20. Ribeiro A. Sequential elimination of pressor mechanisms in severe hypertension in humans. Hypertension 1986; 8 (Suppl I): I169–I173.
21. De Paula RB, Plavnik FL, Rodrigues CIS et al. Age and race determine vasopressin participation in upright blood pressure control in essential hypertension. Ann NY Acad Sci 1993; 689: 534–6.
22. Thibonnier M, Kilani A, Rahman M et al. Effects of the nonpeptide V1 vasopressin receptor antagonist SR49059 in hypertensive patients. Hypertension 1999; 34: 1293–300.
23. Thibonnier M, Graves MK, Wagner MS, Auzan C, Clauser E, Willard HF. Structure, sequence, expression, and chromosomal localization of the human V1a vasopressin receptor gene. Genomics 1996; 31: 327–34.
24. Thibonnier M, Jeunemaitre X, Graves MK et al. Structure of the human V1a vasopressin receptor gene. In: Saito T, Kurokawa T, Yoshida S (eds). Neurohypophysis: recent progress of vasopressin and oxytocin research. Amsterdam: Elsevier, 1995, pp 553–71.
25. Kotchen TA, Kotchen JM, Grim CE et al. Genetic determinants of hypertension – identification of candidate phenotypes. Hypertension 2000; 36: 7–13.
26. Province MA, Kardia SL, Ranade K et al. A meta-analysis of genome-wide linkage scans for hypertension: the National Heart, Lung and Blood Institute Family Blood Pressure Program. Am J Hypertens 2003; 16: 144–7.
27. Jessup M, Brozena S. Heart failure. N Engl J Med 2003; 348: 2007–18.
28. Goldsmith SR. Congestive heart failure: potential role of arginine vasopressin antagonists in the therapy of heart failure. Congest Heart Fail 2002; 8: 251–6.
29. Price JF, Towbin JA, Denfield SW et al. Arginine vasopressin levels are elevated and correlate with functional status in infants

and children with congestive heart failure. Circulation 2004; 109: 2550–3.
30. Xu Y, Hopfner R, McNeill R, Gopalakrishnan V. Vasopressin accelerates protein synthesis in neonatal rat cardiomyocytes. Mol Cell Biochem 1999; 195: 183–90.
31. Francis GS, Benedict C, Johnstone DE et al. Comparison of neuroendocrine activation in patients with left ventricular dysfunction with and without congestive heart failure. A substudy of the Studies of Left Ventricular Dysfunction (SOLVD). Circulation 1990; 82: 1724–9.
32. Rouleau JL, Packer M, Moye L et al. Prognostic value of neurohumoral activation in patients with an acute myocardial infarction: effect of captopril. J Am Coll Cardiol 1994; 24: 583–91.
33. Goldsmith SR. Vasopressin antagonists in CHF: ready for clinical trials? Cardiovasc Res 2002; 54: 13–15.
34. Naitoh M, Risvanis J, Balding LC, Johnston CI, Burrell LM. Neurohormonal antagonism in heart failure; beneficial effects of vasopressin V(1a) and V(2) receptor blockade and ACE inhibition. Cardiovasc Res 2002; 54: 51–7.
35. Clair MJ, King MK, Goldberg AT et al. Selective vasopressin, angiotensin II, or dual receptor blockade with developing congestive heart failure. J Pharmacol Exp Ther 2000; 293: 852–60.
36. Burrell LM, Phillips PA, Risvanis J, Chan RK, Aldred KL, Johnston CI. Long-term effects of nonpeptide vasopressin V2 antagonist OPC-31260 in heart failure in the rat. Am J Physiol 1998; 275 (1 Pt 2): H176–H182.
37. Yatsu T, Kusayama T, Tomura Y et al. Effect of conivaptan, a combined vasopressin V(1a) and V(2) receptor antagonist, on vasopressin-induced cardiac and haemodynamic changes in anaesthetised dogs. Pharmacol Res 2002; 46: 375–81.
38. Yatsu T, Tomura Y, Tahara A et al. Cardiovascular and renal effects of conivaptan hydrochloride (YM087), a vasopressin V1A and V2 receptor antagonist, in dogs with pacing-induced congestive heart failure. Eur J Pharmacol 1999; 376: 239–46.
39. Wada K, Tahara A, Arai Y et al. Effect of the vasopressin receptor antagonist conivaptan in rats with heart failure following myocardial infarction. Eur J Pharmacol 2002; 450: 169–77.
40. Chan PS, Coupet J, Park HC et al. VPA-985, a nonpeptide orally active and selective vasopressin V_2 receptor antagonist. In: Zingg HH, Bourque CW, Bichet D (eds). Vasopressin and oxytocin. Molecular, cellular, and clinical advances. Montréal, Canada: Plenum Press, 1998, pp 439–43.
41. Wong F, Blei AT, Blendis LM, Thuluvath PJ. A vasopressin receptor antagonist (VPA-985) improves serum sodium concentration in patients with hyponatremia: a multicenter, randomized, placebo-controlled trial. Hepatology 2003; 37: 182–91.
42. Yamamura Y, Nakamura S, Ito S et al. OPC-41061, a highly potent human vasopressin V_2-receptor antagonist: pharmacological profile and aquaretic effect by single and multiple oral dosing in rats. J Pharmacol Exp Ther 1998; 287: 860–7.
43. Gheorghiade M, Niazi I, Ouyang J et al. Vasopressin V_2-receptor blockade with Tolvaptan in patients with chronic heart failure. Circulation 2003; 107: 2690–6.
44. Gheorghiade M, Gattis WA, O'Connor CM et al. Effects of tolvaptan, a vasopressin antagonist, in patients hospitalized with worsening heart failure: a randomized controlled trial. JAMA 2004; 291: 1963–71.
45. Tahara A, Tomura Y, Wada KI et al. Pharmacological profile of YM087, a novel potent nonpeptide vasopressin V1a and V2 receptor antagonist, in vitro and in vivo. J Pharmacol Exp Ther 1997; 282: 301–8.
46. Burnier M, Fricker AF, Hayoz D, Nussberger J. Pharmacokinetic and pharmacodynamic effects of YM087, a combined V_1/V_2 vasopressin receptor antagonist in normal subjects. Eur J Clin Pharmacol 1999; 55: 633–7.
47. Udelson JE, Smith WB, Hendrix GH et al. Acute hemodynamic effects of conivaptan, a dual V(1A) and V(2) vasopressin receptor antagonist, in patients with advanced heart failure. Circulation 2001; 104: 2417–23.
48. Laugwitz KL, Ungerer M, Schoneberg T et al. Adenoviral gene transfer of the human V2 vasopressin receptor improves contractile force of rat cardiomyocytes. Circulation 1999; 99: 925–33.
49. Weig HJ, Laugwitz KL, Moretti A et al. Enhanced cardiac contractility after gene transfer of V2 vasopressin receptors in vivo by ultrasound-guided injection or transcoronary delivery. Circulation 2000; 101: 1578–85.
50. Schrier RW, Wang W. Acute renal failure and sepsis. N Engl J Med 2004; 351: 159–69.
51. Landry DW, Levin HR, Gallant EM et al. Vasopressin deficiency contributes to the vasodilation of septic shock. Circulation 1997; 95: 1122–5.
52. Reid IA. Role of vasopressin deficiency in the vasodilation of septic shock. Circulation 1997; 95: 1108–10.
53. Obritsch MD, Jung R, Fish DN, MacLaren R. Effects of continuous vasopressin infusion in patients with septic shock. Ann Pharmacother 2004; 38: 1117–22.
54. Dunser MW, Mayr AJ, Ulmer H et al. Arginine vasopressin in advanced vasodilatory shock: a prospective, randomized, controlled study. Circulation 2003; 107: 2313–19.

20

Neuropeptide Y, calcitonin, calcitonin gene-related peptide and adrenomedullin

Tatsuo Shimosawa, Toshiro Fujita, Ralph Watson, Scott Supowit and Donald DiPette

INTRODUCTION

More than 100 years have passed since conventional blood pressure measurements became available.[1] Soon after the method was reported, the existence of a hypertensive agent, now known as renin, was reported.[2] Since then laboratory investigations as well as clinical and epidemiological studies have been carried out in hypertension research and have been advancing in an exponential fashion.[3] Since the 1950s, several circulating regulatory peptides, both hypertensive and hypotensive, have been discovered. Blood circulates by the pressure force generated by the cardiac output and peripheral resistance. Each of these primary determinants of the blood pressure is determined by the interaction of an exceedingly complex array of factors including vasoactive peptides. Several peptides directly regulate peripheral resistance such as angiotensin II (Ang II),[4] endothelin,[5] vasopressin,[6] and neuropeptide Y (NPY)[7] which are vasoconstrictive, and atrial natriuretic peptide,[8] calcitonin gene-related peptide (CGRP),[9] vasoactive intestinal peptide,[10] and adrenomedullin (ADM),[11] which are vasodilators. Also, there are volume-regulating peptides such as atrial natriuretic peptide,[12] vasopressin,[13] and ADM.[14] Besides these direct actions, peptides may regulate peripheral resistance and cardiac output indirectly. Peptides may interact with each other as well as regulate humoral factors such as sympathetic nerve activity, nitric oxide (NO), steroid hormones and prostaglandins. It is critical to determine the mosaic of interactions between these agents to determine the physiological role of newly found factors. In this chapter we will focus on NPY, calcitonin, CGRP, and ADM and their mechanism(s) in regulating blood pressure and their effects on end organ damage produced by hypertension.

GENERAL PROPERTIES OF NPY, CALCITONIN, CGRP, AND ADM

NPY, a 36-amino acid peptide was originally isolated from porcine brain and is highly conserved throughout evolution.[15,16] NPY-containing neurons are found in the hypothalamic paraventricular and arcuate nuclei, as well as in the catecholamine neurons of the central adrenergic cell groups. NPY is also found in the bed nucleus of the stria terminalis and the nucleus of the tractus solitarius.[17] Peripheral localization is mainly in adrenergic, norepinephrine (NE)-containing nerve fibers supplying arteries.[18] NPY binds to six Gi/o protein-coupled receptors that inhibit adenylyl cyclase, increase intracellular calcium, and activates (PKC), PLC, and MAP kinase. These receptors are found not only in the brain but also in blood vessels (predominantly Y1 and Y2 receptor). NPY is a very potent vasoconstrictor and systemic administration increases blood pressure.[19]

Calcitonin is a 32-amino acid peptide synthesized and secreted by the parafollicular C cells of the thyroid as well as extrathyroidal sites.[20] The gene for calcitonin generates two discrete messages encoding the precursor peptides for both calcitonin and CGRP.[21] Calcitonin acts directly on osteoclasts to decrease bone resorption and the removal of calcium and phosphorus from bone. The relation between calcium homeostasis and blood pressure regulation has been widely studied; however, calcitonin itself does not regulate blood pressure at physiological doses.[22,23]

CGRP is the most potent endogenous vasodilator peptide known to date.[22,23] There are two forms of CGRP, α and β, which differ in only two amino acids in rats and three in humans. α-CGRP is derived from the tissue-specific splicing of the calcitonin/CGRP gene. Whereas calcitonin is produced mainly in the C cells of the thyroid, CGRP synthesis is limited almost exclusively to specific regions of the central and peripheral nervous systems.[22,23] The β-CGRP gene that is located on the same chromosome as the calcitonin/α-CGRP gene does not produce calcitonin and is also synthesized primarily in neuronal tissues. α-CGRP is prevalent in the central nervous system and in the peripheral sensory neural network. β-CGRP is also prevalent in the central nervous system, but peripherally is common in intestinal neurons. However, the biological activities of both peptides are similar in most vascular beds.

Both forms of CGRP belong to a superfamily of closely related genes that include calcitonin, adrenomedullin, and amylin.[22,23] The α and β forms of CGRP, calcitonin, and ADM are all found on human chromosome 11, whereas amylin is located on chromosome 12. ADM, calcitonin, and amylin share structural and functional homology with CGRP, although they are less potent. Moreover, all of these genes are further related to the insulin superfamily of peptides. The agonist properties of all of the calcitonin/CGRP superfamily peptides reside at the N-terminal end (residues 1–8) and are dependent on a disulfide bridge between two cystein residues in positions 2 and 7 and an arginine at position 11 is important for receptor interactions. The highest degree of homology of these proteins that have vasodilator activity (CGRP, ADM, amylin) is found within the sequence 1–13. The C-terminal CGRP sequence 8–37 is a potent high affinity antagonist for the CGRP (and ADM) receptor and for years has been the primary antagonist used to characterize the functions of CGRP and its receptor(s). All members of the CGRP superfamily discoved to date interact with seven-transmembrane domain G protein receptors.

Immunoreactive CGRP (iCGRP) and its receptors are widely distributed in the nervous and cardiovascular systems.[22,23] In the peripheral sensory nervous system, prominent sites of CGRP synthesis are the dorsal root ganglia (DRG). These structures contain the cell bodies of sensory nerves that terminate peripherally on blood vessels and all other tissues innervated by sensory nerves and centrally in laminae I/II of the dorsal horn of the spinal cord. A dense perivascular CGRP neural network is seen around the blood vessels in all vascular beds. In these vessels CGRP-containing nerves are found at the junction of the adventitia and the media passing into the muscle layer. It is thought that circulating CGRP is largely derived from these perivascular nerve terminals and represents a spillover phenomenon related to the release of these peptides to promote vasodilation or other tissue functions. Receptors for CGRP have been identified in the media and intima of resistance vessels as well as the endothelial layer.

ADM is a 52-amino acid peptide and was originally isolated from pheochromocytoma cells but is also produced and secreted in endothelial cells.[11,24] It is a 52-amino acid peptide with a unique 6-amino acid ring structure formed by an intramolecular disulfide bond between residues 16 and 21. It also has a C-terminal amide structure. Both of these features are similar to structures found in CGRP and amylin (a 37-amino acid peptide packaged with insulin in pancreatic beta cell secretory granules that inhibits glycogen synthesis and glucose utilization). Thus ADM is considered a member of the CGRP/amylin/calcitonin superfamily of peptides. ADM has a potent and long-lasting hypotensive effect. The ADM gene is situated in a single locus of chromosome 11. ADM antagonists like ADM-(22–52) and ADM-(40–52) do not contain the ring and lack agonist activity. ADM exhibits hypotensive action by direct vasodilation via both elevating intracellular cAMP and altering calcium sensitivity in vascular smooth muscle cells.[25,26]

Preproadrenomedullin consists of 185 amino acids, and cleavage at the signal peptide between Thr^{21} and Ala^{22} yields a truncated propeptide with 164 peptides which contains ADM. Three proteolytic processing sites are found in the proadrenomedullin. The first, paired basic amino acids Lys^{43}-Arg^{44}, is a representative site for proteolytic cleavage and is preceded by Arg^{41}-Gly^{42} residue for the possible C-terminal amidation, giving the product named as proadrenomedullin N-terminal 20 peptide (PAMP).[27,28] The binding sites for ADM are abundant in a variety of tissues such as kidney, brain, spleen, heart, and adrenal glands.[29–32]

CGRP AND ADM RECEPTORS

CGRP and ADM have been shown to selectively dilate multiple vascular beds, with the coronary vasculature being a particularly sensitive target of CGRP.[33] Systemic administration of CGRP decreases blood pressure in a dose-dependent manner in normotensive and hypertensive animals and humans. The primary mechanism responsible for this reduction in blood pressure is peripheral arterial dilation. The CGRP (and ADM) receptor(s) are coupled to G proteins and in a number of tissues, including vascular smooth muscle, CGRP increases intracellular cAMP. Other reports indicate that CGRP is capable of activating K-ATP channels of vascular smooth muscle. There is additional evidence that the vasodilator response evoked by CGRP is mediated, in part, by NO release and that various vascular beds differ in their dependence on the endothelium for the dilator response to CGRP. Therefore, CGRP can dilate blood vessels through endothelium-dependent and -independent mechanisms. Originally, two types of CGRP receptors were identified. The CGRP1 receptor was characterized by high affinity binding to the aforementioned CGRP antagonist $CGRP_{8-37}$, and the CGRP2 receptor was characterized by binding to the linear agonist analog diacetoaminomethylcysteine CGRP.

The identification and characterization of the functional CGRP receptor(s) has since become very controversial, especially following the publication of the 'RAMP' (receptor activity modifying protein) hypothesis.[33] This hypothesis states that both ADM and CGRP signal through the common receptor CLR (calcitonin-like receptor). Ligand specificity is determined by co-expression of either of two chaperone proteins RAMP1 (CGRP) or RAMP2 (ADM). Another RAMP (RAMP3) has also been postulated to confer ADM specificity to the CLR. So far, three biological functions for RAMPs have been defined: they transport CLR to the cell surface, define its pharmacology, and determine its glycosylation state. In light of more recent studies, it now appears that a functional CGRP (or ADM) receptor must include three proteins in a complex: the ligand-binding, membrane-spanning protein (CLR); a chaperone (RAMP1 or 2); and a third peptide, the receptor component protein (RCP), that couples the receptor to the cellular signal transduction pathway.[33] This story has been complicated further by the cloning of a canine orphan receptor (RDC-1) that was later identified as the putative CGRP1 receptor.[33] Indeed, several pharmacologic and functional studies suggest that there are additional CGRP and/or ADM receptors that have yet to be discovered.

REGULATION OF BLOOD PRESSURE

NPY is co-stored with NE and co-released by Y1 receptor stimulation but NPY does not appear to regulate basal vascular tone. NPY transgenic rats or NPY receptor knockout mice did not show differences in basal blood pressure.[34–38] However, NPY potentiates the effects of NE and contributes to stress-induced vasoconstriction.[37] Supporting this, selective Y1 receptor blockade or genetic deletion of Y1 receptor attenuates stress-induced vasoconstriction. NPY or Y2 or Y4 receptor knockout mice studies revealed that NPY alters autonomic balance primarily by inhibiting vagal tone to regulate cardiac function.[35,36] In addition, NPY transgenic rats showed enhanced responsiveness to NE.[34] Clinically, in panic disorder, NPY is released from cardiac sympathetic nerve terminals and leads to coronary vasospasms.[39] In contrast, NPY interacts at the prejunctional level to inhibit the release of NE and when injected intracisternally, it induces hypotension and sedation.[40] Moreover in a transgenic rat study, it was shown that the lower blood pressure was associated with reduced catecholamines, lower decrease in pressure after autonomic ganglionic blockade, and increased longevity.[41]

α-CGRP has been shown to inhibit the effects of NE on the vasculature. However, it elevates blood pressure and heart rate when administered into the central amygdaloid nucleus.[42] Also, systemic administration increases catecholamine levels in humans.[43] The long-term effect of α-CGRP on blood pressure was revealed by developing α-CGRP knockout mice which are hypertensive.[43–45] α-CGRP null mice display higher basal blood pressure and heart rate together with elevated catecholamine levels. Pharmacological studies showed that α-CGRP null mice have increased sympathetic tone and diminished vagal tone. This autonomic nerve regulation by α-CGRP may be explained by α-CGRP effects on the rostral ventrolateral medulla that provides feedback to suppress the discharge and decreases sympathetic activity.[46]

Although CGRP administration can markedly decrease high blood pressure in humans, it is not clear what role CGRP plays in human hypertension. Data concerning circulating levels of iCGRP in hypertensive humans have been conflicting.[23] These results have been attributed to several factors including the assay itself, heterogeneity of the disease, severity and duration of the hypertension, the degree of end organ damage, and the variety of treatment regimens used in these patients. In contrast, a direct role for CGRP in experimental hypertension has now been established.[47] Earlier reports demonstrated that CGRP can attenuate chronic hypoxic pulmonary hypertension and we have, for the first time, demonstrated that CGRP acts as a compensatory depressor mechanism to partially attenuate the blood pressure increase in three models of experimental hypertension: 1) deoxycorticosterone acetate (DOCA-salt), 2) subtotal nephrectomy (SN-salt), and 3) L-NAME-induced hypertension during pregnancy. A similar role for CGRP has also been shown in the two-kidney one-clip model. In contrast, in the spontaneously hypertensive rat (SHR), CGRP may contribute to the development and maintenance of high blood pressure in this genetic model of hypertension.

ADM directly dilates peripheral vasculature and, moreover, when this peptide is administered centrally, it inhibits water and salt appetite.[47] It also attenuates aldosterone secretion, increases renal blood flow, and stimulates sodium excretion. These physiological effects contribute significantly to the role of ADM in regulating blood pressure.[47,48] Plasma ADM levels are increased in hypertensive patients compared with normotensive controls, especially if there is an increase in serum creatinine or renin levels. There is a progressive rise in ADM proportionate to the severity of the hypertension and the end organ damage. This suggests that ADM is released to compensate for the elevated blood pressure. After control of blood pressure with antihypertensive medication plasma ADM levels did not come down. Plasma ADM levels are directly proportional to serum creatinine levels and inversely related to glomerular filtration rates in hypertensive patients. Neither acute nor chronic salt loading changed plasma ADM levels in normotensives or essential hypertensives.

In Dahl salt-sensitive rats plasma ADM, cardiac ventricle ADM concentration, and ADM mRNA levels were higher in rats on high-salt than low-salt intake.[48] Also plasma ADM correlates well with the weight of the left ventricle. This suggests that ADM participates in the pathophysiology of salt-dependent hypertension and plays a role in cardiac hypertrophy. Also, in DOCA-treated SHRs which developed malignant hypertension, plasma ADM and renal tissue ADM are significantly higher than the levels in control rats. In addition, chronic ADM infusion in Dahl salt-sensitive rats significantly improved renal function (serum creatinine, creatinine clearance, and urinary protein excretion) and histological findings (glomerular injury score) without changing mean arterial pressure compared to untreated Dahl salt-sensitive rats. This suggests that ADM has renoprotective effects in this experimental model of hypertension. In this same model chronic infusion of ADM significantly prolonged life. Human ADM gene delivery delays the blood pressure rise and protects against cardiovascular remodeling and renal injury in several rat models of hypertension.

Although PAMP and ADM are derived from the same precursor, PAMP does not dilate the vasculature but inhibits sympathetic tone. In vivo, PAMP showed the hypotensive effect to the same extent as ADM. The hypotension evoked by PAMP was accompanied by less reflex tachycardia than that evoked by AM in the conscious, unrestrained rat. In the pithed rat, ADM but not PAMP evoked hypotension.[31] These results indicate that an interaction between PAMP and sympathetic nerve activity plays a role in the hypotensive effect of PAMP but not that of ADM. Using a mesenteric artery perfusion model, we showed that PAMP decreased NE overflow in a dose-dependent fashion, indicating that it possesses sympathoinhibitory actions.[30] PAMP inhibited α-conotoxin-sensitive calcium influx in nerve growth factor (NGF)-treated PC12 cells.[49] Thus, it has been suggested that PAMP decreases NE release from nerve endings via inhibiting calcium influx from N-type calcium channels and thus causes hypotension.

PLEIOTROPIC EFFECTS OF NPY, CALCITONIN, CGRP, AND ADM

NPY biological activities have been extensively studied using NPY transgenic, NPY null, and NPY receptor null rodents. These studies revealed that NPY is one of the major regulators of food consumption and energy homeostasis. NPY, when overexpressed in the hypothalamus, induces metabolic syndrome-like phenotype such as obesity, diabetes, and cardiovascular damage.[50] When NPY or its receptors are knocked out along with leptin (Ob/Ob mice and NPY–/–, Y1–/– or Y2–/–), they did not gain weight nor develop metabolic syndrome.[50–52] However, these effects were not observed in other obese mouse models such as A^y or agouti related peptide lacking mice.[53,54] These data suggest that the central antiobese effect of NPY is downstream of leptin. Recently Y1 knockout mice as well as selective NPY receptor antagonists and agonists demonstrated that NPY is proliferative for nestin-positive, sphere-forming hippocampal precursor cells and beta-tubulin-positive neuroblasts and that NPY has a neuroproliferative effect.[55] NPY also acts on the vasculature as a potent angiogenic factor. Unlike vascular endothelial growth factor (VEGF), microvessels induced by NPY have distinct vascular tree-like structures. This angiogenic pattern was similar to that induced by fibroblast growth factor-2, and the angiogenic response was dose-dependent. The angiogenic functions were clearly shown by Y2 knockout mice studies.[56,57] This function suggests a therapeutic use of NPY in ischemic conditions and vascular remodeling.

The α-CGRP gene also has significant protective activity against hypertension-induced heart and kidney damage. In a recent study it was shown that the DOCA-salt protocol (21 days) produced a significant 35% MAP increase in both the α-CGRP knockout and wild-type (WT) mice.[58] No pathological changes were observed in sections of aortas and femoral arteries from any of the groups studied. Likewise, heart and kidney sections from the hypertensive WT mice showed no pathological changes compared to their normotensive counterparts. In contrast, marked vasculitis was seen in the heart sections from the DOCA-salt-treated α-CGRP knockout mice. In addition, myocarditis and focal epicarditis with areas of myocardial necrosis were present. The kidneys of these mice exhibited prominent glomerular damage. Urinary microalbumin was significantly higher in the hypertensive α-CGRP knockout compared with the hypertensive WT mice. Additional histopathological, immunohistochemical, and functional studies were performed on days 0, 14, 21, and 42 after initiation of the DOCA-salt protocol. As before, renal sections from DOCA-salt WT mice showed no histopathological changes at any of the time points studied. On days 14, 21, and 42 kidney sections from the DOCA-salt α-CGRP knockout mice displayed progressive increases in the inflammatory markers ICAM-1 and VCAM-1, and MCP-1. There was a significant increase in 24-hour urinary levels including isoprostane, a marker of lipid peroxidation, at days 14, 21, and 42 in the DOCA-salt α-CGRP knockout mice compared with DOCA-salt WT mice. The hypertensive knockout mice also had significantly higher levels of urinary total protein and microalbumin and decreased creatinine clearance compared with the hypertensive WT animals. Heart sections from the DOCA-salt WT mice showed no pathological changes compared to normotensive WT mice at any time point or the CGRP knockout mice at time 0. As described previously there were progressive increases of ICAM-1, VCAM-1, and MCP-1 in coronary vessels. Serum troponin I, a marker for cardiac damage, was significantly elevated fourfold in the 21-day DOCA-salt knockout mice compared with DOCA-salt WT mice.[58] There are three possible mechanisms that underlie these observations. The first is the higher absolute MAPs in the DOCA-salt α-CGRP knockout mice compared with their WT counterparts due to the loss of a potent vasodilator system. The second is due to a direct effect of the lack of α-CGRP. The third is that permanent deletion of the α-CGRP gene may lead to alterations in other neurohumoral systems that may influence blood pressure and hypertension-induced end organ damage.

Although at this point we cannot differentiate between the three potential mechanisms discussed above, there is considerable evidence that increase in reactive oxygen species (ROS) initiates the inflammatory responses observed in a number of cardiovascular disease states including hypertension-induced end organ damage. Oxidative stress and ROS have been demonstrated in several animal models of hypertension including spontaneous hypertension, renovascular hypertension, DOCA-salt-induced hypertension, and obesity-related hypertension. DOCA-salt hypertension produced a significant increase in urinary markers of lipid peroxidation in both the α-CGRP knockout and WT mice; however, the increase was much more pronounced in the α-CGRP knockout mice. Oxidative stress leads to activation of transcription factors such as NF-κB, which in turn activate genes that trigger inflammation, including ICAM-1, VCAM-1, and MCP-1. The presence of all three markers was detectable at day 14 in the DOCA-salt α-CGRP knockout mice. This inflammatory response was progressive and by day 21 there was marked inflammation as seen by the localization and staining intensity in comparison to the absence or minimal expression of these markers in DOCA-salt WT mice.

These data demonstrate that the deletion of the α-CGRP gene enhances hypertension-induced end organ renal and cardiac damage. The mechanism of this increased tissue damage may be through the loss of α-CGRP-mediated vasodilator activity, resulting in higher blood pressure and reduced renal blood flow, leading to an increase in local tissue production of oxidative and inflammatory mediators or the loss of a direct protective effect of α-CGRP, among others. This is the first report of a sensory nerve-mediated protective effect against hypertension-induced end organ damage. Traditionally, sensory nerves were defined as purely afferent neurons that monitor changes in their chemical and physical environment and convey this information to the central nervous system. The capacity to act in an efferent manner is mediated by the release of neuropeptides, including α-CGRP, from their peripheral terminals that regulate vasodilation and other activities independently of sensation. Thus, this organ-protective activity of α-CGRP may reflect another significant function of the efferent arm of the sensory nervous system.

Homozygous ADM/PAMP knockout mice and ADM knockout mice are embryonic lethal.[59–61] So far the precise mechanism of this lethality is still unclear; however, exogenous supplementation of ADM failed to rescue the fetuses. Therefore, it has been necessary to use heterozygous ADM knockout mice for other studies as well as the rat models of acquired or genetic hypertension. For example, gene delivery to SHRs, DOCA-salt rats or Dahl salt-sensitive rats revealed that ADM decreased blood pressure and cardiac and renal end organ damage was significantly attenuated.[62–65] It has been suggested that the direct vasodilator actions of ADM plays a key role in end organ protection from hypertension. Besides this direct action, there are reports that ADM protects organs from several types of stress in an indirect fashion. In ischemic heart or kidney models,[66,67] pulmonary hypertension model[68–70] or a septic shock model,[71] ADM could protect organs from damage by inhibiting apoptosis, cell proliferation, or by inducing NO synthesis.

Numerous studies clearly demonstrate that oxidative stress is a primary cause of organ damage in a variety of pathological conditions. Specially, ischemia-reperfusion, hypertension, or diabetic conditions increase oxidative stress, thereby initiating inflammatory reactions which in turn induces vascular damage, that extends injuries throughout a number of organ systems. ADM expression is increased by oxidative stress.[70,71] At the same time, ADM inhibits formation of ROS.[72,73] Using an ADM-deficient mouse model, it appears that ADM has intrinsic antioxidant activity. Ang II and salt loading, hypoxia and mechanical stress models revealed that local oxidative stress is clearly higher in ADM-deficient mice. Concomitantly the vascular damage in coronary arteries, pulmonary arteries, and other vascular beds is more severe in ADM-deficient mice and this damage can be attenuated by administration of exogenous ADM or known antioxidants.[74–76] Moreover, in a metabolic syndrome model and also in aged mice there were markedly higher levels of oxidative stress together with insulin resistance that were reversible by SOD mimetics or ADM administration.[77–79] From these studies, it appears that like CGRP, ADM is a vascular protective peptide that may have therapeutic potential in preventing organ damage, not only by lowering blood pressure, but also by inhibiting oxidative stress in a variety of disease states.

REFERENCES

1. Riva-Rocci S. Un sfigmomanometro nuovo. Gaz Med Torino 1896; 47: 981–96.
2. Tigerstedt R, Bergman PG. Niere und Kreislauf. Skand Ark Physiol 1898; 7–8: 223–71.
3. Dickinson CJ. Neurogenic hypertension: a synthesis and review. London: Chapman & Hall, 1991.
4. Marsden PA, Brenner BM, Ballermann BJ. Mechanisms of angiotensin action on vascular smooth muscle, the adrenal, and the kidney. New York: Raven Press, 1990.
5. Yanagisawa M, Kurihara H, Kimura S et al. A novel potent vasoconstrictor peptide produced by vascular endothelial cells. Nature 1988; 332: 411–15.
6. Cowley AWJ. Vasopressin and cardiovascular regulation. Baltimore: University Park Press, 1982.
7. Pernow J. Co-release and functional interactions of neuropeptide Y and noradrenaline in peripheral sympathetic vascular control. Acta Physiol Scand 1988; Suppl 568: 1–58.
8. Fujita T, Ito Y, Noda H et al. Vasodilatory actions of alpha-human atrial natriuretic peptide and high Ca2+ effects in normal man. J Clin Invest 1987; 80: 832–40.
9. Brain SD, Williams TJ, Tippins JR, Morris HR, MacIntyre I. Calcitonin gene-related peptide is a potent vasodilator. Nature 1985; 313: 54–6.
10. Said SI. Vasoactive peptides. State-of-the-art review. Hypertension 1983; 5: I17–I26.
11. Kitamura K, Kangawa K, Kawamoto M et al. Adrenomedullin: a novel hypotensive peptide isolated from human pheochromocytoma. Biochem Biophys Res Commun 1993; 192: 553–60.
12. Blaine EH. Atrial natriuretic factor plays a significant role in body fluid homeostasis. Hypertension 1990; 15: 2–8.
13. Hall JE, Montani JP, Woods LL, Mizelle HL. Renal escape from vasopressin: role of pressure natriuresis. Am J Physiol 1986; 250: F907–F916.
14. Vari RC, Adkins SD, Samson WK. Renal effects of adrenomedullin in the rat. Proc Soc Exp Biol Med 1996; 211: 178–83.
15. Tatemoto K, Carlquist M, Mutt V. Neuropeptide Y: complete amino acid sequence of the brain peptide neuropeptide Y – a novel brain peptide with structural similarities to peptide YY and pancreatic polypeptide. Proc Natl Acad Sci U S A 1982; 79: 5485–9.
16. Tatemoto K, Carlquist M, Mutt V. Neuropeptide Y – a novel brain peptide with structural similarities to peptide YY and pancreatic polypeptide. Nature 1982; 296: 659–60.
17. Chronwall BM, DiMaggio DA, Massari VJ, Pickel VM, Ruggiero DA, O'Donohue TL. The anatomy of neuropeptide-Y-containing neurons in rat brain. Neuroscience 1985; 15: 1159–81.
18. Edvinsson L, Hakanson R, Steen S et al. Innervation of human omental arteries and veins and vasomotor response to noradrenaline, neuropeptide Y, substance P and vasoactive intestinal peptide Neuropeptide Y co-exists and co-operates with noradrenaline in perivascular nerve fibers. Regul Pept 1985; 12: 67–79.
19. Chronwall BM, Zukowska Z. Neuropeptide Y, ubiquitous and elusive. Peptides 2004; 25: 359–63.
20. Austin LA, Heath H 3rd. Calcitonin: physiology and pathophysiology. N Engl J Med 1981; 304: 269–78.
21. Amara SG, Jonas V, Rosenfeld MG, Ong ES, Evans RM. Alternative RNA processing in calcitonin gene expression generates mRNAs encoding different polypeptide products. Nature 1982; 298: 240–4.
22. Wimalawansa SJ. Calcitonin gene-related peptide and its receptors: molecular genetics, physiology, pathophysiology, and therapeutic potentials. Endocr Rev 1996; 17: 533–85.
23. DiPette DJ, Wimalawansa SJ. Cardiovascular actions of calcitonin gene-related peptide. In: Crass J, Avioli L (eds). Calicum regulating hormones and cardiovascular function. Ann Arbor, NY: CRC Press, 1994: 239.
24. Sugo S, Minamino N, Kangawa K et al. Endothelial cells actively synthesize and secrete adrenomedullin. Biochem Biophys Res Commun 1994; 201: 1160–6.
25. Kureishi Y, Kobayashi S, Nishimura J, Nakano T, Kanaide H. Adrenomedullin decreases both cytosolic Ca^{2+} concentration and Ca^{2+}-sensitivity in pig coronary arterial smooth muscle. Biochem Biophys Res Commun 1995; 212: 572–9.
26. Nuki C, Kawasaki H, Kitamura K et al. Vasodilator effect of adrenomedullin and calcitonin gene-related peptide receptors in rat mesenteric vascular beds. Biochem Biophys Res Commun 1993; 196: 245–51.
27. Kitamura K, Sakata J, Kangawa K, Kojima M, Matsuo H, Eto T. Cloning and characterization of cDNA encoding a precursor for human adrenomedullin. Biochem Biophys Res Commun 1993; 194: 720–5.
28. Sakata J, Shimokubo T, Kitamura K et al. Molecular cloning and biological activities of rat adrenomedullin, a hypotensive peptide. Biochem Biophys Res Commun 1993; 195: 921–7.

29. Iwasaki H, Hirata Y, Iwashina M, Sato K, Marumo F. Specific binding sites for proadrenomedullin N-terminal 20 peptide (PAMP) in the rat. Endocrinology 1996; 137: 3045–50.
30. Shimosawa T, Ito Y, Ando K, Kitamura K, Kangawa K, Fujita T. Proadrenomedullin NH_2-terminal 20 peptide, a new product of the adrenomedullin gene, inhibits norepinephrine overflow from nerve endings. J Clin Invest 1995; 96: 1672–6.
31. Shimosawa T, Fujita T. Hypotensive effect of newly identified peptide, proadrenomedullin N-terminal 20 peptide. Hypertension 1996; 28: 325–9.
32. Shimosawa T, Ando K, Fujita T. Newly identified peptide, proadrenomedullin N-terminal 20 peptide induces hypotensive action via pertussis toxin-sensitive G-proteins. Hypertension 1997; 30: 1009–14.
33. Brain SD, Grant AD. Vascular actions of calcitonin gene-related peptide and adrenomedullin. Physiol Rev 2004; 84: 903–34.
34. Michalkiewicz M, Michalkiewicz T, Kreulen DL, McDougall SJ. Increased blood pressure responses in neuropeptide Y transgenic rats. Am J Physiol Regul Integr Comp Physiol 2001; 281: R417–26.
35. Pedrazzini T, Seydoux J, Kunstner P et al. Cardiovascular response, feeding behavior and locomotor activity in mice lacking the NPY Y1 receptor. Nat Med 1998; 4: 722–6.
36. Naveilhan P, Hassani H, Canals JM et al. Normal feeding behavior, body weight and leptin response require the neuropeptide Y Y2 receptor. Nat Med 1999; 5: 1188–93.
37. Smith-White MA, Herzog H, Potter EK. Cardiac function in neuropeptide Y Y4 receptor-knockout mice. Regul Pept 2002; 110: 47–54.
38. Zukowska Z, Wahlestedt C. Origin and actions of neuropeptide Y in the cardiovascular system. In: Colmers WF, Wahlestedt C (eds). The biology of neuropeptide Y and related peptides. Totowa, NJ: Human Press, 1993, pp. 315–88.
39. Esler M, Alvarenga M, Lambert G et al. Cardiac sympathetic nerve biology and brain monoamine turnover in panic disorder. Ann N Y Acad Sci 2004; 1018: 505–14.
40. Edvinsson L, Hakanson R, Wahlstedt C, Uddman R. Effects of neuropeptide Y on the cardiovascular system. TIPS 1987; 8: 231–5.
41. Michalkiewicz M, Knestaut KM, Bytchkova EY, Michalkiewicz T. Hypotension and reduced catecholamines in neuropeptide Y transgenic rats. Hypertension 2003; 41: 1056–62.
42. Nguyen KQ, Sills MA, Jacobowitz DM. Cardiovascular effects produced by microinjection of calcitonin gene-related peptide into the rat central amygdaloid nucleus. Peptides 1986; 7: 337–9.
43. Howden CW, Logue C, Gavin K, Collie L, Rubin PC. Haemodynamic effects of intravenous human calcitonin-gene-related peptide in man. Clin Sci (Lond) 1988; 74: 413–18.
44. Gangula PR, Zhao H, Supowit SC et al. Increased blood pressure in alpha-calcitonin gene-related peptide/calcitonin gene knockout mice. Hypertension 2000; 35: 470–5.
45. Oh-hashi Y, Shindo T, Kurihara Y et al. Elevated sympathetic nervous activity in mice deficient in alphaCGRP. Circ Res 2001; 89: 983–90.
46. Kim S, Ouchi Y, Sekiguchi H, Fujikawa H, Shimada K, Yagi K. Endogenous calcitonin gene-related peptide modulates tachycardiac but not bradycardiac baroreflex in rats. Am J Physiol 1998; 274: H1489–H494.
47. Watson RE, Supowit SC, Zhao H, Katki KA, DiPette DJ. Role of sensory nervous system vasoactive peptides in hypertension. Br J Med Biol Res 2002; 35: 1033–45.
48. Taylor M, Shimosawa T, Samson W. Endocrine and metabolic action of adrenomedullin. Endocrinologist 2001; 11: 171–7.
49. Takano K, Yamashita N, Fujita T. Proadrenomedullin N-terminal 20 peptide inhibits the voltage-gated Ca^{2+} channel current through a pertussis toxin-sensitive G protein in rat pheochromocytoma-derived PC 12 cells. J Clin Invest 1996; 98: 14–17.
50. Kaga T, Inui A, Okita M et al. Modest overexpression of neuropeptide Y in the brain leads to obesity after high-sucrose feeding. Diabetes 2001; 50: 1206–10.
51. Erickson JC, Hollopeter G, Palmiter RD. Attenuation of the obesity syndrome of ob/ob mice by the loss of neuropeptide Y. Science 1996; 274: 1704–7.
52. Pralong FP, Gonzales C, Voirol MJ et al. The neuropeptide Y Y1 receptor regulates leptin-mediated control of energy homeostasis and reproductive functions. FASEB J 2002; 16: 712–14.
53. Sainsbury A, Schwarzer C, Couzens M, Herzog H. Y2 receptor deletion attenuates the type 2 diabetic syndrome of ob/ob mice. Diabetes 2002; 51: 3420–7.
54. Hollopeter G, Erickson JC, Palmiter RD. Role of neuropeptide Y in diet-, chemical- and genetic-induced obesity of mice. Int J Obes Relat Metab Disord 1998; 22: 506–12.
55. Qian S, Chen H, Weingarth D et al. Neither agouti-related protein nor neuropeptide Y is critically required for the regulation of energy homeostasis in mice. Mol Cell Biol 2002; 22: 5027–35.
56. Howell OW, Scharfman HE, Herzog H, Sundstrom LE, Beck-Sickinger A, Gray WP. Neuropeptide Y is neuroproliferative for post-natal hippocampal precursor cells. J Neurochem 2003; 86: 646–59.
57. Ekstrand AJ, Cao R, Bjorndahl M et al. Deletion of neuropeptide Y (NPY) 2 receptor in mice results in blockage of NPY-induced angiogenesis and delayed wound healing. Proc Natl Acad Sci U S A 2003; 100: 6033–8.
58. Supowit SC, Rao A, Bowers MC et al. Calcitonin gene-related peptide protects against hypertension induced heart and kidney damage. Hypertension 2005; 45: 109–14.
59. Lee EW, Michalkiewicz M, Kitlinska J et al. Neuropeptide Y induces ischemic angiogenesis and restores function of ischemic skeletal muscles. J Clin Invest 2003; 111: 1853–62.
60. Caron KM, Smithies O. Extreme hydrops fetalis and cardiovascular abnormalities in mice lacking a functional adrenomedullin gene. Proc Natl Acad Sci U S A 2001; 98: 615–19.
61. Shindo T, Kurihara Y, Nishimatsu H et al. Vascular abnormalities and elevated blood pressure in mice lacking adrenomedullin gene. Circulation 2001; 104: 1964–71.
62. Shimosawa T, Matsui H, Xing G, Itakura K, Ando K, Fujita T. Organ-protective effects of adrenomedullin. Hypertens Res 2003; 26: S109–S112.
63. Chao J, Jin L, Lin KF, Chao L. Adrenomedullin gene delivery reduces blood pressure in spontaneously hypertensive rats. Hypertens Res 1997; 20: 269–77.
64. Dobrzynski E, Wang C, Chao J, Chao L. Adrenomedullin gene delivery attenuates hypertension, cardiac remodeling, and renal injury in deoxycorticosterone acetate-salt hypertensive rats. Hypertension 2000; 36: 995–1001.
65. Zhang JJ, Yoshida H, Chao L, Chao J. Human adrenomedullin gene delivery protects against cardiac hypertrophy, fibrosis, and renal damage in hypertensive dahl salt-sensitive rats. Hum Gene Ther 2000; 11: 1817–27.
66. Wang C, Dobrzynski E, Chao J, Chao L. Adrenomedullin gene delivery attenuates renal damage and cardiac hypertrophy in Goldblatt hypertensive rats. Am J Physiol Renal Physiol 2001; 280: F964–F971.
67. Kato K, Yin H, Agata J, Yoshida H, Chao L, Chao J. Adrenomedullin gene delivery attenuates myocardial infarction and apoptosis after ischemia and reperfusion. Am J Physiol Heart Circ Physiol 2003; 12: 12.

68. Nishimatsu H, Hirata Y, Shindo T et al. Role of endogenous adrenomedullin in the regulation of vascular tone and ischemic renal injury: studies on transgenic/knockout mice of adrenomedullin gene. Circ Res 2002; 90: 657–63.
69. Yoshihara F, Nishikimi T, Horio T et al. Chronic infusion of adrenomedullin reduces pulmonary hypertension and lessens right ventricular hypertrophy in rats administered monocrotaline. Eur J Pharmacol 1998; 355: 33–9.
70. Nagaya N, Okumura H, Uematsu M et al. Repeated inhalation of adrenomedullin ameliorates pulmonary hypertension and survival in monocrotaline rats. Am J Physiol Heart Circ Physiol 2003; 285: H2125–H2131.
71. Chun T, Itoh H, Saito T et al. Oxidative stress augments secretion of endothelium-derived relaxing peptides, C-type natriuretic peptide and adrenomedullin. J Hypertens 2000; 18: 575–80.
72. Ando K, Ito Y, Kumada M, Fujita T. Oxidative stress increases adrenomedullin mRNA levels in cultured rat vascular smooth muscle cells. Hypertens Res 1998; 21: 187–91.
73. Chini E, Chini C, Bolliger C et al. Cytoprotective effects of adrenomedullin in glomerular cell injury: central role of cAMP signaling pathway. Kidney Int 1997; 52: 917–25.
74. Yoshimoto T, Fukai N, Sato R et al. Antioxidant effect of adrenomedullin on angiotensin II-induced reactive oxygen species generation in vascular smooth muscle cells. Endocrinology 2004; 145: 3331–7.
75. Shimosawa T, Shibagaki Y, Ishibashi K et al. Adrenomedullin, an endogenous peptide, counteracts cardiovascular damage. Circulation 2002; 105: 106–11.
76. Matsui H, Shimosawa T, Itakura K, Guanqun X, Ando K, Fujita T. Adrenomedullin can protect against pulmonary vascular remodeling induced by hypoxia. Circulation 2004; 109: 2246–51.
77. Kawai J, Ando K, Tojo A et al. Endogenous adrenomedullin protects against vascular response to injury in mice. Circulation 2004; 109: 1147–53.
78. Shimosawa T, Ogihara T, Matsui H, Asano T, Ando K, Fujita T. Deficiency of adrenomedullin induces insulin resistance by increasing oxidative stress. Hypertension 2003; 41: 1080–5.
79. Xing G, Shimosawa T, Ogihara T et al. Angiotensin II-induced insulin resistance is enhanced in adrenomedullin-deficient mice. Endocrinology 2004; 145: 3647–51.

21

Leptin and obesity-associated hypertension

Alexei V Agapitov and William G Haynes

INTRODUCTION

Obesity in humans is associated with the development of hypertension,[1] coronary atherosclerosis and myocardial hypertrophy,[2] and increased cardiovascular morbidity and mortality.[3–5] In the United States, approximately 300 000 deaths each year are associated with overweight and obesity. Obesity is also associated with increased risk for diabetes and renal failure. Since the discovery of leptin in 1994, major advances have been made in understanding of neuroendocrine mechanisms regulating appetite, metabolism, adiposity, sympathetic tone, and blood pressure.

ROLE OF LEPTIN

Leptin, a 167-amino acid protein secreted by adipocytes, circulates in proportion to the adipose tissue mass and relays a satiety signal to the hypothalamus (Figure 21.1). Leptin is transported to the central nervous system from plasma by a saturable, unidirectional system,[6] involving binding of leptin to the short form of the leptin receptor located at the endothelium of the vasculature and the epithelium of choroid plexus.[7] In addition to adipocytes, many additional sites of leptin production have recently been identified, including placenta, stomach, ovary, skeletal muscle, mammary gland, pituitary, and brain. The brain appears to make a particularly large contribution to plasma leptin in women and obese men.[8,9] Leptin acts in the hypothalamus to regulate appetite, energy expenditure, and sympathetic nervous system outflow. Leptin transduction mechanisms have been delineated over the last several years (Figure 21.2). The identification of leptin has led to the identification of novel neuroendocrine circuitry that controls appetite, energy homeostasis, sympathetic nervous system, and blood pressure.

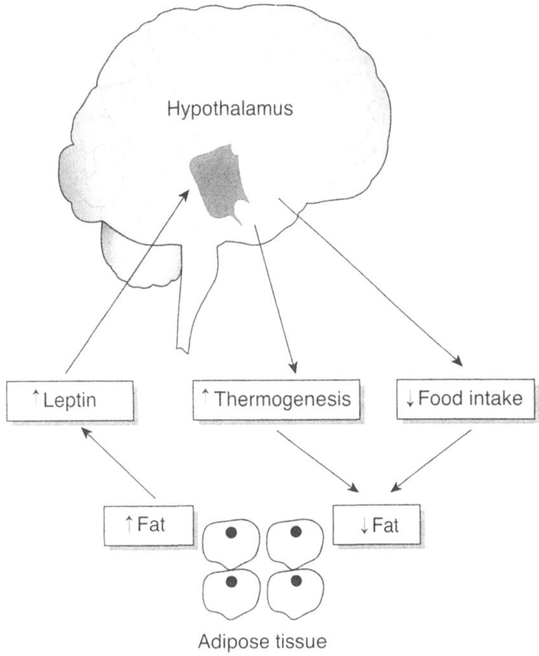

Figure 21.1 Role of leptin in the regulation of adipose tissue mass. Leptin is secreted by adipocytes and circulates in the blood in concentrations proportional to fat mass content. Leptin interaction with its receptor in the hypothalamus inhibits food intake and increases energy expenditure through stimulation of sympathetic nerve activity (SNA). This leads to a reduction in adipose tissue mass

INTRACELLULAR LEPTIN TRANSDUCTION MECHANISMS

The leptin receptor is a single transmembrane protein from the cytokine receptor superfamily. After binding to the leptin receptor, the signal is conducted via the janus kinase/signal transducer and activator of transcription

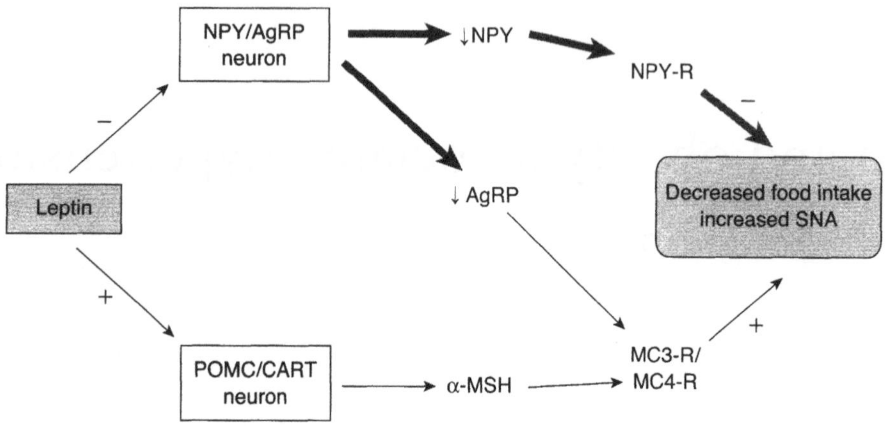

Figure 21.2 Interaction of leptin with neuropeptide Y (NPY)/agouti-related protein (AgRP)- and proopiomelanocortin (POMC)/cocaine- and amphetamine-regulated transcript (CART)-containing neurons in the hypothalamic arcuate nucleus. Leptin stimulates the POMC/CART catabolic pathway and inhibits the NPY/AgRP anabolic pathway, leading to an increase in sympathetic nerve activity (SNA) and reduced food intake

(JAK/STAT) pathway. This pathway is essential for transduction of leptin signal via the melanocortin system, and interruption of the JAK/STAT pathway in mice results in increased food intake and accumulation of adipose tissue.[10] However, compared to db/db mice lacking the long form of the leptin receptor, these mice are less prone to diabetes and their fertility is not affected, probably because of the preserved action of leptin on the neurons containing neuropeptide Y.[10] Another important signaling pathway for the control of food intake by leptin is phosphoinositol-3 kinase, because the effect of leptin on appetite is reversed by blockade of this enzyme.[11–13] Third, AMP-activated protein kinase (AMPK) has been implicated in leptin signal transduction.[13] Activation of this pathway reduces the feeding and weight-reducing actions of leptin, and leptin has been shown to decrease AMPK activity in the hypothalamus.[14]

Besides its effects in the central nervous system, there is evidence that leptin can exert various direct peripheral effects that alter metabolism. Leptin directly stimulates catecholamine synthesis in bovine adrenal medullary cells through activation and phosphorylation of tyrosine hydroxylase, activation of mitogen-activated protein kinases, and possibly altering function of Ca^{2+} channels.[15]

MECHANISMS OF LEPTIN ACTION IN THE BRAIN

The leptin receptor is expressed in several hypothalamic nuclei including the arcuate nucleus, ventromedial hypothalamus, paraventricular nucleus, and dorsomedial hypothalamus.[16,17] The arcuate nucleus is thought to be the major site of transduction of the signal from circulating leptin into a neuronal response. Local injection of leptin in this area reduces food intake. Central neural administration of leptin does not affect food intake or sympathetic nerve activity after destruction of the arcuate nucleus.[18–20] Arcuate nucleus neurons project into the paraventricular nucleus and lateral hypothalamus, which are the locations of the second order neurons in leptin signal transduction.[17] The anorexigenic, metabolic, and sympathetic actions of leptin seem to involve different neuronal circuits.[21–24]

INTERACTION OF LEPTIN AND NEUROPEPTIDES IN THE HYPOTHALAMUS

At least two main neuronal pathways account for leptin action in the brain. Leptin activates the catabolic pathway represented by proopiomelanocortin (POMC)/cocaine- and amphetamine-regulated transcript (CART) neurons and inhibits the anabolic pathway represented by the neuropeptide Y (NPY)/agouti-related protein (AgRP) neurons (Figure 21.2). Both populations of neurons (POMC/CART and NPY/AgRP) project to the paraventricular nucleus and lateral hypothalamic area.[25] The POMC/CART neurons also project to the sympathetic preganglionic neurons in the medulla and spinal cord.[25] Mice lacking leptin receptors in POMC neurons develop obesity and hyperleptinemia.[26]

Neuropeptide Y

In the hypothalamus, NPY is synthesized by neurons of the arcuate nucleus and released from their terminals in the paraventricular nucleus and lateral hypothalamus. NPY increases food intake and promotes obesity.[27,28] These effects of NPY on appetite and body weight are mediated by the NPY-Y1 and NPY-Y5 receptors in the hypothalamus.[29] Leptin-deficient mice have markedly decreased levels of NPY in the hypothalamus.[30] In addition, leptin inhibits NPY gene expression, and knockout of the NPY gene reduces obesity by about 50% in ob/ob mice.[31] Total hypothalamic NPY content negatively correlates with plasma leptin in Sprague-Dawley rats fed a high-fat diet.[32] Intracerebroventricular administration of NPY to animals decreases sympathetic activity to interscapular brown adipose tissue (BAT)[33] and kidney.[34,35] Pretreatment with leptin prevents the renal sympathoinhibitory response to NPY.[35] In obese men, higher leptin and NPY release is observed in the brain.[9] Weight loss decreases cerebrospinal fluid NPY level in obese women.[36] Therefore, inhibition of the NPY pathway appears to be an important component of central leptin action to control energy homeostasis.

Melanocortin system

The melanocortin system is also important in mediating many of leptin's actions in the central nervous system.[17] The melanocortins are peptides (such as alpha-melanocyte stimulating hormone or α-MSH) that are processed from the polypeptide precursor POMC, which is produced by neurons in the arcuate nucleus of the hypothalamus and the nucleus of the tractus solitarius. POMC deficiency leads to hyperphagia and obesity, and the effects of leptin on food intake and body weight are blunted in obese POMC (–/–) knockout mice.[37] Leptin binding to the leptin receptor on POMC neurons leads to the secretion of α-MSH, which subsequently binds to a number of a family of melanocortin receptors.[21,22,38] Five melanocortin receptors (MC-1R to MC-5R) have been described. MC-3R and MC-4R are highly expressed in the central nervous system. MC-4R has an important role in energy balance, because disruption of the MC-4R gene induces hyperphagia and obesity in mice.[39]

In addition, stimulation of hypothalamic MC-4R by central administration of MTII produces a dose-dependent increase in sympathetic nerve activity to BAT and kidney.[40] Surprisingly, MC-4R blockade prevents the sympathoexcitatory effects of leptin to the kidneys, but not to BAT.[40] These results suggest that leptin controls sympathetic nerve activity in a tissue-specific manner through different neuronal pathways.

The neurons in the arcuate nucleus that express NPY also produce a potent antagonist of MC-3R and MC-4R. This molecule is known as agouti-related peptide (AgRP).[41,42] The production of AgRP is increased by fasting and by leptin deficiency. AgRP exerts actions similar to NPY, increasing appetite and decreasing energy expenditure. Intracerebroventricular administration of AgRP causes increased food intake and obesity in mice, an effect blocked by MC-4R knockout.[43]

Other mechanisms of leptin action

Leptin-dependent sympathetic activation to BAT appears to be mediated by corticotropin releasing factor (CRF) because the sympathoexcitatory effect of leptin to this tissue was substantially inhibited by the CRF receptor antagonist.[44] Leptin down-regulates expression of CRF in the paraventricular hypothalamic nucleus in mice.[45] CRF (–/–) knockout mice have a lower leptin level, which is normalized by continuous peripheral CRF infusion.[46] These findings support the concept that leptin controls sympathetic nerve activity in a tissue-specific manner through different pathways. Multiple other anabolic and catabolic pathways are likely to be involved in leptin signal transduction.[17]

ROLE OF SYMPATHOACTIVATION IN OBESITY-ASSOCIATED HYPERTENSION

Several lines of evidence suggest that increased sympathetic nervous system activity plays a major role in obesity-associated hypertension. Plasma and urinary catecholamines are increased in animal models of obesity and in obese humans.[47–49] Obese human subjects have increased muscle sympathetic nerve activity (mSNA) compared with lean individuals.[50] In addition, body fat content is positively correlated with mSNA.[51] Furthermore, reduction in body weight from a hypocaloric diet decreases both mSNA and plasma norepinephrine.[52] Norepinephrine spillover to the kidney is increased in obese humans.[53] Elevated renal SNA is also present in animal models of obesity.[54–56] Adrenoreceptor blockade markedly decreases obesity-induced hypertension in dogs fed a high-fat diet.[57] In addition, bilateral renal denervation attenuates the antinatriuresis and the increase in arterial pressure produced by diet-induced obesity in dogs.[58] Therefore, leptin-mediated sympathoactivation likely plays a major role in obesity-induced hypertension and cardiovascular disease.

PHYSIOLOGIC AND PATHOPHYSIOLOGIC ROLES OF LEPTIN

Leptin promotes weight loss by reducing appetite and by increasing energy expenditure through stimulation of sympathetic nerve activity. Increasing leptin expression by hydrodynamics-based gene delivery leads to marked reductions in food intake and body weight in mice.[59] In animal studies, leptin caused a significant and dose-dependent increase in SNA to the kidneys, hindlimb and adrenal glands,[60,61] which suggests that leptin contributes not only to regulation of energy homeostasis, but also to the control of cardiovascular function. Indeed, chronic infusion of leptin increases arterial pressure and heart rate in conscious rats.[62] Moreover, agouti obese mice[55,63] with hyperleptinemia have elevated arterial pressure. In contrast, leptin-deficient ob/ob mice have low arterial pressure,[63] which strongly suggests a critical physiological role for leptin in maintenance of arterial pressure. Transgenic mice overexpressing leptin have elevated arterial pressure that is fully reversed by sympathetic inhibition.[64]

In humans, renal norepinephrine spillover and blood pressure correlate with plasma leptin.[65–68] Obese subjects have a higher low frequency/high frequency ratio (LF/HF), a measure of heart rate variability representing cardiac modulation by the sympathetic nervous system, and a significant correlation between LF/HF and leptin has been observed.[69] A high leptin level independently predicts stroke in men[70] and myocardial infarction in hypertensive humans.[71] Abnormalities in placental production of leptin and hyperleptinemia have been implicated in the pathogenesis of preeclampsia, although further research in this area is needed.[72] Therefore, leptin might represent one of the major links between obesity and hypertension.

RENAL EFFECTS OF LEPTIN

In humans, renal norepinephrine spillover correlates with plasma leptin, after adjustment for adiposity.[73] In addition, spectral analysis of heart rate variability in non-obese subjects demonstrated that higher fasting plasma leptin concentrations are associated with a progressive increase in sympathoactivation at rest and in response to orthostatic stimulus.[74] Despite some studies showing natriuretic effect of leptin, leptin may elevate blood pressure without increasing natriuresis, thereby adversely shifting the pressure-natriuresis curve.[75,76] Leptin administration increased blood pressure and decreased natriuresis.[77,78] Leptin-induced sodium retention may be mediated by up-regulating Na^+, K^+-ATPase.[77] Rats homozygous for a null mutation of the leptin receptor develop a significantly greater increase in systolic blood pressure in response to a high-salt diet, which is ameliorated by bosentan, an endothelin A and B receptor antagonist.[79] In addition, leptin has been shown to decrease urinary excretion of nitric oxide (NO) metabolites, possibly because of degradation of NO by reactive oxygen species.[78] Increased renal sympathetic activity combined with decreased natriuresis is likely to produce hypertension.[77,80]

DIRECT VASCULAR EFFECTS OF LEPTIN

Leptin increases NO release from endothelial cells in anesthetized Wistar rats but not in leptin receptor-deficient Zucker rats.[81] Leptin correlates with plasma NO metabolites in normotensive but not in hypertensive men.[82] In addition, leptin abolished the pressor effect of N(G)-nitro-L-arginine methyl ester in Wistar rats, suggesting additional hypotensive mechanisms.[83] High doses of leptin increase forearm blood flow[84] and cause coronary vasodilatation[85] in humans independently of NO. However, only sympathectomized rats have a depressor response to leptin, which suggests that leptin-induced sympathoexcitation opposes the direct vasodilatory effect of leptin in vivo.[81,86] However, given the strong association of leptin and hypertension, demonstrated by multiple studies, the in vivo vasodilator effects of leptin seem to be minimal compared with its sympathetic pressor effects (Figure 21.3).

SELECTIVE LEPTIN RESISTANCE

Studies in humans have shown that plasma leptin levels are significantly elevated in obese individuals relative to lean subjects.[87,88] Therefore, it appears that most obese humans are resistant to the metabolic actions of leptin, because hyperleptinemia fails to normalize adipose tissue mass in these subjects. If leptin were to contribute to obesity-related hypertension, then there would have to be preservation of its sympathoexcitatory and pressor actions in obese subjects, despite resistance to its anorexic and thermogenic weight reducing effects (i.e. selective leptin resistance).

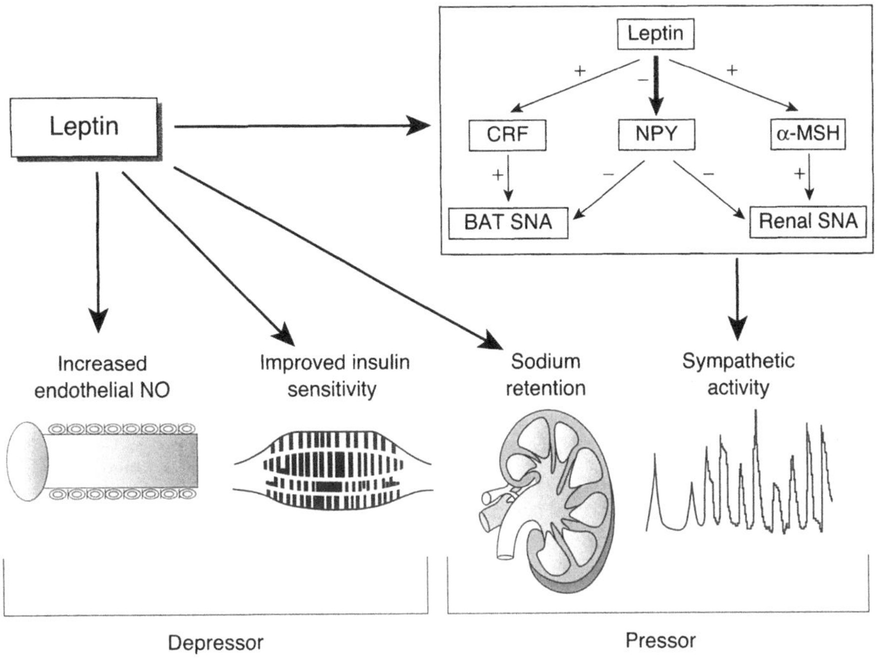

Figure 21.3 Central and peripheral leptin effects on blood pressure. Despite the potential vasodilatory effects of leptin, sympathetically mediated pressor effects predominate in vivo. The metabolic and renal sympathetic actions of leptin are mediated by different neuronal pathways. α-MSH, α-melanocyte-stimulating hormone; BAT, brown adipose tissue; CRF, corticotrophin releasing hormone; NO, nitric oxide; SNA, sympathetic nerve activity

In support of the concept of selective leptin resistance, there is evidence that leptin resistance in genetic and acquired murine obesity models is selective to the metabolic leptin actions, sparing its sympathetic pressor actions.[89] Yellow obese agouti mice, a model of monogenic obesity due to overexpression of agouti protein (endogenous melanocortin receptor inhibitor), are resistant to the anorexigenic effect of leptin but have intact sympathoexcitatory response to systemic and central neural leptin administration.[90,91] Similar results were demonstrated in mice with diet-induced obesity.[92] Mice with diet-induced obesity demonstrate preserved renal but reduced lumbar sympathoexcitation to systemic leptin administration.[93] This preserved renal sympathoactivation could contribute to the pressor effects of leptin while the reduced lumbar SNA may represent reduced thermogenic action of leptin.

Several mechanisms have been suggested to underlie leptin resistance. Saturation in the transport of leptin into the central nervous system represents one potential mechanism of leptin resistance in obesity. In support of this idea is the observation of decreased cerebrospinal fluid (CSF)/serum ratio for leptin with increasing obesity in humans.[36,87,88,94] However, obese humans still have higher CSF leptin concentrations than lean subjects. Another potential mechanism of leptin resistance involves alteration in intracellular leptin signaling pathways in the hypothalamus. It is well known that the leptin receptor, belonging to the cytokine receptor superfamily, signals via the JAK/STAT pathway. The ability of leptin to stimulate the JAK/STAT pathway is impaired in mice with high-fat diet-induced obesity.[95] In addition, a member of the suppressors of the cytokine signaling family (SOCS-3) is activated in the obese mice and potently inhibits leptin signaling.[96] SOCS-3 protein acts intracellularly to inhibit STAT phosphorylation induced by the leptin receptor. Another potential mechanism of leptin resistance is the protein tyrosine phosphatase 1b (PTP1b). This system exerts an inhibitory effect on leptin signaling, because PTP1b-deficient mice are resistant to diet-induced obesity and have increased leptin sensitivity.[97,98] Defects in the leptin receptor can lead to leptin resistance,[38] but leptin receptor mutations are rare in humans.

A dichotomy between metabolic and cardiovascular sympathetic actions of leptin is also supported by the response of leptin-induced sympathetic baroreflex activation. Baroreflex activation selectively inhibits leptin-induced renal sympathoactivation but has no effect on leptin-dependent BAT SNA.[99] Therefore, it seems that leptin-dependent renal sympathoexcitation is involved in the pressor effect of leptin and is modulated by the baroreflex, whereas leptin-induced BAT sympathoactivation is responsible for metabolic actions of leptin. The metabolic and pressor components of leptin-induced sympathoactivation seem to involve different neuronal pathways. Microinjections of leptin into the dorsomedial hypothalamic nucleus caused significant increases in arterial pressure and heart rate, but not renal sympathetic nerve activity, whereas microinjections of leptin into the ventromedial hypothalamic nucleus caused significant increases in arterial pressure and renal SNA, but not heart rate.[23] Antagonists to the melanocortin-4 receptor inhibit renal sympathoactivation to intracerebral administration of leptin but do not affect BAT sympathoactivation.[21] However, leptin-induced BAT sympathoexcitation is inhibited by a CRF receptor antagonist (Figure 21.3).[22]

It seems plausible that obese individuals could have different relative degrees of metabolic versus sympathetic leptin resistance. This could explain the fact that overweight hypertensive women have higher leptin levels than normotensive women with the same total body and abdominal fat mass.[100] In this study, weight loss led to a decrease in blood pressure and 24-hour norepinephrine excretion in hypertensive, but not in the normotensive women, despite a reduction in leptin in both groups.[100] A significant correlation was observed between the changes in the leptin and the changes in the mean blood pressure, after adjusting for the total abdominal fat and 24-hour norepinephrine excretion.[100] In addition, a graded positive relationship between plasma leptin levels and blood pressure was observed in human subjects independent of body mass index (BMI), abdominal adiposity, and insulin resistance.[101]

IMPLICATIONS FOR TREATMENT OF HYPERTENSION

Selective leptin resistance could be the crucial mechanism linking adiposity and hypertension. As humans become obese, leptin levels increase due to adipocyte accumulation. However, this hyperleptinemia fails to cause weight loss because resistance develops to leptin's anorexic and thermogenic actions (likely at the post-receptor neuronal level). However, if there is selective resistance and the sympathoexcitatory actions of leptin are preserved, then hyperleptinemia will increase arterial pressure in obese subjects. Given the strong associations between leptin, sympathoactivation, and hypertension, further research on leptin signaling is expected to lead to development of safe and effective pharmacologic treatments of obesity and subsequent reductions in obesity-induced hypertension and cardiovascular disease. In addition, measurement of leptin could become an important marker of future risk of cardiovascular disease.

REFERENCES

1. Cox BD, Whichelow MJ, Ashwell M et al. Association of anthropometric indices with elevated blood pressure in British adults. Int J Obes 1997; 21: 674–80.
2. Kortelainen ML, Sarkioja T. Coronary atherosclerosis and myocardial hypertrophy in relation to body fat distribution in healthy women: an autopsy study on 33 violent deaths. Int J Obes Relat Metab Disord 1997; 21: 43–9.
3. Lapidus L, Bengtsson C, Larsson B et al. Distribution of adipose tissue and risk of cardiovascular disease and death: a 12-year follow-up of participants in the population study of women in Gothenburg, Sweden. BMJ 1984; 289: 1257–61.
4. Hall JE. The kidney, hypertension, and obesity. Hypertension 2003; 41: 625–33.
5. Sironi AM, Gastaldelli A, Mari A et al. Visceral fat in hypertension: influence on insulin resistance and beta-cell function. Hypertension 2004; 44: 127–33.
6. Banks WA, Kastin AJ, Huang W, Jaspan JB, Maness LM. Leptin enters the brain by a saturable system independent of insulin. Peptides 1996; 17: 305–11.
7. Bjorbaek C, Elmquist JK, Michl P et al. Expression of leptin receptor isoforms in rat brain microvessels. Endocrinology 1998; 139: 3485–91.
8. Wiesner G, Vaz M, Collier G et al. Leptin is released from the human brain: influence of adiposity and gender. J Clin Endocrinol Metab 1999; 84: 2270–4.
9. Eikelis N, Lambert G, Wiesner G et al. Extra-adipocyte leptin release in human obesity and its relation to sympathoadrenal function. Am J Physiol Endocrinol Metab 2004; 286: E744–E752.
10. Bates SH, Stearns WH, Dundon TA et al. STAT3 signalling is required for leptin regulation of energy balance but not reproduction. Nature 2003; 421: 856–9.
11. Niswender KD, Schwartz MW. Insulin and leptin revisited: adiposity signals with overlapping physiological and intracellular signaling capabilities. Front Neuroendocrinol 2003; 24: 1–10.
12. Rahmouni K, Haynes WG, Morgan DA, Mark AL. Intracellular mechanisms involved in leptin regulation of sympathetic outflow. Hypertension 2003; 41: 763–7.
13. Bjorbaek C, Kahn BB. Leptin signaling in the central nervous system and the periphery. Recent Prog Horm Res 2004; 59: 305–31.
14. Minokoshi Y, Alquier T, Furukawa N et al. AMP-kinase regulates food intake by responding to hormonal and nutrient signals in the hypothalamus. Nature 2004; 428: 569–74.
15. Shibuya I, Utsunomiya K, Toyohira Y et al. Regulation of catecholamine synthesis by leptin. Ann N Y Acad Sci 2002; 971: 522–7.
16. Elmquist JK, Elias CF, Saper CB. From lesions to leptin: hypothalamic control of food intake and body weight. Neuron 1999; 22: 221–32.
17. Schwartz MW, Woods SC, Porte D Jr et al. Central nervous system control of food intake. Nature 2000; 404: 661–71.

18. Satoh N, Ogawa Y, Katsuura G et al. The arcuate nucleus as a primary site of satiety effect of leptin in rats. Neurosci Lett 1997; 224: 149–52.
19. Dawson R, Pelleymounter MA, Millard WJ et al. Attenuation of leptin-mediated effects by monosodium glutamate-induced arcuate nucleus damage. Am J Physiol 1997; 273: E202–E206.
20. Haynes WG. Interaction between leptin and sympathetic nervous system in hypertension. Curr Hypertens Rep 2000; 2: 311–18.
21. Haynes WG, Morgan DA, Djalali A et al. Interactions between the melanocortin system and leptin in control of sympathetic nerve traffic. Hypertension 1999; 33: 542–7.
22. Correia ML, Morgan DA, Mitchell JL et al. Role of corticotrophin-releasing factor in effects of leptin on sympathetic nerve activity and arterial pressure. Hypertension 2001; 38: 384–8.
23. Marsh AJ, Fontes MA, Killinger S, Pawlak DB, Polson JW, Dampney RA. Cardiovascular responses evoked by leptin acting on neurons in the ventromedial and dorsomedial hypothalamus. Hypertension 2003; 42: 488–93.
24. Bagnasco M, Dube MG, Kalra PS, Kalra SP. Evidence for the existence of distinct central appetite, energy expenditure, and ghrelin stimulation pathways as revealed by hypothalamic site-specific leptin gene therapy. Endocrinology 2002; 143: 4409–21.
25. Elmquist JK, Elias CF, Saper CB. From lesions to leptin: hypothalamic control of food intake and body weight. Neuron 1999; 22: 221–32.
26. Balthasar N, Coppari R, McMinn J et al. Leptin receptor signaling in POMC neurons is required for normal body weight homeostasis. Neuron 2004; 42: 983–91.
27. Inui, A. Transgenic approach to the study of body weight regulation. Pharmacol Rev 2000; 52: 35–61.
28. Stanley BG, Kyrkouli SE, Lampert S, Leibowitz SF. Neuropeptide Y chronically injected into the hypothalamus: a powerful neurochemical inducer of hyperphagia and obesity. Peptides 1986; 7: 1189–92.
29. Parker E, Van Heek M, Stamford A. Neuropeptide Y receptors as targets for anti-obesity drug development: perspective and current status. Eur J Pharmacol 2002; 440: 173–87.
30. Wilding JP, Gilbery SG, Bailey CJ et al. Increased neuropeptide-Y messenger ribonucleic acid (mRNA) and decreased neurotensin mRNA in the hypothalamus of the obese (ob/ob) mouse. Endocrinology 1993; 132: 1939–44.
31. Erickson JC, Hollopeter G, Palmiter RD. Attenuation of the obesity syndrome of ob/ob mice by the loss of neuropeptide Y. Science 1996; 274: 1704–7.
32. Hansen MJ, Jovanovska V, Morris MJ. Adaptive responses in hypothalamic neuropeptide Y in the face of prolonged high-fat feeding in the rat. J Neurochem 2004; 88: 909–16.
33. Egawa M, Yoshimatsu H, Bray GA. Neuropeptide Y suppresses sympathetic activity to interscapular brown adipose tissue in rats. Am J Physiol 1991; 260: R328–R334.
34. Chen XL, Knuepfer MM, Westfall TC. Hemodynamic and sympathetic effects of spinal administration of neuropeptide Y in rats. Am J Physiol 1990; 259: H1674–H1680.
35. Matsumura K, Tsuchihashi T, Abe I. Central cardiovascular action of neuropeptide Y in conscious rabbits. Hypertension 2000; 36: 1040–4.
36. Nam SY, Kratzsch J, Kim KW, Kim KR, Lim SK, Marcus C. Cerebrospinal fluid and plasma concentrations of leptin, NPY, and alpha-MSH in obese women and their relationship to negative energy balance. J Clin Endocrinol Metab 2001; 86: 4849–53.
37. Challis BG, Coll AP, Yeo GS et al. Mice lacking pro-opiomelanocortin are sensitive to high-fat feeding but respond normally to the acute anorectic effects of peptide-YY(3–36). Proc Nat Acad Sci U S A 2004; 101: 4695–700.
38. Clement K, Vaisse C, Lahlou N et al. A mutation in the human leptin receptor gene causes obesity and pituitary dysfunction. Nature 1998; 392: 398–401.
39. Huszar D, Lynch CA, Fairchild-Huntress V et al. Targeted disruption of the melanocortin-4 receptor results in obesity in mice. Cell 1997; 88: 131–41.
40. Haynes WG, Morgan DA, Djalali A et al. Interactions between the melanocortin system and leptin in control of sympathetic nerve traffic. Hypertension 1999; 33: 542–7.
41. Graham M, Shutter JR, Sarmiento U et al. Overexpression of Agrt leads to obesity in transgenic mice. Nat Genet 1997; 17: 273–4.
42. Ollmann MM, Wilson BD, Yang YK et al. Antagonism of central melanocortin receptors in vitro and in vivo by agouti-related protein. Science 1997; 278: 135–8.
43. Fekete C, Marks DL, Sarkar S et al. Effect of agouti-related protein in regulation of the hypothalamic-pituitary-thyroid axis in the melanocortin 4 receptor knockout mouse. Endocrinology 2004; 145: 4816–21.
44. Correia MLG, Morgan DA, Mitchell JL et al. Role of corticotrophin-releasing factor in effects of leptin on sympathetic nerve activity and arterial pressure. Hypertension 2001; 38: 384–8.
45. Arvaniti K, Huang Q, Richard D. Effects of leptin and corticosterone on the expression of corticotropin-releasing hormone, agouti-related protein, and proopiomelanocortin in the brain of ob/ob mouse. Neuroendocrinology 2001; 73: 227–36.
46. Jeong KH, Sakihara S, Widmaier EP, Majzoub JA. Impaired leptin expression and abnormal response to fasting in corticotropin-releasing hormone-deficient mice. Endocrinology 2004; 145: 3174–81.
47. Rocchini AP, Moorhead CP, Deremer S, Bondi D. Pathogenesis of weight-related pressure changes in blood pressure in dogs. Hypertension 1989; 13: 922–8.
48. Sowers JR, Whitfield LA, Catania RA et al. Role of the sympathetic nervous system in blood pressure maintenance in obesity. J Clin Endocrinol Metab 1982; 54: 1181–6.
49. Young JB, Landsberg L. Diet-induced changes in sympathetic nervous system activity: possible implications for obesity and hypertension. J Chronic Dis 1982; 35: 879–86.
50. Grassi G, Servalle G, Cattaneo BM et al. Sympathetic activation in obese normotensive subjects. Hypertension 1995; 25: 560–3.
51. Jones PP, Snitker S, Skinner JS et al. Gender differences in muscle sympathetic nerve activity: effect of body fat distribution. Am J Physiol 1996; 33: E363–E366.
52. Grassi G, Seravalle G, Colombo M et al. Body weight reduction, sympathetic nerve traffic, and arterial baroreflex in obese normotensive humans. Circulation 1998; 97: 2037–42.
53. Vaz M, Jennings G, Turner A et al. Regional sympathetic nervous activity and oxygen consumption in obese normotensive human subjects. Circulation 1997; 96: 3423–9.
54. Iwashita S, Tanida M, Terui N et al. Direct measurement of renal sympathetic nervous activity in high-fat diet-related hypertensive rats. Life Sci 2002; 71: 537–46.
55. Rahmouni K, Haynes WG, Morgan DA, Mark AL. Selective resistance to central neural administration of leptin in agouti obese mice. Hypertension 2002; 39: 486–90.
56. Morgan DA, Anderson EA, Mark AL. Renal sympathetic nerve activity is increased in obese Zucker rats. Hypertension 1995; 25: 834–8.
57. Hall JE, Hildebrandt DA, Kuo J, Fitzgerald S. Role of sympathetic nervous system and neuropeptides in obesity hypertension. Braz J Med Biol Res 2000; 33: 605–18.
58. Kassab S, Kato T, Wilkins C et al. Renal denervation attenuates the sodium retention and hypertension associated with obesity. Hypertension 1995; 25: 893–7.

59. Jiang J, Yamato E, Miyazaki J. Long-term control of food intake and body weight by hydrodynamics-based delivery of plasmid DNA encoding leptin or CNTF. J Gene Med 2003; 5: 977–83.
60. Haynes WG, Morgan DA, Walsh SA et al. Receptor-mediated regional sympathetic nerve activation by leptin. J Clin Invest 1997; 100: 270–8.
61. Dunbar JC, Hu Y, Lu H. Intracerebroventricular leptin increases lumbar and renal sympathetic nerve activity and blood pressure in normal rats. Diabetes 1997; 46: 2040–3.
62. Shek EW, Brands MW, Hall JE. Chronic leptin infusion increases arterial pressure. Hypertension 1998; 32: 376–7.
63. Mark AL, Shaffer RA, Correia ML et al. Contrasting blood pressure effects of obesity in leptin-deficient ob/ob mice and agouti yellow obese mice. J Hypertens 1999; 17: 1949–53.
64. Aizawa-Abe M, Ogawa Y, Masuzaki H et al. Pathophysiological role of leptin in obesity-related hypertension. J Clin Invest 2000; 105: 1243–52.
65. Agata J, Masuda A, Takada M et al. High plasma immunoreactive leptin level in essential hypertension. Am J Hypertens 1997; 10: 1171–4.
66. Canatan H, Bakan I, Akbulut M, Baydas G, Halifeoglu I, Gursu MF. Comparative analysis of plasma leptin levels in both genders of patients with essential hypertension and healthy subjects. Endocr Res 2004; 30: 95–105.
67. Nishina M, Kikuchi T, Yamazaki H, Kameda K, Hiura M, Uchiyama M. Relationship among systolic blood pressure, serum insulin and leptin, and visceral fat accumulation in obese children. Hypertens Res 2003; 26: 281–8.
68. Eikelis N, Schlaich M, Aggarwal A, Kaye D, Esler M. Interactions between leptin and the human sympathetic nervous system. Hypertension 2003; 41: 1072–9.
69. Amador N, Perez-Luque E, Malacara JM, Guizar JM, Paniagua R, Lara S. Leptin and heart sympathetic activity in normotensive obese and non-obese subjects. Ital Heart J 2004; 5: 29–35.
70. Soderberg S, Stegmayr B, Stenlund H et al. Leptin, but not adiponectin, predicts stroke in males. J Intern Med 2004; 256: 128–36.
71. Wallerstedt SM, Eriksson AL, Niklason A, Ohlsson C, Hedner T. Serum leptin and myocardial infarction in hypertension. Blood Press 2004; 13: 243–6.
72. Anderson CM, Ren J. Leptin, leptin resistance and endothelial dysfunction in pre-eclampsia. Cell Mol Biol 2002; 48: OL323–9.
73. Eikelis N, Schlaich M, Aggarwal A et al. Interactions between leptin and the human sympathetic nervous system. Hypertension 2003; 41: 1072–9.
74. Paolisso G, Manzella D, Montano N et al. Plasma leptin concentrations and cardiac autonomic nervous system in healthy subjects with different body weights. J Clin Endocrinol Metab 2000; 85: 1810–14.
75. Jackson EK, Li P. Human leptin has natriuretic activity in the rat. Am J Physiol Renal Physiol 1997; 272: F333–F338.
76. Carlyle M, Jones OB, Kuo JJ, Hall JE. Chronic cardiovascular and renal actions of leptin: role of adrenergic activity. Hypertension 2002; 39: 496–501.
77. Beltowski J, Jamroz-Wisniewska A, Borkowska E, Wojcicka G. Up-regulation of renal Na(+), K(+) ATPase: the possible novel mechanism of leptin-induced hypertension. Pol J Pharmacol 2004; 56: 213–22.
78. Beltowski J, Wojcicka G, Marciniak A, Jamroz A. Oxidative stress, nitric oxide production, and renal sodium handling in leptin-induced hypertension. Life Sci 2004; 74: 2987–3000.
79. Radin MJ, Holycross BJ, Hoepf TM, McCune SA. Increased salt sensitivity secondary to leptin resistance in SHHF rats is mediated by endothelin. Mol Cell Biochem 2003; 242: 57–63.
80. Coatmellec-Taglioni G, Dausse JP, Giudicelli Y, Ribiere C. Sexual dimorphism in cafeteria diet-induced hypertension is associated with gender-related difference in renal leptin receptor down-regulation. J Pharmacol Exp Ther 2003; 305: 362–7.
81. Fruhbeck G. Pivotal role of nitric oxide in the control of blood pressure after leptin administration. Diabetes 1999; 48: 903–8.
82. Tsuda K, Nishio I. Leptin and nitric oxide production in normotensive and hypertensive men. Obes Res 2004; 12: 1223–37.
83. Beltowski J, Wojcicka G, Borkowska E. Human leptin stimulates systemic nitric oxide production in the rat. Obes Res 2002; 10: 939–46.
84. Nakagawa K, Higashi Y, Sasaki S et al. Leptin causes vasodilation in humans. Hypertens Res 2002; 25: 161–5.
85. Matsuda K, Teragawa H, Fukuda Y et al. Leptin causes nitric-oxide independent coronary artery vasodilation in humans. Hypertens Res 2003; 26:147–52.
86. Lembo G, Vecchione C, Fratta L et al. Leptin induces direct vasodilation through distinct endothelial mechanisms. Diabetes 2000; 49: 293–7.
87. Considine RV, Sinha MK, Heiman ML et al. Serum immunoreactive-leptin concentrations in normal-weight and obese humans. N Engl J Med 1996; 334: 292–5.
88. Halaas JL, Boozer C, Blair-West J et al. Physiological response to long-term peripheral and central leptin infusion in lean and obese mice. Proc Natl Acad Sci U S A 1997; 94: 8878–83.
89. Mark AL, Correia ML, Rahmouni K, Haynes WG. Selective leptin resistance: a new concept in leptin physiology with cardiovascular implications. J Hypertens 2002; 20: 1245–50.
90. Correia ML, Haynes WG, Rahmouni K et al. The concept of selective leptin resistance: evidence from agouti yellow obese mice. Diabetes 2002; 51: 439–42.
91. Rahmouni K, Haynes WG, Morgan DA, Mark AL. Selective resistance to central neural administration of leptin in agouti obese mice. Hypertension 2002; 39: 486–90.
92. Morgan DA, Rahmouni K, Mark AL et al. Selective leptin resistance during high fat diet in mice: preservation of sympathetic activation despite attenuation of metabolic responses [abstract]. Hypertension 2001; 38: 34.
93. Rahmouni K, Morgan DA, Morgan GM et al. Renal-specific preservation of sympathoexcitatory effect of leptin in diet-induced obese mice [abstract]. Hypertension 2003; 42: 421.
94. Van Heek M, Compton DS, France CF et al. Diet-induced obese mice develop peripheral, but not central, resistance to leptin. J Clin Invest 1997; 99: 385–90.
95. El-Haschimi K, Pierroz DD, Hileman SM et al. Two defects contribute to hypothalamic leptin resistance in mice with diet-induced obesity. J Clin Invest 2000; 105: 1827–32.
96. Bjorbaek C, El-Haschimi K, Frantz JD, Flier JS. The role of SOCS-3 in leptin signaling and leptin resistance. J Biol Chem 1999; 274: 30059–65.
97. Zabolotny JM, Bence-Hanulec KK, Stricker-Krongrad A et al. PTP1B regulates leptin signal transduction in vivo. Dev Cell 2002; 2: 489–95.
98. Cheng A, Uetani N, Simoncic PD et al. Attenuation of leptin action and regulation of obesity by protein tyrosine phosphatase 1B. Dev Cell 2002; 2: 497–503.
99. Hausberg M, Morgan DA, Chapleau MA et al. Differential modulation of leptin-induced sympathoexcitation by baroreflex activation. J Hypertens 2002; 20: 1633–41.
100. Itoh K, Imai K, Masuda T et al. Relationship between changes in serum leptin levels and blood pressure after weight loss. Hypertens Res 2002; 25: 881–6.
101. Barba G, Russo O, Siani A et al. Plasma leptin and blood pressure in men: graded association independent of body mass and fat pattern. Obes Res 2003; 11: 160–6.

22

Molecular aspects of the natriuretic peptide system

David G Gardner, Songcang Chen, Dolkun Rahmutula, Feng Wang and Keith Olsen

INTRODUCTION

The natriuretic peptides (NPs) collectively constitute a family of hormonal peptides that play important roles in the control of renal, cardiovascular, and skeletal homeostasis. Atrial natriuretic peptide (ANP), the first member of the group to be identified, is a 28-amino peptide in humans that assumes a hairpin structure by virtue of a cysteine bridge linking residues 7 and 23 (Figure 22.1). This hairpin structure typifies each of the natriuretic peptides. It is conserved across species and is required for functional activity. Brain natriuretic peptide (BNP), also known as the B-type natriuretic peptide, is 32 amino acids long in the human. It demonstrates considerably more heterogeneity across species than ANP. CNP is a 22-amino acid peptide which has a truncated carboxy-terminus distal to the second cysteine residue in the bridge.

ANP and BNP are produced primarily in the myocardium of the heart. ANP is preferentially expressed and secreted from the cardiac atria vs ventricle, while chamber-specific expression is less marked for BNP. ANP is also expressed in a variety of extra-cardiac locations, including the hypothalamus, where it is thought to participate in regulation of blood pressure and cardiovascular homeostasis. Ironically, BNP is produced in the brains of only a limited number of species (pig and dog predominantly). CNP is produced in the central nervous system, the reproductive tract, bone, and the endothelium of blood vessels.

There are three types of NP receptors and all three span the membrane bilayer as a single transmembrane segment. The type A natriuretic peptide receptor (NPR-A), also known as guanylyl cyclase A (GC-A), is the high affinity receptor for both ANP and BNP. It has a large extracellular domain followed by the transmembrane spanning segment, a noncatalytic, ATP-binding, kinase-like domain (KLD) in the proximal intracellular portion of the molecule, which is thought to function in an autoregulatory mode, and a short

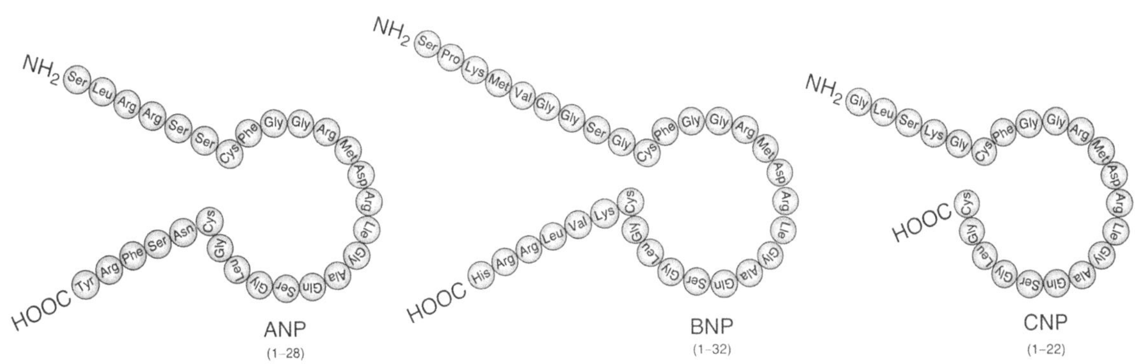

Figure 22.1 Structure of human natriuretic peptides

hinge region (Figure 22.1). The carboxy-terminus of NPR-A harbors a particulate guanylyl cyclase which provides the catalytic effector of the receptor. Association of NPR-A with ANP or BNP results in a conformational change in the molecule, likely involving the KLD, which releases a tonic inhibition of guanylyl cyclase activity and increases production of cyclic guanosine 3′,5′ monophosphate (cyclic GMP). NPR-B is similar to NPR-A in terms of its overall structure and it shares 44% sequence homology at the amino acid level in the extracellular (ligand binding) domain and 74% homology in the intracellular domain.[1] It binds selectively to CNP. NPR-C, the so-called clearance receptor, has a large extracellular domain followed by a single transmembrane-spanning segment, but it harbors only 37 amino acids in its intracellular domain. It binds with relatively high affinity to all three natriuretic peptides, as well as to a variety of other peptides which have only limited structural similarity to the NPs. It is thought to function largely in a clearance mode, removing NPs from the extracellular compartment and processing them for subsequent degradation; however, it may also possess signaling activity that does not directly involve cyclic GMP production, but rather a G protein transducer like G_i.

This chapter will focus on the molecular underpinnings of the NP systems and the role that each plays in contributing to normal homeostasis.

TRANSCRIPTIONAL REGULATION OF THE NP GENES

Expression of the ANP and BNP genes in the heart is often controlled in parallel by a variety of factors extrinsic to the cardiac myocyte. These include α adrenergic agonists, endothelin (ET), prostaglandin $F_{2\alpha}$, growth factors, vitamin D, retinoids, glucocorticoids, mechanical strain, and hypoxia, among others. Coincidentally, there is a close correlation between those factors that lead to up-regulation of ANP and BNP gene expression and those that lead to myocyte hypertrophy. The link between hypertrophic growth and NP expression has led to identification of the latter as among the most highly conserved markers of hypertrophy-dependent gene transcription across different pathophysiological paradigms and different species. Detailed descriptions of NP gene expression have been provided in earlier reviews;[2,3] this chapter will focus on more recent investigations.

The rat ANP gene is controlled by members of the GATA transcription factor family (factors that bind to the sequence WGATAR where W is A/T and R is A/G), particularly GATA 4 and 6. There are paired GATA sites located at −280 and −120 relative to the transcription start site of the rat ANP gene.[4] Similarly positioned GATA sites are shared with the mouse and human genes. Transient transfection of a GATA 4 expression vector along with an ANP promoter-driven reporter resulted in a moderate induction of reporter activity.[5] GATA sites have also been identified in the rat[5] and human[6–8] BNP gene promoters. Paired sites are positioned at roughly −96 and −84 in both species. Mutation of these sites leads to a reduction in promoter activity[7–9] and forced expression of GATA-4 leads to increased expression.[5,7,10] A third GATA site is positioned at −30 in both rat and human genes and represents a TATA box equivalent. Mutation of this site leads to a predictable reduction in hBNP promoter activity. It is noteworthy, however, that mutation of the GATA to a more conventional TATA motif results in an increase in promoter activity[11] (D.G. Gardner, unpublished observations), implying that this GATA site may have a unique function in this promoter. GATA has been shown to be phosphorylated on Ser_{105} by p38 mitogen activated protein kinase (MAPK), resulting in increased binding of the factor to DNA and activation of contiguous gene transcription.[12,13] GATA sites in the BNP gene promoter have been linked to the stimulatory activity of lipolysaccharide,[9] β adrenergic agonists,[7] endothelin, operating through a Rho kinase signaling pathway,[13] and mechanical strain/hemodynamic overload.[14,15] GATA-4 has been shown to physically contact and synergize functionally with GATA-6,[16] MEF-2,[17] dHAND,[18] SRF,[19] Nkx2.5[20,21] and YY1.[22] In the case of dHAND[18] and YY1[22] and GATA-5,[23] the functional synergy appears to occur by virtue of recruitment of the coactivators p300 and CBP into the transcriptional complex. The friend of GATA (FOG-2), a corepressor that binds specifically to GATA-4, directly interacts with chicken ovalbumin upstream promoter transcription factor 2 (COUP-TF2) and blocks its stimulation of the chicken ANP promoter.[24] *Jumonjii* is thought to mediate its inhibition of rANP gene transcription through direct interaction with and subsequent inhibition of GATA-4 and Nkx2.5.[25] GATA-independent interactions (e.g. between dHAND and MEF-2c and between PITX2 and MEF2A) can also occur at the level of the ANP promoter.[26,27]

AP1 binding elements, which associate with various members of the *jun/fos* transcription factor family, have been identified in both the human ANP and BNP genes. The site in the hANP gene promoter has been shown to be required for maintenance of basal promoter activity.[28] Importantly, different members of the

Jun and *Fos* families display differential activity at the level of the hANP promoter[28,29] with c-*Fos* inhibiting and *fra1* stimulating activity. For undefined reasons, the rat ANP gene appears to be negatively regulated by both *c-Jun* and *c-Fos*.[30] It does, however, harbor a *Fos*- but not *Jun*-activatable AP1 binding element (*Jun* is thought to tether *Fos* to the promoter) which is potentiated by activated MAPK.[29] Similar AP1 sites have been identified at −394 in the rBNP gene and at −109 in the hBNP gene.[14] Mutation of each has been shown to lead to a significant reduction in basal promoter activity[14] (F. Wang and D.G. Gardner, unpublished observations).

Transcription enhancing factor (TEF)-binding sites or M-CAT sites have been identified in the proximal promoter (−110 in the rat with paired sites at −123 and −94 in human). Mutation of these sites leads to a pronounced decrease in basal promoter activity.[8,31] Mutation of the rat M-CAT site has been linked to loss of α adrenergic agonist-dependent rBNP promoter activity.[31]

Pikkarainen et al. recently identified an Ets binding site at position -498 in the rBNP gene that traffics ET-dependent promoter activity through a p38 MAPK pathway.[32]

Kuwahara et al.[33] identified a neuron restrictive silencer element (NRSE) in the 3′ untranslated region of the rat ANP gene which regulates both basal and ET-dependent gene transcription in ventricular myocytes. A similar NRSE has been identified in the hBNP 5′ FS.[8,34] Mutation of this site reduces basal promoter activity and blunts the response to fibronectin. NRSF (neuron restrictive silencer factor), which binds to the NRSE, is believed to control expression of the fetal gene program during hypertrophy.[35] Transgenic mice that overexpress a dominant negative mutant of NRSF display dilated cardiomyopathy, and increased susceptibility to arrhythmias and sudden death. An E box motif upstream (−1152) in the hBNP gene has also been shown to harbor transcriptional repressor activity.[11]

A serum response factor-binding site (SRE) has been identified in both the rat and human ANP genes.[8,36] Mutation of this site at −241 in the human promoter reduces basal activity and impairs the response to ET operating through a Src-[36] and p130 Cas-dependent pathway.[37]

The BNP gene transcriptional response to mechanical strain has been linked to three shear stress response element-like structures in the 5′ FS of that gene (located at −650, −641, and −160). Mutation of these sites reduces strain-dependent promoter activation by ~50%, as does inhibition of p38 MAPK and NF-κB-dependent signaling pathways, suggesting that the latter ultimately signal through the SSREs.[38,39] Mutation of an NF-AT site at −927 in the human BNP gene leads to a reduction in ET-dependent activation of the BNP promoter.[40] This, in concert with parallel studies, has implicated the calcineurin/NF-AT pathway in signaling the hypertrophic response in the cardiac myocyte.[41] As noted above, the strain response has also been linked to the presence of intact GATA binding sites in the proximal promoter.[14,15]

Members of the extended nuclear receptor hormone family – e.g. vitamin D receptor (VDR), peroxisome proliferator activated receptor (PPAR), retinoic acid and retinoid X receptors – have been shown to reduce basal and agonist-stimulated ANP and BNP gene transcription. While the inhibitory promoter loci for the VDR[42–45] and PPARα[8] appear to track to proximal 5′FS, there has yet to be a definitive identification of the critical DNA binding element(s). On the other hand a thyroid hormone receptor binding element (TRE) has been identified at ~1 kb upstream from the transcription start site. This element binds to liganded thyroid hormone receptor in vitro and appears to traffic the bulk of thyroid hormone-dependent stimulation of hBNP promoter activity.[46] A schematic diagram depicting the known transcriptional regulatory elements in the human ANP and BNP genes is presented in Figure 22.2.

Of note, Deschepper and colleagues have recently determined that sequence differences in the proximal rat ANP promoter are linked to reduced promoter activity and, consequently, diminished ANP gene expression in the WKHA vs WKY rat.[47,48] WKHA rats have exaggerated cardiac hypertrophy relative to the WKY. The nature of the transcription factor(s) that interacts with this site remains undefined; however, these studies add to a growing body of data[49–55] suggesting that the NPs exert protective, anti-hypertrophic activity in the myocardium.

Relatively little is known of the transcriptional regulation of the CNP gene promoter. Like that of its cognate receptor,[56] the CNP gene appears to require GC-rich regions in the proximal promoter to support basal transcriptional activity.[57] Subsequent analyses have suggested that TSC-22, a transforming growth factor (TGF)-β-stimulated transcription factor, is likely to play a role in controlling CNP gene transcription.[58]

REGULATION OF THE NP RECEPTORS

As noted above, NP receptors differ to some degree in structure, signaling capacity and ligand specificity

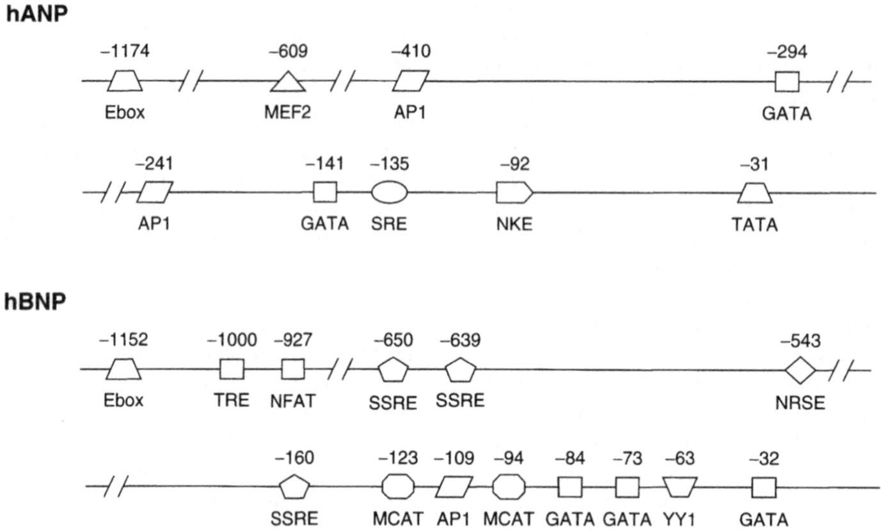

Figure 22.2 Overview of the 5′ flanking region of human atrial natriuretic peptide (ANP) and brain natriuretic peptide (BNP) genes. Documented functional elements are shown. Numbers are relative to the transcription start site

(Figure 22.3). Partial structures of NPR-A[59] and NPR-C[60] have been solved, revealing important details of receptor–ligand interactions. The genomic structures of mouse,[61] rat[62] and human[63,64] NPR-A, human NPR-B,[56,65] and mouse[66] and human[67] NPR-C have been reported; however, only a limited amount of information has been reported about the specific regulatory elements that govern their transcriptional activity. Regulation of rat NPR-A gene transcriptional activity is governed by three Sp1 binding sites (at −341, −282 and −56) in the promoter.[68,69] Mutation of these sites led to >90% reduction in promoter activity. These Sp1 sites synergistically interact with an NF-Y site (at −141) to control >95% of basal promoter activity.[69] A contiguous series of Sp1 sites positioned between −118 and −83 in the human NPR-B gene also play a dominant role in the regulation of basal promoter activity.[56]

NPR-A activity, gene expression and promoter activity are negatively regulated by its cognate ligand ANP through a mechanism that appears to require cyclic GMP.[70,71] Promoter inhibition is conveyed by sequence positioned between −1575 and −1290 relative to the transcription start site, a region which has been shown to harbor the sequence AaAtRKaNTTCaAcAkTY that is thought to represent the cyclic GMP-dependent regulatory element in this gene.[72] NPR-A is also regulated by 1,25-dihydroxyvitamin D through a single vitamin D response element in the 5′ flanking sequence of the gene.[73] This effect may account for at least some of the salutary effects of vitamin D in the cardiovascular system. 1,25-dihydroxyvitamin D has also been shown to up-regulate NPR-C gene expression in mouse osteoblasts.[74] TGF-β decreases levels of both NPR-A and NPR-B mRNA, but the precise mechanism(s) underlying these reductions remains undefined.[75] Glucocorticoids have been shown to up-regulate[76,77] or down-regulate[78,79] NPR-A, -B or -C mRNA levels in different cellular contexts. NPR-C expression is also down-regulated by beta 2-adrenergic stimulation in vascular smooth muscle cells,[80] an action that enhances the response to ANP by reducing clearance of the latter. NPR-A has also been shown to be negatively regulated by angiotensin II[81] and positively regulated by osmotic stimuli[82] through a signaling pathway that involves the endothelial nitric oxide synthase and p38 MAPK.[83]

The NPRs are also regulated at a post-transcriptional level. Desensitization of NPR-A activity is observed following exposure to ANP[84] or activation of protein kinase C.[85] ANP-dependent desensitization requires dephosphorylation of six phosphoserines or phosphothreonines (Ser_{497}, Thr_{500}, Ser_{502}, Ser_{506}, Ser_{510} and Thr_{513}) in the kinase homology domain of the receptor.[86] Similar dephosphorylation of five residues (Ser_{513}, Thr_{516}, Ser_{518}, Ser_{523} and Ser_{526}) in NPR-B was found to be responsible for desensitization of NPR-B by CNP.[87,88] Interestingly, in contrast to the CNP-dependent desensitization, activation of protein kinase C largely resulted in dephosphorylation of a single site at Ser_{523}.[89] NPR-B desensitization by hyperosmotic

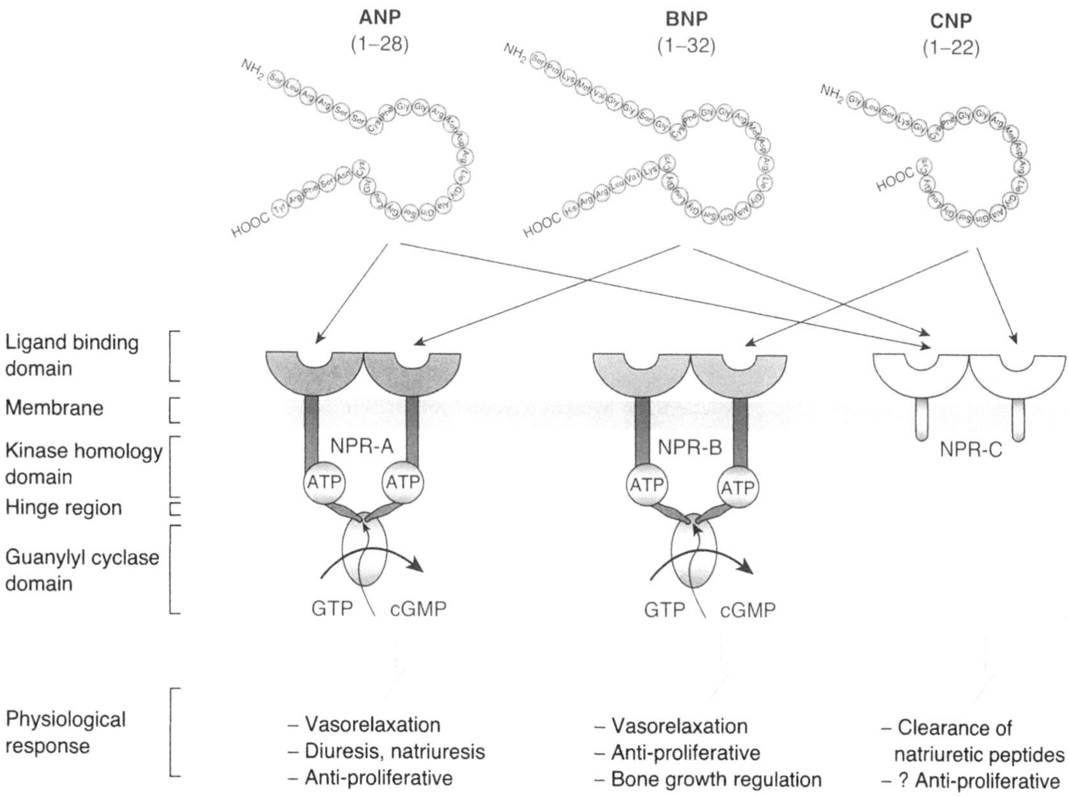

Figure 22.3 Structure and function of the natriuretic peptide receptors

stimuli or lysophosphatidic acid appears to require calcium-dependent dephosphorylation of the receptor.

Thus, as pointed out by Foster and Garbers[90] adenine nucleotides exert two separate regulatory functions in controlling NPR activity – the first as a substrate for phosphorylation (and activation) of the receptors and the second as an allosteric regulator of receptor activity through noncatalytic interactions with the kinase homology domain.

GENETIC MANIPULATION OF THE NP SYSTEMS

A number of laboratories have taken advantage of newer technologies to manipulate the natriuretic peptide systems genetically (see Table 22.1). These studies have provided extraordinary insights into the physiology of these systems. Steinhelper and colleagues[91] overexpressed the mouse ANP gene in the livers (using the transthyretin gene promoter) of transgenic mice. Plasma ANP levels were increased more than eightfold. Blood pressure fell by almost 30 mm Hg, albeit without accompanying natriuresis or diuresis. Elevated ANP levels inhibit the development of hypoxic pulmonary hypertension in these mice,[92] but at least in this instance, did not reduce endogenous ANP expression under normoxic or chronic hypoxic conditions. These mice maintain normal salt excretion despite reduction in blood pressure,[93] presumably reflecting direct effects of ANP on glomerular hemodynamics or tubular transport. Volume challenge was accompanied by a dramatic increase in urinary volume and sodium excretion relative to the controls. These animals also demonstrated increased water intake and excretion, which is inferred to be due to ANP-dependent antagonism of vasopressin-induced water permeability in the terminal nephron.[94]

Genetic deletion of the ANP gene locus was first reported by John et al.[95] The homozygous knockout mice had no circulating or atrial ANP. BPs were increased by 8 and 23 mm Hg when animals were fed standard (0.5%) or intermediate (2%) NaCl diets. Heterozygotes had normal blood pressure on standard diet but blood pressure increased by 27 mm Hg on 8% NaCl. This salt-sensitive hypertension may reflect, at

Table 22.1 Summary of the phenotypes associated with genetic manipulation of the natriuretic peptide system

Gene Disruption	*Phenotype/Physiology*	*References*
ANP overexpression	Hypotension, decrease in hypoxic hypertension, normal salt excretion, increased H_2O intake and excretion	91–94
ANP knockout ($Nppa^{-/-}$)	Salt-sensitive hypertension, blood pressure-independent right and left ventricular hypertrophy, impaired Na and Cl excretion	95, 97–99, 101
BNP overexpression	Hypotension, skeletal overgrowth, resistance to immune-mediated renal injury	102–104
BNP knockout ($Nppb^{-/-}$)	Load-dependent ventricular fibrotic lesions, no hypertrophy, no hypertension	106, 107
CNP knockout ($Nppc^{-/-}$)	Dwarfism, early death	108
CNP overexpression (chondrocyte targeted)	Rescue of dwarfism phenotype	109
NPR-A (GC-A) overexpression	Hypotension, protection against salt-sensitive hypertension	111
NPR-A (GC-A) knockout ($Npr1^{-/-}$)	Salt-resistant hypertension, blood pressure-independent ventricular hypertrophy, increase in sudden death	51, 54, 55, 110
Targeted knockout		
cardiomyocyte	Hypertrophy, increase in hypertrophy markers, hypotension	114
smooth muscle	Loss of ANP response, volume-dependent hypertension	115
NPR-A (GC-A) overexpression in cardiac myocytes in $Npr^{-/-}$	Reduction in myocyte size and ANP gene expression, no effect on blood pressure	55
NPR-B (GC-B) knockout ($Npr2^{-/-}$)	Dwarfism, neuronal disorders, female infertility	117
NPR-C knockout ($Npr3^{-/-}$)	Hypotension, bone overgrowth, reduced blood volume	119

least in part, the inability of these mice to completely suppress plasma renin activity.[96] It was shown subsequently that the homozygous mutants have increased right and left ventricular hypertrophy under normal conditions[97,98] and this is exaggerated (relative to controls) in response to transverse aortic constriction.[98] This was associated with enhanced expression of a variety of extracellular matrix proteins (e.g. osteopontin) and metalloproteinases (e.g. matrix metalloproteinase-2), suggesting that ANP negatively regulates those signaling pathways involved in matrix remodeling in the myocardium. Right and Left ventricular hypertrophy, peripheral pulmonary vessel muscularization and right ventricular peak pressure in homozygous ANP knockout mice were increased relative to heterozygous knockouts or wild-type mice[97] following 3 weeks of hypoxia. Importantly, Feng et al.[99] showed that normalization of blood pressure in the ANP knockout animals through administration of a low salt diet failed to reverse the hypertrophy in these animals, suggesting that ANP exerts a direct anti-hypertrophic effect on the cardiac myocyte, a hypothesis that has subsequently been supported by a combination of in vitro[49,50] and in vivo studies.[51–55] ANP knockout mice also displayed an impaired diuretic response to acute saline infusion.[100] Blood pressures were higher in the knockouts but there were no differences in glomerular filtration rate. Despite this the knockouts had an impaired ability to excrete Na and Cl, suggesting inappropriate reabsorption of these ions in the medullary collecting duct.[101] Collectively, these studies demonstrate that ANP reduces blood pressure without significantly altering urinary sodium excretion at steady-state and that ANP is not essential for maintenance of normal salt balance but is essential for the natriuresis that accompanies acute expansion of intravascular volume.

Transgenic overexpression of the mouse BNP gene under the control of the liver-specific human serum amyloid P component promoter led to plasma BNP levels that were 10–100-fold elevated above normal and a significant increase in plasma cyclic GMP levels.[102] This resulted in a reduction in blood pressure relative to their non-transgenic littermates. Over the longer term these animals developed pronounced skeletal overgrowth resulting in marked kyphosis of the spine, elongation of limbs and crooked tails.[103] In vitro analyses revealed that BNP increased the height of the cartilaginous primordium leading to increased longitudinal bone growth. Subsequent studies from Suganami et al.[104] showed that the BNP transgenic mice are somewhat resistant to immune-mediated renal injury. These animals displayed less albuminuria and improved histological and functional scores relative to wild-type animals following renal injury. Also of note, BNP transgenic mice displayed increased neutrophil infiltration and cardiac matrix metalloproteinase-9 expression after acute myocardial infarction,[105] implying a potential role for the peptide in myocardial remodeling.

Mice with BNP gene deletion, unlike their ANP-deleted counterparts, displayed no hypertension or ventricular hypertrophy.[106] They did display multifocal fibrotic lesions in the ventricles, which increased in size and number in response to ventricular overload, suggesting that BNP subserves a role as an antifibrotic factor in vivo.[106,107]

Deletion of CNP results in somatic dwarfism and early death.[108] The bone lesion is characterized by impaired endochondral ossification; the skeletal phenotypes were similar to those seen in human achondroplasia. Importantly, targeted expression of CNP to the growth plate chondrocytes both rescued the skeletal phenotype of the *Nppc–/–* mice and prolonged their survival. Targeted overexpression of CNP in chondrocytes was subsequently shown to rescue the dwarfed phenotype in a mouse model of achondroplasia with activated fibroblast growth factor receptor 3 in cartilage.[109]

Deletion of the type A natriuretic peptide receptor (NPR-A or guanylyl cyclase-A/GC-A receptor) resulted in salt-resistant hypertension, cardiac hypertrophy, and an increased incidence of cardiac sudden death.[51,110] Subsequently blood pressures were shown to be directly proportional to the number of copies of the NPR-A gene present.[111] Virtually all cardiovascular effects of ANP and BNP were lost in the NPR-A knockout mouse, suggesting that these peptides signal physiological activity almost exclusively through the NPR-A receptor.[52] As with the ANP knockouts described above, NPR-A knockout mice have a normal ability to respond to changes in dietary sodium concentration but impaired ability to generate a natriuretic response to acute iso-oncotic volume expansion.[112,113] Similarly, NPR-A gene deletion worsens right ventricular hypertrophy and causes left ventricular hypertrophy in response to chronic hypoxia.[53] The cardiac hypertrophy seen in these mice appears to reflect, in large part, the loss of a direct anti-hypertrophic effect of the liganded NPR-A in the heart. Pharmacological control of blood pressure in these animals failed to reverse left ventricular hypertrophy and the mice hyper-responded to transverse aortic constriction with an increase in left venticular mass and activation of ANP gene expression relative to wild-type controls.[54] Overproduction of NPR-A selectively in the hearts of the NPR-A knockout mice resulted in reductions in myocyte size and ANP gene expression.[55] Finally, selective inactivation of the NPR-A gene locus in the heart resulted in mild hypertrophy and significantly increased expression of the hypertrophic marker genes ANP, α skeletal actin and β myosin heavy chain. Interestingly, blood pressures were lower in these animals, presumably reflecting the peripheral hormonal effects of increased levels of circulating ANP.[114] Selective deletion of NPR-A in smooth muscle cells had no effect on systemic blood pressure but it did eliminate the hypotensive response to infused ANP.[115] Acute vascular expansion in these animals led to a rapid and significant increase in blood pressure in the gene-deleted but not in the wild-type mice. Presumably blood pressure elevations in the latter were blocked by endogenous ANP.[115] Interestingly, inactivation of the NPR-A gene locus appears to alleviate ischemia/reperfusion injury through suppression of NF-κB-mediated P-selectin induction, as does the NPR-A antagonist HS-142–1, implying that blockade of this system may prove useful in limiting reperfusion injury clinically.[116]

NPR-B gene knockout mice display significant impairment of endochondral ossification and diminished longitudinal growth in vertebra and limbs.[117] Developmental abnormalities in the female reproductive tract which resulted in female infertility were also seen. The mice were not hypertensive under a variety of salt loading paradigms. Interestingly, mutations in the human NPR-B gene have been associated with

Maroteaux-type acromesomelic dysplasia,[118] further supporting the link between the CNP/NPR-B system and normal longitudinal bone growth.

Deletion of the NPR-C gene leads to low blood pressure (8 mm Hg below normal), mild diuresis, and reduced blood volume, presumably reflecting the longer half-life of endogenous NPs. Noteworthy, these animals also have a bone phenotype which is similar to that seen in the BNP transgenics. In this case, it is thought to reflect failure to clear and, thereby control, the effects of locally synthesized CNP.[119]

ACKNOWLEDGMENTS

Supported by HL45637 and HL35753 from the NIH and grants from the American Heart Association and American Diabetes Association. D.R. is supported by a postdoctoral fellowship from the AHA Western Affiliate. F.W. is supported by an NRSA.

REFERENCES

1. Chang MS, Lowe DG, Lewis M, Hellmiss R, Chen E, Goeddel DV. Differential activation by atrial and brain natriuretic peptides of two different receptor guanylate cyclases. Nature 1989; 341: 68–72.
2. Levin ER, Gardner DG, Samson WK. Natriuretic peptides. N Engl J Med 1998; 339: 321–8.
3. Gardner D, Wu J, Kovacic-Milivojevic B. Cellular and molecular aspects of A-type natriuretic peptide. In: Samson WK, Levin ER (eds). Natriuretic peptides in health and disease. Totowa: Humana Press; 1997, pp 71–94.
4. McBride K, Nemer M. Regulation of the ANF and BNP promoters by GATA factors: lessons learned for cardiac transcription. Can J Physiol Pharmacol 2001; 79: 673–81.
5. Grepin C, Dagnino L, Robitaille L, Haberstroh L, Antakly T, Nemer M. A hormone-encoding gene identifies a pathway for cardiac but not skeletal muscle gene transcription. Mol Cell Biol 1994; 14: 3115–29.
6. LaPointe MC, Wu G, Garami M, Yang XP, Gardner DG. Tissue-specific expression of the human brain natriuretic peptide gene in cardiac myocytes. Hypertension 1996; 27: 715–22.
7. He Q, Mendez M, LaPointe MC. Regulation of the human brain natriuretic peptide gene by GATA-4. Am J Physiol Endocrinol Metab 2002; 283: E50–E57.
8. Liang F, Wang F, Zhang S, Gardner DG. Peroxisome proliferator activated receptor (PPAR)alpha agonists inhibit hypertrophy of neonatal rat cardiac myocytes. Endocrinology 2003; 144: 4187–94.
9. Tomaru Ki K, Arai M, Yokoyama T et al. Transcriptional activation of the BNP gene by lipopolysaccharide is mediated through GATA elements in neonatal rat cardiac myocytes. J Mol Cell Cardiol 2002; 34: 649–59.
10. Liang Q, Wiese RJ, Bueno OF, Dai YS, Markham BE, Molkentin JD. The transcription factor GATA4 is activated by extracellular signal-regulated kinase 1- and 2-mediated phosphorylation of serine 105 in cardiomyocytes. Mol Cell Biol 2001; 21: 7460–9.
11. Garami M, Gardner DG. An E-box motif conveys inhibitory activity on the atrial natriuretic peptide gene. Hypertension 1996; 28: 315–9.
12. Liang Q, De Windt LJ, Witt SA, Kimball TR, Markham BE, Molkentin JD. The transcription factors GATA4 and GATA6 regulate cardiomyocyte hypertrophy in vitro and in vivo. J Biol Chem 2001; 276: 30245–53.
13. Charron F, Tsimiklis G, Arcand M et al. Tissue-specific GATA factors are transcriptional effectors of the small GTPase RhoA. Genes Dev 2001; 15: 2702–19.
14. Marttila M, Hautala N, Paradis P et al. GATA4 mediates activation of the B-type natriuretic peptide gene expression in response to hemodynamic stress. Endocrinology 2001; 142: 4693–700.
15. Pikkarainen S, Tokola H, Majalahti-Palviainen T et al. GATA-4 is a nuclear mediator of mechanical stretch-activated hypertrophic program. J Biol Chem 2003; 278: 23807–16.
16. Charron F, Paradis P, Bronchain O, Nemer G, Nemer M. Cooperative interaction between GATA-4 and GATA-6 regulates myocardial gene expression. Mol Cell Biol 1999; 19: 4355–65.
17. Morin S, Charron F, Robitaille L, Nemer M. GATA-dependent recruitment of MEF2 proteins to target promoters. Embo J 2000; 19: 2046–55.
18. Dai YS, Cserjesi P, Markham BE, Molkentin JD. The transcription factors GATA4 and dHAND physically interact to synergistically activate cardiac gene expression through a p300-dependent mechanism. J Biol Chem 2002; 277: 24390–8.
19. Morin S, Paradis P, Aries A, Nemer M. Serum response factor-GATA ternary complex required for nuclear signaling by a G-protein-coupled receptor. Mol Cell Biol 2001; 21: 1036–44.
20. Durocher D, Charron F, Warren R, Schwartz RJ, Nemer M. The cardiac transcription factors Nkx2-5 and GATA-4 are mutual cofactors. Embo J 1997; 16: 5687–96.
21. Shiojima I, Komuro I, Oka T et al. Context-dependent transcriptional cooperation mediated by cardiac transcription factors Csx/Nkx-2.5 and GATA-4. J Biol Chem 1999; 274: 8231–9.
22. Bhalla SS, Robitaille L, Nemer M. Cooperative activation by GATA-4 and YY1 of the cardiac B-type natriuretic peptide promoter. J Biol Chem 2001; 276: 11439–45.
23. Kakita T, Hasegawa K, Morimoto T, Kaburagi S, Wada H, Sasayama S. p300 protein as a coactivator of GATA-5 in the transcription of cardiac-restricted atrial natriuretic factor gene. J Biol Chem 1999; 274: 34096–102.
24. Huggins GS, Bacani CJ, Boltax J, Aikawa R, Leiden JM. Friend of GATA 2 physically interacts with chicken ovalbumin upstream promoter-TF2 (COUP-TF2) and COUP-TF3 and represses COUP-TF2-dependent activation of the atrial natriuretic factor promoter. J Biol Chem 2001; 276: 28029–36.
25. Kim TG, Chen J, Sadoshima J, Lee Y. Jumonji represses atrial natriuretic factor gene expression by inhibiting transcriptional activities of cardiac transcription factors. Mol Cell Biol 2004; 24: 10151–60.
26. Zang MX, Li Y, Xue LX, Jia HT, Jing H. Cooperative activation of atrial naturetic peptide promoter by dHAND and MEF2C. J Cell Biochem 2004; 93: 1255–66.
27. Toro R, Saadi I, Kuburas A, Nemer M, Russo AF. Cell-specific activation of the atrial natriuretic factor promoter by PITX2 and MEF2A. J Biol Chem 2004; 279: 52087–94.
28. Kovacic-Milivojevic B, Gardner DG. Regulation of the human atrial natriuretic peptide gene in atrial cardiocytes by the transcription factor AP-1. Am J Hypertens 1993; 6: 258–63.
29. McBride K, Nemer M. The C-terminal domain of c-fos is required for activation of an AP-1 site specific for jun-fos heterodimers. Mol Cell Biol 1998; 18: 5073–81.

30. McBride K, Robitaille L, Tremblay S, Argentin S, Nemer M. fos/jun repression of cardiac-specific transcription in quiescent and growth-stimulated myocytes is targeted at a tissue-specific cis element. Mol Cell Biol 1993; 13: 600–12.
31. Thuerauf DJ, Glembotski CC. Differential effects of protein kinase C, Ras, and Raf-1 kinase on the induction of the cardiac B-type natriuretic peptide gene through a critical promoter-proximal M-CAT element. J Biol Chem 1997; 272: 7464–72.
32. Pikkarainen S, Tokola H, Kerkela R, Majalahti-Palviainen T, Vuolteenaho O, Ruskoaho H. Endothelin-1-specific activation of B-type natriuretic peptide gene via p38 mitogen-activated protein kinase and nuclear ETS factors. J Biol Chem 2003; 278: 3969–75.
33. Kuwahara K, Saito Y, Ogawa E et al. The neuron-restrictive silencer element-neuron-restrictive silencer factor system regulates basal and endothelin 1-inducible atrial natriuretic peptide gene expression in ventricular myocytes. Mol Cell Biol 2001; 21: 2085–97.
34. Ogawa E, Saito Y, Kuwahara K et al. Fibronectin signaling stimulates BNP gene transcription by inhibiting neuron-restrictive silencer element-dependent repression. Cardiovasc Res 2002; 53: 451–9.
35. Kuwahara K, Saito Y, Takano M et al. NRSF regulates the fetal cardiac gene program and maintains normal cardiac structure and function. Embo J 2003; 22: 6310–21.
36. Kovacic B, Ilic D, Damsky CH, Gardner DG. c-Src activation plays a role in endothelin-dependent hypertrophy of the cardiac myocyte. J Biol Chem 1998; 273: 35185–93.
37. Kovacic-Milivojevic B, Roediger F, Almeida EA, Damsky CH, Gardner DG, Ilic D. Focal adhesion kinase and p130Cas mediate both sarcomeric organization and activation of genes associated with cardiac myocyte hypertrophy. Mol Biol Cell 2001; 12: 2290–307.
38. Liang F, Gardner DG. Mechanical strain activates BNP gene transcription through a p38/NF-kappaB-dependent mechanism. J Clin Invest 1999; 104: 1603–12.
39. Liang F, Lu S, Gardner DG. Endothelin-dependent and -independent components of strain-activated brain natriuretic peptide gene transcription require extracellular signal regulated kinase and p38 mitogen-activated protein kinase. Hypertension 2000; 35: 188–92.
40. Molkentin JD, Lu JR, Antos CL et al. A calcineurin-dependent transcriptional pathway for cardiac hypertrophy. Cell 1998; 93: 215–28.
41. Wilkins BJ, De Windt LJ, Bueno OF et al. Targeted disruption of NFATc3, but not NFATc4, reveals an intrinsic defect in calcineurin-mediated cardiac hypertrophic growth. Mol Cell Biol 2002; 22: 7603–13.
42. Li Q, Gardner DG. Negative regulation of the human atrial natriuretic peptide gene by 1,25-dihydroxyvitamin D3. J Biol Chem 1994; 269: 4934–9.
43. Chen S, Wu J, Hsieh JC et al. Suppression of ANP gene transcription by liganded vitamin D receptor: involvement of specific receptor domains. Hypertension 1998; 31: 1338–42.
44. Chen S, Cui J, Nakamura K, Ribeiro RC, West BL, Gardner DG. Coactivator-vitamin D receptor interactions mediate inhibition of the atrial natriuretic peptide promoter. J Biol Chem 2000; 275: 15039–48.
45. Chen S, Costa CH, Nakamura K, Ribeiro RC, Gardner DG. Vitamin D-dependent suppression of human atrial natriuretic peptide gene promoter activity requires heterodimer assembly. J Biol Chem 1999; 274: 11260–6.
46. Liang F, Webb P, Marimuthu A, Zhang S, Gardner DG. Triiodothyronine increases brain natriuretic peptide (BNP) gene transcription and amplifies endothelin-dependent BNP gene transcription and hypertrophy in neonatal rat ventricular myocytes. J Biol Chem 2003; 278: 15073–83.
47. Masciotra S, Picard S, Deschepper CF. Cosegregation analysis in genetic crosses suggests a protective role for atrial natriuretic factor against ventricular hypertrophy. Circ Res 1999; 84: 1453–8.
48. Deschepper CF, Masciotra S, Zahabi A, Boutin-Ganache I, Picard S, Reudelhuber TL. Functional alterations of the Nppa promoter are linked to cardiac ventricular hypertrophy in WKY/WKHA rat crosses. Circ Res 2001; 88: 223–8.
49. Ito T, Yoshimura M, Nakamura S et al. Inhibitory effect of natriuretic peptides on aldosterone synthase gene expression in cultured neonatal rat cardiocytes. Circulation 2003; 107: 807–10.
50. Calderone A, Thaik CM, Takahashi N, Chang DL, Colucci WS. Nitric oxide, atrial natriuretic peptide, and cyclic GMP inhibit the growth-promoting effects of norepinephrine in cardiac myocytes and fibroblasts. J Clin Invest 1998; 101: 812–8.
51. Oliver PM, Fox JE, Kim R et al. Hypertension, cardiac hypertrophy, and sudden death in mice lacking natriuretic peptide receptor A. Proc Natl Acad Sci U S A 1997; 94: 14730–5.
52. Lopez MJ, Garbers DL, Kuhn M. The guanylyl cyclase-deficient mouse defines differential pathways of natriuretic peptide signaling. J Biol Chem 1997; 272: 23064–8.
53. Klinger JR, Warburton RR, Pietras L et al. Targeted disruption of the gene for natriuretic peptide receptor-A worsens hypoxia-induced cardiac hypertrophy. Am J Physiol Heart Circ Physiol 2002; 282: H58–H65.
54. Knowles JW, Esposito G, Mao L et al. Pressure-independent enhancement of cardiac hypertrophy in natriuretic peptide receptor A-deficient mice. J Clin Invest 2001; 107: 975–84.
55. Kishimoto I, Rossi K, Garbers DL. A genetic model provides evidence that the receptor for atrial natriuretic peptide (guanylyl cyclase-A) inhibits cardiac ventricular myocyte hypertrophy. Proc Natl Acad Sci U S A 2001; 98: 2703–6.
56. Rahmutula D, Cui J, Chen S, Gardner DG. Transcriptional regulation of type B human natriuretic peptide receptor gene promoter: dependence on Sp1. Hypertension 2004; 44: 283–8.
57. Ohta S, Shimekake Y, Nagata K. Cell-type-specific function of the C-type natriuretic peptide gene promoter in rat anterior pituitary-derived cultured cell lines. Mol Cell Biol 1993; 13: 4077–86.
58. Ohta S, Shimekake Y, Nagata K. Molecular cloning and characterization of a transcription factor for the C-type natriuretic peptide gene promoter. Eur J Biochem 1996; 242: 460–6.
59. van den Akker F, Zhang X, Miyagi M, Huo X, Misono KS, Yee VC. Structure of the dimerized hormone-binding domain of a guanylyl-cyclase-coupled receptor. Nature 2000; 406: 101–4.
60. He X, Chow D, Martick MM, Garcia KC. Allosteric activation of a spring-loaded natriuretic peptide receptor dimer by hormone. Science 2001; 293: 1657–62.
61. Garg R, Oliver PM, Maeda N, Pandey KN. Genomic structure, organization, and promoter region analysis of murine guanylyl cyclase/atrial natriuretic peptide receptor-A gene. Gene 2002; 291: 123–33.
62. Yamaguchi M, Rutledge LJ, Garbers DL. The primary structure of the rat guanylyl cyclase A/atrial natriuretic peptide receptor gene. J Biol Chem 1990; 265: 20414–20.
63. Takahashi Y, Nakayama T, Soma M, Izumi Y, Kanmatsuse K. Organization of the human natriuretic peptide receptor A gene. Biochem Biophys Res Commun 1998; 246: 736–9.
64. Nakayama T, Soma M, Takahashi Y, Rehemudula D, Kanmatsuse K, Furuya K. Functional deletion mutation of the 5′-flanking region of type A human natriuretic peptide receptor gene and its association with essential hypertension and left ventricular hypertrophy in the Japanese. Circ Res 2000; 86: 841–5.

65. Rehemudula D, Nakayama T, Soma M et al. Structure of the type B human natriuretic peptide receptor gene and association of a novel microsatellite polymorphism with essential hypertension. Circ Res 1999; 84: 605–10.
66. Yanaka N, Kotera J, Taguchi I, Sugiura M, Kawashima K, Omori K. Structure of the 5′-flanking regulatory region of the mouse gene encoding the clearance receptor for atrial natriuretic peptide. Eur J Biochem 1996; 237: 25–34.
67. Yanaka N, Kotera J, Omori K. Isolation and characterization of the 5'-flanking regulatory region of the human natriuretic peptide receptor C gene. Endocrinology 1998; 139: 1389–400.
68. Liang F, Schaufele F, Gardner DG. Sp1 dependence of natriuretic peptide receptor A gene transcription in rat aortic smooth muscle cells. Endocrinology 1999; 140: 1695–701.
69. Liang F, Schaufele F, Gardner DG. Functional interaction of NF-Y and Sp1 is required for type A natriuretic peptide receptor gene transcription. J Biol Chem 2001; 276: 1516–22.
70. Cao L, Wu J, Gardner DG. Atrial natriuretic peptide suppresses the transcription of its guanylyl cyclase-linked receptor. J Biol Chem 1995; 270: 24891–7.
71. Cao L, Chen SC, Cheng T, Humphreys MH, Gardner DG. Ligand-dependent regulation of NPR-A gene expression in inner medullary collecting duct cells. Am J Physiol 1998; 275: F119–F125.
72. Hum D, Besnard S, Sanchez R et al. Characterization of a cGMP-response element in the guanylyl cyclase/natriuretic peptide receptor A gene promoter. Hypertension 2004; 43: 1270–8.
73. Chen S, Ni XP, Humphreys MH, Gardner DG. 1,25 dihydroxyvitamin D amplifies type A natriuretic peptide receptor expression and activity in target cells. J Am Soc Nephrol 2005; 16: 329–39.
74. Yanaka N, Akatsuka H, Kawai E, Omori K. 1,25-Dihydroxyvitamin D3 upregulates natriuretic peptide receptor-C expression in mouse osteoblasts. Am J Physiol 1998; 275: E965–E973.
75. Fujio N, Gossard F, Bayard F, Tremblay J. Regulation of natriuretic peptide receptor A and B expression by transforming growth factor-beta 1 in cultured aortic smooth muscle cells. Hypertension 1994; 23: 908–13.
76. Nuglozeh E, Mbikay M, Stewart DJ, Legault L. Rat natriuretic peptide receptor genes are regulated by glucocorticoids in vitro. Life Sci 1997; 61: 2143–55.
77. Ardaillou N, Blaise V, Placier S, Amestoy F, Ardaillou R. Dexamethasone upregulates ANP C-receptor protein in human mesangial cells without affecting mRNA. Am J Physiol 1996; 270: F440–F446.
78. Suda M, Komatsu Y, Tanaka K et al. C-Type natriuretic peptide/guanylate cyclase B system in rat osteogenic ROB-C26 cells and its down-regulation by dexamethazone. Calcif Tissue Int 1999; 65: 472–8.
79. Herman JP, Dolgas CM, Marcinek R, Langub MC Jr. Expression and glucocorticoid regulation of natriuretic peptide clearance receptor (NPR-C) mRNA in rat brain and choroid plexus. J Chem Neuroanat 1996; 11: 257–65.
80. Kishimoto I, Yoshimasa T, Suga S et al. Natriuretic peptide clearance receptor is transcriptionally down-regulated by beta 2-adrenergic stimulation in vascular smooth muscle cells. J Biol Chem 1994; 269: 28300–8.
81. Garg R, Pandey KN. Angiotensin II-mediated negative regulation of Npr1 promoter activity and gene transcription. Hypertension 2003; 41: 730–6.
82. Chen S, Gardner DG. Osmoregulation of natriuretic peptide receptor signaling in inner medullary collecting duct. A requirement for p38 MAPK. J Biol Chem 2002; 277: 6037–43.
83. Chen S, Cao L, Intengan HD, Humphreys M, Gardner DG. Osmoregulation of endothelial nitric-oxide synthase gene expression in inner medullary collecting duct cells. Role in activation of the type A natriuretic peptide receptor. J Biol Chem 2002; 277: 32498–504.
84. Potter LR, Garbers DL. Dephosphorylation of the guanylyl cyclase-A receptor causes desensitization. J Biol Chem 1992; 267: 14531–4.
85. Potter LR, Garbers DL. Protein kinase C-dependent desensitization of the atrial natriuretic peptide receptor is mediated by dephosphorylation. J Biol Chem 1994; 269: 14636–42.
86. Potter LR, Hunter T. Phosphorylation of the kinase homology domain is essential for activation of the A-type natriuretic peptide receptor. Mol Cell Biol 1998; 18: 2164–72.
87. Potter LR, Hunter T. Identification and characterization of the major phosphorylation sites of the B-type natriuretic peptide receptor. J Biol Chem 1998; 273: 15533–9.
88. Potter LR. Phosphorylation-dependent regulation of the guanylyl cyclase-linked natriuretic peptide receptor B: dephosphorylation is a mechanism of desensitization. Biochemistry 1998; 37: 2422–9.
89. Potter LR, Hunter T. Activation of protein kinase C stimulates the dephosphorylation of natriuretic peptide receptor-B at a single serine residue: a possible mechanism of heterologous desensitization. J Biol Chem 2000; 275: 31099–106.
90. Foster DC, Garbers DL. Dual role for adenine nucleotides in the regulation of the atrial natriuretic peptide receptor, guanylyl cyclase-A. J Biol Chem 1998; 273: 16311–18.
91. Steinhelper ME, Cochrane KL, Field LJ. Hypotension in transgenic mice expressing atrial natriuretic factor fusion genes. Hypertension 1990; 16: 301–7.
92. Klinger JR, Petit RD, Curtin LA et al. Cardiopulmonary responses to chronic hypoxia in transgenic mice that overexpress ANP. J Appl Physiol 1993; 75: 198–205.
93. Field LJ, Veress AT, Steinhelper ME, Cochrane K, Sonnenberg H. Kidney function in ANF-transgenic mice: effect of blood volume expansion. Am J Physiol 1991; 260: R1–R5.
94. Veress AT, Chong CK, Field LJ, Sonnenberg H. Blood pressure and fluid-electrolyte balance in ANF-transgenic mice on high- and low-salt diets. Am J Physiol 1995; 269: R186–R192.
95. John SW, Krege JH, Oliver PM et al. Genetic decreases in atrial natriuretic peptide and salt-sensitive hypertension. Science 1995; 267: 679–81.
96. Melo LG, Veress AT, Chong CK, Pang SC, Flynn TG, Sonnenberg H. Salt-sensitive hypertension in ANP knockout mice: potential role of abnormal plasma renin activity. Am J Physiol 1998; 274: R255–R261.
97. Klinger JR, Warburton RR, Pietras LA, Smithies O, Swift R, Hill NS. Genetic disruption of atrial natriuretic peptide causes pulmonary hypertension in normoxic and hypoxic mice. Am J Physiol 1999; 276: L868–L874.
98. Wang D, Oparil S, Feng JA et al. Effects of pressure overload on extracellular matrix expression in the heart of the atrial natriuretic peptide-null mouse. Hypertension 2003; 42: 88–95.
99. Feng JA, Perry G, Mori T, Hayashi T, Oparil S, Chen YF. Pressure-independent enhancement of cardiac hypertrophy in atrial natriuretic peptide-deficient mice. Clin Exp Pharmacol Physiol 2003; 30: 343–9.
100. John SW, Veress AT, Honrath U et al. Blood pressure and fluid-electrolyte balance in mice with reduced or absent ANP. Am J Physiol 1996; 271: R109–R114.
101. Honrath U, Chong CK, Melo LG, Sonnenberg H. Effect of saline infusion on kidney and collecting duct function in atrial natriuretic peptide (ANP) gene 'knockout' mice. Can J Physiol Pharmacol 1999; 77: 454–7.

102. Ogawa Y, Itoh H, Tamura N et al. Molecular cloning of the complementary DNA and gene that encode mouse brain natriuretic peptide and generation of transgenic mice that overexpress the brain natriuretic peptide gene. J Clin Invest 1994; 93: 1911–21.
103. Suda M, Ogawa Y, Tanaka K et al. Skeletal overgrowth in transgenic mice that overexpress brain natriuretic peptide. Proc Natl Acad Sci U S A 1998; 95: 2337–42.
104. Suganami T, Mukoyama M, Sugawara A et al. Overexpression of brain natriuretic peptide in mice ameliorates immune-mediated renal injury. J Am Soc Nephrol 2001; 12: 2652–63.
105. Kawakami R, Saito Y, Kishimoto I et al. Overexpression of brain natriuretic peptide facilitates neutrophil infiltration and cardiac matrix metalloproteinase-9 expression after acute myocardial infarction. Circulation 2004; 110: 3306–12.
106. Tamura N, Ogawa Y, Chusho H et al. Cardiac fibrosis in mice lacking brain natriuretic peptide. Proc Natl Acad Sci U S A 2000; 97: 4239–44.
107. Ogawa Y, Tamura N, Chusho H, Nakao K. Brain natriuretic peptide appears to act locally as an antifibrotic factor in the heart. Can J Physiol Pharmacol 2001; 79: 723–9.
108. Chusho H, Tamura N, Ogawa Y et al. Dwarfism and early death in mice lacking C-type natriuretic peptide. Proc Natl Acad Sci U S A 2001; 98: 4016–21.
109. Yasoda A, Komatsu Y, Chusho H et al. Overexpression of CNP in chondrocytes rescues achondroplasia through a MAPK-dependent pathway. Nat Med 2004; 10: 80–6.
110. Lopez MJ, Wong SK, Kishimoto I et al. Salt-resistant hypertension in mice lacking the guanylyl cyclase-A receptor for atrial natriuretic peptide. Nature 1995; 378: 65–8.
111. Oliver PM, John SW, Purdy KE et al. Natriuretic peptide receptor 1 expression influences blood pressures of mice in a dose-dependent manner. Proc Natl Acad Sci U S A 1998; 95: 2547–51.
112. Dubois SK, Kishimoto I, Lillis TO, Garbers DL. A genetic model defines the importance of the atrial natriuretic peptide receptor (guanylyl cyclase-A) in the regulation of kidney function. Proc Natl Acad Sci U S A 2000; 97: 4369–73.
113. Shi SJ, Vellaichamy E, Chin SY, Smithies O, Navar LG, Pandey KN. Natriuretic peptide receptor A mediates renal sodium excretory responses to blood volume expansion. Am J Physiol Renal Physiol 2003; 285: F694–F702.
114. Holtwick R, van Eickels M, Skryabin BV et al. Pressure-independent cardiac hypertrophy in mice with cardiomyocyte-restricted inactivation of the atrial natriuretic peptide receptor guanylyl cyclase-A. J Clin Invest 2003; 111: 1399–407.
115. Holtwick R, Gotthardt M, Skryabin B et al. Smooth muscle-selective deletion of guanylyl cyclase-A prevents the acute but not chronic effects of ANP on blood pressure. Proc Natl Acad Sci U S A 2002; 99: 7142–7.
116. Izumi T, Saito Y, Kishimoto I et al. Blockade of the natriuretic peptide receptor guanylyl cyclase-A inhibits NF-kappaB activation and alleviates myocardial ischemia/reperfusion injury. J Clin Invest 2001; 108: 203–13.
117. Tamura N, Doolittle LK, Hammer RE, Shelton JM, Richardson JA, Garbers DL. Critical roles of the guanylyl cyclase B receptor in endochondral ossification and development of female reproductive organs. Proc Natl Acad Sci U S A 2004; 101: 17300–5.
118. Bartels CF, Bukulmez H, Padayatti P et al. Mutations in the transmembrane natriuretic peptide receptor NPR-B impair skeletal growth and cause acromesomelic dysplasia, type Maroteaux. Am J Hum Genet 2004; 75: 27–34.
119. Matsukawa N, Grzesik WJ, Takahashi N et al. The natriuretic peptide clearance receptor locally modulates the physiological effects of the natriuretic peptide system. Proc Natl Acad Sci U S A 1999; 96: 7403–8.

23

Vascular growth mechanisms in hypertension

Haruhiko Ohtsu and Satoru Eguchi

REMODELING OF VASCULAR SMOOTH MUSCLE CELLS UNDER HYPERTENSION

In hypertension, small arteries undergo functional, structural, and mechanical changes, resulting in increased lumen size and peripheral resistance. The change in structure of resistance arteries referred to as 'remodeling' involves a combination of eutrophic remodeling and hypertrophic remodeling.[1] Eutrophic remodeling is an increase in lumen diameter without change in the amount or characteristics of the vessel. In contrast, hypertrophic remodeling involves a thickening of the media that encroaches on the lumen. The narrowed lumen is thus associated with an increased media–lumen ratio and medial cross-sectional area. At cellular levels, the structural changes with hypertension are characterized by enhanced cell number (proliferation), cell size (hypertrophy), cell migration, extracellular matrix (ECM) deposition, and inflammation. Proliferation of vascular smooth muscle cells (VSMCs) is usually observed in intermediate and large arterioles that are also associated with many other vascular diseases including atherosclerosis and restenosis (response to vascular injury).[2] VSMC hypertrophy is also a noteworthy structural change, because it accounts for the increase in thickness of large capacitance arteries. In hypertrophy, VSMCs enlarge through increases in protein synthesis with minimal hyperplasia. VSMC hypertrophy is associated with polyploidization during hypertension.[3] The VSMC phenotypic modulations induced by hypertension such as VSMC proliferation and hypertrophy are caused by both humoral and mechanical factors that modulate intracellular signaling events, resulting in abnormal growth of VSMCs as described below.

HUMORAL FACTORS INVOLVED IN VASCULAR REMODELING

Several autocrine, paracrine, and endocrine humoral factors have been implicated in vascular remodeling under hypertension. These factors are generally divided into growth factors, cytokines, and G protein-coupled receptor (GPCR) agonists (Table 23.1).[4,5] Under hypertension, expression and secretion of these humoral factors are enhanced in the circulation (endocrine), or at the site of remodeling consisting of VSMCs (autocrine), endothelial cells or activated monocytes (paracrine). Several growth factors such as platelet-derived growth factor (PDGF) and fibroblast growth factor (FGF) induce proliferation, and the epidermal growth factor ligand family (HB-EGF and epiregulin) stimulate proliferation and/or hypertrophy of VSMCs. These growth factors have their cognate tyrosine kinase receptors that undergo autophosphorylation and catalyze the phosphorylation of multiple downstream signal proteins. As a cytokine family, interleukins such as interleukin (IL)-1, IL-6 and transforming growth factor (TGF-β) are most implicated in vascular growth. Interleukins such as IL-6 mediate downstream signals through an IL receptor coupled to a JAK tyrosine kinase, whereas IL-1β signals through the IKK/NFκβ pathway. TGF-β may mediate its vascular effects through a transcriptional factor, SMAD. It is known that low concentrations of TGF-β promote growth of VSMCs, whereas at high concentrations, TGF-β inhibits the proliferation. GPCR agonists, angiotensin II (Ang II), endothelin (ET), and thrombin stimulate VSMC proliferation and/or hypertrophy through their seven-transmembrane receptors, AT_1, ET_A, and protease activated receptor-1 (PAR1), expressed in VSMCs, respectively (Table 23.1). In the

Table 23.1 Growth-promoting factors implicated in VSMC remodeling under hypertension

Growth factors	*Source/origin*	*Receptor*
PDGF-AA, AB, BB	Platelet/VSMC	PDGFRα, PGDFRβ
HB-EGF, epiregulin, BTC (EGF family)	VSMC	EGFR, ErbB2, 3, 4
aFGF, bFGF	Endothelial cell, VSMC	FGF receptor (FGFR-1, 2)
IGF-I	Multiple cells	IGF-I receptor
		Insulin receptor
GPCR agonists		
Ang II	VSMC/endothelial cell	AT_1
Endothelin	Endothelial cell	ET_A/ET_B
Thrombin	Plasma	PAR1/4
Cytokines		
IL-1, IL-6	Endothelial cell/VSMC, macrophage	IL-1 receptor, gp130
TGF-β	Multiple cells	ALK-2, 3, 5, 6

Data from references 4 and 5.

signal transduction pathways of these GPCR agonists, tyrosine kinases such as EGFR, PDGFR, JAK, PYK2, FAK, and Src are activated through mechanisms that are not yet fully characterized. Moreover, there is cross-talk between these VSMC remodeling factors and mechanical stress. For example, expression of HB-EGF and PDGF is induced by Ang II and thrombin, and mechanical strain induces expression of Ang II and HB-EGF.[4] The latter could be a key mechanism by which mechanical stress contributes to vascular remodeling.

Similar to cardiac myocytes and skeletal muscle myocytes, VSMCs share the ability to undergo hypertrophy under certain conditions including hypertension. Importantly, hypertrophic factors utilize common signal transduction pathways in VSMCs. Generally, hypertrophy is induced by a progression of cellular protein synthesis. In the signaling pathway of protein synthesis in VSMCs, phosphatidylinositol 3-kinase (PI3-K), Akt/protein kinase B (PKB), and p70 S6 kinase (p70S6K) play an important role.[6] Phosphorylation and activation of Akt/PKB is catalyzed by phosphatidylinositol (3,4,5)-trisphosphate (PIP_3)-dependent protein kinase-1 (PDK-1). PIP_3 is the product of the reaction catalyzed by PI3-K. Activation of Akt/PKB leads to p70S6K activation in VSMCs[7] through the mammalian target of rapamysin (mTOR).[8] p70S6K phosphorylates the ribosomal protein S6 and thereby participates in the translation of a class of mRNA transcripts which contain an oligopyrimidine tract at their transcriptional start site. In addition, regulation of eIF4E (eukaryotic initiation factor-4E) and its inhibitory protein PHAS-1, also called eIF4E binding protein (4EBP), has been shown to be critical for translation initiation, the rate-limiting step for protein synthesis.[6] Several Ser/Thr kinases have been implicated in the phosphorylation of PHAS-1 in different cell types, including mitogen activated protein kinases (MAPKs), extracellular signal regulated kinase (ERK) and p38MAPK, mTOR, and Akt/PKB.[9] Furthermore, it has been reported that MAPK signal-integrating kinase-1 (Mnk1), an effector kinase of ERK and p38-MAPK, phosphorylates eIF4E in VSMCs. A signaling mechanism leading to VSMC hypertrophy is illustrated in Figure 23.1.

In addition to the above-mentioned protein synthesis signaling, three major MAPKs – ERK, c-Jun NH_2-terminal kinase (JNK), and p38MAPK – have been implicated in VSMC proliferation. Among these MAPKs, ERK has been most studied. In the ERK activation signal transduction pathway, Raf-1, MAPK kinase kinase, and a small G protein, Ras, exist upstream. Ras is activated by extracellular signals and recruits the Raf-1 to the membrane. Raf-1 specifically phosphorylates and activates the MAPK kinases, MEK-1 and MEK-2, which are immediately upstream of ERK and leads to ERK phosphorylation and activation. VSMC mitogens including growth factors, cytokines, and GPCR agonists activate this Ras/Raf/ERK pathway. Interestingly, GPCR agonists, such as Ang II, ET-1, and thrombin activate ERK through EGFR 'trans'-activation. The signaling pathway of EGFR transactivation induced by Ang II or thrombin requires a growth factor, proHB-EGF, shedding by a

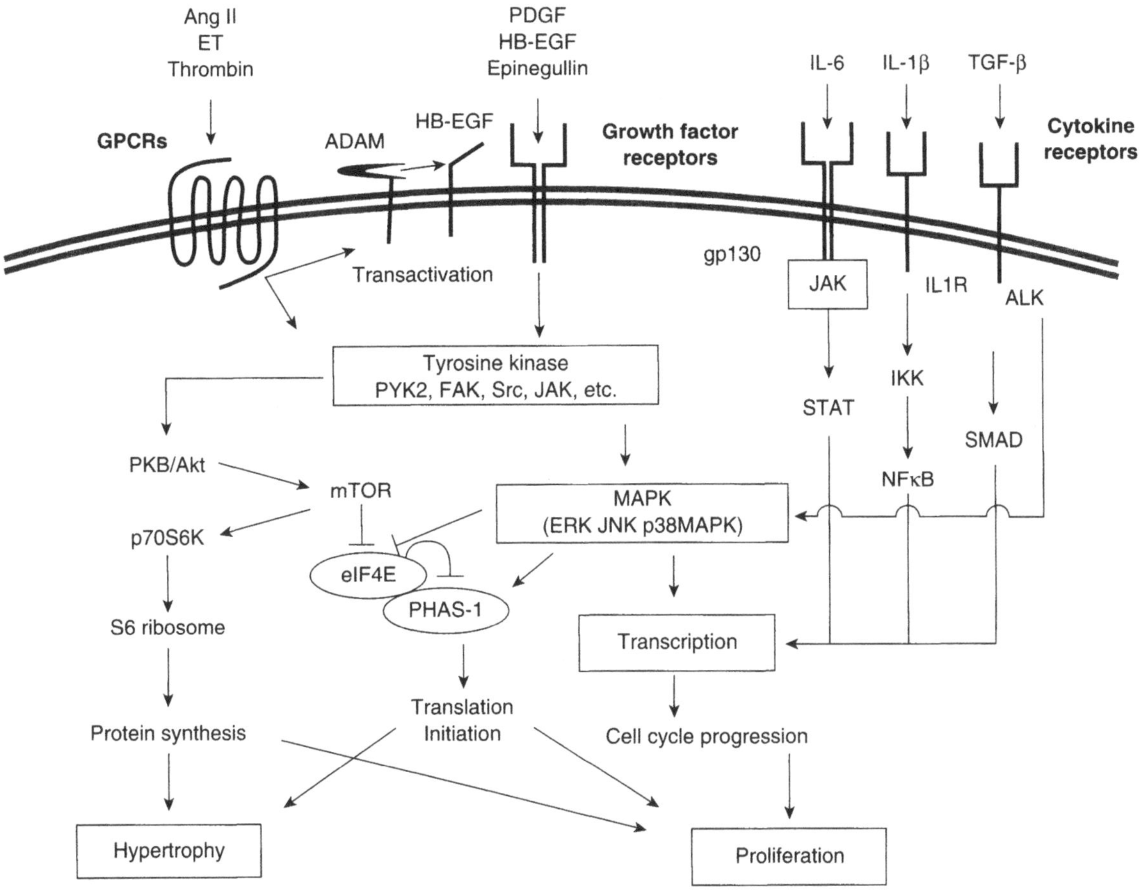

Figure 23.1 Proposed signal transduction mechanisms leading to vascular remodeling by growth factors, GPCR agonists, and cytokines under hypertension

metalloprotease.[10] A disintegrin and metalloprotease (ADAM) is responsible for this HB-EGF shedding. Upon activation, the ERK pathway increases cyclin D1 mRNA leading to the progression of the cell cycle as described below. Also, ERK phosphorylates and activates various transcription factors such as AP-1, ELK-1, c-Myc, and Sap-1, which may lead to VSMC proliferation. For instance, c-Jun and AP-1 contribute to PDGF-induced G_1/S transition through down-regulation of $p27^{Kip}$ and activation of the CDK2 in VSMCs.[11]

The mammalian cell cycle is controlled by holoenzymes composed of a catalytic cyclin-dependent protein kinase (CDK) and a regulatory cyclin. Different CDK/cyclin complexes are activated in specific phases of the cell cycle. CDK activity is attenuated by the interaction with CDK inhibitory proteins (CKIs) such as $p21^{Cip1}$, $p27^{Kip1}$, and $p57^{Kip2}$. Numerous studies have implicated $p27^{Kip1}$ and $p21^{Cip1}$ in the control of vascular cell proliferation in vitro and neointimal thickening in vivo.[12] For example, IL-1β induced $p27^{Kip1}$ and $p21^{Cip1}$ down-regulation, thereby promoting neointimal VSMC proliferation.[13] The down-regulation of $p27^{Kip1}$ also participates in PDGF-induced VSMC proliferation.[14]

MECHANICAL STRESS MEDIATES VASCULAR REMODELING

In addition to humoral factors, VSMCs are exposed to mechanical stretch stress or tension created by blood pressure. Mechanical stress has been proven to contribute to the vascular remodeling associated with hypertension.[15] Mechanical stress has been shown to induce production of various hormonal factors implicated in vascular remodeling. In this regard, expression and secretion of Ang II, IGF, PDGF-A, PDGF-B, and TGF-β by mechanical stretch were demonstrated in VSMCs.[4] Although detailed signal transduction pathways by which the mechanostress induces VSMCs remodeling have not been fully characterized, several signal transduction pathways are known to be involved in this process.[15] Hormonal factors induced by mechanical stress and/or receptors that are sensitive to the mechanical stress may mediate downstream activation of tyrosine kinases, protein kinase C (PKC) and MAPKs. Receptor tyrosine kinases, including EGFR,[16] ErbB2, and PDGFR[15] have been shown to be activated in response to mechanical stretch in cultured VSMCs. Among them, both EGFR and PDGFR are implicated in stretch-dependent MAPK activation in VSMCs. However, the upstream process required for activation of these receptor tyrosine kinases needs to be determined. Mechanical stretch also activates a GPCR in VSMCs. PARs are a recently characterized class of G protein-coupled receptors activated by certain proteases such as thrombin and trypsin. PAR-1, a thrombin receptor, was found to be activated in VSMCs in response to mechanical stress.[17]

Alternatively, mechanostress could induce VSMC growth through activation of the integrin system. VSMCs are surrounded by basement membranes consisting largely of ECM. Integrins are heterodimers composed of non-covalently bound transmembrane α and β subunits, and mediate cell attachment to ECM proteins at sites called focal contacts. Integrin is a receptor for numerous ECM ligands including vitronectin, fibronectin, fibrinogen, thrombospondin, proteolyzed collagens, and osteopontin. Integrins function not only as cell adhesion mediators, but also as transmitters of mechanical stress to induce intracellular signaling events.[18,19] Thus, integrins create numerous downstream signals involved in cytoskeleton reorganization as well as cell growth. In this regard, mechanical stress increases DNA synthesis when the culture substrate is collagen, fibronectin, or vitronectin in VSMCs and these responses were blocked by a specific integrin antibody.[20,21] This indicates that the mechanical stress sensed via specific cell–ECM interactions alters myosin isoform expression as well.

Mechanical stress also activates membrane ion channels such as Ca^{2+} channels and Na^+ channels. In VSMCs, mechanical stress induces an increase in intracellular Ca^{2+} not only from extracellular sources, but also from intracellular reserves. Calcium influx across the plasma membrane occurs via a stretch-activated channel and/or voltage-gated Ca^{2+} channel. Elevation of intracellular Ca^{2+} by mechanical stress probably contributes to vascular remodeling in hypertension.[15]

OTHER FACTORS CONTRIBUTE TO THE VSMC PHENOTYPE CHANGES UNDER HYPERTENSION AND POTENTIAL DEFENSE MECHANISMS AGAINST REMODELING

Additional factors are known to contribute to or accelerate VSMC remodeling in cardiovascular diseases. Some of these factors are associated with other cardiovascular and metabolic diseases/risks such as high glucose, glucosylated protein, oxidized LDL, and hypoxia. Importantly, reactive oxygen species (ROS) have been greatly implicated as a central player among the factors in mediating vascular remodeling. ROS production and/or defect of the reduction systems are considered to be enhanced in virtually all kinds of cardiovascular diseases, including hypertension. A majority of the vascular pathogenic factors such as Ang II, PDGF, and cytokines stimulate ROS production in VSMCs. ROS not only stimulate induction of the hormonal remodeling factors (growth factors, cytokines, GPCR agonists) but also act as cellular signaling second messengers that activate or enhance a variety of protein kinases.[22] In addition, ROS transactivates EGFR and PDGFR in VSMCs, which may be involved in the downstream kinase activation as well.[23]

There are several potential defense mechanisms against vascular remodeling. Most importantly, endothelial dysfunction characterized by decreases in nitric oxide (NO) bioavailability is strongly associated with the incidence of many cardiovascular diseases including hypertension.[24] As a potent vasodialator, NO counter-regulates excess vasoconstriction, whereas ROS inhibit NO function by forming peroxynitrate, which acts as a form of ROS. NO also inhibits growth and migration of VSMCs, preventing vascular remodeling. Therefore, the balance between ROS and NO is of particular importance. Vascular pathogens such as Ang II have been shown to disrupt this balance by producing excess ROS from VSMC NA(D)PH oxidase as well as by inducing endothelial NO synthesis uncoupling.[9] Interestingly, in addition to NO, many vasodilators are believed to inhibit vascular remodeling under hypertension. Natriuretic peptides (ANP, BNP, and CNP) share signal transduction with NO by binding and stimulating their guanylate cyclase-coupled receptors to elevate intracellular cyclic GMP. ANP and BNP inhibit VSMC proliferation.[25] In addition, several GPCR agonists whose receptors preferentially couple to the Gs/cyclic AMP pathway generally act as vasodilators and potentially prevent vascular remodeling by inhibiting growth and/or migration of VSMCs. This is demonstrated by GPCR agonists such as prostacyclin and adrenomedullin.[26]

SUMMARY

Abnormal vascular growth, a key mechanism of vascular remodeling under hypertension, is induced by many (hormonal or mechanical) factors, along with their interactions with specific receptors and sensors. These extracellular events initiate activation of the intracellular signal transduction cascades leading to translational events, cell cycle progression and subsequent cellular hypertrophy/proliferation. The balance between ROS and NO is critical in accelerating and preventing vascular remodeling. In this regard, the molecular mechanisms underlying their regulation are of particular interest. Further studies focusing on this area will contribute to the development of better strategies to prevent vascular incidents under hypertension.

ACKNOWLEDGMENTS

We thank Dr Gerald D. Frank for critical reading of this chapter. This work was supported in part by NIH grant HL076770.

REFERENCES

1. Mulvany MJ, Baumbach GL, Aalkjaer C et al. Vascular remodeling. Hypertension 1996; 28: 505–6.
2. Dzau VJ, Braun-Dullaeus RC, Sedding DG. Vascular proliferation and atherosclerosis: new perspectives and therapeutic strategies. Nat Med 2002; 8: 1249–56.
3. Hixon ML, Gualberto A. Vascular smooth muscle polyploidization. Cell Cycle 2003; 2: 105–10.
4. Berk BC. Vascular smooth muscle growth: autocrine growth mechanisms. Physiol Rev 2001; 81: 999–1030.
5. Kofler S, Nickel T, Weis M. Role of cytokines in cardiovascular diseases: a focus on endothelial responses to inflammation. Clin Sci (Lond) 2005; 108: 205–13.
6. Toker A. Protein kinases as mediators of phosphoinositide 3-kinase signaling. Mol Pharmacol 2000; 57: 652–8.
7. Eguchi S, Iwasaki H, Ueno H et al. Intracellular signaling of angiotensin II-induced p70 S6 kinase phosphorylation at Ser(411) in vascular smooth muscle cells. Possible requirement of epidermal growth factor receptor, Ras, extracellular signal-regulated kinase, and Akt. J Biol Chem 1999; 274: 36843–51.
8. Mourani PM, Garl PJ, Wenzlau JM, Carpenter TC, Stenmark KR, Weiser-Evans MC. Unique, highly proliferative growth phenotype expressed by embryonic and neointimal smooth muscle cells is driven by constitutive Akt, mTOR, and p70S6K signaling and is actively repressed by PTEN. Circulation 2004; 109: 1299–306.
9. Suzuki H, Motley ED, Frank GD, Utsunimiya H, Eguchi S. Recent progress in signal transduction research of the angiotensin II type-1 receptor: protein kinases, vascular dysfunction, and structural requirement. Curr Med Chem Cardiovasc Hematol Agents 2005; 3: 305–22.
10. Eguchi S, Frank GD, Mifune M, Inagami T. Metalloprotease-dependent ErbB ligand shedding in mediating EGFR transactivation and vascular remodelling. Biochem Soc Trans 2003; 31: 1198–202.
11. Zhan Y, Kim S, Yasumoto H, Namba M, Miyazaki H, Iwao H. Effects of dominant-negative c-Jun on platelet-derived growth factor-induced vascular smooth muscle cell proliferation. Arterioscler Thromb Vasc Biol 2002; 22: 82–8.
12. Sriram V, Patterson C. Cell cycle in vasculoproliferative diseases: potential interventions and routes of delivery. Circulation 2001; 103: 2414–19.
13. Nathe TJ, Deou J, Walsh B, Bourns B, Clowes AW, Daum G. Interleukin-1beta inhibits expression of p21(WAF1/CIP1) and p27(KIP1) and enhances proliferation in response to platelet-derived growth factor-BB in smooth muscle cells. Arterioscler Thromb Vasc Biol 2002; 22: 1293–8.
14. Servant MJ, Coulombe P, Turgeon B, Meloche S. Differential regulation of p27(Kip1) expression by mitogenic and hypertrophic factors: involvement of transcriptional and posttranscriptional mechanisms. J Cell Biol 2000; 148: 543–56.
15. Shaw A, Xu Q. Biomechanical stress-induced signaling in smooth muscle cells: an update. Curr Vasc Pharmacol 2003; 1: 41–58.
16. Iwasaki H, Eguchi S, Ueno H, Marumo F, Hirata Y. Mechanical stretch stimulates growth of vascular smooth muscle cells via epidermal growth factor receptor. Am J Physiol Heart Circ Physiol 2000; 278: H521–H529.
17. Nguyen KT, Frye SR, Eskin SG, Patterson C, Runge MS, McIntire LV. Cyclic strain increases protease-activated receptor-1 expression in vascular smooth muscle cells. Hypertension 2001; 38: 1038–43.
18. Ross R. The pathogenesis of atherosclerosis: a perspective for the 1990s. Nature 1993; 362: 801–9.
19. Aplin AE, Howe A, Alahari SK, Juliano RL. Signal transduction and signal modulation by cell adhesion receptors: the role of integrins, cadherins, immunoglobulin-cell adhesion molecules, and selectins. Pharmacol Rev 1998; 50: 197–263.
20. Wilson E, Sudhir K, Ives HE. Mechanical strain of rat vascular smooth muscle cells is sensed by specific extracellular matrix/integrin interactions. J Clin Invest 1995; 96: 2364–72.
21. Sudhir K, Wilson E, Chatterjee K, Ives HE. Mechanical strain and collagen potentiate mitogenic activity of angiotensin II in rat vascular smooth muscle cells. J Clin Invest 1993; 92: 3003–7.
22. Griendling KK, Sorescu D, Lassegue B, Ushio-Fukai M. Modulation of protein kinase activity and gene expression by reactive oxygen species and their role in vascular physiology and pathophysiology. Arterioscler Thromb Vasc Biol 2000; 20: 2175–83.
23. Frank GD, Eguchi S. Activation of tyrosine kinases by reactive oxygen species in vascular smooth muscle cells: significance and involvement of EGF receptor transactivation by angiotensin II. Antioxid Redox Signal 2003; 5: 771–80.
24. Cai H, Harrison DG. Endothelial dysfunction in cardiovascular diseases: the role of oxidant stress. Circ Res 2000; 87: 840–4.
25. Ahluwalia A, MacAllister RJ, Hobbs AJ. Vascular actions of natriuretic peptides. Basic Res Cardiol 2004; 99: 83–9.
26. Bunton DC, Petrie MC, Hillier C, Johnston F, McMurray JJV. The clinical relevance of adrenomedullin: a promising profile? Pharmacol Therap 2004; 103: 179–201.

24

The adrenal medulla in hypertension

Ryan S Friese, Fangwen Rao and Daniel T O'Connor

INTRODUCTION

The adrenal gland is a compelling target in the study of hypertension because its secretory products, both medullary and cortical, directly influence endocrine, cardiovascular, and sympathetic function. The adrenal medulla is highly innervated with preganglionic sympathetic fibers and is capable of biosynthesis and secretion of catecholamines (i.e. dopamine, norepinephrine, epinephrine) directly into the circulation through the adrenal vein. The chromaffin cell is the principal cell type of the adrenal medulla and is specialized for biosynthesis, vesicular storage, and regulated secretion of catecholamines. The adrenal cortex envelops the medulla and is the site of biosynthesis and secretion of several classes of steroid hormones, including mineralocorticoids, glucocorticoids, and sex steroids. The zona glomerulosa, zona fasiculata, and zona reticularis constitute the adrenal cortex, and each zone contains histologically and functionally distinct cells that synthesize and secrete mineralocorticoids, glucocorticoids, and sex steroids, respectively. The entire adrenal gland is richly vascularized with a generally centripetal circulation (cortex → medulla), and all medullary and cortical secretory products exit the gland through the single, large adrenal vein.

CATECHOLAMINE BIOSYNTHESIS, ACTION, AND METABOLISM

Catecholamines function as both neurotransmitters and circulating, endocrine hormones. Norepinephrine serves as the neurotransmitter in noradrenergic neurons of the central nervous system (CNS) as well as in post-ganglionic neurons of the sympathetic branch of the autonomic nervous system. In the adrenal medulla, both norepinephrine and epinephrine are synthesized and released into the circulation as endocrine hormones. Catecholamines are stored for regulated exocytotic secretion in secretory vesicles, which are known as chromaffin granules in chromaffin cells. In addition to catecholamines, chromaffin granules contain a variety of soluble proteins and bioactive peptides that are co-released with the catecholamines.[1]

Catecholamine biosynthesis

Catecholamine biosynthesis begins in the cytosol with the conversion of phenylalanine, an essential dietary amino acid, to the amino acid tyrosine by the enzyme phenylalanine hydroxylase. Tyrosine hydroxylase then catalyzes the rate-limiting step in catecholamine biosynthesis: conversion of tyrosine to dihydroxyphenylalanine (DOPA). The enzyme DOPA decarboxylase converts DOPA to dopamine, which is shuttled into catecholamine storage vesicles via vesicular monoamine transporters. Inside the storage vesicles, dopamine β-hydroxylase catalyzes the conversion of dopamine to norepinephrine. Norepinephrine is the final catecholamine product in noradrenergic neurons of the CNS, in post-ganglionic sympathetic neurons, and in ~15–20% of chromaffin cells. In the remaining 80–85% of chromaffin cells, phenylethanolamine-N-methyltransferase, a cytosolic enzyme, coverts norepinephrine to epinephrine.[1]

Catecholamine action

Catecholamines act through adrenergic receptors, which differ in their ligand binding specificity and affinity, predominant tissue distribution, mode of action, and physiological effects, and as such, are classified as subtypes of the α ($\alpha_{1a,b,c}$, $\alpha_{2a,b,c}$) and β ($\beta_{1,2,3}$) classes. The adrenergic receptors are G protein-coupled receptors characterized by 7-transmembrane α-helical domains and elicit their effects through alterations in intracellular calcium, cyclic nucleotides, inositol phosphates, and/or protein phosphorylation. Norepinephrine is an effective agonist at the α_1 (vascular, vasoconstrictive), α_2 (neuronal and vascular), and β_1 (cardiac inotropic and chronotropic effects) receptors, but a weaker agonist at the β_2 (vascular, vasodilatory) receptor. Epinephrine is a stronger agonist of the α_1 and α_2 receptors than norepinephrine and also functions as an agonist at the β_1 and β_2 receptors. In general, activation of the adrenergic receptors increases the rate and force of contraction of the heart, and causes cardiac and vascular hypertrophy, bronchodilation, and vasoconstriction. Inhibition of the adrenergic receptors leads to a decrease in the rate and force of contraction of the heart, vasodilation, and relaxation of smooth muscle.

Catecholamine metabolism

The main mechanism of catecholamine inactivation in synaptic clefts of noradrenergic neurons is uptake (or 'reuptake') through NET, the norepinephrine transporter. Catecholamines transported by NET at neuronal sites can also be recycled for re-release, thus eliciting additional effects without the need for *de novo* catecholamine biosynthesis. Extraneuronal uptake of catecholamines is possible and is usually mediated by the organic cation transporter (OCT) family, especially OCT3. Neuronal uptake is important for termination of catecholamine effects at sympathetic effector junctions as well as clearance of circulating catecholamines; extraneuronal uptake functions primarily as a mechanism for clearance of circulating catecholamines.

Neuronal reuptake of catecholamines is followed by either transport into storage vesicles for re-release or enzymatic degradation. Catecholamine enzymatic degradation is initiated by the action of monoamine oxidase (MAO) or catechol-O-methyltransferase (COMT). MAO, a mitochondrial enzyme, deaminates catecholamines to the unstable intermediate dihydroxyphenylglycoaldehyde, which is metabolized to dihydroxyphenylglycol (DHPG). COMT, a cytosolic enzyme expressed primarily in the liver, kidney, and chromaffin cells, can convert DHPG to MHPG, which is oxidized by alcohol dehydrogenase in the liver to form vanillylmandelic acid (VMA), the major urinary metabolite of adrenal and sympathetic catecholamines. Alternatively, COMT can act directly on catecholamines through methylation of a hydroxyl oxygen of the dihydroxyphenyl ring of catecholamines to yield normetanephrine (i.e. methoxynorepinephrine from norepinephrine) or metanephrine (i.e. methoxyepinephrine from epinephrine). The metanephrines can then be deaminated by MAO to produce VMA. Circulating catecholamines have a short half-life, approximately 1–2 minutes, and are cleared mainly by neuronal uptake. Direct renal excretion and sulfoconjugation in the gastrointestinal tract by a monoamine-preferring sulfotransferase provide additional mechanisms of catecholamine clearance from the circulation.[1]

THE CHROMOGRANINS OR SECRETOGRANINS

Vesicles present in neurons and adrenal neuroendocrine cells store and release a group of acidic and soluble secretory proteins known as the chromogranins/secretogranins, or 'granins.' The granin family currently consists of seven proteins: chromogranin A, chromogranin B, secretogranin II (or chromogranin C), secretogranin III (or 1B1075), secretogranin IV (or HISL-19), secretogranin V (or 7B2), and secretogranin VI (or NESP55). The granins have roles in vesiculogenesis but also serve as pro-hormones that can be proteolytically processed to yield bioactive peptides with a wide variety of effects, including regulation of catecholamine secretion. Granins are ubiquitously distributed in neuroendocrine and nervous tissue and are co-secreted with catecholamines – these properties make the granins useful indicators of sympathoadrenal activity and secretion. Chromogranin A measurements in particular have proved clinically useful and have even provided clues to the pathogenesis of essential hypertension. Chromogranin A was the first granin discovered and has been studied the most extensively. Bioactive peptides of chromogranin A include catestatin (an inhibitor of nicotinic receptor-induced catecholamine secretion), vasostatin (a vascular smooth muscle relaxant), pancreastatin (a peptide capable of elevating blood glucose through inhibition of glucose-stimulated insulin release from pancreatic islet beta cells), and chromacin and prochromacin (antimicrobial peptides that may play a role in the neuroendocrine response to systemic infection).[1]

GENETICS OF HYPERTENSION

Blood pressure is a continuously distributed, quantitative trait. Variation in blood pressure results from the contribution of many genes, i.e. blood pressure is a polygenic trait. It is this complex, multifactorial nature of essential hypertension that has obfuscated genetic and pathogenic analyses of the trait. Indeed, in each case of essential hypertension, it is likely that the subset of genes responsible for increases in blood pressure is different from individual to individual.

Candidate gene sequence comparison of human essential hypertensive patients has revealed great diversity in the type (e.g. single nucleotide transition/transversion, insertion/deletion, duplication) and location (e.g. promoter, exon) of polymorphisms, even with the same gene in different patients, and with phenotypic consequences likely involving a variety of epistatic and pleiotropic effects. Furthermore, environmental factors such as diet and exercise play major roles in ultimate trait penetrance and further complicate and confound genetic analyses of the disease.

ANIMAL MODELS OF ESSENTIAL (HEREDITARY) HYPERTENSION

The use of animal models of essential hypertension circumvents many of the problems faced when studying the genetically heterogeneous and environmentally uncontrolled human population. Genetically/hereditarily hypertensive rat and mouse strains have been developed with selective breeding paradigms based on elevated blood pressure. Within each species, after the elevated blood pressure trait is fixed by many generations of selective breeding, the hypertensive rodents are inbred to homozygosity, i.e. both paternal and maternal chromosomes contain the same alleles for all genes. Examples of these types of rodent models of human essential hypertension include the spontaneously hypertensive rat (SHR) and the blood pressure high mouse (BPH). Studying inbred models has several advantages over studying human populations, such as the homogeneity of the genomes and the ability to strictly control environmental factors.

Friese et al. used microarrays to perform a genome-wide, interspecies (rat/mouse) gene expression comparison of the adrenal glands of juvenile, 4-week-old SHR and 5-week-old BPH.[2] Gene expression values for SHR and BPH were compared to their respective inbred control strains (control for the SHR is the Wistar-Kyoto Rat, WKY; control for BPH is the blood pressure low mouse, BPL) to determine which genes are overexpressed and underexpressed in the adrenal gland in rodent hereditary hypertension. Computation of the statistically significant differentially expressed genes was followed by an interspecies (rat/mouse) ortholog comparison between the SHR and BPH strains – orthologs exhibiting shared expression patterns (i.e. overexpressed or underexpressed in both SHR and BPH) may represent fundamental mechanisms of blood pressure elevation across mammalian species and, therefore, might provide clues to the pathology of human essential hypertension.

Figure 24.1 provides an overview of gene expression alterations in catecholamine biosynthesis, degradation, and receptor biochemical pathways in 4-week-old SHR and 5-week-old BPH. Global, widespread gene expression changes are observed in both SHR and BPH, yet the direction of change, i.e. overexpressed versus underexpressed, differs between the hypertensive rat and hypertensive mouse.

The pattern of gene expression within the catecholamine biosynthetic pathway suggests fundamentally different effects on biosynthetic enzyme transcription on catecholamine biosynthesis in SHR and BPH. Catecholamine biosynthetic transcripts appear depressed in the SHR but enhanced in BPH. No change in expression of tyrosine hydroxylase, the rate-limiting enzyme of catecholamine biosynthesis, is observed in SHR, but BPH exhibited overexpression of the enzyme. GTP cyclohydrolase 1 (Gch), the rate-limiting enzyme in synthesis of tetrahydrobiopterin (BH_4), the essential cofactor of tyrosine hydroxylase, is not differentially expressed in SHR but is overexpressed in BPH. Both dopamine beta-hydroxylase (Dbh) and phenylethanolamine-N-methyltransferase (Pnmt) were underexpressed in SHR. The mouse microarray did not contain a probe for Dbh, but Pnmt was overexpressed in BPH. Overall, the expression patterns of the catecholamine biosynthetic enzymes suggest decreased transcriptional activity in SHR and increased transcriptional activity in BPH.

The vesicular monoamine transporters (Slc18a1 and Slc18a2) shuttle dopamine and monoamines between the cytosol and secretory vesicles. The Slc18a1 transporter is specifically located in adrenal chromaffin granules and underexpressed in SHR, which is consistent with depressed biosynthesis and vesicular storage of catecholamines in SHR. Slc18a2 is thought to function primarily in the brain and other noradrenergic neurons. The significance of Slc18a2 differential expression in the adrenal gland of SHR is unclear. The mouse microarray did not contain probes for Slc18a1 and Slca18a2.

SHR displayed underexpression of secretogranin II, which is consistent with a depression of catecholamine biosynthesis. Chromogranin A, chromogranin B, and secretogranin II overexpression in BPH suggests enhanced catecholamine vesicular storage – an increase in catecholamine biosynthesis would tend to increase the steady-state level of catecholamines, perhaps eventuating in an increase in the number and/or size of vesicles.

The largest fold change observed in the SHR was the overexpression of catechol-O-methyltransferase (Comt) by ~40-fold. If large fold changes are indicative of biological importance, then Comt is a compelling

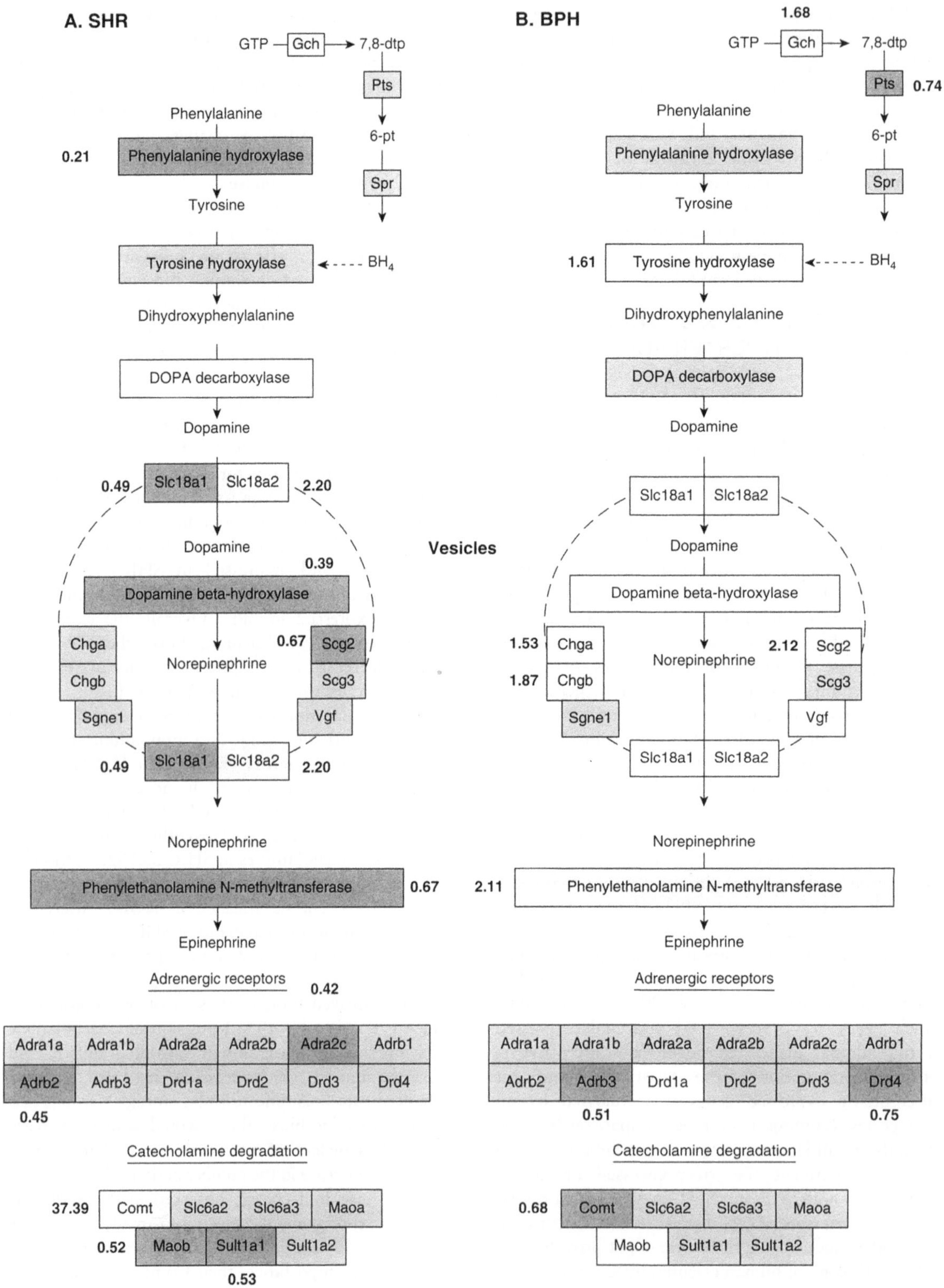
A. SHR
GTP
Gch
7,8-dtp
Pts
6-pt
Spr
Phenylalanine
0.21
Phenylalanine hydroxylase
Tyrosine
Tyrosine hydroxylase
BH4
Dihydroxyphenylalanine
DOPA decarboxylase
Dopamine
0.49
Slc18a1
Slc18a2
2.20
Dopamine
0.39
Dopamine beta-hydroxylase
Chga
Chgb
Sgne1
Norepinephrine
0.67
Scg2
Scg3
Vgf
0.49
Slc18a1
Slc18a2
2.20
Norepinephrine
Phenylethanolamine N-methyltransferase
0.67
Epinephrine
Adrenergic receptors
0.42
Adra1a
Adra1b
Adra2a
Adra2b
Adra2c
Adrb1
Adrb2
Adrb3
Drd1a
Drd2
Drd3
Drd4
0.45
Catecholamine degradation
37.39
Comt
Slc6a2
Slc6a3
Maoa
0.52
Maob
Sult1a1
Sult1a2
0.53
Vesicles
B. BPH
1.68
GTP
Gch
7,8-dtp
Pts
0.74
6-pt
Spr
Phenylalanine
Phenylalanine hydroxylase
Tyrosine
1.61
Tyrosine hydroxylase
BH4
Dihydroxyphenylalanine
DOPA decarboxylase
Dopamine
Slc18a1
Slc18a2
Dopamine
Dopamine beta-hydroxylase
1.53
Chga
1.87
Chgb
Sgne1
Norepinephrine
2.12
Scg2
Scg3
Vgf
Slc18a1
Slc18a2
Norepinephrine
2.11
Phenylethanolamine N-methyltransferase
Epinephrine
Adrenergic receptors
Adra1a
Adra1b
Adra2a
Adra2b
Adra2c
Adrb1
Adrb2
Adrb3
Drd1a
Drd2
Drd3
Drd4
0.51
0.75
Catecholamine degradation
0.68
Comt
Slc6a2
Slc6a3
Maoa
Maob
Sult1a1
Sult1a2

candidate for or indicator of aberrant catecholaminergic responses in SHR. The significance of underexpression of Comt in BPH is not clear.

Overall, gene expression patterns suggest depressed catecholamine production in the SHR, while BPH might suffer from increased catecholamine action. Further investigation of catecholamine concentrations and activity in the adrenal gland and circulation of SHR and BPH will improve the understanding of the impact of the gene expression changes observed in SHR and BPH. Nonetheless, aberrant adrenal catecholamine physiology may underlie hypertensive pathology in both SHR and BPH.

HUMAN HYPERTENSION

Common strategies to dissect human polygenic traits such as hypertension include sib-pair analysis, genome scans, association studies, and the classic twin study. The power of the twin study design lies in the fact that it enables calculation of trait heritability ($h^2 = V_G/V_P$), the fraction of total trait phenotypic variance (V_P) that results from additive genetic variance (V_G). Heritability provides a concrete measure of the tractability of a trait to genetic analyses. Estimates of blood pressure heritability typically range from ~20 to 40%.

Tyrosine hydroxylase: genetic variation and autonomic 'intermediate phenotypes'

Zhang et al. employed the classic twin study design to probe the influence of tyrosine hydroxylase polymorphisms on autonomic traits.[3] Previous studies have shown associations between the microsatellite tetranucleotide repeat $(TCAT)_n$ polymorphism within intron A of the human tyrosine hydroxylase gene, hypertension,[4] and blood pressure regulation.[5,6] Zhang et al. investigated the relationship between biochemical (catecholamine) and physiological autonomic phenotypes, heritability estimates, and $(TCAT)_n$ genotypes within the twin population. The twin study consisted of 103 monozygotic (MZ) and 45 dizygotic (DZ) twin pairs of European ancestry (white) from urban southern California (San Diego). Thirty subjects were hypertensive (29 treated with antihypertensive medications; 1 untreated) while the remaining individuals were normotensive.

Biochemical and physiological autonomic phenotypes measured included plasma and urinary catecholamines (norepinephrine and epinephrine), basal blood pressure, pulse interval (R-R interval or heart period, in msec/beat), and blood pressure and pulse interval responses to cold stress (i.e. the 'cold pressor test': immersion of one hand in ice-water for 60 seconds). Heritability for each of the autonomic phenotypes was determined and each subject was genotyped for the $(TCAT)_n$ microsatellite. Sequencing revealed six alleles of the $(TCAT)_n$ microsatellite repeat, differing in number of consecutive TCAT repeats: $(TCAT)_6$, $(TCAT)_7$, $(TCAT)_8$, $(TCAT)_9$, $(TCAT)_{10}$, and the imperfect repeat $(TCAT)_4CAT(TCAT)_5$, also known as $(TCAT)_{10i}$. The two most common alleles observed were $(TCAT)_6$ and $(TCAT)_{10i}$.

Biochemical phenotypes showed substantial heritability (h^2): plasma norepinephrine (NE) = 55.3 ± 8.0%, $p < 0.0001$; plasma epinephrine (EPI) = 61.4 ± 9.8%, $p = 0.0460$; urinary NE = 32.5 ± 9.6%, $p = 0.001$; urinary EPI = 47.1 ± 8.8%, $p < 0.0001$. Basal heart rate and basal blood pressure also showed significant heritability,

---

Figure 24.1 Catecholamines and sympathetic function in SHR and BPH. Gene expression of the catecholamine biosynthetic and target (receptor) pathway is shown in the SHR hypertensive rat strain (A) and BPH hypertensive mouse strain (B). Light gray indicates an overexpressed gene, dark gray indicates an underexpressed gene, white indicates no data (i.e. no probe on chip), and medium gray indicates lack of statistical significance. The **bold** number listed next to significantly ($p < 0.05$) differentially expressed genes is the fold change (BPH/BPL or SHR/WKY). Abbreviations: 6-pt, 6-pyruvoyl-tetrahydropterin; 7,8-dtp, 7,8-dihydroneopterin triphosphate; Adra1a, adrenergic receptor, alpha 1a; Adra1b, adrenergic receptor, alpha 1b; Adra2a, adrenergic receptor, alpha 2a; Adra2b, adrenergic receptor, alpha 2b; Adra2c, adrenergic receptor, alpha 2c; Adrb1, adrenergic receptor, beta 1; Adrb2, adrenergic receptor, beta 2; Adrb3, adrenergic receptor, beta 3; BH_4, tetrahydrobiopterin; Chga, chromogranin A; Chgb, chromogranin B; Comt, catechol-O-methyltransferase; Drd1a, dopamine receptor 1a; Drd2, dopamine receptor 2; Drd3, dopamine receptor 3; Drd4, dopamine receptor 4; Gch, GTP cyclohydrolase 1; GTP, guanosine triphosphate; Maoa, monoamine oxidase A; Maob, monoamine oxidase B; Pts, 6-pyruvoyl-tetrahydrobiopterin synthase; Scg2, sececretogranin II; Scg3, secretogranin III; Sgne1, secretory granule neuroendocrine protein 1; Slc6a2, solute carrier family 6 (neurotransmitter transporter, noradrenalin), member 2; Slc6a3, solute carrier family 6 (neurotransmitter transporter, dopamine), member 3; Slc18a1, solute carrier family 18 (vesicular monoamine transporter) member 1; Slc18a2, solute carrier family 18 (vesicular monoamine transporter) member 2; Spr, sepiapterin reductase; Sult1a1, sulfotransferase family 1A, phenol-preferring, member 1; Sult1a2, sulfotransferase family 1A, member 2; Vgf, VGF nerve growth factor-inducible. (Reproduced from Friese et al. Am J Hypertens 2005; 18: 633–52[2] with permission from American Journal of Hypertension, Ltd.)

with heart rate ($h^2=61\pm6\%$, $p<0.0001$) showing substantially more heritability than either systolic blood pressure (SBP) ($h^2=26\pm8\%$, $p=0.0016$) or diastolic blood pressure (DBP) ($h^2=18\pm9\%$, $p=0.0359$). Cold stress-induced changes in heart rate (ΔHR $h^2=36\pm8\%$, $p<0.0001$) and blood pressure (ΔSBP $h^2=23\pm9\%$, $p=0.0098$; ΔDBP $h^2=32\pm8\%$) were also heritable. As positive controls, the heritability of weight ($h^2=87\pm2\%$, $p<0.0001$) and height ($h^2=93\pm1\%$, $p<0.0001$) were computed to verify the reliability of the heritability estimates.

Significant correlations between biochemical and physiological traits with mechanistic implications for autonomic control of blood pressure were reported: 1) a positive correlation between renal NE excretion and resting SBP (Pearson $R=0.48$, $R^2=0.23$, $n=111$, $p<10^{-7}$), and 2) a positive correlation between renal NE excretion and SBP increase in response to cold stress ($R=0.30$, $R^2=0.09$, $n=112$, $p=0.001$).

Zhang et al. used a variance components method to determine the effect of variation of individual $(TCAT)_n$ microsatellite alleles on autonomic trait heritability. To maximize statistical power, the variance components analysis focused only on the most common alleles: $(TCAT)_6$ and $(TCAT)_{10i}$. An increase in $(TCAT)_6$ copy number (from 0 to 1 to 2 alleles) was associated with increased basal pulse interval ($p=0.007$), as well as basal ($p=0.0003$) and post cold-stress ($p=0.0001$) heart rate. In contrast, an increase in $(TCAT)_{10i}$ copy number was associated with decreased pulse interval ($p=0.0349$), increased plasma epinephrine ($p=0.0133$), and increased renal NE excretion ($p=0.0309$). The $(TCAT)_6$ and $(TCAT)_{10i}$ alleles exerted directionally opposite effects on pulse interval.

The $(TCAT)_6/(TCAT)_6$ homozygous, $(TCAT)_6/(TCAT)_{10i}$ heterozygous, and $(TCAT)_{10i}/(TCAT)_{10i}$ homozygous diploid genotypes also exerted effects on autonomic phenotypes, specifically basal and post-stress heart rate. Within the diploid genotypes, the $(TCAT)_6$ allele exerted a dose-dependent direct effect on basal pulse interval and inverse effect on pre- and post-stress heart rate. Conversely, the $(TCAT)_{10i}$ allele displayed a dose-dependent inverse effect on basal pulse interval, and a direct effect on pre- and post-stress heart rate. Finally, Zhang et al. suggested that the $(TCAT)_n$ polymorphisms of tyrosine hydroxylase exhibit pleiotropy (i.e. one gene influences multiple phenotypes), since $(TCAT)_{10i}$ allele copy number predicted both pulse interval (inverse relationship) and renal norepinephrine excretion (direct relationship) in a dose-dependent fashion (MANOVA: Pillai $F=3.30$, $p=0.012$).

Zhang et al. thus presented compelling evidence for the role of allelic variation at the tyrosine hydroxylase locus in regulation of biochemical and physiological autonomic phenotypes, with mechanistic implications for regulation of blood pressure and, ultimately, the development of hypertension.

Chromogranin A: human genetic variation

Chromogranin A (CHGA) expression and activity have been proposed as 'intermediate phenotypes' in human essential hypertension. Family studies have shown substantial heritability of hypertension, yet the specific genes leading to chronic, pathological increases in blood pressure remain poorly understood. Genetic analyses of complex traits such as hypertension are complemented by the use of intermediate phenotypes – simpler, often monogenic traits with earlier penetrance than the ultimate disease phenotype. The CHGA locus likely controls intermediate phenotypes that contribute to hypertension.[7] CHGA is overexpressed in chromaffin cells of genetic (SHR)[8,9] and acquired (renovascular)[10] rodent models of human essential hypertension, and twin studies have shown significant heritability of circulating CHGA in humans.[11] Furthermore, circulating levels of the CHGA catestatin fragment, which inhibits nicotinic receptor-induced secretion of catecholamines, are decreased in hypertensive patients as well as in normotensive patients at genetic risk (i.e. one or both parents have hypertension) of developing the disease.[7,12,13]

Wen et al. studied the effect of sequence variation within the chromogranin A gene to identify genetic variants that might quantitatively and/or qualitatively alter the protein and its bioactive peptide products.[14] The investigators resequenced all eight exons and adjacent intronic regions, ~1.2 kilobases of 5′ promoter region, and two highly conserved intronic regions from 180 ethnically diverse (white, African American, Hispanic, Asian) human subjects living in urban southern California (San Diego). Wen et al. identified 53 single nucleotide polymorphisms (SNPs) and 2 single-base insertion/deletions in the resequenced regions. Seventeen of the polymorphisms occurred in the coding region of the gene, while 11 of the 17 encoded amino acid substitutions. Two of these non-synonymous coding SNPs, Gly364Ser and Pro370Leu, are uncommon (minor allele frequency 0.6–3.1%) variants of the catestatin region, where they affect the ability of the peptide to inhibit catecholamine secretion.

The functional significance of individual SNPs on the expression of CHGA and its peptide products was examined. One-way ANOVA with Bonferroni correction for multiple comparisons identified three SNPs in the promoter region that were significantly associated with plasma CHGA concentrations. These three SNPs were in absolute linkage disequilibrium with each other, thus indicating possible haplotype-specific effects. The authors tested the functional significance of inferred promoter haplotypes by placing the haplotypes upstream of a luciferase reporter and assaying expression in PC12 rat chromaffin cells. The promoter SNPs resolved into six relatively common haplotypes, each differing in the ability to promote transcription and regulate gene expression. To determine the functional significance of the two amino acid substitution SNPs occurring in the catestatin peptide, the authors synthesized wild-type and variant synthetic peptides and assayed their potency for inhibition of nicotinic cholinergic-stimulated catecholamine release from PC12 chromaffin cells. The two SNPs resulted in ~10.8-fold differences in the ability of catestatin to inhibit catecholamine release. Thus, genetic variation within the chromogranin A locus can quantitatively and qualitatively affect the protein and its bioactive peptide products, further supporting the role of CHGA as an important contributor to and intermediate phenotype for hypertension.

CHROMOGRANIN A IN PHEOCHROMOCYTOMA

Rao et al.[15] studied plasma concentrations of chromaffin granule transmitters (chromogranin A, norepinephrine, and epinephrine) in patients with pheochromocytoma ($n=27$), both benign ($n=13$) and malignant ($n=14$). Patients with benign pheochromocytoma were studied before and after surgical removal ($n=6$), while patients with malignant pheochromocytoma were evaluated before and after chemotherapy cycles of cyclophosphamide/dacarbazine/vincristine (non-randomized trial in $n=9$).

In the diagnosis of pheochromocytoma (benign or malignant), Rao et al. found a progressive rise ($p<0.0001$) in plasma chromogranin A, from control subjects (48.0±3.0 ng/ml) to benign pheochromocytoma (188±40.5 ng/ml) to malignant pheochromocytoma (2932±960 ng/ml). Parallel changes were seen for plasma norepinephrine ($p<0.0001$). When stepwise linear regression was allowed to select the model, the independent variable best predicting the distinction of pheochromocytoma versus control was norepinephrine (multiple $R=0.417$, $R^2=0.174$, adjusted $R^2=0.149$, $T=2.67$, $F=7.14$, $p=0.011$).

Both plasma chromogranin A ($p=0.0003$) and norepinephrine ($p=0.0344$) were higher in malignant than benign pheochromocytoma, although plasma epinephrine was actually lower ($p=0.0182$) in malignant tumors. In a stepwise multivariate analysis, plasma chromogranin A elevation proved to be the most significant difference between benign and malignant tumors (adjusted $R^2=0.202$, $F=7.56$, $p=0.011$).

In the treatment of pheochromocytoma, Rao et al. found that after excision of benign pheochromocytomas, chromogranin A ($p=0.028$), norepinephrine ($p=0.047$), and epinephrine ($p=0.037$) all fell to values near normal. During chemotherapy of malignant pheochromocytoma ($n=9$), plasma chromogranin A ($p=0.047$) and norepinephrine ($p=0.02$) fell, but not epinephrine. After chemotherapy, five clinical 'responders' showed declines in chromogranin A (by ~91%, $p=0.03$) and norepinephrine (also by ~91%, $p=0.03$) but not epinephrine ($p=0.31$). By contrast, four 'non-responders' showed no significant decline in any of the transmitters (all $p=0.13$).

Rao et al. concluded that plasma chromogranin A is an effective tool in the diagnosis of pheochromocytoma, and markedly elevated chromogranin A may point to malignant pheochromocytoma.[15] During chemotherapy of malignant pheochromocytoma, chromogranin A can be used to gauge tumor response and relapse.

REFERENCES

1. Taupenot L, Harper KL, O'Connor DT. The chromogranin-secretogranin family. N Engl J Med 2003; 348: 1134–49.
2. Friese RS, Mahboubi P, Mahapatra NR et al. Common genetic mechanisms of blood pressure elevation in two independent rodent models of human essential hypertension. Am J Hypertens 2005; 18(5 Pt1): 633–52.
3. Zhang L, Rao F, Wessel J et al. Functional allelic heterogeneity and pleiotropy of a repeat polymorphism in tyrosine hydroxylase: prediction of catecholamines and response to stress in twins. Physiol Genomics 2004; 19: 277–91.
4. Sharma P, Hingorani A, Jia H et al. Positive association of tyrosine hydroxylase microsatellite marker to essential hypertension. Hypertension 1998; 32: 676–82.
5. Barbeau P, Litaker MS, Jackson RW, Treiber FA. A tyrosine hydroxylase microsatellite and hemodynamic response to stress in a multi-ethnic sample of youth. Ethn Dis 2003; 13: 186–92.
6. Jindra A, Jachymova M, Horky K et al. Association analysis of two tyrosine hydroxylase gene polymorphisms in normotensive offspring from hypertensive families. Blood Press 2000; 9: 250–4.
7. O'Connor DT, Kailasam MT, Kennedy BP, Ziegler MG, Yanaihara N, Parmer RJ. Early decline in the catecholamine release-inhibitory peptide catestatin in humans at genetic risk of hypertension. J Hypertens 2002; 20: 1335–45.
8. Schober M, Howe PR, Sperk G, Fischer-Colbrie R, Winkler H. An increased pool of secretory hormones and peptides in adrenal medulla of stroke-prone spontaneously hypertensive rats. Hypertension 1989; 13: 469–74.

9. O'Connor DT, Takiyyuddin MA, Printz MP et al. Catecholamine storage vesicle protein expression in genetic hypertension. Blood Press 1999; 8: 285–95.
10. Takiyyuddin MA, De Nicola L, Gabbai FB et al. Catecholamine secretory vesicles. Augmented chromogranins and amines in secondary hypertension. Hypertension 1993; 21: 674–9.
11. Takiyyuddin MA, Parmer RJ, Kailasam MT et al. Chromogranin A in human hypertension. Influence of heredity. Hypertension 1995; 26: 213–20.
12. Kennedy BP, Mahata SK, O'Connor DT, Ziegler MG. Mechanism of cardiovascular actions of the chromogranin A fragment catestatin in vivo. Peptides 1998; 19: 1241–8.
13. Mahata SK, Mahata M, Wakade AR, O'Connor DT. Primary structure and function of the catecholamine release inhibitory peptide catestatin (chromogranin A(344–364)): identification of amino acid residues crucial for activity. Mol Endocrinol 2000; 14: 1525–35.
14. Wen G, Mahata SK, Cadman P et al. Both rare and common polymorphisms contribute functional variation at CHGA, a regulator of catecholamine physiology. Am J Hum Genet 2004; 74: 197–207.
15. Rao F, Keiser HR, O'Connor DT. Malignant pheochromocytoma: chromaffin granule transmitters and response to treatment. Hypertension 2000; 36: 1045–52.

25

Clinical characteristics of pheochromocytoma

William F Young Jr

INTRODUCTION

Although catecholamine-secreting tumors are rare (annual incidence of 2–8 cases per million people),[1] it is important to suspect, confirm, localize, and resect these tumors because: the associated hypertension is curable with surgical removal of the tumor, risk of a lethal paroxysm exists, and at least 10% of the tumors are malignant. Catecholamine-secreting tumors that arise from chromaffin cells of the adrenal medulla and the sympathetic ganglia are termed *pheochromocytomas* and *extra-adrenal catecholamine-secreting paragangliomas* ('extra-adrenal pheochromocytomas'), respectively. Many clinicians use the term 'pheochromocytoma' to refer to both adrenal pheochromocytomas and extra-adrenal catecholamine-secreting paragangliomas because the tumors have similar clinical presentations and are treated with similar approaches.

Catecholamine-secreting tumors occur with equal frequency in men and women, primarily in the third, fourth, and fifth decades. Patients harboring catecholamine-secreting tumors may be asymptomatic. However, symptoms usually are present and are due to the pharmacologic effects of excess circulating catecholamine concentrations. The resulting hypertension may be sustained or paroxysmal. Episodic symptoms that may occur in spells, or paroxysms, can be extremely variable, but typically include forceful heartbeat, pallor, tremor, and diaphoresis. Spells may be either spontaneous or precipitated by postural change, anxiety, medications (e.g. metoclopramide, anesthetic agents), exercise, or maneuvers that increase intra-abdominal pressure. Although the types of spells experienced across the patient population are highly variable, spells tend to be stereotypical for each patient. However, the clinician must recognize that most patients with spells do not have a pheochromocytoma (Box 25.1).[2]

Additional clinical signs of catecholamine-secreting tumors include hypertension, hypertensive retinopathy, orthostatic hypotension, constipation (megacolon may be the presenting symptom),[3] painless hematuria and paroxysmal attacks induced by micturition (associated with urinary bladder paragangliomas), hyperglycemia and diabetes mellitus, hypercalcemia, and erythrocytosis. Thus, the presentation of patients with catecholamine-secreting tumors may mimic other disorders (Box 25.2). Some of the co-secreted hormones that may dominate the clinical presentation include adrenocorticotropin (Cushing's syndrome), parathyroid hormone-related peptide (hypercalcemia), vasoactive intestinal peptide (watery diarrhea), and growth hormone releasing hormone (acromegaly) (Box 25.2).[4–7] Cardiomyopathy and congestive heart failure are the symptomatic presentations that are perhaps most frequently unrecognized by clinicians to be caused by pheochromocytoma.[8–10] Many physical exam findings can be associated with genetic syndromes that predispose to pheochromocytoma; these findings include retinal angiomas, marfanoid body habitus, café au lait spots, axillary freckling, subcutaneous neurofibromas, and mucosal neuromas on the eyelids and tongue.

A 'rule of 10' has been quoted for describing the characteristics of catecholamine-secreting tumors: 10% are extra-adrenal, 10% occur in children, 10% are multiple or bilateral, 10% recur after surgical removal, 10% are malignant, 10% are familial, and 10% of benign sporadic adrenal pheochromocytoma present as adrenal incidentalomas.[11,12] None of these 'rules' is precisely 10%. For example, recent studies

Box 25.1 Differential diagnosis of pheochromocytoma-type spells

Endocrine
- Pheochromocytoma
- 'Hyperadrenergic spells'
- Thyrotoxicosis
- Primary hypogonadism (menopausal syndrome)
- Medullary thyroid carcinoma
- Pancreatic tumors (e.g. insulinoma)
- Hypoglycemia
- Carbohydrate intolerance

Cardiovascular
- Labile essential hypertension
- Cardiovascular deconditioning
- Pulmonary edema
- Syncope
- Orthostatic hypotension
- Paroxysmal cardiac arrhythmia and torsade de pointes
- Angina
- Renovascular disease

Psychologic
- Anxiety and panic attacks
- Somatization disorder
- Hyperventilation
- Factitious (e.g. drugs, valsalva)

Pharmacologic
- Withdrawal of adrenergic inhibitor
- MAO inhibitor + decongestant
- Sympathomimetic ingestion
- Illegal drug ingestion (cocaine, PCP, LSD)
- Chlorpropamide-alcohol flush
- Vancomycin ('red man syndrome')

Neurologic
- Postural orthostatic tachycardia syndrome (POTS)
- Autonomic neuropathy
- Migraine headache
- Diencephalic epilepsy (autonomic seizures)
- Stroke
- Cerebrovascular insufficiency

Other
- Unexplained flushing spells
- Mast cell disease
- Carcinoid syndrome
- Recurrent idiopathic anaphylaxis

Box 25.2 Conditions that pheochromocytoma may mimic or cause

- Resistant essential hypertension
- Renovascular hypertension
- Myocardial ischemia
- Dilated cardiomyopathy
- Hypertrophic obstructive cardiomyopathy
- Pulmonary edema – cardiogenic and non-cardiogenic
- Adult respiratory distress syndrome (ARDS)
- Syncope
- Cardiac arrhythmia
- Apical LVH
- Stroke
- Vasculitis
- Multiple organ failure with DIC
- Hemobilia, jaundice, and pancreatic infarction
- Hypermetabolism with weight loss and fever (IL-6)
- Hyperthyroidism
- Diabetes mellitus
- Orthostatic hypotension (adrenomedullin)
- Cushing's syndrome (ectopic CRH/ACTH)
- Primary aldosteronism (? ASF)
- Acromegaly (GHRH)
- Hyperparathyroidism (PTH-RP)
- Watery diarrhea (VIP)
- Constipation/ostipation (adrenomedullin)
- Acute abdomen
- Psychiatric disorders (e.g. panic attacks)

ACTH, corticotropin; ASF, aldosterone-stimulating factor; CRH, corticotropin-releasing hormone; DIC, disseminated intravascular coagulation; GHRH, growth hormone releasing hormone; IL-6, interleukin 6; LVH, left ventricular hypertrophy; PTH-RP, parathyroid-related peptide; VIP, vasoactive intestinal polypeptide.

suggest that up to 20% of catecholamine-secreting tumors are familial.[13]

Pheochromocytomas are localized to the adrenal glands and have an average size of 4.5 cm.[14] Paragangliomas are found where chromaffin tissue exists: along the paraaortic sympathetic chain, within the organs of Zuckerkandl (at the origin of the inferior mesenteric artery), in the wall of the urinary bladder, and in the sympathetic chain in the neck or mediastinum.[15,16] In early postnatal life, the extra-adrenal sympathetic paraganglionic tissues are prominent; these tissues then degenerate, leaving residual foci associated with the vagal nerves, carotid vessels, aortic arch, pulmonary vessels, and mesenteric arteries. Odd locations for paragangliomas include the neck, intra-atrial cardiac septum,[17] spermatic cord, vagina, scrotum, and sacrococcygeal region.

Approximately 10–20% of patients with catecholamine-secreting tumors have associated germline mutations (inherited mutations present in all cells of the body) in genes known to cause genetic disease.[13,18,19] The familial neurocristopathic syndromes associated with adrenal pheochromocytoma include familial pheochromocytoma; multiple endocrine neoplasia type 2A (MEN 2A) (pheochromocytoma, medullary thyroid carcinoma, and hyperparathyroidism) and type 2B (MEN 2B) (pheochromocytoma, medullary thyroid carcinoma, mucosal neuromas, thickened corneal nerves, intestinal ganglioneuromatosis, and marfanoid body habitus); neurofibromatosis type 1 (NF1); von Hippel-Lindau disease (VHL) (pheochromocytoma, retinal angiomas, cerebellar hemangioblastoma, renal and pancreatic cysts, and renal cell carcinoma); and familial paraganglioma.[20–24] Additional neurocutaneous syndromes associated with catecholamine-secreting tumors include ataxia-telangiectasia, tuberous sclerosis, and Sturge-Weber syndrome. Other diagnoses associated with catecholamine-secreting tumors that do not appear to be inherited are Carney triad (gastric leiomyosarcoma, pulmonary chondroma, and extra-adrenal pheochromocytoma),[25] cholelithiasis, and renal artery stenosis.

Catecholamine-secreting paragangliomas may be associated with familial paraganglioma, NF1, VHL, Carney triad, and rarely MEN 2. Genetic testing is available for nearly all of these disorders. Families should be offered genetic counseling prior to performing genetic testing. To obtain informative genetic testing results, a symptomatic family member should always be tested first.

DIAGNOSTIC INVESTIGATION

Case finding

Pheochromocytoma should be suspected in patients with hypertension accompanied by one or more of the following: hyperadrenergic spells (e.g. self-limited episodes of non-exertional palpitations, diaphoresis, headache, tremor, and pallor); resistant hypertension; a familial syndrome that predisposes to catecholamine-secreting tumors (e.g. MEN 2); an incidentally discovered adrenal mass; or a history of gastric stromal tumor or pulmonary chondromas (Carney triad). The diagnosis must be confirmed biochemically by the presence of increased urine or plasma concentrations of catecholamines and/or metanephrines.

Most laboratories now measure catecholamines and metanephrines by high pressure liquid chromatography with electrochemical detection or with tandem mass spectroscopy.[26] These techniques have overcome the problems with fluorometric analysis (e.g. false positive results caused by α-methyldopa and other drugs with high native fluorescence).

At the Mayo Clinic, the single most reliable screening method for identifying catecholamine-secreting tumors is measuring metanephrines in a 24-hour urine collection[12,27] this finding is shared by other groups.[28,29] If clinical suspicion is high, then urinary catecholamines (epinephrine, norepinephrine, and dopamine) are measured in addition to the 24-hour urine metanephrines. Fractionated plasma free metanephrines, which are products of intra-pheochromocytoma catecholamine metabolism, are also obtained in high suspicion cases.[30] Some groups have advocated that fractionated plasma free metanephrines should be a first-line test for pheochromocytoma.[31,32] However, we have found that fractionated plasma free metanephrines lack the necessary specificity to be recommended as a first-line test; therefore, this measurement should be reserved for high suspicion cases.[27,33,34] High suspicion cases include patients who have one or more of the following: resistant hypertension; spells; a family history of pheochromocytoma; a genetic syndrome that predisposes to pheochromocytoma (e.g. MEN 2); a past history of resected pheochromocytoma and now have recurrent hypertension or spells; or an incidentally discovered adrenal mass that has imaging characteristics consistent with pheochromocytoma (e.g. marked enhancement with intravenous contrast medium on CT, high signal intensity on T2-weighted MRI imaging, cystic and hemorrhagic changes, larger size (e.g. >4 cm), or bilaterality).[12] In addition, measuring fractionated plasma free metanephrines is a good first-line test in pediatric patients since obtaining a complete 24-hour urine collection is difficult in children.

A recent review of the literature that examined the diagnostic efficacy of measuring fractionated plasma free metanephrines in the biochemical investigation for pheochromocytoma found that a normal result adequately ruled out pheochromocytoma;[33] however, a positive result only moderately increased the likelihood of disease, especially when sporadic pheochromocytoma is suspected. The plasma normetanephrine fraction is responsible for most false positive results, and the amount of plasma normetanephrine increases with age.[27] When screening for sporadic pheochromocytoma, the false positive rate of fractionated plasma free metanephrines can be significantly reduced by using age-dependent cut-offs in result interpretation.[34] Reducing the false positive rate may save expenditures related to confirmatory imaging.[35] Since fractionated plasma free metanephrines are highly specific, their true value comes from normal results that rule out pheochromocytoma.

For patients with episodic hypertension, the 24-hour urine collection should be started with the onset of a spell. When the 24-hour urine is collected in this manner, patients with pheochromocytoma have one or both the following findings: (1) levels of 24-hour urine catecholamines are increased more than twofold above the upper normal limit (e.g. norepinephrine >170 mcg, or epinephrine >35 mcg, or dopamine >700 mcg), or (2) levels of urinary metanephrines (e.g. >400 mcg) or normetanephrine (e.g. >900 mcg) are significantly increased above the upper normal limit. In 130 patients with benign sporadic adrenal pheochromocytomas who were surgically treated at the Mayo Clinic from 1978 to 1995: (1) 24-hour urinary total metanephrines (metanephrines + normetanephrine) were increased above the upper normal limit in 94% of patients, and (2) 24-hour urinary norepinephrine or epinephrine was increased more than twofold above the upper normal limit in 93% of patients, and (3) diagnostic increases occurred in either 24-hour urine metanephrines or catecholamines in 99% of patients.[12]

Although it is preferred that patients not receive any medication during the diagnostic evaluation, treatment with most medications may be continued, with some exceptions (Box 25.3). Tricyclic antidepressants are the agents that interfere most frequently with the interpretation of 24-hour urine catecholamines and metabolites. To effectively screen for catecholamine-secreting tumors, treatment with tricyclic antidepressants and other psychoactive agents listed in Box 25.3 should be tapered and discontinued at least 2 weeks before any hormonal assessments. In addition, catecholamine secretion may be appropriately increased in situations of physical stress or illness (e.g. stroke, obstructive sleep apnea). Therefore, the clinical circumstances under which measurements of catecholamines and metanephrines are made must be assessed in each case.

Box 25.3 Medications that may increase measured levels of catecholamines and metanephrines

Tricyclic antidepressants
Levodopa
Drugs containing catecholamines
(e.g. decongestants)
Amphetamines
Buspirone, and most psychoactive agents
Withdrawal from clonidine and other drugs
Ethanol
Acetaminophen and phenoxybenzamine
(may increase measured levels of fractionated plasma metanephrines in some assays)

Renal failure

Measurements of urinary catecholamines and metabolites may be invalid in patients with advanced renal insufficiency.[36] Serum chromogranin A levels have poor diagnostic specificity in these patients.[37] In non-pheochromocytoma, hemodialyzed patients, plasma norepinephrine and dopamine concentrations are increased threefold and twofold, respectively, above the upper normal limit.[38,39] However, standard normal ranges can be used for interpreting plasma epinephrine concentrations.[40] Therefore, when patients with renal failure have plasma norepinephrine concentrations that are increased more than threefold above the upper normal limit or epinephrine that is increased above the upper normal limit, pheochromocytoma should be suspected.[36] One study found that plasma concentrations of free metanephrines are increased approximately twofold in patients with renal failure; this finding may be useful in the biochemical evaluation of patients with marked renal insufficiency or renal failure.[41] However, a prior study suggested that concentrations of fractionated plasma free metanephrines could not distinguish between 10 patients with pheochromocytoma and 11 patients with end-stage renal disease who required long-term hemodialysis.[42]

Factitious pheochromocytoma

As with other factitious disorders, factitious pheochromocytoma can be difficult to confirm.[43] The patient usually has a medical background. The patient may 'spike' the 24-hour urine container or self-administer catecholamines.[44,45]

Localization

Localization studies should not be initiated until biochemical studies have confirmed the diagnosis of a catecholamine-secreting tumor (Figure 25.1). The

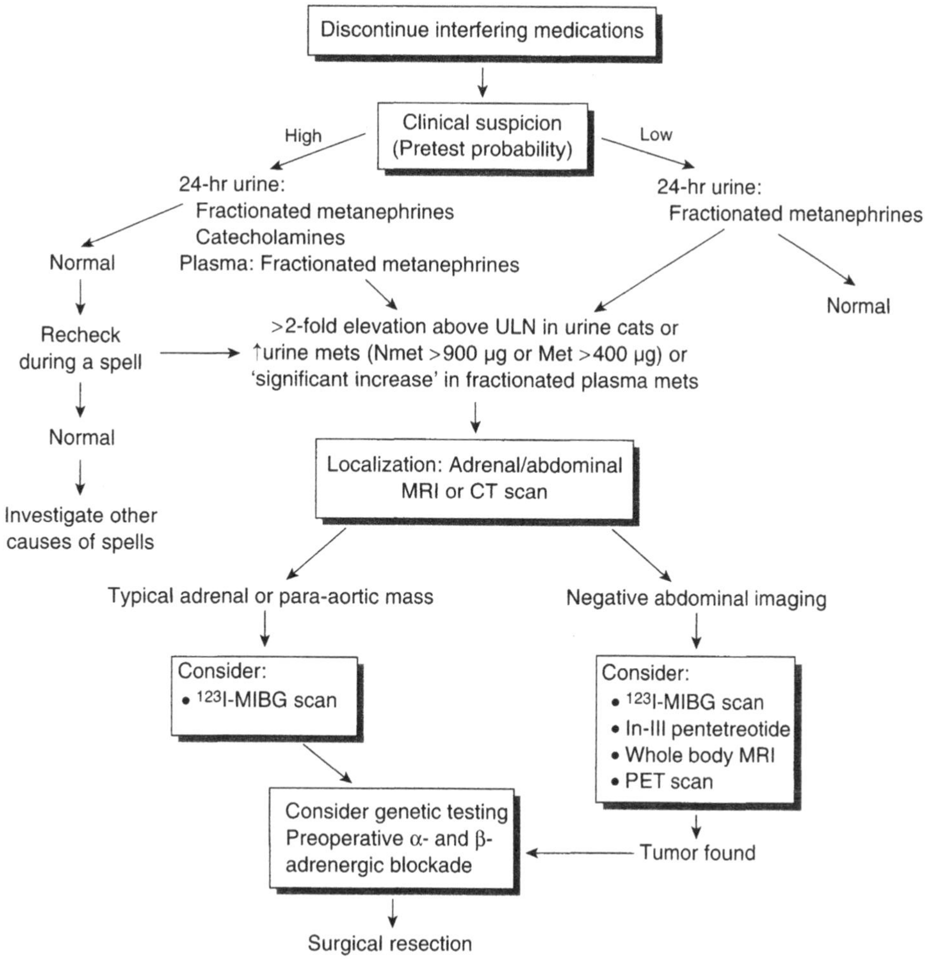

Figure 25.1 Evaluation and treatment of catecholamine-secreting tumors. Clinical suspicion is triggered by the following: paroxysmal symptoms (especially hypertension); hypertension that is intermittent, unusually labile, or resistant to treatment; family history of pheochromocytoma or associated conditions; or incidentally discovered adrenal mass. The details are discussed in the text. CT, computed tomography; ^{123}I-MIBG, ^{123}I-metaiodobenzylguanidine; MRI, magnetic resonance imaging. (Modified from Young WF Jr: Pheochromocytoma: 1926–1993. *Trends Endocrinol Metab* 4: 122, 1993; with permission from Elsevier Science.[61])

first localization test should be computer-assisted imaging of the adrenal glands and abdomen (magnetic resonance imaging, MRI, or computed tomography, CT) (sensitivity >95%; specificity >65%).[46] Approximately 90% of these tumors are found in the adrenal glands and 98% are found in the abdomen.[47] If the results of abdominal imaging are negative, scintigraphic localization with ^{123}I-metaiodobenzylguanidine (^{123}I-MIBG) is indicated. This radiopharmaceutical agent accumulates preferentially in catecholamine-secreting tumors; however, this procedure is not as sensitive as initially hoped (sensitivity 80%; specificity 99%).[48] In a study of 282 patients with catecholamine-secreting tumors that were surgically confirmed, the sensitivities of imaging studies were 89% for CT, 98% for MRI, and 81% for ^{131}I-MIBG.[49] Catecholamine-secreting paragangliomas are found where chromaffin tissue is located (e.g. along the para-aortic sympathetic chain, within the organs of Zuckerkandl at the origin of the inferior mesenteric artery, in the wall of the urinary bladder, and in the sympathetic chain in the neck or mediastinum).[15] Tumor size is correlated with the degree of increase in plasma free metanephrine concentration[50] but not with the degree of increase in catecholamine concentration.[51] In one study, tumor diameter was strongly correlated with summed plasma concentrations and urinary outputs of metanephrine and normetanephrine ($r=0.81$ and 0.77; $p<0.001$).[50]

All the tumors associated with a plasma metanephrine concentration that was >15% of the combined increases of normetanephrine and metanephrine were either located in the adrenal glands or appeared to be recurrences of previously resected adrenal tumors.

If a typical (<10 cm) unilateral adrenal pheochromocytoma is found on CT or MRI, ^{123}I-MIBG scintigraphy is superfluous, and the results may confuse the clinician.[52,53] However, if a paraganglioma is identified on CT or MRI, then ^{123}I-MIBG scintigraphy is indicated because the patient has increased risk of having additional paragangliomas and malignant disease. Performing preoperative ^{123}I-MIBG scintigraphy in patients with large (>10 cm) adrenal pheochromocytomas may be indicated to identify metastatic disease; however, finding metastatic disease preoperatively does not usually change the surgical treatment plan.

Localizing procedures that can also be used, but are rarely required, include central venous sampling and computer-assisted imaging of the chest, neck, and head. Results of selective venous sampling for catecholamines are frequently misleading because of periodic secretion; however, some medical centers have had successful results.[54,55] Other localizing studies, such as somatostatin-receptor imaging with indium In-111-labeled pentetreotide, may also be considered.[56,57] Positron emission tomography (PET) scanning[58] with ^{18}F-fluorodeoxyglucose (FDG) or ^{11}C-hydroxyephedrine or 6-[^{18}F]fluorodopamine is capable of identifying paragangliomas that may be detected with less expensive techniques, but this procedure should be reserved for identifying sites of metastatic disease in ^{123}I-MIBG-negative patients.[59,60]

TREATMENT

The treatment of choice for pheochromocytoma is complete surgical resection. Careful preoperative pharmacologic preparation is crucial to successful treatment. Most catecholamine-secreting tumors are benign and can be totally excised. Tumor excision usually cures hypertension. Some form of preoperative pharmacologic preparation is indicated in all patients with catecholamine-secreting neoplasms. Combined α- and β-adrenergic blockade is one approach to control the patient's blood pressure and to prevent intraoperative hypertensive crises.[61] α-Adrenergic blockade with phenoxybenzamine should be started 7–10 days preoperatively to normalize blood pressure and expand the contracted blood volume. Target blood pressures are <120/80 mm Hg (seated), with systolic blood pressure >90 mm Hg (standing); both targets should be modified on the basis of patient age and comorbid disease. On the second or third day of α-adrenergic blockade, patients are encouraged to start a diet high in sodium content because of the catecholamine-induced volume contraction and the orthostasis associated with α-adrenergic blockade. Once adequate α-adrenergic blockade is achieved, β-adrenergic blockade is initiated, which typically occurs 2–3 days preoperatively. Calcium channel blockers, which block norepinephrine-mediated calcium transport into vascular smooth muscle, have been used successfully at several medical centers to preoperatively prepare patients with pheochromocytoma.[62–64] Acute hypertensive crises may occur before or during operation, and they should be treated intravenously with sodium nitroprusside, phentolamine, or nicardipine.

In the past, an anterior midline abdominal surgical approach was usually used for resecting adrenal pheochromocytoma. However, the procedure of choice for patients with solitary intra-adrenal pheochromocytomas that are <8 cm in diameter is now the laparoscopic approach.[65] If the pheochromocytoma is in the adrenal gland, the entire gland should be removed. Laparoscopic adrenalectomy for pheochromocytoma should be converted to open adrenalectomy for difficult dissection, invasion, adhesions, or surgeon inexperience.[66] If the tumor is malignant, as much of the tumor should be removed as possible. An anterior midline abdominal surgical approach is indicated for abdominal paragangliomas. The midline abdomen should be inspected carefully. Paragangliomas of the neck, chest, and urinary bladder require specialized approaches. 'Unresectable' cardiac pheochromocytomas may require cardiac transplantation.[67]

Approximately 1–2 weeks after surgery, catecholamines and metanephrines should be measured by collecting a 24-hour urine. If the levels are normal, the resection of the pheochromocytoma should be considered complete. The survival rate after removal of a benign pheochromocytoma is nearly that of age- and sex-matched normal controls. Increased levels of catecholamines and metanephrines detected postoperatively are consistent with residual tumor, either a second primary lesion or occult metastases. If bilateral adrenalectomy was performed, lifelong glucocorticoid and mineralocorticoid replacement therapy should be prescribed. Twenty-four-hour urinary excretion of catecholamines and metanephrines or plasma metanephrines should be checked annually for life. The annual biochemical testing assesses for metastatic disease, tumor recurrence in the adrenal bed, or delayed appearance of multiple primary tumors.[68] The highest tumor recurrence rates are found in patients that have one or more of the following: a positive family history, a right-sided adrenal tumor, or a paraganglioma.[69] Follow-up computerized imaging is not needed unless the metanephrine and/or catecholamine levels become elevated or the original tumor was associated with minimal catecholamine excess.

Genetic testing should be considered for patients with one or more of the following: a family history of pheochromocytoma, a paraganglioma, or any signs that suggest a genetic etiology (e.g. retinal angiomas, axillary freckling, café au lait spots, cerebellar tumor, MTC, hyperparathyroidism). In addition, all first-degree relatives of the pheochromocytoma/paraganglioma patient should have biochemical testing (e.g. 24-hour urine for fractionated metanephrines and catecholamines). When a patient has an identified mutation, genetic testing of first-degree relatives should proceed in a stepwise fashion (i.e. parents first).

REFERENCES

1. Stenstrom G, Svardsudd K. Phaechromocytoma in Sweden, 1958–81. An analysis of the National Cancer Registry Data. Acta Med Scand 1986; 220: 225–32.
2. Young WF Jr, Maddox DE. Spells: in search of a cause. Mayo Clin Proc 1995; 70: 757–65.
3. Sweeney AT, Malabanan AO, Blake MA et al. Megacolon as the presenting feature in pheochromocytoma. J Clin Endocrinol Metab 2000; 85: 3968–72.
4. O'Brien TO, Young WF Jr, Davila DG et al. Cushing' syndrome associated with ectopic production of corticocotrophin-releasing hormone, corticotrophin, and vasopressin by a phaeochromocytoma. Clin Endocrinol (Oxf) 1992; 37: 460–7.
5. Mune T, Katakami H, Kato Y et al. Production and secretion of parathyroid hormone-related protein in pheochromocytoma: participation of an alpha-adrenergic mechanism. J Clin Endocrinol Metab 1993; 76: 757–62.
6. Smith SL, Slappy AL, Fox TP et al. Pheochromocytoma producing vasoactive intestinal peptide. Mayo Clin Proc 2002; 77: 97–100.
7. Saito H, Sano T, Yamasaki R et al. Demonstration of biological activity of growth hormone-releasing hormone-like substance produced by a pheochromocytoma. Acta Endocrinol (Copenh) 1993; 129: 246–50.
8. Schifferdecker B, Kodali D, Hausner E et al. Adrenergic shock – an overlooked clinical entity? Cardiol Rev 2005; 13: 69–72.
9. Gordon RY, Fallon JT, Baran DA. Case report: a 32-year-old woman with familial paragangliomas and acute cardiomyopathy. Transplant Proc 2004; 36: 2819–22.
10. Kim J, Reutrakul S, Davis DB et al. Multiple endocrine neoplasia 2A syndrome presenting as peripartum caridiomyopathy due to catecholamine excess. Eur J Endocrinol 2004; 151: 771–7.
11. Manger WM, Gifford RW Jr. Diagnosis. In: Clinical and experimental Pheochromocytoma. Cambridge, MA: Blackwell Science, 1996.
12. Kudva YC, Sawka AM, Young WF Jr. Clinical review 164: the laboratory diagnosis of adrenal pheochromocytoma: the Mayo Clinic experience. J Clin Endocrinol Metab 2003; 88: 4533–9.
13. Neumann HP, Bausch B, McWhinney SR et al. Germ-line mutations in nonsyndromeic pheochromocytoma. N Engl J Med 2002; 346: 1459–66.
14. Kinney MA, Warner ME, vanHeerden JA et al. Perianesthetic risks and outcomes of pheochromocytoma and paraganglioma resection. Anesth Analg 2000; 91: 1118–23.
15. O'Riordain DS, Young WF Jr, Grant CS et al. Clinical spectrum and outcome of functional extraadrenal paraganglioma. World J Surg 1996; 20: 916–22.
16. Erickson D, Kudva YC, Ebersold MJ et al. Benign paragangliomas: clinical presentation and treatment outcomes in 236 patients. J Clin Endocrinol Metab 2001; 86: 5210–16.
17. Osranek M, Bursi F, Gura GM et al. Echocardiographic features of pheochromocytoma of the heart. Am J Cardiol 2003; 91: 640–3.
18. Elder EE, Elder G, Larsson C. Pheochromocytoma and functional paraganglioma syndrome: no longer the 10% tumor. J Surg Oncol 2005; 89: 193–201.
19. Gimm O, Koch CA, Januszewicz A et al. The genetic basis of pheochromocytoma. Front Horm Res 2004; 31: 45–60.
20. Gross DJ, Avishai N, Meiner V et al. Familial pheochromocytoma associated with a novel mutation in the von Hippel-Lindau gene. J Clin Endocrinol Metab 1996; 81: 147–9.
21. Atuk NO, McDonald T, Wood T et al. Familial pheochromocytoma, hypercalcemia, and von Hippel-Lindau disease: a ten year study of a large family. Medicine 1979; 58: 209–18.
22. Brauch H, Kishida T, Glavac D et al. von Hippel-Lindau (VHL) disease with pheochromocytoma in the Black Forest region of Germany: evidence for a founder effect. Hum Genet 1995; 95: 551–6.
23. Eng C, Clayton D, Schuffenecker I et al. The relationship between specific RET proto-oncogene mutations and disease phenotype in multiple endocrine neoplasia type 2: international RET mutation consortium analysis. JAMA 1996; 276: 1575–9.
24. Atuk NO, Stolle C, Owen JA Jr et al. Pheochromocytoma in von Hippel-Lindau disease: clinical presentation and mutation analysis in a large multigenerational kindred. J Clin Endocrinol Metab 1998; 83: 117–20.
25. Carney JA. The triad of gastric epithelioid leiomyosarcoma, pulmonary chondroma, and functioning extra-adrenal paraganglioma: a five-year review. Medicine 1983; 62: 159–69.
26. Taylor RL, Singh RJ. Validation of liquid chromatography-tandem mass spectrometry method for analysis of urinary conjugated metanephrine and normetanephrine for screening of pheochromocytoma. Clin Chem 2002; 48: 533–9.
27. Sawka AM, Jaeschke R, Singh RJ et al. A comparison of biochemical tests for pheochromocytoma: measurement of fractionated plasma metanephrines compared with the combination of 24-hour urinary metanephrines and catecholamines. J Clin Endocrinol Metab 2003; 88: 553–8.
28. Hernandez FC, Sanchez M, Alvarez A et al. A five-year report on experience in the detection of pheochromocytoma. Clin Biochem 2000; 33: 649–55.
29. Witteles RM, Kaplan EL, Roizen MF. Sensitivity of diagnostic and localization tests for pheochromocytoma in clinical practice. Arch Intern Med 2000; 160: 2521–4.
30. Eisenhofer G, Keiser H, Friberg P et al. Plasma metanephrines are markers of pheochromocytoma produced by catechol-O-methyltransferase within tumors. J Clin Endocrinol Metab 1998; 83: 2175–85.
31. Raber W, Raffesberg W, Bischof M et al. Diagnostic efficacy of unconjugated plasma metanephrines for the detection of pheochromocytoma. Arch Intern Med 2000; 160: 2957–63.
32. Lenders JW, Pacak K, Walther MM et al. Biochemical diagnosis of pheochromocytoma: which test is best? JAMA 2002; 287: 1427–34.

33. Sawka AM, Prebtani AP, Thabane L et al. A systematic review of the literature examining the diagnostic efficacy of measurement of fractionate plasma free metanephrines in the biochemical diagnosis of pheochromocytoma. BMC Endocr Disord 2004; 4: 2.
34. Sawka AM, Thabane L, Gafni A et al. Measurement of fractionated plasma metanephrines for exclusion of pheochromocytoma: can specificity be improved by adjustment for age? BMC Endocr Disord 2005; 5: 1.
35. Sawka AM, Gafni A, Thabane L et al. The economic implications of three biochemical screening algorithms for pheochromocytoma. J Clin Endocrinol Metab 2004; 89: 2859–66.
36. Godfrey JA, Rickman OB, Williams AW et al. Pheochromocytoma in a patient with end-stage renal disease. Mayo Clin Proc 2001; 76: 953–7.
37. Canale MP, Bravo EL. Diagnostic specificity of serum chromogranin-A for pheochromocytoma in patients with renal dysfunction. J Clin Endocrinol Metab 1994; 78: 1139–44.
38. Chauveau D, Martinez F, Houhou S et al. Malignant hypertension secondary to pheochromocytoma in a hemodialyzed patient. Am J Kidney Dis 1993; 21: 52–3.
39. Stumvoll M, Radjaipour M, Seif F. Diagnostic considerations in pheochromocytoma and chronic hemodialysis: case report and review of the literature. Am J Nephrol 1995; 15: 147–51.
40. Morioka M, Yuihama S, Nakajima T et al. Incidentally discovered pheochromocytoma in long-term hemodialysis patients. Int J Urol 2002; 9: 700–3.
41. Eisenhofer G, Huysmans F, Pacak K et al. Plasma metanephrines in renal failure. Kidney Int 2005; 67: 668–77.
42. Marini M, Fathi M, Ballotton M. [Determination of serum metanephrines in the diagnosis of pheochromocytoma.] Ann Endocrinol (Paris) 1994; 54: 337–42.
43. Stern TA, Cremens CM. Factitious pheochromocytoma. One patient history and literature review. Psychosomatics 1998; 39: 283–7.
44. Spitzer D, Bongartz D, Ittel TH et al. Simulation of a pheochromocytoma – Munchausen syndrome. Eur J Med Res 1998; 3: 549–53.
45. Sawka AM, Singh RJ, Young WF Jr. False positive biochemical testing for pheochromocytoma caused by surreptitious catecholamine addition to urine. Endocrinologist 2001; 11: 421–3.
46. Jackson JA, Kleerekoper M, Mendlovic D. Endocrine grand rounds: a 51-year-old man with accelerated hypertension, hypercalcemia, and right adrenal and paratracheal masses. Endocrinologist 1993; 3: 5.
47. van Gils APG, Falke THM, van Erkel AR et al. MR imaging and MIBG scintigraphy of pheochromocytomas and extra-adrenal functioning paragangliomas. Radiographics 1991; 11: 37–57.
48. Shapiro B, Gross MD, Fig L et al. Localization of functioning sympathoadrenal lesions. In: Biglieri EG, Melby JC (eds). Endocrine hypertension. New York: Raven Press, 1990, pp 235–55.
49. Jalil ND, Pattou FN, Combemale F et al. Effectiveness and limits of preoperative imaging studies for the localisation of pheochromocytomas and paragangliomas: a review of 282 cases. French Association of Surgery (AFC), and The French Association of Endocrine Surgeons (AFCE). Eur J Surg 1998; 164: 23–8.
50. Eisenhofer G, Lenders JW, Goldstein DS et al. Pheochromocytoma catecholamine phenotypes and prediction of tumor size and location by use of plasma free metanephrines. Clin Chem 2005; 51: 735–44.
51. Ito Y, Fujimoto Y, Obara T. The role of epinephrine, norepinephrine, and dopamine in blood pressure disturbances in patients with pheochromocytoma. World J Surg 1992; 16: 759–63.
52. Miskulin J, Shulkin BL, Doherty GM et al. Is preoperative iodine 123 meta-iodobenzylguanidine scintigraphy routinely necessary before initial adrenalectomy for pheochromocytoma? Surgery 2003; 134: 918–22.
53. Taieb D, Sebag F, Hubbard JG et al. Does iodine-131 meta-iodobenzylguanidine (MIBG) scintigraphy have an impact on the management of sporadic and familial phaeochromocytoma? Clin Endocrinol (Oxf) 2004; 61: 102–8.
54. Newbould EC, Ross GA, Dacie JE et al. The use of venous catheterization in the diagnosis and localization of bilateral phaeochromocytomas. Clin Endocrinol (Oxf) 1991; 35: 55–9.
55. Walker IA. Selective venous catheterization and plasma catecholamine analysis in the diagnosis of phaeochromocytoma. J R Soc Med 1996; 89: 216P–8P.
56. Lamberts SW, Bakker WH, Reubi JC et al. Somatostatin-receptor imaging in the localization of endocrine tumors. N Engl J Med 1990; 323: 1246–9.
57. Tenenbaum F, Lumbroso J, Schlumberger M et al. Comparison of radiolabeled octreotide and meta-iodobenzylguanidine (MIBG) scintigraphy in malignant pheochromocytoma. J Nucl Med 1995; 36: 1–6.
58. Pacak K, Eisenhofer G, Carrasquillo JA et al. Diagnostic localization of pheochromocytoma: the coming of age of positron emission tomography. Ann N Y Acad Sci 2002; 970: 170–6.
59. Hwang JJ, Uchio EM, Patel SV et al. Diagnostic localization of malignant bladder pheochromocytoma using 6–18F fluorodopamine positron emission tomography. J Urol 2003; 169: 274–5.
60. Shulkin BL, Wieland DM, Schwaiger M et al. PET scanning with hydroxyephedrine: an approach to the localization of pheochromocytoma. J Nucl Med 1992; 33: 1125–31.
61. Young WF Jr. Pheochromocytoma: 1926–1993. Trends Endocrinol Metab 1993; 4: 122–7.
62. Bravo EL. Pheochromocytoma: an approach to antihypertensive management. Ann N Y Acad Sci 2002; 970: 1–10.
63. Combemale F, Carnaille B, Tavernier B et al. Exclusive use of calcium channel blockers and cardioselective beta-blockers in the pre- and per-operative management of pheochromocytomas. 70 cases. Ann Chir 1998; 52: 341–5.
64. Ulchaker JC, Goldfarb DA, Bravo EL et al. Successful outcomes in pheochromocytoma surgery in the modern era. J Urol 1999; 161: 764–7.
65. Assalia A, Gagner M. Laparoscopic adrenalectomy. Br J Surg 2004; 91: 1259–74.
66. Shen WT, Sturgeon C, Clark OH et al. Should pheochromocytoma size influence surgical approach? A comparison of 90 malignant and 60 benign pheochromocytomas. Surgery 2004; 136: 1129–37.
67. Jeevanandam V, Oz MC, Shapiro B et al. Surgical management of cardiac pheochromocytoma. Resection versus transplantation. Ann Surg 1995; 221: 415–19.
68. van Heerden JA, Roland JA, Carney JA et al. Long-term evaluation following resection of apparently benign pheochromocytoma(s)/paraganglioma(s). World J Surg 1990; 14: 325–9.
69. Amar L, Servais A, Gimeniz-Roqueplo AP et al. Year of diagnosis, features at presentation, and risk of recurrence in patients with pheochromocytoma or secreting paraganglioma. J Clin Endocrinol Metab 2005; 90: 2110–16.

26

Microarray analysis of models of hypertension

Henry L Keen and Curt D Sigmund

INTRODUCTION

Hypertension is a prevalent disease and is one of the leading risk factors for end organ damage.[1] Elucidation of the molecular mechanisms underlying the maintenance of elevated blood pressure and the associated increase in cardiovascular risk should greatly enhance the search for therapeutic agents for this disease. Microarray technology permits the simultaneous measurement of thousands of mRNA transcripts, and has proven to be an invaluable resource in the study of biological systems, particularly in the area of cancer research.[2] Recent technological advances in microarray chip design now allow expression of almost all genes to be assessed in a single hybridization experiment. By examining the global gene expression changes occurring during various physiological perturbations or in disease models we can begin to form an integrative view of transcriptional regulation in a particular cell type or tissue. Moreover, due to the highly parallel nature of the microarray experiment, its use as an initial screening step combined with appropriate prioritization algorithms will lead to the more rapid identification of critical genes and pathways than could be achieved by examining genes one by one.

IDENTIFICATION OF THE CAUSATIVE GENETIC VARIANTS IN HYPERTENSION MODELS

The causative factors in several single-gene (monogenic) hypertensive syndromes have been successfully elucidated by the use of genetic linkage studies followed by positional cloning techniques.[3] Identification of these genes has greatly increased our understanding about the pathways involved in sustaining an elevated blood pressure. These disorders, however whilst severe, are usually rare, affecting only a very small percentage of the population. In contrast, essential hypertension is believed to be caused by combined effects of multiple genes (polygenic), with each gene contributing a small amount to the overall magnitude of the blood pressure increase.[4] Quantitative trait locus (QTL) analysis has been used to localize chromosomal locations that may play a role in complex diseases. In QTL analyses, it is possible to associate chromosomal regions with a specific phenotype. However, these genomic intervals can be very large, containing hundreds of genes, thus necessitating additional approaches such as haplotype analysis and generation of congenic animals, to narrow the QTL interval.[5] Even after application of these techniques, the list of potential candidate genes remains daunting.

The causative variant in a QTL location can alter downstream pathways ultimately effecting the quantitative trait of interest (e.g. blood pressure), either by modulating the expression of one or more of the genes in the interval or by generating a functional change in a protein. In cases involving a change in gene expression, it should be possible to prioritize the list of differentially expressed candidate genes in a non-biased manner through microarray analysis. Experimentally, the gene expression profile from a tissue known to be important in the regulation of blood pressure (e.g. kidney, brain, vasculature) is compared between a hypertensive model and its normotensive control. The ideal control is one with minimal genetic differences compared to the hypertensive model, making it easier to detect the variants that are responsible for the increased blood pressure. The experimental comparison often used is between a parental strain (such as spontaneously hypertensive rat, SHR) and a congenic strain that is

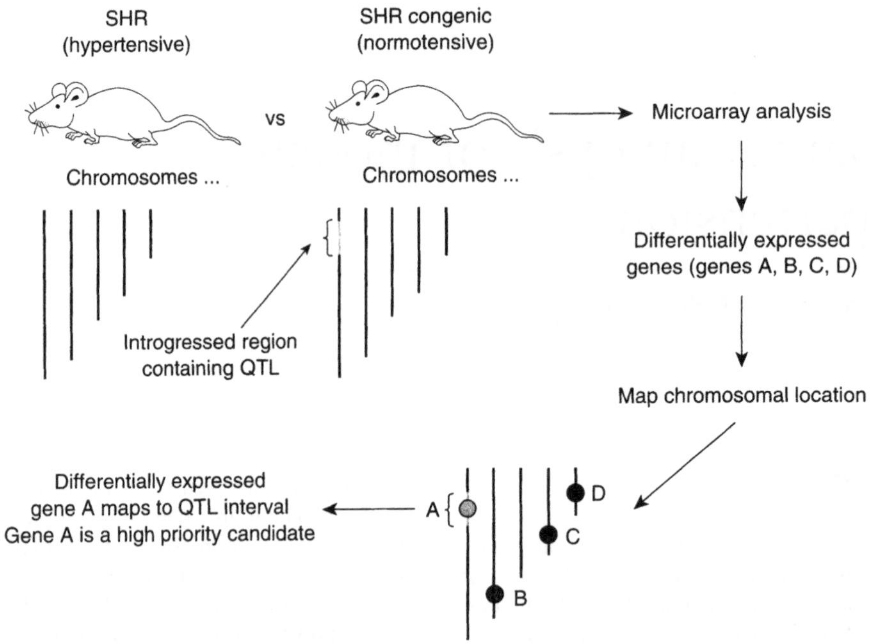

Figure 26.1 Schematic illustrating the use of microarray analysis to prioritize hypertension candidate genes. Microarray hybridizations are performed on RNA extracted from a tissue of interest (e.g. kidney) from a hypertensive strain (SHR) and from its normotensive control (SHR congenic). Note that the SHR parent and congenic are genetically identical except in a small region of the first chromosome (gray line). Genes differentially expressed between the two groups (A, B, C, D) are then mapped to their respective chromosomal locations. Gene A maps to a blood pressure QTL interval and is a high priority candidate for further study. Genes B, C, and D are differentially expressed but map to other locations. Altered expression of these genes is likely secondary to the primary causative genetic variant

genetically identical except for an introgressed genomic region thought to contain the QTL. An investigator then determines which differentially expressed genes are present in the QTL interval. A differentially expressed gene that is also located on a region of a chromosome where a QTL has been mapped will become a high priority candidate gene (Figure 26.1).

Using this approach, Aitman et al. identified a gene (CD36) that was decreased by approximately 90% in the SHR compared with its congenic control.[6] CD36 mapped to the putative blood pressure QTL interval on rat chromosome 4 and sequencing of multiple rat strains revealed a mutation in the CD36 gene in the SHR. Functional analysis confirmed that loss of CD36 contributes to the defective fatty acid metabolism and insulin resistance observed in the SHR. There are other examples as well. In another study, renal expression of a gene (glutathione S-transferase) located in a hypertension QTL interval on rat chromosome 2, was found to be significantly reduced in the SHR stroke-prone rat compared with its congenic control.[7] In an attempt to identify candidate genes on chromosome 13 responsible for salt sensitivity of blood pressure in the Dahl salt-sensitive (Dahl S) rat, Liang et al. performed a time-course study to detect genes whose expression in the renal medulla was regulated in a differential manner in the Dahl S rat compared with its salt-resistant congenic control, Dahl S with chromosome 13 from the Brown Norway strain.[8] Most of the genes found to have distinct patterns of expression were not located on chromosome 13, suggesting that the causative genetic variant (or variants) on chromosome 13 exerts part of its phenotypic action by altering the expression of downstream genes.

ANALYSIS OF TRANSCRIPTIONAL PATHWAYS DOWNSTREAM OF HYPERTENSION-RELATED GENES

Another approach to identify genes involved in the development of hypertension is to directly stimulate or inhibit systems already known to be important to the regulation of blood pressure and then observe the resulting changes in downstream genes or pathways. The renin-angiotensin system, of which angiotensin II (Ang II) is the active component, is an important regulator of sodium homeostasis and blood pressure. Larkin et al. performed a time-course study of cardiac gene expression in mice infused with a pressor dose of Ang II.[9] After performing statistical tests to evaluate the significance of expression changes in molecular pathways or functional categories, several pathways including mitochondrial metabolism and ribosomal activity were shown to be consistently modulated by Ang II at all time points, whereas other functional groups such as cytoskeletal and extracellular matrix genes were only altered by chronic (14 day) Ang II infusion. Non-pressor doses of Ang II have also been reported to have profound changes on gene expression including activation of groups of genes likely to increase oxidative stress and interstitial fibrosis in the renal outer medulla.[10] In addition to animals, cell culture models have been utilized to examine specific molecular pathways in greater detail. Using rat aortic vascular smooth muscle cells and pharmacological antagonists of various intracellular signaling pathways, Campos et al. identified a cluster of six genes up-regulated by Ang II by a mechanism dependent on the ERK and p38 pathways.[11] Importantly, two genes (Calpactin I LC, Calpactin II) not previously known to be Ang II responsive were among those identified. The other four genes, including osteopontin and plasminogen activator inhibitor-1, appear to be involved in regulation of the extracellular matrix. Hong et al. demonstrated in cardiac fibroblasts that Ang II activates the transcription factor AP-1, and that an AP-1 binding site located in the promoter region was crucial for Ang II inducement of the endothelin-1 gene.[12]

This serves to illustrate that because altered gene expression is usually the result of a change in transcriptional activity, identification of differentially expressed transcription factors may be needed to form a complete picture of the regulatory pathways in hypertension. An example of this is a recent study from our group examining peroxisome proliferator-activated receptor-gamma (PPARγ) response genes in the blood vessel. PPARγ, a transcription factor of the nuclear hormone receptor subfamily, exerts significant vascular protective actions including lowering of blood pressure and reduction of expression of proinflammatory molecules in the blood vessel wall.[13] In humans, naturally occurring loss-of-function mutations in PPARγ are associated with severe glucose intolerance and hypertension.[14] We performed microarray analysis and extensive real-time quantitative RT-PCR on aortic RNA from mice treated with an activator of PPARγ (rosiglitazone) to generate, in a non-biased manner, a list of PPARγ target genes in the vasculature.[15] Among the genes that were differentially expressed were six transcription factors, suggesting that the actions of PPARγ probably depend on a secondary cascade of transcription factors. We next integrated the microarray results with several computational approaches including comparative genomic analysis to identify potential regulatory elements and to construct plausible transcriptional networks. Some of these approaches include: 1) comparative genomics to look for conserved sequences across species, and 2) a search for PPARγ response elements (PPRE) in sequences upstream of the differentially expressed genes. Interestingly, some of the other 175 differentially regulated genes appear to be targets of one or more of these 6 transcription factors. Experiments are currently underway in our laboratory to test the hypotheses generated from these analyses.

IDENTIFICATION OF THE DETERMINANTS OF GENE EXPRESSION VARIATION

Another approach toward dissecting the mechanisms underlying the development or maintenance of hypertension involves elucidation of the naturally occurring genetic variants that alter the expression of genes important to the normal regulation of blood pressure. These variants have been the subject of much recent investigation and are referred to as expression level polymorphisms.[16] This basic approach is to combine genetic mapping with gene expression, by employing large panels of genetic markers spread throughout the genome and microarrays to interrogate the expression of thousands of genes. This procedure is very analogous to standard QTL mapping between genetic markers and a quantitative trait such as blood pressure. The only difference is that the gene expression values generated from the microarray experiments are the traits, and the QTL interval is referred to as an expression QTL or eQTL.[17]

Using expression data from liver tissue derived from an F_2 population of 111 mice generated from two common inbred strains (C57BL/6J and DBA/2J), Schadt et al. were able to identify 784 eQTLs with a LOD score >7.0.[18] Co-localization of eQTLs and genes occurred 71% of the time, suggesting that for these genes, the genetic variation strongly influencing their expression was near the gene, perhaps in the gene itself or in the promoter region. As you might expect, the differential expression of a gene might map to the promoter of that gene. This leads to the hypothesis that genetic variation in that gene's promoter may be responsible for its differential expression. eQTLs that are located at the same chromosomal locus as the linked gene are termed cis-acting eQTLs. It has been proposed that the presence of a strong linkage to cis-acting eQTLs should be among the criteria used to prioritize gene candidates from conventional QTL intervals.[19] The remaining 29% of eQTLs were located at physically distinct locations, most often on different chromosomes, and are therefore, termed trans-acting eQTLs. In contrast to cis eQTLs, the QTL responsible for the differential expression of a gene or set of genes might map to an unexpected location. This becomes interesting when that location corresponds to another transcription factor. The differential expression of this transcription factor could then influence the expression of its target genes.

The primary limitation with this method, as with conventional QTL mapping, is the difficulty in finding the causative genetic variation within the eQTL interval, as regulatory elements such as enhancers are sometimes located at a relatively large distance from the gene being regulated. Rubin et al. have demonstrated that a comparative genomics approach can be used to narrow the genomic interval to search for important regulatory sequences.[20] High similarity between orthologous genomic sequences from distantly related species suggests that the sequence is under selective pressure and likely to contain important regulatory elements (Figure 26.2). Even without identifying the genetic variation underlying the eQTL, much insight can be gained by examining the group of genes whose trans-acting eQTLs co-localize. In other words, genes whose expression is strongly influenced by the same genetic variation are likely to be part of a common pathway or to be, in some way, functionally related. In the study from Schadt et al., eQTLs from many genes known to be important in obesity or metabolism were clustered onto a region of chromosome 2.[18] Other genes whose expression was linked to this region included a group of major urinary protein genes including Mup-1, suggesting the possibility that this protein family known to participate in pheromone binding might also play a role in obesity.[21] In a recent report, Hubner et al. performed genetic and microarray analysis on 30 recombinant inbred strains (BXH/HXB) generated from a cross between SHR/Ola and Brown-Norway congenic (BN-Lx) rats and identified a set of genes whose expression in kidney was genetically linked to an eQTL.[22] Whether any of these are causally related to hypertension will require additional testing.

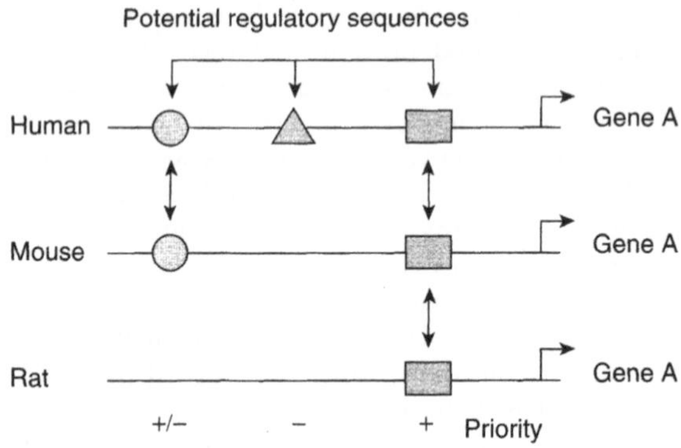

Figure 26.2 Schematic illustrating the use of comparative genomics to identify important regulatory sequences. Three potential regulatory sequences are illustrated by the shapes in the promoter region of hypothetical gene A from human. The corresponding orthologs from mouse and rat are shown as well. The sequence indicated by the square box is highly conserved across each of these species and is likely to be functionally important. Conservation between only two species (circles) suggests potential importance, whereas areas with no conservation (triangle) would be the lowest priority candidates for further study

GENE EXPRESSION PROFILING AS A DIAGNOSTIC TOOL IN HUMAN ESSENTIAL HYPERTENSION

Both the underlying mechanisms of essential hypertension and the end organ damage in response to the chronic elevation in blood pressure are quite heterogeneous in the general population. Moreover, it is difficult to predict the clinical outcome or optimal therapeutic regimen for patients using standard diagnostic measures. Gene expression profiles combined with clustering techniques have been used effectively to classify cancer subtypes (e.g. metastatic) in situations in which it was not possible to make such distinctions based on histological or biochemical analysis.[23] Clustering analysis is a set of mathematical tools used to detect similar patterns of gene expression. Recent studies suggest that similar methods might be useful in systemic disorders such as hypertension as well. In a study of patients with acute renal allograft rejection, three distinct gene expression patterns were found in kidney biopsy samples that were otherwise indistinguishable by light microscopic examination.[24] These patterns were associated with differences in clinical outcome. Using expression profiling from lung tissue, Geraci et al. were able to distinguish between sporadic and familial forms of primary pulmonary hypertension.[25] In a heterogeneous group of patients with focal segmental glomerulosclerosis (FSGS), a leading cause of chronic renal failure, Schwab et al. identified a set of genes and pathways that were consistently differently regulated in patients with this disease.[26] Importantly, many of these pathways were not previously known to be altered in FSGS.

While tissue biopsies are not routinely taken in hypertensive patients (except those with clinically significant end-stage disease), several reports suggest that microarray analysis of blood cell-derived RNA could provide clinical and mechanistic insight into systemic diseases. Moreover, this technique is relatively non-invasive, possibly allowing for therapeutic interventions to be made earlier than would have occurred otherwise. In a study of 75 healthy individuals, Whitney et al. demonstrated using whole blood samples (i.e. all cell types) that the gene expression profiles within non-diseased individuals had relatively low variability but were clearly and significantly different compared with individuals with leukemia or acute bacterial infection.[27] In patients with systemic lupus erythematosus (SLE), microarray analysis of RNA from leukocytes revealed 10 genes that were highly correlated with the SLE disease activity index.[28] In a study using peripheral blood mononuclear cells, it was demonstrated that a subset of 106 genes was able to accurately discriminate between normal individuals and those with primary pulmonary hypertension.[29] With regard to essential hypertension, Chon et al. recently reported that there were significant alterations in gene expression in leukocytes from a small group of untreated hypertensive patients with no evidence of end organ damage.[30] These changes were almost completely absent in hypertensive patients whose blood pressure was adequately controlled by treatment with β-blockers or angiotensin converting enzyme (ACE) inhibitors. There was a significant activation of leukocyte inflammatory and oxidative stress pathways, and increased expression of two genes with known important roles in blood pressure regulation, the angiotensin AT_1 receptor and the atrial natriuretic peptide receptor A, in the untreated patients. An important area of future investigation will be to determine if there is a leukocyte gene expression pattern predictive of those patients likely to develop end organ damage. It would be advantageous to identify these patients early and start antihypertensive medications before severe end organ damage occurs. This is particularly significant considering that the increased cardiovascular risk associated with hypertension is not ameliorated in many patients with pre-existing damage even after normalization of blood pressure.

INTEGRATION OF PUBLICLY AVAILABLE REPOSITORIES OF MICROARRAY DATA

Several publicly available repositories including the Gene Expression Omnibus[31] (GEO, http://www.ncbi.nih.gov/geo) at the NCBI and Array Express[32] at the European Bioinformatics Institute (http://www.ebi.ac.uk/arrayexpress) have been established to store and disseminate array results to the scientific community. It is hoped that investigators will be able to integrate these results with those from their laboratory in order to gain additional insights. While the ability to accurately compare results across different experimental platforms remains a challenge, recent reports suggest that with appropriate statistical algorithms it is possible to perform comprehensive meta-analysis across disparate datasets. Wang et al. used Bayesian statistical methods to combine results from three different array platforms, and generated a list of genes differentially expressed in leukemia.[33] In another study, data from two different array platforms were used to determine a subset of genes useful for classifying lung adenocarcinoma tumors.[34] Other investigators have used array-based data from a wide range of samples and conditions to generate hypotheses regarding genetic regulatory networks.[35,36] A recent paper provided evidence that the expression patterns of transcription factors tend to cluster with their respective downstream targets.[37] In other words, they found that if a transcription factor directly regulates a particular target gene, then the expression level of that gene varies with the expression level of the transcription factor. Publicly available gene expression datasets can also be useful to help prioritize the list of differentially expressed genes generated from an individual experiment. For example, if a particular gene shows consistent changes across similar but different experimental models, including across multiple species, this gene would be a higher priority candidate for further experimental study than a gene whose expression was altered in only one array experiment. This approach is particularly important considering that there is often little prior knowledge or published reports about many of the differentially expressed genes in an experiment.

FUTURE DIRECTIONS

Gene expression microarrays along with genotyping arrays and new proteomic methods will be at the forefront of future advances in basic and clinical research. Improvements in gene annotation and probe selection should improve the quality and utility of microarrays. Additional informatic and statistical methods will allow investigators to more fully utilize the vast amounts of available data. In addition, development of additional types of array platforms is needed in response to new genomic discoveries. For example, it is now appreciated that alternative splicing of human genes is common, and is regulated by appropriate developmental and physiological stimuli.[38] In a recent study, Gerzanich et al. provided evidence that alternative splicing of cGMP-dependent protein kinase I is, at least partially, responsible for the reduction in nitric oxide-mediated vasodilation during chronic infusion of Ang II.[39] However, with existing microarrays, only limited insight can be gained regarding the differential expression of splice variants. In conclusion, although significant achievements have already been made in hypertension research, we believe that systematic approaches that integrate high-throughput technologies and computational methods with traditional laboratory techniques and novel experimental models of cardiovascular disease are essential for continued progress.

REFERENCES

1. Chobanian AV, Bakris GL, Black HR et al. Seventh report of the Joint National Committee on Prevention, Detection, Evaluation, and Treatment of High Blood Pressure. Hypertension 2003; 42: 1206–52.
2. Gerhold DL, Jensen RV, Gullans SR. Better therapeutics through microarrays. Nat Genet 2002; 32: 547–51.
3. Lifton RP, Gharavi AG, Geller DS. Molecular mechanisms of human hypertension. Cell 2001; 104: 545–56.
4. Smithies O, Kim HS, Takahashi N et al. Importance of quantitative genetic variations in the etiology of hypertension. Kidney Int 2000; 58: 2265–80.
5. DiPetrillo K, Tsaih SW, Sheehan S et al. Genetic analysis of blood pressure in C3H/HeJ and SWR/J mice. Physiol Genomics 2004; 17: 215–20.
6. Aitman TJ, Glazier AM, Wallace CA et al. Identification of Cd36 (Fat) as an insulin-resistance gene causing defective fatty acid and glucose metabolism in hypertensive rats. Nat Genet 1999; 21: 76–83.
7. McBride MW, Carr FJ, Graham D et al. Microarray analysis of rat chromosome 2 congenic strains. Hypertension 2003; 41: 847–53.
8. Liang M, Yuan B, Rute E et al. Insights into Dahl salt-sensitive hypertension revealed by temporal patterns of renal medullary gene expression. Physiol Genomics 2003; 12: 229–37.
9. Larkin JE, Frank BC, Gaspard RM et al. Cardiac transcriptional response to acute and chronic angiotensin II treatments. Physiol Genomics 2004; 18: 152–66.
10. Yuan B, Liang M, Yang Z et al. Gene expression reveals vulnerability to oxidative stress and interstitial fibrosis of renal outer medulla to nonhypertensive elevations of ANG II. Am J Physiol Regul Integr Comp Physiol 2003; 284: R1219–R1230.
11. Campos AH, Zhao Y, Pollman MJ et al. DNA microarray profiling to identify angiotensin-responsive genes in vascular smooth muscle cells: potential mediators of vascular disease. Circ Res 2003; 92: 111–18.
12. Hong HJ, Chan P, Liu JC et al. Angiotensin II induces endothelin-1 gene expression via extracellular signal-regulated kinase pathway in rat aortic smooth muscle cells. Cardiovasc Res 2004; 61: 159–68.
13. Diep QN, El Mabrouk M, Cohn JS et al. Structure, endothelial function, cell growth, and inflammation in blood vessels of angiotensin II-infused rats: role of peroxisome proliferator-activated receptor-gamma. Circulation 2002; 105: 2296–302.
14. Barroso I, Gurnell M, Crowley VE et al. Dominant negative mutations in human PPARgamma associated with severe insulin resistance, diabetes mellitus and hypertension. Nature 1999; 402: 880–3.
15. Keen HL, Ryan MJ, Beyer A et al. Gene expression profiling of potential PPARgamma target genes in mouse aorta. Physiol Genomics 2004; 18: 33–42.
16. Knight JC. Regulatory polymorphisms underlying complex disease traits. J Mol Med 2004; 9: 9.
17. Schadt EE, Monks SA, Friend SH. A new paradigm for drug discovery: integrating clinical, genetic, genomic and molecular phenotype data to identify drug targets. Biochem Soc Trans 2003; 31: 437–43.
18. Schadt EE, Monks SA, Drake TA et al. Genetics of gene expression surveyed in maize, mouse and man. Nature 2003; 422: 297–302.
19. Allayee H, Ghazalpour A, Lusis AJ. Using mice to dissect genetic factors in atherosclerosis. Arterioscler Thromb Vasc Biol 2003; 23: 1501–9.
20. Pennacchio LA, Rubin EM. Genomic strategies to identify mammalian regulatory sequences. Nat Rev Genet 2001; 2: 100–9.
21. Beynon RJ, Hurst JL. Multiple roles of major urinary proteins in the house mouse, Mus domesticus. Biochem Soc Trans 2003; 31: 142–6.
22. Hubner N, Wallace CA, Zimdahl H et al. Integrated gene expression profiling and linkage mapping in rat recombinant inbred strains. Hypertension 2004; 44: 544.
23. Greer BT, Khan J. Diagnostic classification of cancer using DNA microarrays and artificial intelligence. Ann N Y Acad Sci 2004; 1020: 49–66.
24. Sarwal M, Chua MS, Kambham N et al. Molecular heterogeneity in acute renal allograft rejection identified by DNA microarray profiling. N Engl J Med 2003; 349: 125–38.
25. Geraci MW, Moore M, Gesell T et al. Gene expression patterns in the lungs of patients with primary pulmonary hypertension: a gene microarray analysis. Circ Res 2001; 88: 555–62.
26. Schwab K, Witte DP, Aronow BJ et al. Microarray analysis of focal segmental glomerulosclerosis. Am J Nephrol 2004; 24: 438–47.
27. Whitney AR, Diehn M, Popper SJ et al. Individuality and variation in gene expression patterns in human blood. Proc Natl Acad Sci U S A 2003; 100: 1896–901.
28. Bennett L, Palucka AK, Arce E et al. Interferon and granulopoiesis signatures in systemic lupus erythematosus blood. J Exp Med 2003; 197: 711–23.
29. Bull TM, Coldren CD, Moore M et al. Gene microarray analysis of peripheral blood cells in pulmonary arterial hypertension. Am J Respir Crit Care Med 2004; 170: 911–19.
30. Chon H, Gaillard CA, van der Meijden BB et al. Broadly altered gene expression in blood leukocytes in essential hypertension is absent during treatment. Hypertension 2004; 43: 947–51.

31. Barrett T, Suzek TO, Troup DB et al. NCBI GEO: mining millions of expression profiles – database and tools. Nucleic Acids Res 2005; 33: D562–D566.
32. Parkinson H, Sarkans U, Shojatalab M et al. ArrayExpress – a public repository for microarray gene expression data at the EBI. Nucleic Acids Res 2005; 33: D553–D555.
33. Wang J, Coombes KR, Highsmith WE et al. Differences in gene expression between B-cell chronic lymphocytic leukemia and normal B cells: a meta-analysis of three microarray studies. Bioinformatics 2004; 20: 3166–78.
34. Jiang H, Deng Y, Chen HS et al. Joint analysis of two microarray gene-expression data sets to select lung adenocarcinoma marker genes. BMC Bioinformatics 2004; 5: 81.
35. Haverty PM, Hansen U, Weng Z. Computational inference of transcriptional regulatory networks from expression profiling and transcription factor binding site identification. Nucleic Acids Res 2004; 32: 179–88.
36. Qian J, Lin J, Luscombe NM et al. Prediction of regulatory networks: genome-wide identification of transcription factor targets from gene expression data. Bioinformatics 2003; 19: 1917–26.
37. Zhu Z, Pilpel Y, Church GM. Computational identification of transcription factor binding sites via a transcription-factor-centric clustering (TFCC) algorithm. J Mol Biol 2002; 318: 71–81.
38. Brett D, Pospisil H, Valcarcel J et al. Alternative splicing and genome complexity. Nat Genet 2002; 30: 29–30.
39. Gerzanich V, Ivanov A, Ivanova S et al. Alternative splicing of cGMP-dependent protein kinase I in angiotensin-hypertension: novel mechanism for nitrate tolerance in vascular smooth muscle. Circ Res 2003; 93: 805–12.

27

Genetics of human essential hypertension – from single mutations to quantitative trait loci

Maciej Tomaszewski, Nick JR Brain, Fadi J Charchar and Anna F Dominiczak

INTRODUCTION

Essential hypertension is a typical example of a complex, heterogeneous, polygenic trait.[1] Multiple genes and at least several environmental factors (such as alcohol consumption or lack of physical activity) interact together contributing to high blood pressure. The contribution of genetic factors to blood pressure variation is estimated to be about 30%. However, the number of loci responsible for essential hypertension, precise mechanisms of gene–gene and gene–environment interactions, as well as the functional significance of these effects at a protein level are not known. Although the pathogenesis of high blood pressure has not been elucidated fully yet, the achievements of cardiovascular genetics should not be underestimated.

The studies on hypertension discussed below illustrate how exploring of the human genome facilitated the identification of new disorders, verified the utility of common genetic strategies, and contributed to our understanding of all complex traits.

WHAT HAVE WE LEARNED FROM CANDIDATE GENE STUDIES?

The candidate gene approach has been the most common strategy in studies on essential hypertension. This method is based on a logical assumption that genes associated with essential hypertension encode proteins involved in blood pressure regulation. Consistent with this pathophysiological rationale genetic polymorphisms in several candidate loci have been genotyped in subjects representing two contrasting phenotypes (case-control study) or in families with affected offspring (family-based analysis). Depending on the number of polymorphisms used in a given study, single locus or haplotype analyses are employed in interpretation of the results. Over/under-representation of a genetic variant in affected subjects is interpreted as evidence of its association with hypertension. Although both case-control and family-based studies seek associations between the candidate and hypertension, the latter strategy is much more robust to false positive results due to population admixture.[2] Family-based studies are also superior to case-control comparisons in the reconstruction of haplotypes in multilocus investigations.[3]

The most obvious candidates such as components of the renin-angiotensin-aldosterone system,[4] adrenergic receptors,[5] enzymes involved in nitric oxide metabolism,[6,7] endothelin,[8] water and sodium handling[9] and many others have been tested in numerous studies on hypertension (Figure 27.1). In addition, candidate genes that encode proteins involved in insulin resistance, obesity, and diabetes have also been investigated for association with hypertension[10] in view of the common co-existence of these traits and their pathophysiological similarities. Despite more than 100 relevant candidate genes,[11] the development of new statistical strategies[2,3] and thousands of investigations, none of the candidates have been consistently associated with hypertension in all populations.[12] Several associations between hypertension and candidate loci have not been replicated in other studies and this discrepancy is apparent not only across populations of different ethnic origin but even within ethnically identical samples. Among many candidate genes, β_2-adrenergic receptor gene is one of the

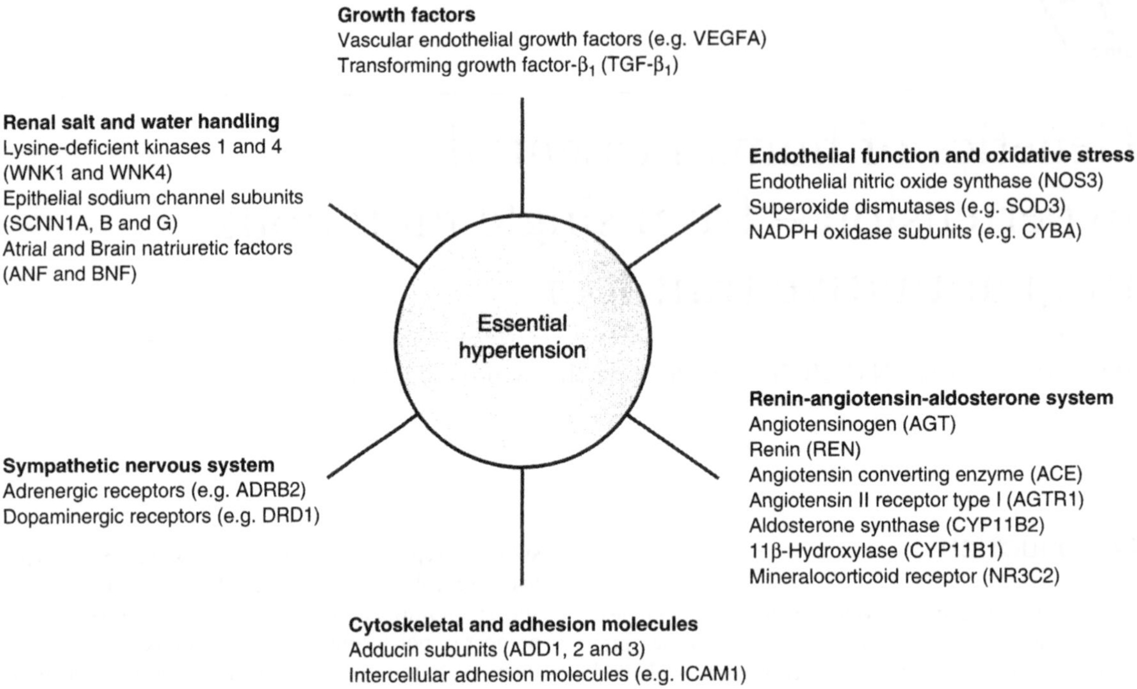

Figure 27.1 Selected candidate genes grouped by physiological function

most striking examples of a locus with a relatively equal number of negative and positive results from association studies on blood pressure-related phenotypes.[13] The only exception to this overwhelming inconsistency among studies on the same candidate locus is a series of investigations on the human Y chromosome.[14] These studies were undertaken to verify the hypothesis that higher prevalence of cardiovascular morbidity and mortality in men than women could be attributed to the influence of genes located on the human Y chromosome.[14] Markers within the non-recombining region of the human Y chromosome were investigated for association with cardiovascular phenotypes in several studies.[14] Most of them have provided consistent evidence for the association between the Y chromosome and blood pressure,[15,16] as well as cholesterol levels.[14,17]

The general lack of consistency in investigations on autosomal candidate genes and hypertension may be explained by differences in methodology and, in particular, phenotyping.[18] Arbitrary definition of hypertension based on several blood pressure measurements, natural diurnal changes in blood pressure and confounding influence of antihypertensive treatment may contribute to difficulties in precise phenotyping. In addition, late onset of hypertension can lead to potential misclassification of cases and controls. This may explain why discrepancy among the results from studies on the same locus is most apparent in candidate gene association investigations.

One of the most important lessons learnt from the lack of reproducibility in candidate gene studies is that major causative loci can reside outside classical pathways of blood pressure control. This hypothesis is supported by the identification of novel candidate loci whose pathophysiological potential to affect blood pressure is less obvious than that of angiotensinogen or β_2-adrenergic receptor gene. Solute bicarbonate transporter gene that encodes a protein involved in acid-base balance is a good example of such a novel positional candidate.[19]

Moreover, multiple genes and haplotypes rather than single polymorphisms should be investigated, as most of the genetic effects on hypertension are based on additive and epistatic intergenic (between different genes) and intragenic (between different polymorphisms within the same genes) interactions.[20–22] As a result of such interactions, a variant that has been considered as cardioprotective may turn out to be potentially detrimental in the presence of other loci.[20,21] The candidate gene approach is indeed an excellent strategy in multi-locus analysis as pathophysiologically most important interactions occur between the genes involved in the same regulatory network within the cardiovascular system.[21,22]

Finally, standardization of methodology (including phenotyping) in future candidate gene studies is absolutely essential for comparisons of results across populations. Under uniform criteria, replication of the positive finding in ethnically distinct cohorts will not only provide additional evidence for association of a candidate gene with hypertension but will also support the common disease:common variant hypothesis.[18] This hypothesis assumes that high blood pressure genes represent a few ancient genetic variants present in DNA of our ancestors – subSaharan African founding population.[18] These few common genetic variants were spread around the world with human migration and became detrimental, possibly as a result of interaction with the environment (alcohol, obesity, lack of physical activity). The contrary common disease: rare variant hypothesis proposes that numerous rare, evolutionarily younger and more population-specific genetic variants are responsible for high blood pressure.[23,24] Both hypotheses represent two equally important extreme views on the genetics of hypertension, but the common variant:common disease alternative seems to have more supporters,[22,25] and will be easier to prove using available association strategies.[22] Therefore, it may be more successful in uncovering genetic determinants of high blood pressure.

INSIGHT INTO PATHOGENESIS OF HIGH BLOOD PRESSURE FROM GENOME-WIDE SCANS

The genome-wide screen is a relatively new strategy – the first comprehensive genome-wide linkage analysis of systolic blood pressure was published in 1999.[26] This launched an era of cardiovascular genome-wide scans – tens of screens of human genome were performed in pursuit of genes predisposing to hypertension and related disorders.[11] Screening of the human genome is based on genotyping of related subjects (usually sib-pairs) for several hundreds of microsatellite markers distributed evenly through the chromosomes. The genetic markers selected for this type of analysis are usually located outside genes. Significant genetic polymorphism of these markers guarantees high heterozygosity rates that are essential in linkage analysis.[13] Most of the linkage strategies search for chromosomal regions defined by microsatellite markers with higher than expected allelic identity among hypertensive offspring.[22] Such regions of linkage travelling through generations together with high blood pressure are called quantitative trait loci (QTLs). QTLs usually span tens of centiMorgans (millions of base-pairs) (Figure 27.2) and may contain one, a few or more genes predisposing to hypertension.[22]

The results from scans of the human genome have created a dense map of regions linked to blood pressure – QTLs are present on each chromosome with a possible exception of chromosome 13. The QTL map is slightly different in populations of different ethnicity, underscoring the genetic heterogeneity of essential hypertension. Nevertheless, several of these QTLs overlap across at least two ethnically different populations, suggesting that these regions may indeed contain common variants responsible for predisposition to hypertension in many populations.[27] In addition, several of these QTLs map to chromosomal regions linked to blood pressure in rodents. One such example is the distal portion in the long arm of human chromosome 5. Linked to both systolic[26] and post-exercise diastolic[28] blood pressure this human chromosomal segment maps to the region containing blood pressure QTL on rat chromosome 18.[29] Such conservation among the species underscores the potential significance of this region in blood pressure regulation.

Stringent criteria of significance have been established for uniform interpretation of findings from a genome scan.[30] In line with these guidelines, suggestive linkage corresponds to a LOD score of 1.9 and is expected to occur once at random in a genome scan.[30] Significant linkage corresponding to a LOD score of 3.3 is statistically more convincing, as it is expected to occur 0.05 times in a genome scan.[30] Interestingly, most of the regions linked to blood pressure (or hypertension) reached only suggestive rather than significant levels of linkage,[27] confirming that the genetic effects of each locus on inter-individual variation in blood pressure are moderate. Consistent with this hypothesis, loci with major effect (reaching a threshold of genome-wide significance)[30] on blood pressure have been detected only in four analyses.[27] This dominance of QTLs with suggestive linkage to blood pressure over loci that reached the threshold of genome-wide significance suggests the existence of several common variants with a moderate effect on blood pressure rather than a few major genes. Therefore, QTLs with suggestive

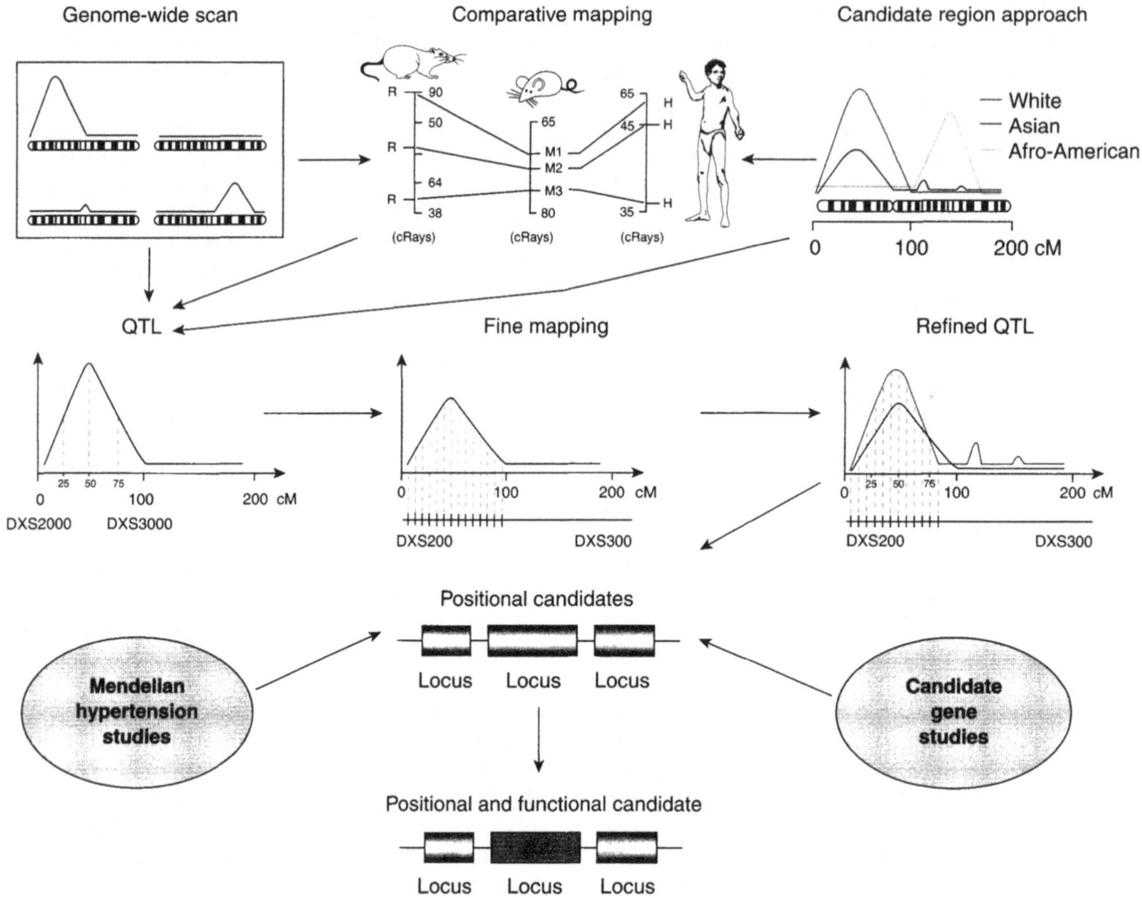

Figure 27.2 From genome-wide scans to positional and functional candidates – basic genetic strategies complement each other in the search for hypertension genes

linkage to blood pressure, in particular overlapping across populations and rich in pathophysiological candidate genes, are currently being dissected in search of common variants predisposing to hypertension. This candidate region approach benefits from advantages of both genome-wide scan and candidate gene strategies.[13] Recent studies using the candidate region approach have provided evidence for the utility of this strategy in dissecting QTLs for blood pressure.[13,31]

The limited number of QTLs in each genome-wide analysis indicates that instead of a truly polygenic disorder, hypertension may in fact be, an oligogenic disease.[11] This hypothesis is also supported by fine mapping and positional studies in regions linked to blood pressure. Although theoretically all genes within the QTL may mediate linkage to blood pressure, the recent data from dissected QTLs suggest that usually one gene under the linkage peak exerts a dominant effect.[19] Recent modifications of the linkage analysis that evaluate the contribution of each locus under the QTL to the observed linkage[19] will certainly help to verify these observations. If, indeed hypertension is an oligogenic disorder, genome-wide screening and candidate region strategy will make major contributions to this discovery.

There are several limitations of a genome-wide scanning strategy. First, narrowing down a QTL by genotyping additional microsatellite markers may go only as far as a couple of centiMorgans due to limited recombination events in sib-pairs.[22] Therefore, genome-wide scanning will not be able to identify hypertension genes without additional approaches. Second, genome-wide screening provides no information about the Y chromosome (due to its haploid

Table 27.1 Comparison of Mendelian and essential hypertension

Mendelian	*Essential*
Rare Minimal contribution to global disease burden	*Common* Affects about 20% of subjects in industrialized societies
Monogenic Mutations in one gene are necessary and sufficient	*Oligogenic or polygenic* Subtle polymorphisms in multiple – possibly many – genes increase susceptibility
Simple genetic syndrome Effect of causative gene is large; interactions with other genes are of secondary importance	*Complex genetic trait* Gene–gene interactions are important and result in clinically relevant effects on blood pressure
Unifactorial Gene defect is highly penetrant	*Multifactorial* Effects of genes are important in the context of environmental and dietary factors
Relative risk is high Risk of syndrome in first degree relative of affected person is much higher than in the general population	*Relative risk is lower* Risk of hypertension in first degree relative of affected person is about 2–5-fold higher than in the general population

nature) and many of the genome-wide scans also exclude the X chromosome from analysis. This, in turn suggests that this strategy will be practically of no use in explanation of the apparent sexual dimorphism in cardiovascular risk.[14]

Despite these limitations, genome-wide screens have contributed significantly to our understanding of the genetics of hypertension. Firstly, they have confirmed that essential hypertension has a truly polygenic or, at least, oligogenic nature. Although cardiovascular disorders were recognized as polygenic before the era of genomics, compelling evidence for the existence of multiple loci linked to blood pressure has been provided by genome-wide scans. Moreover, genome-wide screening has shown that although different genes may predispose to hypertension in ethnically distinct cohorts, there are also at least a few common loci that may be responsible for high blood pressure in most of the populations. Overlapping of several QTLs across ethnically distinct cohorts implicates these chromosomal regions as the most relevant parts of the human genome in terms of predisposition to essential hypertension.

LESSONS FROM MENDELIAN FORMS OF HYPERTENSION

Successful identification of genes responsible for monogenic forms of hypertension is one of the most impressive achievements of cardiovascular genetics. At least six monogenic forms of hypertension have been reported and new data suggest that there may be more hypertensive syndromes caused by single mutations.[32] Nevertheless, as the Mendelian forms of hypertension are extremely rare, their cumulative contribution to the prevalence of high blood pressure in the general population is small even when compared to the unique secondary forms of hypertension. Phenotypically most of the monogenic hypertension syndromes differ from essential hypertension by early onset,[33,34] stronger predisposition to life-threatening complications,[35] and pronounced metabolic disturbances.[36] Most frequently, abnormal serum and urine concentrations of different ion fractions are associated with high blood pressure.[36] Capture of these specific phenotypic characteristics was, in fact, a key step to the identification of causative genetic variants.

Genetically, Mendelian forms of hypertension are caused by single, rare genetic mutations exerting large effect on blood pressure[34] (see Table 27.1 for a comparison between essential and Mendelian hypertension). The causative genetic defects include a wide spectrum of abnormalities from chimeric genes,[36] to missense, frameshift and aberrant splicing mutations caused by single nucleotide substitutions or insertions.[37,38] In addition, different mutations within a single gene are responsible for the same phenotype, i.e. several types of rare genetic variants within the gene encoding beta and gamma subunit of epithelial sodium channel lead to Liddle syndrome.[37] On the other hand, penetrance of these mutations is frequently incomplete – subjects with the same genetic variant differ in terms of the phenotype characteristics.[39] Interactions with environmental exposure are also evident, at least in certain monogenic disorders.[36] Collectively, these data underscore the substantial genetic heterogeneity and possible environmental component of at least some of Mendelian forms of hypertension.

Interestingly, although mutations responsible for Mendelian hypertension affect different types of proteins including enzymes, receptors, and ion transporters,[36] dysregulation of the same physiological pathway is a common ultimate abnormality. Specifically, tubular reabsorption of sodium is altered either directly by affected ion channels or indirectly by abnormal activity of hormonal regulators.[12] Targeting the defective proteins by specific, direct treatment (such as thiazides in pseudohypoaldosteronism type II[40] or amiloride in Liddle syndrome[41]) usually corrects metabolic disturbances and lowers blood pressure in affected subjects.

Despite identification of causative genetic mutations, elucidation of molecular mechanisms and tailoring drug therapies for Mendelian forms of hypertension, the contribution of this knowledge to identification of the loci responsible for essential hypertension has been modest. Most of the genes leading to Mendelian hypertension are located outside the most consistent blood pressure QTLs implicated by genome-wide scans. In addition, although preliminary results from single studies testing for associations between these rare variants and essential hypertension provide some positive data,[42] it is too early to speculate about the possible implications of these findings.

Nevertheless, studies on human Mendelian hypertension are among the most important lessons learnt from genetics over the last decade. Firstly, they have provided evidence that precise definition of a hypertensive phenotype based on a combination of clinical, biochemical, hormonal, and renal examination is the most critical step to success in genetic analysis. Such an approach, called 'phenomics',[43] should become a uniform phenotyping strategy in studies on essential hypertension. Secondly, the studies on Mendelian forms of hypertension have clearly shown that even monogenic disorders are genetically heterogeneous. Consequently, heterogeneity of essential hypertension as an oligogenic or polygenic trait may be substantially higher then we expect. Thirdly, implication of renal tubular epithelium as a major site of abnormal blood pressure regulation has confirmed the role of the kidney not only as a victim but also as a villain of high blood pressure.[44] Finally, by showing that target antihypertensive therapy is possible after dissecting of underlying genetic mechanisms, studies on Mendelian hypertension have provided evidence that pharmacogenetics is not a matter of elusive future but is close to the bed-side.

PERSPECTIVE

Genome-wide scans and the candidate region approach will remain important strategies in pursuit of hypertension genes. However, the availability of accurate public databases and decreasing costs of SNP genotyping will enable us to replace microsatellite screens with dense genome-wide SNP scans. In addition, genome-wide expression studies based on already available microarray platforms will complement the available strategies. Whatever analytical method and markers are used, genome-wide analysis will remain a first-step method in screening of the human chromosomes in pursuit of loci predisposing to cardiovascular disorders. The candidate gene strategy will be an important approach used in the studies on cardiovascular genetics, in particular in investigations of gene–gene interactions. However, new criteria for identification and selection of a candidate gene will be used. Instead of focusing on pathophysiological criteria only, a positional potential to mediate a linkage within QTL will be taken into consideration. We should also expect identification of new Mendelian syndromes that will provide additional insight into molecular mechanisms of hypertension.

ACKNOWLEDGMENTS

Research in Professor Dominiczak's laboratory is supported by the British Heart Foundation Chair and Programme Grant (BHF/CI/04/001), the Wellcome Trust Cardiovascular Genomics Initiative (06678/Z/01/Z) and the EURNETGEN Project QLG1–2000–01137. Dr Tomaszewski is supported by the Wellcome Trust International Research Development Award (067827/Z/02/Z) and NIH Fogarty International Collaboration Award (RO3TW 007165).

REFERENCES

1. Dominiczak AF, Negrin DC, Clark JS et al. Genes and hypertension: from gene mapping in experimental models to vascular gene transfer strategies. Hypertension 2000; 35: 164–72.
2. Thomson G. Mapping disease genes: family-based association studies. Am J Hum Genet 1995; 57: 487–98.
3. Horvath S, Xu X, Lake SL et al. Family-based tests for associating haplotypes with general phenotype data: application to asthma genetics. Genet Epidemiol 2004; 26: 61–9.
4. Miller JA, Scholey JW. The impact of renin-angiotensin system polymorphisms on physiological and pathophysiological processes in humans. Curr Opin Nephrol Hypertens 2004; 13: 101–6.
5. Kirstein SL, Insel PA. Autonomic nervous system pharmacogenomics: a progress report. Pharmacol Rev 2004; 56: 31–52.

6. Rossi GP, Taddei S, Virdis A et al. The T-786C and Glu298Asp polymorphisms of the endothelial nitric oxide gene affect the forearm blood flow responses of Caucasian hypertensive patients. J Am Coll Cardiol 2003; 41: 938–45.
7. Rutherford S, Johnson MP, Curtain RP et al. Chromosome 17 and the inducible nitric oxide synthase gene in human essential hypertension. Hum Genet 2001; 109: 408–15.
8. Sharma P, Hingorani A, Jia H et al. Quantitative association between a newly identified molecular variant in the endothelin-2 gene and human essential hypertension. J Hypertens 1999; 17: 1281–87.
9. Cho Y, Somer BG, Amatya A. Natriuretic peptides and their therapeutic potential. Heart Dis 1999; 1: 305–28.
10. Gibbons GH, Liew CC, Goodarzi MO et al. Genetic markers: progress and potential for cardiovascular disease. Circulation 2004; 109 (Suppl 1): IV47–58.
11. Tomaszewski M, Charchar FJ, Padmanabhan S et al. Cardiovascular diseases and G-protein beta3 subunit gene (GNB3) in the era of genomewide scans. J Hum Hypertens 2003; 17: 379–80.
12. Turner ST, Boerwinkle E. Genetics of blood pressure, hypertensive complications, and antihypertensive drug responses. Pharmacogenomics 2003; 4: 53–65.
13. Tomaszewski M, Brain NJ, Charchar FJ et al. Essential hypertension and beta2-adrenergic receptor gene: linkage and association analysis. Hypertension 2002; 40: 286–91.
14. Charchar FJ, Tomaszewski M, Strahorn P et al. Y is there a risk to being male? Trends Endocrinol Metab 2003; 14: 163–8.
15. Charchar FJ, Tomaszewski M, Padmanabhan S et al. The Y chromosome effect on blood pressure in two European populations. Hypertension 2002; 39: 353–56.
16. Ellis JA, Stebbing M, Harrap SB. Association of the human Y chromosome with high blood pressure in the general population. Hypertension 2000; 36: 731–33.
17. Charchar FJ, Tomaszewski M, Lacka B et al. Association of the human Y chromosome with cholesterol levels in the general population. Arterioscler Thromb Vasc Biol 2004; 24: 308–12.
18. Doris PA. Hypertension genetics, single nucleotide polymorphisms, and the common disease:common variant hypothesis. Hypertension 2002; 39: 323–31.
19. Barkley RA, Chakravarti A, Cooper RS et al. Positional identification of hypertension susceptibility genes on chromosome 2. Hypertension 2004; 43: 477–82.
20. Tomaszewski M, Charchar FJ, Lacka B et al. Epistatic interaction between beta2-adrenergic receptor and neuropeptide Y genes influences LDL-cholesterol in hypertension. Hypertension 2004; 44: 689–94.
21. Tsai CT, Fallin D, Chiang FT et al. Angiotensinogen gene haplotype and hypertension: interaction with ACE gene I allele. Hypertension 2003; 41: 9–15.
22. Carlson CS, Eberle MA, Kruglyak L et al. Mapping complex disease loci in whole-genome association studies. Nature 2004; 429: 446–52.
23. Pritchard JK. Are rare variants responsible for susceptibility to complex diseases? Am J Hum Genet 2001; 69: 124–37.
24. Harrap SB. Where are all the blood-pressure genes? Lancet 2003; 361: 2149–51.
25. Lohmueller KE, Pearce CL, Pike M et al. Meta-analysis of genetic association studies supports a contribution of common variants to susceptibility to common disease. Nat Genet 2003; 33: 177–82.
26. Krushkal J, Ferrell R, Mockrin SC et al. Genome-wide linkage analyses of systolic blood pressure using highly discordant siblings. Circulation 1999; 99: 1407–10.
27. Samani NJ. Genome scans for hypertension and blood pressure regulation. Am J Hypertens 2003; 16: 167–71.
28. Rankinen T, An P, Rice T et al. Genomic scan for exercise blood pressure in the Health, Risk Factors, Exercise Training and Genetics (HERITAGE) Family Study. Hypertension 2001; 38: 30–7.
29. Cowley AW Jr, Stoll M, Greene AS et al. Genetically defined risk of salt sensitivity in an intercross of Brown Norway and Dahl S rats. Physiol Genomics 2000; 2: 107–15.
30. Lander E, Kruglyak L. Genetic dissection of complex traits: guidelines for interpreting and reporting linkage results. Nat Genet 1995; 11: 241–7.
31. Tomaszewski M, Charchar FJ, Lacka B et al. Genetic variation within the acidic fibroblast growth factor gene is associated with essential hypertension – from identification of new polymorphisms to family based haplotype analysis. Hypertension 2004; 44: 545.
32. Wilson FH, Hariri A, Farhi A et al. A cluster of metabolic defects caused by mutation in a mitochondrial tRNA. Science 2004; 306: 1190–4.
33. Dluhy RG, Anderson B, Harlin B et al. Glucocorticoid-remediable aldosteronism is associated with severe hypertension in early childhood. J Pediatr 2001; 138: 715–20.
34. Pradervand S, Vandewalle A, Bens M et al. Dysfunction of the epithelial sodium channel expressed in the kidney of a mouse model for Liddle syndrome. J Am Soc Nephrol 2003; 14: 2219–28.
35. Litchfield WR, Anderson BF, Weiss RJ et al. Intracranial aneurysm and hemorrhagic stroke in glucocorticoid-remediable aldosteronism. Hypertension 1998; 31: 445–50.
36. Lifton RP, Gharavi AG, Geller DS. Molecular mechanisms of human hypertension. Cell 2001; 104: 545–56.
37. Nakano Y, Ishida T, Ozono R et al. A frameshift mutation of beta subunit of epithelial sodium channel in a case of isolated Liddle syndrome. J Hypertens 2002; 20: 2379–82.
38. Lavery G, Ronconi V, Draper N et al. Late-onset apparent mineralocorticoid excess caused by novel compound heterozygous mutations in the HSD11B2 gene. Hypertension 2003; 42: 123–29.
39. Gates LJ, MacConnachie AA, Lifton RP et al. Variation of phenotype in patients with glucocorticoid remediable aldosteronism. J Med Genet 1996; 33: 25–8.
40. Mayan H, Vered I, Mouallem M et al. Pseudohypoaldosteronism type II: marked sensitivity to thiazides, hypercalciuria, normomagnesemia, and low bone mineral density. J Clin Endocrinol Metab 2002; 87: 3248–54.
41. Genest J. Progress in hypertension research: 1900–2000. Hypertension 2001; 38: E13–E18.
42. Erlich PM, Cui J, Chazaro I et al. Genetic variants of WNK4 in whites and African Americans with hypertension. Hypertension 2003; 41: 1191–5.
43. Hegele RA. Phenomics, lipodystrophy, and the metabolic syndrome. Trends Cardiovasc Med 2004; 14: 133–7.
44. Klahr S. The kidney in hypertension – villain and victim. N Engl J Med 1989; 320: 731–3.

PART III

28

Nitric oxide: molecular mechanisms in hypertension and cardiovascular disease

Ivonne Hernandez Schulman, Ming-Sheng Zhou and Leopoldo Raij

INTRODUCTION

Endothelium-derived nitric oxide (NO) is a major cardiovascular and renoprotective molecule. NO is a labile free radical gas that is generated continuously and on demand and functions as an endogenous mediator in the control of systemic and microvascular tone, the glomerular microcirculation, renal sodium excretion, and inflammatory and growth responses in the vasculature and kidney. Some of the most important effects that NO exerts in the vascular wall are potentially vasoprotective, because these effects maintain important physiological functions such as vasodilatation, anticoagulation, leukocyte adhesion, smooth muscle proliferation, and antioxidative capacity.[1] The link between NO and cardiovascular and renal health is likely due to the pleiotropic effects of NO on the vascular wall.

NO production by NO synthases (NOS) is under complex, tight control to dictate specificity of its signaling and to limit toxicity to other cellular components, due to its potent chemical reactivity and high diffusibility. The three major NOS isoforms described are neuronal NOS (nNOS or NOS 1), inducible NOS (iNOS or NOS 2), and endothelial NOS (eNOS or NOS 3). They share a common basic structural organization and requirement for substrate cofactors for enzymatic activity. NOS activity requires binding of calmodulin and tetrahydrobiopterin (BH_4) and the formation of a homodimer. Calmodulin binding is triggered by transient elevations in intracellular calcium levels and serves as an allosteric modulator of the three NOS isoforms. nNOS is expressed in neural tissues, skeletal muscle, and macula densa as well as other tubule segments and is a calcium/calmodulin-dependent enzyme that is also subject to transcriptional and other posttranslational controls.[2,3] Transcription of iNOS is induced in nearly all tissues in response to cytokines, endotoxin, or other proinflammatory stimuli. iNOS is less responsive to intracellular calcium transients owing to tight calmodulin binding at ambient intracellular calcium levels.[4] eNOS is expressed predominantly in the endothelium and is the NOS isoform responsible for maintaining systemic blood pressure, vascular remodeling, and angiogenesis, and thus a fundamental determinant of cardiovascular homeostasis. eNOS is subject to rapid regulation by calcium/calmodulin as well as a variety of transcriptional, posttranscriptional, and posttranslational controls.[5,6]

By virtue of its molecular targeting, eNOS is a peripheral membrane protein. N-Myristoylation of eNOS targets the protein to the Golgi apparatus, where it undergoes cysteine palmitoylation.[6–8] The myristoylated and palmitoylated eNOS is then targeted to the caveolae, the major plasma membrane vesicle structure in endothelial cells.[9] Caveolin-1, the major coat protein responsible for assembly of caveolae, directly interacts with and inhibits eNOS in endothelial cells.[9] In the resting state, eNOS appears to be tethered to caveolin-1 and inactive. Agonists that raise intracellular calcium levels promote calmodulin binding to eNOS and caveolin dissociation from the enzyme, resulting in an activated eNOS-calmodulin complex. The cycle is reversed when intracellular calcium levels return to the resting state, with calmodulin dissociating and caveolin reassociating with eNOS. G protein-coupled receptors resident in caveolae also contribute to the eNOS-membrane complex and regulate eNOS activity.[10] The membrane-proximal regions of intracellular domain 4 of the bradykinin B2, angiotensin (Ang) II type 1 (AT_1), and endothelin ET_B receptors are capable of binding and inhibiting eNOS and these interactions are modulated by receptor phosphorylation.[10] For example, the B2 receptor is transiently phosphorylated on tyrosine residues in cultured endothelial cells in response to bradykinin stimulation. This leads to a transient dissociation of eNOS from the receptor accompanied by an increase in NO production.

In endothelial cells, eNOS is expressed constitutively, but its rate of transcription and translation can be modulated by numerous factors. Blood flow-induced shear stress on endothelial cells is the major physiologic stimulus for vascular NO production by eNOS.[11] Increased vascular flow and fluid shear stress promote eNOS dissociation from caveolin and association with calmodulin to activate the enzyme.[12,13] This activation of eNOS has been shown to be directly dependent on phosphorylation by serine/threonine protein kinase Akt/PKB, and not primarily mediated by a rise in intracellular calcium.[14] Bradykinin, vascular endothelial growth factor, and estrogen also trigger Akt-mediated phosphorylation of eNOS, leading to eNOS activation in vitro and in vivo.[6,15–17] In addition to activating eNOS, laminar shear stress increases eNOS mRNA expression.[18] The tyrosine kinase c-Src has been shown to modulate eNOS expression in response to shear stress via divergent pathways involving a short-term increase in eNOS transcription, via activation of Ras/Raf and ERK1/2, and a longer-term stabilization of eNOS mRNA, independent of Ras/Raf/ERK.[18] Expression of eNOS is also increased by Ang II,[19] glucose,[20] hydrogen peroxide,[21] and transforming growth factor-β (TGF-β).[22] Mediators that decrease eNOS expression include RhoA/Rho-kinase,[23] oxidized LDL,[24] lipopolysaccharide,[25] and tumor necrosis factor-α (TNF-α).[25,26] Ignarro's group has shown that NO itself can act as a negative feedback modulator of eNOS catalytic activity by interacting with the heme iron in the enzyme.[27]

ROLE OF NO IN THE REGULATION OF VASCULAR TONE

Endothelium-derived NO may contribute to the overall regulation of arterial blood pressure by virtue of its ability to relax vascular smooth muscle.[1] NO activates the enzyme soluble guanylate cyclase (sGC) to generate the second messenger cyclic guanosine monophosphate (cGMP).[28] Activation of this enzyme is mediated by the binding of NO to the heme moiety of sGC to form the nitrosyl-heme adduct of sGC.[29] As a result, the heme iron is shifted out of the plane of the porphyrin ring configuration, which initiates the binding of GTP and the formation of cGMP. Cyclic GMP activates two specific cGMP-dependent protein kinases, PKG I and II. PKG I is the main kinase mediating vasodilatation and inhibition of platelet aggregation.[30]

The mechanisms by which NO causes vasodilatation of vascular smooth muscle involve the lowering of intracellular calcium and down-regulation of the contractile apparatus. These effects are mediated by increased intracellular cGMP and activation of PKG.[31,32] The reduction of intracellular calcium by cGMP/PKG is accomplished in several ways, which include inhibition of calcium influx, reduction in calcium mobilization through the inositol 1,4,5,-trisphosphate (IP3) receptor, down-regulation of IP3 formation, enhancement of calcium efflux, and augmentation of calcium sequestration in the sarcoplasmic reticulum.

Voltage- and receptor-operated calcium channels of the plasma membrane are directly phosphorylated and inactivated by cGMP/PKG.[33] In addition, cGMP/PKG phosphorylates and activates calcium-sensitive potassium channels of the plasma membrane, causing hyperpolarization and consequently reducing calcium influx through the voltage-operated calcium channels.[34,35]

IP3 produced by activation of phospholipase C (PLC) binds to its receptor located in the membrane of the sarcoplasmic reticulum. The IP3 receptor is a channel protein that opens when bound to IP3 and permits calcium efflux into the cytoplasm, thereby increasing calcium concentration. cGMP/PKG phosphorylates the IP3 receptor and reduces channel activity, leading to a decrease in calcium concentration and smooth muscle relaxation.[36,37] Moreover, NO and cGMP/PKG negatively regulate IP3 formation by direct inhibition of PLC activity.[38,39]

Enhanced calcium extrusion from the cytoplasm into the extracellular space also contributes to the vasodilatory effect of cGMP/PKG. Calcium efflux is mediated by activation of the membrane calcium-pumping ATPase (mCa^{2+}-ATPase) and the sodium-calcium (Na^+/Ca^{2+}) exchanger. cGMP/PKG stimulates the plasma membrane mCa^{2+}-ATPase, possibly via phosphorylation of an intermediate protein responsible for the activation of mCa^{2+}-ATPase.[40] Extrusion of calcium through the Na^+/Ca^{2+} exchanger is dependent upon depletion of intracellular sodium via activation of Na^+/K^+-ATPase or hyperpolarization of the cell membrane through activation of potassium channels. Na^+/K^+-ATPase in the plasma membrane is activated by cGMP through PKG, thereby promoting calcium efflux from the cell.[41] Calcium sequestration into the sarcoplasmic reticulum is also potentiated by cGMP/PKG via phosphorylation of the protein phospholamban, which activates the calcium-pumping ATPase of the sarcoplasmic reticulum and induces calcium uptake.[33,42]

Decreasing the calcium sensitivity of contractile proteins is another means by which cGMP/PKG reduces vascular tone. The contractile force of vascular smooth muscle is primarily dependent on the status of myosin light chain phosphorylation, which is regulated by the balance of myosin light chain kinase (MLCK) and myosin light chain phosphatase (MLCP). cGMP induces calcium desensitization by altering the balance between the activities of MLCK and MLCP at a constant calcium concentration. cGMP/PKG induces MLCP activity without affecting MLCK activity.[43,44] PKG may increase MLCP activity by phosphorylation of the myosin-binding subunit of MLCP.[43–45] Furthermore, recent evidence indicates that NO may also induce vasorelaxation through inhibition of the RhoA/Rho-kinase signaling pathway in a cGMP/PKG-dependent manner.[46] PKG has been shown to phosphorylate and inactivate RhoA, thereby inhibiting RhoA-induced calcium sensitization of the contractile apparatus.[46]

The contribution of NO in endothelium-dependent vasodilatation may differ in the conduit and resistant artery. In the conduit artery, NO is a primary mediator of endothelium-dependent relaxation. However, in resistant arteries, including mesenteric arteries, coronary arteries, cerebral arteries and renal arteries, endothelium-derived hyperpolarizing factor (EDHF) appears to be a major mediator of endothelium-dependent relaxation and NO action may be limited.[47] Recently, Freitas et al.[48] reported that in mesenteric arteries of Lyon rats either inhibition of NO or blockade of potassium channels abolished endothelium-dependent relaxation, suggesting that a synergistic interaction between endothelium-derived NO and EDHF participates in the control of vascular tone in some vascular beds.[49] There is evidence from experimental animal models that constitutive production of NO by the endothelium maintains the vasculature in a state of vasodilatation. Mice lacking the eNOS gene have hypertension and a heightened response to injury,[50] whereas mice with overexpression of the eNOS gene exhibit hypotension.[51] Blood pressure is also increased by NOS inhibition,[52] genetic deficiency of the BH_4 cofactor of eNOS,[53] or inhibitors of BH_4 synthesis.[54] Inhibition of NO production stimulates endothelial angiotensin converting enzyme (ACE) activity and generation of Ang II and superoxide anion (O_2^-), induces vasoconstriction, and causes pronounced and sustained hypertension.[55,56]

NO inhibits the production and action of endothelin-1 (ET-1), a powerful vasoconstricting peptide released from the endothelium.[57] In the porcine aorta, NOS inhibition augments the release of ET-1, while 8-bromo cGMP has an inhibitory effect on ET-1 release, suggesting that NO inhibits ET-1 production via a cGMP-dependent mechanism.[58] Selective ET_A or dual ET_A/ET_B receptor antagonists blunt the acute pressor response caused by NOS inhibition,[59] whereas blockade of NO formation magnifies ET-1-induced vasoconstriction of various vascular territories.[60] NO also modulates ACE activity and AT_1 receptor expression. NO donors have been shown to inhibit ACE activity in vitro and in vivo.[61–63] In vascular smooth muscle cells, NO decreases AT_1 receptor mRNA expression.[64] NOS inhibition facilitates Ang II-related effects, which can be inhibited by both AT_1 receptor and ET-1 receptor antagonists. Human and animal studies have suggested that there is a feedback mechanism between Ang II, ET-1, and NO synthesis that acts reciprocally to regulate vascular tone.[65,66] The inhibition of the ET-1 and Ang II systems may be one of the mechanisms by which NO exerts its antihypertensive properties.

ENDOTHELIAL DYSFUNCTION

Impairment in the synthesis or bioactivity of endothelial NO, as manifested by reduced endothelium-dependent relaxation, has been shown to be an independent risk factor for major adverse cardiovascular events.[67,68] The underlying mechanisms of reduced endothelium-dependent relaxation are multifactorial. Accumulating evidence indicates that inactivation of NO by increased reactive oxygen species (ROS), especially O_2^-, plays a vital role in the impaired endothelium-dependent relaxation associated with atherosclerosis and all major cardiovascular risk factors such as hypertension, diabetes, hyperlipidemia, and smoking. The chemical interaction between O_2^- and NO produces peroxynitrite anion ($ONOO^-$), a potent oxidant, and thereby reduces NO bioavailability. $ONOO^-$ is an important mediator of oxidation of LDL, emphasizing its proatherogenic role.[69] Furthermore, both O_2^- and $ONOO^-$ have been demonstrated to oxidize BH_4, a critical eNOS cofactor, and lead to eNOS 'uncoupling'.[70–72] An uncoupled eNOS produces O_2^- rather than NO. There is increasing evidence demonstrating the presence of eNOS dysfunction or uncoupling in hypertension, hyperlipidemia, and atherosclerosis. Dysfunction of eNOS was shown to accelerate atherosclerotic lesion formation in mice,[67] whereas overexpression of eNOS in mice with hypercholesterolemia resulted in increased eNOS-derived O_2^- production and promotion of atherogenesis.[73]

An increased asymmetric dimethylarginine (ADMA) may also be involved in oxidative stress-induced endothelial dysfunction.[74,75] ADMA is an endogenous eNOS inhibitor and increased plasma concentration of ADMA has been demonstrated to be a novel risk factor for development of endothelial dysfunction[75] and a predictor for cardiovascular mortality.[74] Therefore, since the effects of NO on the cardiovascular system are dependent on the concomitant production of O_2^- in the microenvironment where NO is synthesized and released, the changes in the endothelial redox state may have a profound impact on endothelial NO bioavailability and endothelium-dependent relaxation.

Vascular up-regulation of NO is recognized as an adaptive response to elevation of blood pressure that may help in the prevention of end organ damage.[52,76] Studies in spontaneously hypertensive (SHR) and Dahl salt-sensitive (DS) rats, animal models of human salt-resistant and salt-sensitive hypertension, respectively, suggest that individual variability in susceptibility to hypertensive end organ injury may be at least partially explained by genetic differences in vascular eNOS activity in response to hypertension. eNOS activity in the aorta, left ventricle, and kidney of SHR rats significantly increased compared with their normotensive counterpart, Wistar-Kyoto rats, whereas eNOS in the aorta, left ventricle, and kidney of DS rats decreased compared with the normotensive control. At similar blood pressures, hypertensive DS rats showed significantly greater left ventricular hypertrophy, aortic hypertrophy, and several fold more proteinuria than SHR rats.[77,78] Furthermore, therapeutic interventions that normalize eNOS activity, such as atorvastatin or an ACE inhibitor in combination with a diuretic,[77,79] have been shown to attenuate or normalize, respectively, blood pressure and end organ injury in DS rats. Thus, in susceptible individuals, decreased vascular NO bioavailability in response to blood pressure elevation may contribute to cardiovascular injury.

ROLE OF NO IN THE REGULATION OF RENAL HEMODYNAMICS

In vivo studies have suggested that NO plays an important role in maintaining renal hemodynamics near the normal range in response to elevated Ang II levels.[80] Ang II, via the AT_1 receptor, causes a dose-dependent decrease in renal blood flow, a smaller reduction in glomerular filtration rate, and an increase in filtration fraction.[81] These effects are mediated by Ang II-induced vasoconstriction of the afferent and efferent arterioles, thereby increasing both pre- and post-glomerular resistances. This renal hemodynamic response to Ang II is similar to the renal hemodynamic response to acute systemic NOS inhibition, implying that NO may counteract the vascular actions of Ang II.[82]

In normotensive rat kidneys, intrarenal NO regulates afferent and efferent arteriolar tone and modulates both afferent and efferent arteriolar responsiveness to Ang II.[83] The relative degree to which NO affects the afferent and efferent arteriolar responsiveness to Ang II significantly affects renal function. In Ang II-infused hypertensive rats, inhibition of NOS decreased afferent and efferent arteriolar diameters, and the decrease in diameter was significantly greater in afferent than in efferent arterioles. The addition of sodium nitroprusside, an NO donor, to increase local NO concentrations blunted the Ang II response in afferent arterioles but was not sufficient to alter the efferent arteriolar reactivity to Ang II. Thus, NO modulation of Ang II responsiveness is maintained in afferent but not efferent arterioles. The maintained NO-dependent tone and function in afferent arterioles may contribute to maintaining renal hemodynamics during the development of Ang II-dependent hypertension.[84]

NO influences medullary hemodynamics to a greater extent than cortical hemodynamics.[85,86] In normotensive and hypertensive rats, Ang II stimulates medullary NO generation, which in turn prevents its vasoconstricting effects on the medullary circulation.[82,87,88] Moreover, studies have suggested that an increased susceptibility to the hypertensive actions of Ang II may result from an impaired NO counterregulatory system in the medulla.[88,89]

ROLE OF NO IN THE REGULATION OF SODIUM BALANCE

The capability of the kidneys to excrete sodium is considered to be an important determinant of arterial blood pressure. Studies evaluating the effect of intrarenal NOS inhibition indicated that NO plays a key role in the preservation of normal renal excretory function.[86] Furthermore, NO administered intrarenally has been shown to serve as a diuretic and natriuretic agent.[86] Experimental evidence from proximal tubule and cortical collecting duct cells and isolated, perfused proximal tubule and collecting duct segments demonstrated that this effect of NO is mediated by direct inhibition of epithelial transport mechanisms.[90] NO inhibits the sodium/hydrogen (Na^+/H^+) antiporter on the luminal membrane of the proximal tubule and attenuates the sodium/potassium (Na^+/K^+) ATPase activity on the basolateral membrane of the proximal tubule and collecting duct segments.[82] However, accumulating experimental evidence suggests that the effects of intrarenal NOS inhibitors or NO donors on tubular reabsorptive function are also mediated indirectly by the associated changes in peritubular hemodynamics or interstitial pressure.[86,91]

ROLE OF NO IN VASCULAR REMODELING AND ATHEROSCLEROSIS

Increased peripheral vascular resistance is one of the hallmark features of hypertension. The resistance arteries, characterized by a lumen diameter of 100–350 μm, are the major determinants of peripheral resistance.[92,93] Structural changes in these resistance arteries are commonly observed in experimental animal models of hypertension and in human hypertension. The two alterations in vascular structure most commonly described are eutrophic and hypertrophic remodeling. Eutrophic remodeling describes the increased media to lumen ratio that results from a reduced outer diameter that narrows the lumen without net growth. In hypertrophic remodeling, the growth of the media narrows the lumen, resulting in increased media cross-sectional area and media to lumen ratio.[94] There is increasing evidence that vascular remodeling in resistance arteries contributes to the development and complications of hypertension.[94] Furthermore, hypertension-induced remodeling in conduit arteries facilitates development of atherosclerosis and contributes to decreased vessel compliance, which results in elevation of systolic blood pressure.[93] The structural alterations exhibited in conduit arteries include decreased lumen size and thickened media with increased extracellular matrix (ECM) deposition. NO plays a central role in the pathophysiology of vascular remodeling of resistance and conduit arteries through modulation of vascular smooth muscle cell (VSMC) growth and ECM deposition.

NO, generated by both eNOS or NO donors, exerts antiproliferative, antimitogenic and antimigratory effects on cultured VSMC.[1,95] In addition, NO has been shown to inhibit total protein and collagen synthesis in VSMC[96] and to activate certain matrix metalloproteinases,[95] suggesting a role in the modulation of ECM turnover in the vessel wall. The inhibitory effects of NO on vascular wall growth have been verified in in vivo models of vascular injury using NOS inhibitor-treated animals,[55,97,98] mice genetically deficient in eNOS,[95,99,100] transgenic mice that overexpress eNOS in the endothelium,[96] and animals that overexpress eNOS in VSMC and/or the adventitia via eNOS gene transfer.[101,102] The mechanisms underlying these actions of NO have not been fully elucidated. Recent evidence suggests that activation of protein kinase A, at least partially mediated by cGMP-induced inhibition of phosphodiesterase III, contributes to the antiproliferative activity of NO by regulating the expression of cell cycle proteins and by inhibiting Raf-1.[1] The inhibition of arginase and ornithine decarboxylase by NO, independently of cGMP, is another mechanism demonstrated to mediate the antiproliferative effects of NO on VSMC.[1] The phosphorylation of ERK 1/2 is an important mediator of Ang II-induced VSMC growth. Blockade of the AT_1 receptor and the ERK 1/2 pathway have both been shown to attenuate this growth response to Ang II.[103,104] It has been recently reported that NO is an endogenous inhibitor of ERK 1/2 phosphorylation, thus counteracting the growth-promoting effects of Ang II in conduit arteries.[105] In addition, NO down-regulates expression of AT_1 receptors and ACE in vascular tissue and heart and inhibits ET-1 synthesis and release in endothelial cells.[64,106] NO has been shown to down-regulate expression of TGF-β in the mesangium and endothelium.[107] TGF-β has been demonstrated to stimulate pro-fibrotic processes and ECM protein deposition in the vasculature and glomeruli.

NO inhibits vascular smooth muscle and mesangial cell migration and proliferation, platelet aggregation, leukocyte-endothelial adhesion, and plasminogen activator inhibitor-1 activation.[68,108] These findings suggest that NO has anti-inflammatory and anti-atherogenic properties. Tomita et al. reported that Wistar-Kyoto rats treated for 1 week with L-NAME, a specific NOS inhibitor, exhibited a marked infiltration of mononuclear leukocytes and fibroblast-like cells into the coronary vessels and myocardial interstitial areas.[109] These inflammatory changes were associated with increases in mRNA and protein expression of monocyte chemoattractant protein-1 (MCP-1), which is thought to be responsible for the migration of monocytes into the intima at sites of atherosclerotic lesion formation.[110] Long-term (8 weeks) inhibition of NO has been shown to cause coronary microvascular remodeling, characterized by increased wall to lumen ratio and perivascular fibrosis.[97] eNOS-deficient mice manifest an increase in leukocyte adhesion to vascular endothelium and expression of vascular MCP-1.[108] In apolipoprotein E (apoE) knockout mice, which are prone to develop atherosclerosis, deletion of the eNOS gene markedly accelerated atherosclerotic lesion formation in the aorta and coronary arteries.[111] This effect could not be attributed to the hemodynamic effects of elevated blood pressure in apoE/eNOS double knockout mice because a subsequent study showed that despite normalization of blood pressure with hydralazine, these mice developed a similar degree of accelerated atherosclerosis.[112] It has been reported that eNOS is also present in platelets. Indeed, it has been shown that impaired platelet production of NO predicts the presence of acute coronary syndromes.[113] Taken together, these findings provide strong evidence for antiatherosclerotic properties of endothelium-derived NO.

CONCLUSION

In summary, modulating the bioavailability of NO has important implications for the treatment of hypertension and the prevention of end organ damage. Agents that lower blood pressure and concomitantly enhance NO bioavailability may exert cardio- and vasculoprotective effects by preventing the maladaptive changes that accompany hypertension, namely endothelial dysfunction, up-regulation of proinflammatory molecules, VSMC growth and migration, and increased ECM deposition, mechanisms that lead to atherosclerotic cardiovascular disease.

ACKNOWLEDGMENTS

This work was supported by a grant from the Veterans Affairs Administration to Leopoldo Raij.

REFERENCES

1. Gewaltig MT, Kojda G. Vasoprotection by nitric oxide: mechanisms and therapeutic potential. Cardiovasc Res 2002; 55: 250–60.
2. Wilcox CS, Welch WJ, Murad F et al. Nitric oxide synthase in macula densa regulates glomerular capillary pressure. Proc Natl Acad Sci U S A 1992; 89: 11993–7.
3. Boissel JP, Schwarz PM, Forstermann U. Neuronal-type NO synthase: transcript diversity and expressional regulation. Nitric Oxide 1998; 2: 337–49.
4. Abu-Soud HM, Loftus M, Stuehr DJ. Subunit dissociation and unfolding of macrophage NO synthase: relationship between enzyme structure, prosthetic group binding, and catalytic function. Biochemistry 1995; 34: 11167–75.
5. Li H, Wallerath T, Forstermann U. Physiological mechanisms regulating the expression of endothelial-type NO synthase. Nitric Oxide 2002; 7: 132–47.
6. Kone BC, Kuncewicz T, Zhang W et al. Protein interactions with nitric oxide synthases: controlling the right time, the right place, and the right amount of nitric oxide. Am J Physiol Renal Physiol 2003; 285: F178–F190.
7. Garcia-Cardena G, Oh P, Liu J et al. Targeting of nitric oxide synthase to endothelial cell caveolae via palmitoylation: implications for nitric oxide signaling. Proc Natl Acad Sci U S A 1996; 93: 6448–53.
8. Shaul PW, Smart EJ, Robinson LJ et al. Acylation targets endothelial nitric-oxide synthase to plasmalemmal caveolae. J Biol Chem 1996; 271: 6518–22.
9. Gratton JP, Bernatchez P, Sessa WC. Caveolae and caveolins in the cardiovascular system. Circ Res 2004; 94: 1408–17.
10. Marrero MB, Venema VJ, Ju H et al. Endothelial nitric oxide synthase interactions with G-protein-coupled receptors. Biochem J 1999; 343 (Pt 2): 335–40.
11. Pohl U, Holtz J, Busse R et al. Crucial role of endothelium in the vasodilator response to increased flow in vivo. Hypertension 1986; 8: 37–44.
12. Rizzo V, McIntosh DP, Oh P et al. In situ flow activates endothelial nitric oxide synthase in luminal caveolae of endothelium with rapid caveolin dissociation and calmodulin association. J Biol Chem 1998; 273: 34724–9.
13. Garcia-Cardena G, Fan R, Shah V et al. Dynamic activation of endothelial nitric oxide synthase by Hsp90. Nature 1998; 392: 821–4.
14. Dimmeler S, Fleming I, Fisslthaler B et al. Activation of nitric oxide synthase in endothelial cells by Akt-dependent phosphorylation. Nature 1999; 399: 601–5.
15. Fulton D, Gratton JP, McCabe TJ et al. Regulation of endothelium-derived nitric oxide production by the protein kinase Akt. Nature 1999; 399: 597–601.
16. Luo Z, Fujio Y, Kureishi Y et al. Acute modulation of endothelial Akt/PKB activity alters nitric oxide-dependent vasomotor activity in vivo. J Clin Invest 2000; 106: 493–9.
17. Stirone C, Boroujerdi A, Duckles SP et al. Estrogen receptor activation of phosphoinositide-3 kinase, akt, and nitric oxide signaling in cerebral blood vessels: rapid and long-term effects. Mol Pharmacol 2005; 67: 105–13.
18. Davis ME, Cai H, Drummond GR et al. Shear stress regulates endothelial nitric oxide synthase expression through c-Src by divergent signaling pathways. Circ Res 2001; 89: 1073–80.
19. Mollnau H, Wendt M, Szocs K et al. Effects of angiotensin II infusion on the expression and function of NAD(P)H oxidase and components of nitric oxide/cGMP signaling. Circ Res 2002; 90: E58–E65.
20. Ding Q, Hayashi T, Packiasamy AJ et al. The effect of high glucose on NO and O_2^- through endothelial GTPCH1 and NADPH oxidase. Life Sci 2004; 75: 3185–94.
21. Drummond GR, Cai H, Davis ME et al. Transcriptional and posttranscriptional regulation of endothelial nitric oxide synthase expression by hydrogen peroxide. Circ Res 2000; 86: 347–54.
22. Saura M, Zaragoza C, Cao W et al. Smad2 mediates transforming growth factor-beta induction of endothelial nitric oxide synthase expression. Circ Res 2002; 91: 806–13.
23. Lee DL, Webb RC, Jin L. Hypertension and RhoA/Rho-kinase signaling in the vasculature: highlights from the recent literature. Hypertension 2004; 44: 796–9.
24. Mehta JL, Li DY, Chen HJ et al. Inhibition of LOX-1 by statins may relate to upregulation of eNOS. Biochem Biophys Res Commun 2001; 289: 857–61.
25. Cardaropoli S, Silvagno F, Morra E et al. Infectious and inflammatory stimuli decrease endothelial nitric oxide synthase activity in vitro. J Hypertens 2003; 21: 2103–10.
26. Alonso J, Sanchez de Miguel L, Monton M et al. Endothelial cytosolic proteins bind to the 3′ untranslated region of endothelial nitric oxide synthase mRNA: regulation by tumor necrosis factor alpha. Mol Cell Biol 1997; 17: 5719–26.
27. Ignarro LJ. Nitric oxide as a unique signaling molecule in the vascular system: a historical overview. J Physiol Pharmacol 2002; 53 (4 Pt 1): 503–14.
28. Lucas KA, Pitari GM, Kazerounian S et al. Guanylyl cyclases and signaling by cyclic GMP. Pharmacol Rev 2000; 52: 375–414.

29. Ignarro LJ, Cirino G, Casini A et al. Nitric oxide as a signaling molecule in the vascular system: an overview. J Cardiovasc Pharmacol 1999; 34: 879–86.
30. Massberg S, Sausbier M, Klatt P et al. Increased adhesion and aggregation of platelets lacking cyclic guanosine 3′,5′-monophosphate kinase I. J Exp Med 1999; 189: 1255–64.
31. Hampl V, Herget J. Role of nitric oxide in the pathogenesis of chronic pulmonary hypertension. Physiol Rev 2000; 80: 1337–72.
32. Yan C, Kim D, Aizawa T et al. Functional interplay between angiotensin II and nitric oxide: cyclic GMP as a key mediator. Arterioscler Thromb Vasc Biol 2003; 23: 26–36.
33. Andriantsitohaina R, Lagaud GJ, Andre A et al. Effects of cGMP on calcium handling in ATP-stimulated rat resistance arteries. Am J Physiol 1995; 268 (3 Pt 2): H1223–H1231.
34. Archer SL, Huang JM, Hampl V et al. Nitric oxide and cGMP cause vasorelaxation by activation of a charybdotoxin-sensitive K channel by cGMP-dependent protein kinase. Proc Natl Acad Sci U S A 1994; 91: 7583–7.
35. Archer SL, Huang JM, Reeve HL et al. Differential distribution of electrophysiologically distinct myocytes in conduit and resistance arteries determines their response to nitric oxide and hypoxia. Circ Res 1996; 78: 431–42.
36. Komalavilas P, Lincoln TM. Phosphorylation of the inositol 1,4,5-trisphosphate receptor. Cyclic GMP-dependent protein kinase mediates cAMP and cGMP dependent phosphorylation in the intact rat aorta. J Biol Chem 1996; 271: 21933–8.
37. Komalavilas P, Lincoln TM. Phosphorylation of the inositol 1,4,5-trisphosphate receptor by cyclic GMP-dependent protein kinase. J Biol Chem 1994; 269: 8701–7.
38. Hirata M, Kohse KP, Chang CH et al. Mechanism of cyclic GMP inhibition of inositol phosphate formation in rat aorta segments and cultured bovine aortic smooth muscle cells. J Biol Chem 1990; 265: 1268–73.
39. Xia C, Bao Z, Yue C et al. Phosphorylation and regulation of G-protein-activated phospholipase C-beta 3 by cGMP-dependent protein kinases. J Biol Chem 2001; 276: 19770–7.
40. Yoshida Y, Sun HT, Cai JQ et al. Cyclic GMP-dependent protein kinase stimulates the plasma membrane Ca2+ pump ATPase of vascular smooth muscle via phosphorylation of a 240-kDa protein. J Biol Chem 1991; 266: 19819–25.
41. Tamaoki J, Tagaya E, Nishimura K et al. Role of Na(+)-K+ ATPase in cyclic GMP-mediated relaxation of canine pulmonary artery smooth muscle cells. Br J Pharmacol 1997; 122: 112–16.
42. Twort CH, van Breemen C. Cyclic guanosine monophosphate-enhanced sequestration of Ca2+ by sarcoplasmic reticulum in vascular smooth muscle. Circ Res 1988; 62: 961–4.
43. Wu X, Somlyo AV, Somlyo AP. Cyclic GMP-dependent stimulation reverses G-protein-coupled inhibition of smooth muscle myosin light chain phosphate. Biochem Biophys Res Commun 1996; 220: 658–63.
44. Lee MR, Li L, Kitazawa T. Cyclic GMP causes Ca2+ desensitization in vascular smooth muscle by activating the myosin light chain phosphatase. J Biol Chem 1997; 272: 5063–8.
45. Carvajal JA, Germain AM, Huidobro-Toro JP et al. Molecular mechanism of cGMP-mediated smooth muscle relaxation. J Cell Physiol 2000; 184: 409–20.
46. Sauzeau V, Le Jeune H, Cario-Toumaniantz C et al. Cyclic GMP-dependent protein kinase signaling pathway inhibits RhoA-induced Ca2+ sensitization of contraction in vascular smooth muscle. J Biol Chem 2000; 275: 21722–9.
47. Coats P, Johnston F, MacDonald J et al. Endothelium-derived hyperpolarizing factor: identification and mechanisms of action in human subcutaneous resistance arteries. Circulation 2001; 103: 1702–8.
48. Freitas MR, Schott C, Corriu C et al. Heterogeneity of endothelium-dependent vasorelaxation in conductance and resistance arteries from Lyon normotensive and hypertensive rats. J Hypertens 2003; 21: 1505–12.
49. Zhou MS, Raij L. Cross-talk between nitric oxide and endothelium-derived hyperpolarizing factor: synergistic interaction? J Hypertens 2003; 21: 1449–51.
50. Huang PL, Huang Z, Mashimo H et al. Hypertension in mice lacking the gene for endothelial nitric oxide synthase. Nature 1995; 377: 239–42.
51. Ohashi Y, Kawashima S, Hirata K et al. Hypotension and reduced nitric oxide-elicited vasorelaxation in transgenic mice overexpressing endothelial nitric oxide synthase. J Clin Invest 1998; 102: 2061–71.
52. Zhou MS, Schulman IH, Raij L. Nitric oxide, angiotensin II, and hypertension. Semin Nephrol 2004; 24: 366–78.
53. Cosentino F, Barker JE, Brand MP et al. Reactive oxygen species mediate endothelium-dependent relaxations in tetrahydrobiopterin-deficient mice. Arterioscler Thromb Vasc Biol 2001; 21: 496–502.
54. Mitchell BM, Dorrance AM, Webb RC. GTP cyclohydrolase 1 inhibition attenuates vasodilation and increases blood pressure in rats. Am J Physiol Heart Circ Physiol 2003; 285: H2165–H2170.
55. Takemoto M, Egashira K, Usui M et al. Important role of tissue angiotensin-converting enzyme activity in the pathogenesis of coronary vascular and myocardial structural changes induced by long-term blockade of nitric oxide synthesis in rats. J Clin Invest 1997; 99: 278–87.
56. Katoh M, Egashira K, Usui M et al. Cardiac angiotensin II receptors are upregulated by long-term inhibition of nitric oxide synthesis in rats. Circ Res 1998; 83: 743–51.
57. Rubanyi GM, Polokoff MA. Endothelins: molecular biology, biochemistry, pharmacology, physiology, and pathophysiology. Pharmacol Rev 1994; 46: 325–415.
58. Boulanger CM, Luscher TF. Differential effect of cyclic GMP on the release of endothelin-1 from cultured endothelial cells and intact porcine aorta. J Cardiovasc Pharmacol 1991; 17 (Suppl 7): S264–S266.
59. Kramp R, Fourmanoir P, Caron N. Endothelin resets renal blood flow autoregulatory efficiency during acute blockade of NO in the rat. Am J Physiol Renal Physiol 2001; 281: F1132–F140.
60. Qiu C, Baylis C. Endothelin and angiotensin mediate most glomerular responses to nitric oxide inhibition. Kidney Int 1999; 55: 2390–6.
61. Ackermann A, Fernandez-Alfonso MS, Sanchez de Rojas R et al. Modulation of angiotensin-converting enzyme by nitric oxide. Br J Pharmacol 1998; 124: 291–8.
62. Higashi Y, Oshima T, Ono N et al. Intravenous administration of L-arginine inhibits angiotensin-converting enzyme in humans. J Clin Endocrinol Metab 1995; 80: 2198–202.
63. Kumar KV, Das UN. Effect of cis-unsaturated fatty acids, prostaglandins, and free radicals on angiotensin-converting enzyme activity in vitro. Proc Soc Exp Biol Med 1997; 214: 374–9.
64. Ichiki T, Usui M, Kato M et al. Downregulation of angiotensin II type 1 receptor gene transcription by nitric oxide. Hypertension 1998; 31 (1 Pt 2): 342–8.
65. Lavallee M, Takamura M, Parent R et al. Crosstalk between endothelin and nitric oxide in the control of vascular tone. Heart Fail Rev 2001; 6: 265–76.
66. Schiffrin EL. State-of-the-art lecture. Role of endothelin-1 in hypertension. Hypertension 1999; 34 (4 Pt 2): 876–81.
67. Kawashima S, Yokoyama M. Dysfunction of endothelial nitric oxide synthase and atherosclerosis. Arterioscler Thromb Vasc Biol 2004; 24: 998–1005.

68. Landmesser U, Hornig B, Drexler H. Endothelial function: a critical determinant in atherosclerosis? Circulation 2004; 109 (21 Suppl 1): II27–33.
69. Griendling KK, FitzGerald GA. Oxidative stress and cardiovascular injury: Part I: basic mechanisms and in vivo monitoring of ROS. Circulation 2003; 108: 1912–16.
70. Zou MH, Shi C, Cohen RA. Oxidation of the zinc-thiolate complex and uncoupling of endothelial nitric oxide synthase by peroxynitrite. J Clin Invest 2002; 109: 817–26.
71. Alp NJ, McAteer MA, Khoo J et al. Increased endothelial tetrahydrobiopterin synthesis by targeted transgenic GTP-cyclohydrolase I overexpression reduces endothelial dysfunction and atherosclerosis in ApoE-knockout mice. Arterioscler Thromb Vasc Biol 2004; 24: 445–50.
72. Landmesser U, Dikalov S, Price SR et al. Oxidation of tetrahydrobiopterin leads to uncoupling of endothelial cell nitric oxide synthase in hypertension. J Clin Invest 2003; 111: 1201–9.
73. Ozaki M, Kawashima S, Yamashita T et al. Overexpression of endothelial nitric oxide synthase accelerates atherosclerotic lesion formation in apoE-deficient mice. J Clin Invest 2002; 110: 331–40.
74. Sydow K, Munzel T. ADMA and oxidative stress. Atheroscler Suppl 2003; 4: 41–51.
75. Boger RH, Bode-Boger SM, Szuba A et al. Asymmetric dimethylarginine (ADMA): a novel risk factor for endothelial dysfunction: its role in hypercholesterolemia. Circulation 1998; 98: 1842–7.
76. Vaziri ND, Ni Z, Oveisi F. Upregulation of renal and vascular nitric oxide synthase in young spontaneously hypertensive rats. Hypertension 1998; 31: 1248–54.
77. Hayakawa H, Coffee K, Raij L. Endothelial dysfunction and cardiorenal injury in experimental salt-sensitive hypertension: effects of antihypertensive therapy. Circulation 1997; 96: 2407–13.
78. Hayakawa H, Raij L. The link among nitric oxide synthase activity, endothelial function, and aortic and ventricular hypertrophy in hypertension. Hypertension 1997; 29 (1 Pt 2): 235–41.
79. Zhou MS, Jaimes EA, Raij L. Atorvastatin prevents end-organ injury in salt-sensitive hypertension: role of eNOS and oxidant stress. Hypertension 2004; 44: 186–90.
80. Deng X, Welch WJ, Wilcox CS. Role of nitric oxide in short-term and prolonged effects of angiotensin II on renal hemodynamics. Hypertension 1996; 27: 1173–9.
81. Navar LG, Harrison-Bernard LM, Imig JD et al. Renal actions of angiotensin II and AT_1 receptor blockers. In: Murray Epstein BH (ed). Angiotensin II receptor antagonists. Philadelphia, PA: Hanley & Belfus, 2001, pp 189–214.
82. Gabbai FB, Blantz RC. Role of nitric oxide in renal hemodynamics. Semin Nephrol 1999; 19: 242–50.
83. Ohishi K, Carmines PK, Inscho EW et al. EDRF-angiotensin II interactions in rat juxtamedullary afferent and efferent arterioles. Am J Physiol 1992; 263 (5 Pt 2): F900–F906.
84. Ichihara A, Imig JD, Inscho EW et al. Interactive nitric oxide-angiotensin II influences on renal microcirculation in angiotensin II-induced hypertension. Hypertension 1998; 31: 1255–60.
85. Navar LG, Harrison-Bernard LM, Nishiyama A et al. Regulation of intrarenal angiotensin II in hypertension. Hypertension 2002; 39 (2 Pt 2): 316–22.
86. Majid DS, Navar LG. Nitric oxide in the control of renal hemodynamics and excretory function. Am J Hypertens 2001; 14 (6 Pt 2): 74S-82S.
87. Zou AP, Wu F, Cowley AW Jr. Protective effect of angiotensin II-induced increase in nitric oxide in the renal medullary circulation. Hypertension 1998; 31 (1 Pt 2): 271–6.
88. Szentivanyi M Jr, Zou AP, Mattson DL et al. Renal medullary nitric oxide deficit of Dahl S rats enhances hypertensive actions of angiotensin II. Am J Physiol Regul Integr Comp Physiol 2002; 283: R266–R272.
89. Sarkis A, Liu KL, Lo M et al. Angiotensin II and renal medullary blood flow in Lyon rats. Am J Physiol Renal Physiol 2003; 284: F365–72.
90. Stoos BA, Garvin JL. Actions of nitric oxide on renal epithelial transport. Clin Exp Pharmacol Physiol 1997; 24: 591–4.
91. Majid DS, Said KE, Omoro SA et al. Nitric oxide dependency of arterial pressure-induced changes in renal interstitial hydrostatic pressure in dogs. Circ Res 2001; 88: 347–51.
92. Laragh JH. Essential hypertension. In: Brenner BM (ed). Brenner & Rector's The kidney, Vol. 1, 6th edn. Philadelphia, PA: Saunders, 2000, pp 1967–2006.
93. Ernesto L, Schiffrin DH. Role of AT1 angiotensin receptors in vascular remodeling in hypertension. In: Epstein M, Brunner HR (ed). Angiotensin II receptor antagonists. Philadelphia, PA: Hanley & Belfus, 2001, pp 279–94.
94. Intengan HD, Schiffrin EL. Vascular remodeling in hypertension: roles of apoptosis, inflammation, and fibrosis. Hypertension 2001; 38 (3 Pt 2): 581–7.
95. Rudic RD, Shesely EG, Maeda N et al. Direct evidence for the importance of endothelium-derived nitric oxide in vascular remodeling. J Clin Invest 1998; 101: 731–6.
96. Kawashima S, Yamashita T, Ozaki M et al. Endothelial NO synthase overexpression inhibits lesion formation in mouse model of vascular remodeling. Arterioscler Thromb Vasc Biol 2001; 21: 201–7.
97. Numaguchi K, Egashira K, Takemoto M et al. Chronic inhibition of nitric oxide synthesis causes coronary microvascular remodeling in rats. Hypertension 1995; 26 (6 Pt 1): 957–62.
98. Tronc F, Wassef M, Esposito B et al. Role of NO in flow-induced remodeling of the rabbit common carotid artery. Arterioscler Thromb Vasc Biol 1996; 16: 1256–62.
99. Moroi M, Zhang L, Yasuda T et al. Interaction of genetic deficiency of endothelial nitric oxide, gender, and pregnancy in vascular response to injury in mice. J Clin Invest 1998; 101: 1225–32.
100. Yogo K, Shimokawa H, Funakoshi H et al. Different vasculoprotective roles of NO synthase isoforms in vascular lesion formation in mice. Arterioscler Thromb Vasc Biol 2000; 20: E96–E100.
101. von der Leyen HE, Gibbons GH, Morishita R et al. Gene therapy inhibiting neointimal vascular lesion: in vivo transfer of endothelial cell nitric oxide synthase gene. Proc Natl Acad Sci U S A 1995; 92: 1137–41.
102. Varenne O, Pislaru S, Gillijns H et al. Local adenovirus-mediated transfer of human endothelial nitric oxide synthase reduces luminal narrowing after coronary angioplasty in pigs. Circulation 1998; 98: 919–26.
103. Touyz RM, He G, El Mabrouk M et al. p38 Map kinase regulates vascular smooth muscle cell collagen synthesis by angiotensin II in SHR but not in WKY. Hypertension 2001; 37 (2 Part 2): 574–80.
104. Kim S, Iwao H. Molecular and cellular mechanisms of angiotensin II-mediated cardiovascular and renal diseases. Pharmacol Rev 2000; 52: 11–34.
105. Martens FM, Demeilliers B, Girardot D et al. Vessel-specific stimulation of protein synthesis by nitric oxide synthase inhibition: role of extracellular signal-regulated kinases 1/2. Hypertension 2002; 39: 16–21.
106. Usui M, Ichiki T, Katoh M et al. Regulation of angiotensin II receptor expression by nitric oxide in rat adrenal gland. Hypertension 1998; 32: 527–33.

107. Craven PA, Studer RK, Felder J et al. Nitric oxide inhibition of transforming growth factor-beta and collagen synthesis in mesangial cells. Diabetes 1997; 46: 671–81.
108. Lefer DJ, Jones SP, Girod WG et al. Leukocyte-endothelial cell interactions in nitric oxide synthase-deficient mice. Am J Physiol 1999; 276 (6 Pt 2): H1943–H1950.
109. Tomita H, Egashira K, Kubo-Inoue M et al. Inhibition of NO synthesis induces inflammatory changes and monocyte chemoattractant protein-1 expression in rat hearts and vessels. Arterioscler Thromb Vasc Biol 1998; 18: 1456–64.
110. Libby P, Ridker PM, Maseri A. Inflammation and atherosclerosis. Circulation 2002; 105: 1135–43.
111. Kuhlencordt PJ, Gyurko R, Han F et al. Accelerated atherosclerosis, aortic aneurysm formation, and ischemic heart disease in apolipoprotein E/endothelial nitric oxide synthase double-knockout mice. Circulation 2001; 104: 448–54.
112. Chen J, Kuhlencordt PJ, Astern J et al. Hypertension does not account for the accelerated atherosclerosis and development of aneurysms in male apolipoprotein e/endothelial nitric oxide synthase double knockout mice. Circulation 2001; 104: 2391–4.
113. Freedman JE, Ting B, Hankin B et al. Impaired platelet production of nitric oxide predicts presence of acute coronary syndromes. Circulation 1998; 98: 1481–6.

29

Molecular regulation of endothelial nitric oxide synthase

Mariela Garcia Blanes and Jean-Philippe Gratton

INTRODUCTION

Endothelial nitric oxide synthase (eNOS or NOS3) is the NOS isoform responsible for the generation of nitric oxide (NO) from the endothelium of the vascular wall. eNOS-derived NO participates in the regulation of blood pressure, maintenance of a non-thrombogenic endothelium, and inhibition of smooth muscle cell proliferation. eNOS activity is tightly controlled by numerous regulators, indicating that a balance in NO levels is needed to maintain vascular homeostasis. This chapter will deal with the molecular mechanisms that regulate eNOS activity and thus control the extent of NO released from the endothelium.

eNOS CELLULAR LOCALIZATION

Early on, following the purification and cloning of eNOS,[1–4] it was shown that proper cellular distribution of the protein was necessary for efficient NO release. eNOS is anchored to cellular membranes via cotranslational N-myristoylation (glycine 2) and posttranslational palmitoylation (cysteins 15 and 26)[5,6] that direct the protein to discrete pools of cellular membranes. In endothelial cells, eNOS is found both at the plasma membrane and on the cytoplasmic face of the Golgi apparatus. Mutation of the myristic acid acceptor site on eNOS results in the cellular mislocalization of the protein into the cytoplasm and in reduced stimulated NO production from cells.[5] Interestingly, the in vitro catalytic activity of this mutated enzyme remains unaffected, suggesting that membrane association of eNOS is necessary for efficient NO production. In addition, the initial N-myristoylation of eNOS in the trans-Golgi is essential for the subsequent palmitoylation.[6] However, palmitoylation is not necessary for overall membrane association but is essential for eNOS localization in the plasmalemmal caveolae.[7,8] Indeed, dual acylation (myristoylation and palmitoylation) of proteins is considered as a 'molecular zip code' for the targeting to cholesterol-rich domains of the plasma membrane such as the caveolae and lipid rafts.[9,10] Again, mutation of the acceptor cysteins of eNOS, Cys15, and Cys26, results in reduced cellular NO production without affecting the enzymatic activity *per se*, suggesting that eNOS localization to proper membrane microdomains provides some of the regulatory proteins essential for NO production.[11] While cellular localization of eNOS is essential for efficient NO release, the specific cellular pool of eNOS responsible for NO production in cells has been the subject of speculation. Recent evidences suggest that both Golgi and plasmalemmal eNOS participate in overall NO production. However, the relative contribution of both sites is affected by the type of stimulus used and is mostly defined by phosphorylation levels.[12,13]

PROTEIN–PROTEIN INTERACTIONS THAT REGULATE eNOS ACTIVITY

The targeted localization of eNOS to caveolae has prompted the investigation of its association to caveolin, the major coat protein of caveolae. Indeed, caveolin-1 is necessary for the biogenesis of caveolae through an unknown mechanism.[9] Caveolin has the capacity to directly interact with other intracellular signaling proteins such as c-Src and H-Ras through amino acids 82–101, the putative scaffolding domain.[9] Indeed, eNOS was shown to directly interact with caveolin-1[14–16] through a primary binding region of caveolin-1 within amino acids 60–101[16,17] and the association of caveolin and eNOS is disrupted in the presence of caveolin scaffolding peptides (amino acids 82–101).[18,19] Furthermore, eNOS contains a putative caveolin binding motif[20] located within amino acids 350–358 (FSAAPFSGW) which is thought to be responsible for its association to caveolin-1.

The consequence on eNOS activity of caveolin association has been best demonstrated by the incubation of pure eNOS with caveolin scaffolding peptide or glutathione S-transferase (GST)-caveolin fusion protein, which results in inhibition of eNOS.[17] In addition, cotransfection experiments showed that caveolin overexpression resulted in reduced eNOS activity[21] and in reduced NO release.[17] The reduction of eNOS activity by caveolin peptides, or overexpressed caveolin, is reversed by exogenous addition of calmodulin, suggesting a reciprocal regulation by the two proteins.[18]

Collectively, these in vitro results suggested that NO production is negatively regulated by interactions with caveolin and that for NO release to occur, the inhibitory clamp by caveolin must be overcome. Evidence for a physiological relevance of the negative regulation of eNOS by caveolin initially came from work using the caveolin scaffolding domain as a surrogate for caveolin-1. Interestingly, delivery of CSD to permeabilized cells[22] or cell-permeable versions of caveolin-1 scaffolding domain, by fusing it to a cell-permeable leader sequence,[23] can block NO release, inhibit endothelium-dependent responses of isolated blood vessels, inflammation, vascular permeability, angiogenesis, and tumor growth in vivo.[23,24] In addition, the initial publications regarding caveolin-1 null mice also reported that the caveolin-1 and eNOS interaction has functional significance.[25,26] Isolated aortae from caveolin-1 (–/–) mice exhibited blunted responses to vasoconstrictor agents such as phenylephrine and also marked increases in vasodilatory responses to the endothelium-dependent vasodilator, acetylcholine, and both these effects were reversed by treatment of the vessels with the NOS inhibitor L-NAME.[25,26] These results suggest that the absence of caveolin-1 and caveolae in endothelial cells leads to increased eNOS activity and thus NO release resulting in reduced vascular tone.

Other negative regulators of eNOS activity have been uncovered. However, they have not been as extensively studied as the caveolin–eNOS association. The intracellular domain 4 (ID4) of the bradykinin 2 (B2) and the angiotensin AT_1 receptors have been reported to associate with eNOS and negatively regulate its activity in vitro.[27] Indeed, eNOS coprecipitated with the B2 receptor and in vitro interacted with a GST fusion of ID4, and synthetic peptides from ID4 inhibited eNOS activity in a dose-dependent manner in vitro.[28] The concept that a receptor can directly interact with eNOS is interesting; however, direct evidence supporting the physiological relevance of this interaction is presently unavailable.

Recently, two novel interacting proteins have been identified, NOSIP and NOSTRIN.[29,30] Both proteins negatively influence eNOS-derived NO release from cells by influencing eNOS cellular trafficking. NOSIP, a 34-kDa protein, was initially identified as an eNOS C-terminal domain binding protein.[30] Stimulation of cells with calcium ionophore did not change the association of NOSIP and eNOS; however, a peptide derived from the caveolin scaffolding domain was able to displace eNOS from NOSIP. NOSIP overexpression results in reduced NO release from intact cells due to the redistribution of eNOS from the plasma membrane to intracellular compartments. Similarly, NOSTRIN, a 58-kDa protein that binds the eNOS oxygenase domain through an SH3-type sequence was discovered by yeast two-hybrid system.[29] Overexpression of NOSTRIN in Chinese hamster ovary cells results in a profound relocation of eNOS from plasma and Golgi membranes to vesicle-like structures spread over the cytosol. Inhibition of NO production in NOSTRIN-overexpressing cells may be the consequence of this redistribution of eNOS. The identification of NOSIP and NOSTRIN as modulators of eNOS cellular localization demonstrates that membrane compartmentalization of the enzyme is necessary for optimal activity and NO release and that the cytoskeleton is most likely involved in the cellular relocalization of eNOS.[31,32]

The sustained activation of eNOS by a variety of agonists and mechanical forces implies its association with positive regulatory proteins that counterbalance the inhibitory action of caveolins (Figure 29.1). The first protein shown to be involved in eNOS regulation was calmodulin (CaM). Early studies on eNOS[33] demonstrated that purified NOS utilized CaM as an activator of NO synthesis. Mechanistically, CaM binding to a canonical CaM binding motif on eNOS can displace the adjacent autoinhibitory loop, thus facilitating NADPH-dependent electron flux from the reductase domain to the heme located in the oxygenase domain.[34] The heme will permit the insertion of its bound oxygen into the NOS substrate, L-arginine. Nevertheless, there is no evidence currently documenting that CaM can actually be recruited to eNOS in a stimulus-dependent manner. Pharmacological studies using inhibitors of CaM or calcium-free

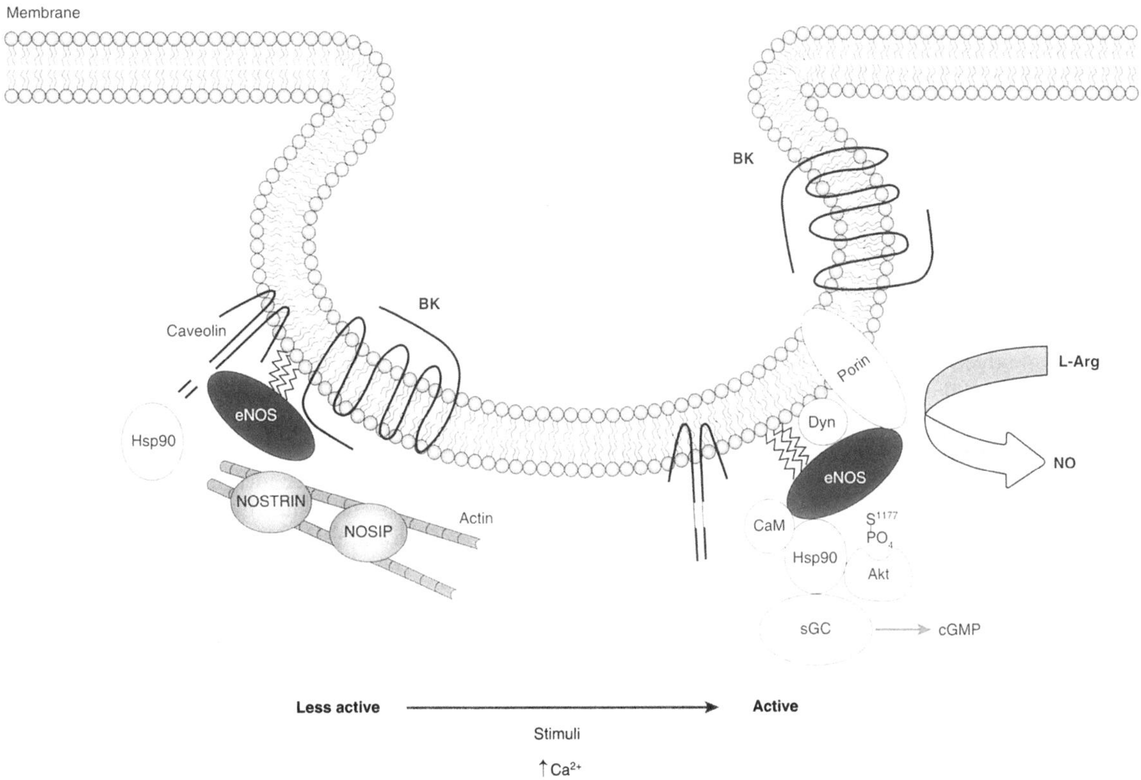

Figure 29.1 eNOS interacting partners. Under basal conditions (less active state), membrane-bound eNOS is associated with the negative regulatory proteins (gray): caveolin, nitric oxide synthase-interacting protein (NOSIP), nitric oxide synthase trafficker (NOSTRIN) and the fourth intracellular domain of the bradykinin (BK) receptor. After endothelial cell stimulation by various stimuli, eNOS associates with the positive regulatory proteins (white): calcium-activated calmodulin (CaM), heat shock protein 90 (Hsp90), Akt, porin, dynamin (Dyn) and soluble guanylyl cyclase (sGC), all interactions associated with increased eNOS activity or NO release

buffers have indirectly shown the requirement of CaM for NO production.[35] In addition, immunoreactive CaM was found bound to eNOS immunoprecipitated from human endothelial cells.[36] Moreover, upon challenge of the cells with estrogen, the amount of CaM recovered in the eNOS immunocomplex did not change. This suggests that CaM may act as a constitutively bound prosthetic group, and that regulation of the affinity of CaM interactions with NOS may occur through subtle changes in free calcium levels.

The second protein found to interact with eNOS and to have a positive influence on its activity is Hsp90. Hsp90 is part of a multicomponent chaperone system that is responsible for the folding of proteins such as steroid receptors and cell cycle-dependent kinases.[37] In addition to this function, Hsp90 can also act as an integral part of numerous signal transduction cascades. Hsp90 can associate with eNOS in resting endothelial cells. Endothelial cell stimulation with vascular endothelial growth factor (VEGF), histamine, fluid shear stress, and estrogen enhances the interaction between Hsp90 and eNOS at the same time that NO production increases.[36,38] The rapid stimulus-dependent formation of the Hsp90-eNOS hetero-complexes suggests that this occurs simultaneously with other signaling events such as the mobilization of intracellular calcium and/or protein phosphorylation. Hsp90 was initially shown to directly activate eNOS in vitro,[38] and coexpression of eNOS with Hsp90 in COS cells increased NOS activity in broken cell lysates. These results suggest that Hsp90 may act as an allosteric modulator of eNOS by inducing a conformational change in the enzyme that results in increased activity.[39] However, a recent study suggested that Hsp90 increases the affinity of neuronal NOS (nNOS) for CaM,[40] and experiments using eNOS have shown that Hsp90 facilitates the CaM-induced displacement of caveolin from eNOS.[19] Moreover, the complexity of Hsp90-mediated activation of eNOS has been further demonstrated by a recent study characterizing the domains of Hsp90 required to bind eNOS. This study also showed that Akt, a kinase involved in eNOS phosphorylation (see later), was recruited to an adjacent region on the M domain of Hsp90, which facilitates eNOS phosphorylation and enzyme activation.[41] Lastly, Hsp90 was shown to function as a scaffold for eNOS and its downstream target, soluble guanylate cyclase,[42] which suggests that Hsp90 also participates in the actions of NO by influencing its effectors.

The physiological relevance of the Hsp90–eNOS interaction came from studies using a specific inhibitor of Hsp90, the ansamycin antibiotic geldanamycin (GA).[43] GA attenuated histamine and VEGF-stimulated cGMP production in cultured endothelial cells and blocked ACh-induced vasorelaxation of rat aortic rings,[38] middle cerebral artery,[44] and flow-induced dilation,[45] indicating that Hsp90 signaling was crucial for NO release and endothelial function.

Recent findings have indicated that dynamin-2 can associate with eNOS. Dynamin-2 belongs to the family of large GTPases, and is believed to be involved in vesicle formation, receptor-mediated endocytosis, caveolae internalization and vesicle trafficking in and out of the Golgi apparatus.[46,47] Dynamin-2 has been shown by confocal microscopy to co-localize with eNOS in the Golgi apparatus and plasma membrane of endothelial cells and to bind eNOS directly through a proline-rich region, both in vivo and in vitro.[48,49] Moreover, in in vitro assays as well as in cultured endothelial cells, an increase in dynamin levels results in enhanced eNOS catalysis.[48] In cells, the association between eNOS and dynamin-2 is increased by calcium ionophore. It has recently been suggested that inhibition of the GTPase activity of dynamin-2 (K44A mutant) prevents bradykinin-induced internalization of eNOS.[50] However, translocation of eNOS upon agonist stimulation remains functionally elusive and a matter of controversy. It is well established that the cellular localization of the enzyme influences NO release as mentioned previously, but the regulation of movement of eNOS between different cellular compartments has yet to be explored.

A recent addition to eNOS positive regulatory proteins is the voltage-dependent anion/cation channel protein porin. Porin was identified by co-immunoprecipitation experiments followed by MS analyses.[51] In vitro binding studies with a GST-porin fusion protein indicated that porin binds directly to eNOS and that this interaction augments eNOS activity. Calcium-mobilizing agonists promote formation of the eNOS/porin complex, which suggests a potential role of intracellular Ca^{2+} mediating this interaction.

REGULATION OF eNOS ACTIVITY BY PHOSPHORYLATION

The role of phosphorylation in the regulation of NO production by endothelial cells has attracted great interest. eNOS phosphorylation, which can occur on serine (S), threonine (T) and tyrosine (Y) residues, is a key regulatory mechanism in the control of eNOS enzyme activity (Figure 29.2). Several potential phosphorylation sites have been identified but eNOS seems to be controlled essentially by the phosphorylation of five residues: the serines 116, 617, 635, 1179 and threonine 497 for the bovine isoform (human eNOS: S114, S615, S633, S1177 and T495).

Serine phosphorylation

Serine 1179 is, without any doubt, the best characterized phosphorylation site on eNOS. It is located on an autoinhibitory loop being part of the C-terminal reductase domain of the enzyme. It is usually not phosphorylated in unstimulated, cultured endothelial cells but can be rapidly phosphorylated in response to various physiological stimuli, including shear stress,[52] estrogen,[53] VEGF,[54] insulin,[55] bradykinin,[56] sphingosine 1-phosphate,[57,58] histamine and thrombin.[59] Several protein kinases have been proposed to be involved in this process: AMP kinase,[60] Akt,[54] protein kinase A (PKA),[61] protein kinase G (PKG),[61] and calmodulin-dependent kinase II (CaMKII).[56] However, the kinase involved depends largely on the stimulus applied. For example, estrogen and VEGF elicit the phosphorylation of Ser1179 through Akt, stimulation by histamine and thrombin requires AMP kinase activation,[59] and bradykinin-mediated phosphorylation occurs through CaMKII.[56] As demonstrated by studies using mutated forms of the enzyme mimicking the non-phosphorylated and phosphorylated state of eNOS (mutations of serine to alanine (A) or serine to aspartate (D), respectively), phosphorylation of the Ser1179 was deduced to result in increased enzymatic activity as well as increased basal and stimulated NO production.[62] It has been proposed that the increase in NO production may be due to a configuration change in the autoinhibitory loop of the enzyme, following Ser1179 phosphorylation,

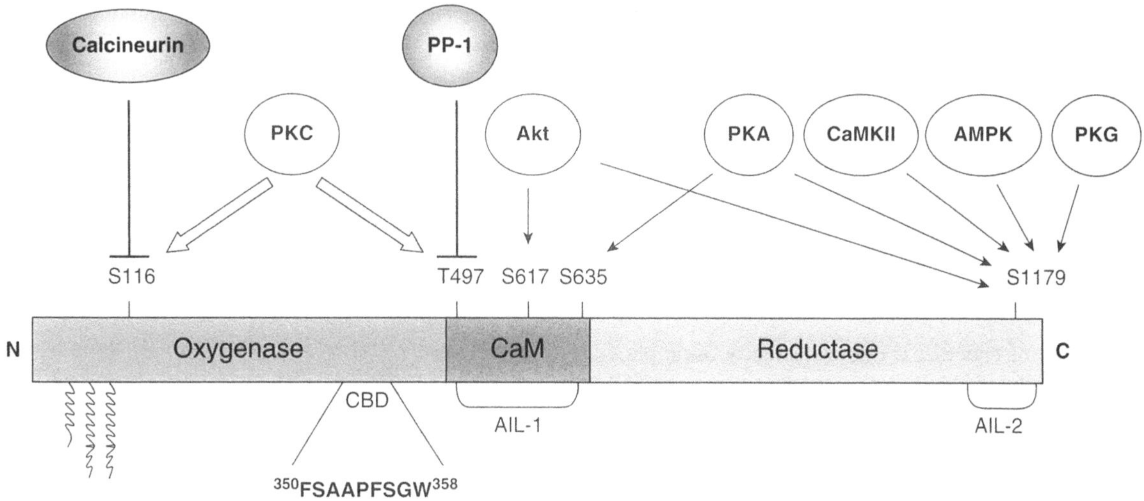

Figure 29.2 Putative phosphorylation sites of eNOS. Schematic representation of eNOS structure showing the N-terminal oxygenase domain (containing the fatty acid acylation sites, the caveolin binding domain (CDB), and phosphorylation site S116) and the C-terminal reductase domain (that contains the calmodulin binding domain (CaM), the autoinhibitory loops 1 and 2 (AIL-1/2) and the phosphorylation sites T497, S617, S635, S1179). PKC, protein kinase C; PP-1, protein phosphatase-1; PKA, protein kinase A; CaMKII, calmodulin kinase II; AMPK, AMP-kinase; PKG, protein kinase G. Grey circle: phosphatases; white circle: kinases; open arrow: inhibitory phosphorylation; black pointed arrow: activating phosphorylation; black blunt arrow: dephosphorylation

which would increase the electron flow from the reductase to the oxygenase domain.[63]

In endothelial cells, bradykinin, ATP, VEGF,[64] and statins[65] are responsible for the phosphorylation of serine 617 and 635. This phosphorylation is mediated by Akt in the case of Ser617 and mediated by PKA for Ser635.[64] These two sites are located in a second autoinhibitory loop within the canonical CaM binding motif. Modification in the phosphorylation status of these sites would thus have an effect on the binding of CaM and the autoinhibition of eNOS activity. Moreover, studies using gain of function mutants of eNOS (mutation of serine to aspartate) at Ser617 and Ser635 resulted in increased enzymatic activity in the case of S635D, whereas with S617D affinity to Ca^{2+}/CaM increased while enzymatic activity remained unchanged in vitro. Phosphorylation of these sites seems to follow different time courses, with a fast and transient phosphorylation for Ser617 and a more sustained phosphorylation for Ser635.[62,64] These data suggest that during eNOS activation, Ser617 is phosphorylated first, making the enzyme more likely to bind CaM. Then, Ser635 is phosphorylated, which increases the maximal activity of eNOS and causes long-term potentiation of NO release.

Ser116, located in the oxygenase domain of eNOS, is always phosphorylated by protein kinase C (PKC) in the basal state in endothelial cells, phosphorylation that can be increased by shear stress[66] and bradykinin. Ser116 can be dephosphorylated by the protein phosphatase calcineurin, under the effect of an agonist such as VEGF.[67] This dephosphorylation process is associated with an increase in enzymatic activity and an increase in the stimulated but not basal NO production.[62]

Interestingly, it was recently shown that the phosphorylation of some serine residues of eNOS might occur by a cooperative mechanism. Indeed, the phosphorylation of Ser1179 is increased in the cells expressing the loss of function mutants eNOS-S116A and eNOS-S617A while the dephosphorylation of Ser116 is increased and the phosphorylation of Ser635 is decreased in cells expressing eNOS-S617A.[62]

Threonine phosphorylation

Thr497 is, together with Ser1179, the second most important site of regulation of eNOS by phosphorylation. It is constitutively phosphorylated in endothelial cells by PKC, but can be dephosphorylated by protein phosphatase-1, in response to several calcium mobilizing stimuli such as bradykinin and histamine.[56] The increase in enzymatic activity observed with the non-phosphorylatable mutant eNOS-T497A establishes this site as a negative regulator of the enzyme.[68] This can be explained by its localization within the CaM binding site where, if phosphorylated, it causes a reduction in the affinity of eNOS for CaM.[56] Recently it was proposed that this site could act as an intrinsic switch that determines the generation of NO versus superoxide.[68]

Tyrosine phosphorylation

Treatment of endothelial cells with the tyrosine phosphatase inhibitor sodium orthovanadate increases eNOS phosphorylation on its tyrosine residues.[15] Moreover, endothelial NO production can be modulated by the use of tyrosine kinase and phosphatase inhibitors.[69,70] The study of eNOS tyrosine phosphorylation has been hampered by the fact that cultured cells rapidly lose the mechanisms that control this phenomenon. Consequently, very little is known on the tyrosine residues that can potentially be phosphorylated, or the kinases implicated in this process. However, it has been suggested that the phosphorylation of the tyrosine residues does not directly modify eNOS enzyme activity but rather modulates its interaction with regulatory proteins such as caveolin-1.[15]

CONCLUSION

The multitude of regulatory events involved in NO production indicates that eNOS is not merely a Ca^{2+}/calmodulin responsive enzyme, and the wide array of interacting proteins and regulatory phosphorylation sites indicates that NO production from endothelial cells needs to be tightly controlled. The cellular availability of interacting proteins and kinases for eNOS in certain intracellular compartments as well as the alteration of these regulators in pathological conditions influences endothelial cell-derived NO. Further characterization of these regulators, and the identification of novel players involved in the regulation of eNOS, can only increase our understanding of mechanisms controlling NO bioavailability, which ultimately influences endothelial cell function.

ACKNOWLEDGMENTS

MGB holds a studentship from the Canadian Institutes of Health Research (CIHR). JPG is a recipient of a Tier II Canada Research Chair. Work performed in JPGs laboratory is supported by grants from the CIHR and the Terry Fox Foundation through the National Cancer Institute of Canada.

REFERENCES

1. Sessa WC, Harrison JK, Barber CM et al. Molecular cloning and expression of a cDNA encoding endothelial cell nitric oxide synthase. J Biol Chem 1992; 267: 15274–6.
2. Janssens SP, Shimouchi A, Quertermous T et al. Cloning and expression of a cDNA encoding human endothelium-derived relaxing factor/nitric oxide synthase. J Biol Chem 1992; 267: 14519–22.
3. Marsden PA, Schappert KT, Chen HS et al. Molecular cloning and characterization of human endothelial nitric oxide synthase. FEBS Lett 1992; 307: 287–93.
4. Nishida K, Harrison DG, Navas JP et al. Molecular cloning and characterization of the constitutive bovine aortic endothelial cell nitric oxide synthase. J Clin Invest 1992; 90: 2092–6.
5. Liu J, Sessa WC. Identification of covalently bound amino-terminal myristic acid in endothelial nitric oxide synthase. J Biol Chem 1994; 269: 11691–4.
6. Liu J, Garcia-Cardena G, Sessa WC. Biosynthesis and palmitoylation of endothelial nitric oxide synthase: mutagenesis of palmitoylation sites, cysteines-15 and/or -26, argues against depalmitoylation-induced translocation of the enzyme. Biochemistry 1995; 34: 12333–40.
7. Shaul PW, Smart EJ, Robinson LJ et al. Acylation targets endothelial nitric-oxide synthase to plasmalemmal caveolae. J Biol Chem 1996; 271: 6518–22.
8. Garcia-Cardena G, Oh P, Liu J et al. Targeting of nitric oxide synthase to endothelial cell caveolae via palmitoylation: implications for nitric oxide signaling. Proc Natl Acad Sci U S A 1996; 93: 6448–53.
9. Smart EJ, Graf GA, McNiven MA et al. Caveolins, liquid-ordered domains, and signal transduction. Mol Cell Biol 1999; 19: 7289–304.
10. Li S, Couet J, Lisanti MP. Src tyrosine kinases, Galpha subunits, and H-Ras share a common membrane-anchored scaffolding protein, caveolin. Caveolin binding negatively regulates the auto-activation of Src tyrosine kinases. J Biol Chem 1996; 271: 29182–90.
11. Liu J, Garcia-Cardena G, Sessa WC. Palmitoylation of endothelial nitric oxide synthase is necessary for optimal stimulated release of nitric oxide: implications for caveolae localization. Biochemistry 1996; 35: 13277–81.
12. Govers R, Oess S. To NO or not to NO: 'where?' is the question. Histol Histopathol 2004; 19: 585–605.
13. Fulton D, Babbitt R, Zoellner S et al. Targeting of endothelial nitric-oxide synthase to the cytoplasmic face of the Golgi complex or plasma membrane regulates Akt- versus calcium-dependent mechanisms for nitric oxide release. J Biol Chem 2004; 279: 30349–57.
14. Feron O, Belhassen L, Kobzik L et al. Endothelial nitric oxide synthase targeting to caveolae. Specific interactions with caveolin isoforms in cardiac myocytes and endothelial cells. J Biol Chem 1996; 271: 22810–14.
15. Garcia-Cardena G, Fan R, Stern DF et al. Endothelial nitric oxide synthase is regulated by tyrosine phosphorylation and interacts with caveolin-1. J Biol Chem 1996; 271: 27237–40.
16. Ju H, Zou R, Venema VJ et al. Direct interaction of endothelial nitric-oxide synthase and caveolin-1 inhibits synthase activity. J Biol Chem 1997; 272: 18522–5.

17. Garcia-Cardena G, Martasek P, Masters BS et al. Dissecting the interaction between nitric oxide synthase (NOS) and caveolin. Functional significance of the nos caveolin binding domain in vivo. J Biol Chem 1997; 272: 25437–40.
18. Michel JB, Feron O, Sase K et al. Caveolin versus calmodulin. Counterbalancing allosteric modulators of endothelial nitric oxide synthase. J Biol Chem 1997; 272: 25907–12.
19. Gratton JP, Fontana J, O'Connor DS et al. Reconstitution of an endothelial nitric-oxide synthase (eNOS), hsp90, and caveolin-1 complex in vitro. Evidence that hsp90 facilitates calmodulin stimulated displacement of eNOS from caveolin-1. J Biol Chem 2000; 275: 22268–72.
20. Couet J, Li S, Okamoto T et al. Identification of peptide and protein ligands for the caveolin-scaffolding domain. Implications for the interaction of caveolin with caveolae-associated proteins. J Biol Chem 1997; 272: 6525–33.
21. Michel JB, Feron O, Sacks D et al. Reciprocal regulation of endothelial nitric-oxide synthase by Ca2+-calmodulin and caveolin. J Biol Chem 1997; 272: 15583–6.
22. Feron O, Dessy C, Opel DJ et al. Modulation of the endothelial nitric-oxide synthase-caveolin interaction in cardiac myocytes. Implications for the autonomic regulation of heart rate. J Biol Chem 1998; 273: 30249–54.
23. Bucci M, Gratton JP, Rudic RD et al. In vivo delivery of the caveolin-1 scaffolding domain inhibits nitric oxide synthesis and reduces inflammation. Nat Med 2000; 6: 1362–7.
24. Gratton JP, Lin MI, Yu J et al. Selective inhibition of tumor microvascular permeability by cavtratin blocks tumor progression in mice. Cancer Cell 2003; 4: 31–9.
25. Drab M, Verkade P, Elger M et al. Loss of caveolae, vascular dysfunction, and pulmonary defects in caveolin-1 gene-disrupted mice. Science 2001; 293: 2449–52.
26. Razani B, Engelman JA, Wang XB et al. Caveolin-1 null mice are viable but show evidence of hyperproliferative and vascular abnormalities. J Biol Chem 2001; 276: 38121–38.
27. Ju H, Venema VJ, Marrero MB et al. Inhibitory interactions of the bradykinin B2 receptor with endothelial nitric-oxide synthase. J Biol Chem 1998; 273: 24025–9.
28. Golser R, Gorren AC, Leber A et al. Interaction of endothelial and neuronal nitric-oxide synthases with the bradykinin B2 receptor. Binding of an inhibitory peptide to the oxygenase domain blocks uncoupled NADPH oxidation. J Biol Chem 2000; 275: 5291–6.
29. Zimmermann K, Opitz N, Dedio J et al. NOSTRIN: a protein modulating nitric oxide release and subcellular distribution of endothelial nitric oxide synthase. Proc Natl Acad Sci U S A 2002; 99: 17167–72.
30. Dedio J, Konig P, Wohlfart P et al. NOSIP, a novel modulator of endothelial nitric oxide synthase activity. FASEB 2001; 15: 79–89.
31. Zharikov SI, Sigova AA, Chen S et al. Cytoskeletal regulation of the L-arginine/NO pathway in pulmonary artery endothelial cells. Am J Physiol Lung Cell Mol Physiol 2001; 280: L465–L473.
32. Su Y, Edwards-Bennett S, Bubb MR et al. Regulation of endothelial nitric oxide synthase by the actin cytoskeleton. Am J Physiol Cell Physiol 2003; 284: C1542–C1549.
33. Forstermann U, Pollock JS, Schmidt HH et al. Calmodulin-dependent endothelium-derived relaxing factor/nitric oxide synthase activity is present in the particulate and cytosolic fractions of bovine aortic endothelial cells. Proc Natl Acad Sci U S A 1991; 88: 1788–92.
34. Roman LJ, Martasek P, Miller RT et al. The C termini of constitutive nitric-oxide synthases control electron flow through the flavin and heme domains and affect modulation by calmodulin. J Biol Chem 2000; 275: 29225–32.
35. Fleming I, Bauersachs J, Schafer A et al. Isometric contraction induces the Ca2+-independent activation of the endothelial nitric oxide synthase. Proc Natl Acad Sci U S A 1999; 96: 1123–8.
36. Russell KS, Haynes MP, Caulin-Glaser T et al. Estrogen stimulates heat shock protein 90 binding to endothelial nitric oxide synthase in human vascular endothelial cells. Effects on calcium sensitivity and NO release. J Biol Chem 2000; 275: 5026–30.
37. Caplan AJ. Hsp90's secrets unfold: new insights from structural and functional studies. Trends Cell Biol 1999; 9: 262–8.
38. Garcia-Cardena G, Fan R, Shah V et al. Dynamic activation of endothelial nitric oxide synthase by Hsp90. Nature 1998; 392: 821–4.
39. Takahashi S, Mendelsohn ME. Calmodulin-dependent and -independent activation of endothelial nitric-oxide synthase by heat shock protein 90. J Biol Chem 2003; 278: 9339–44.
40. Song Y, Zweier JL, Xia Y. Determination of the enhancing action of HSP90 on neuronal nitric oxide synthase by EPR spectroscopy. Am J Physiol Cell Physiol 2001; 281: C1819–C1824.
41. Fontana J, Fulton D, Chen Y et al. Domain mapping studies reveal that the M domain of hsp90 serves as a molecular scaffold to regulate Akt-dependent phosphorylation of endothelial nitric oxide synthase and NO release. Circ Res 2002; 90: 866–73.
42. Venema RC, Venema VJ, Ju H et al. Novel complexes of guanylate cyclase with heat shock protein 90 and nitric oxide synthase. Am J Physiol Heart Circ Physiol 2003; 285: H669–H678.
43. Pratt WB. The hsp90-based chaperone system: involvement in signal transduction from a variety of hormone and growth factor receptors. Proc Soc Exp Biol Med 1998; 217: 420–34.
44. Khurana VG, Feterik K, Springett MJ et al. Functional interdependence and colocalization of endothelial nitric oxide synthase and heat shock protein 90 in cerebral arteries. J Cereb Blood Flow Metab 2000; 20: 1563–70.
45. Viswanathan M, Rivera O, Short BL. Heat shock protein 90 is involved in pulsatile flow-induced dilation of rat middle cerebral artery. J Vasc Res 1999; 36: 524–7.
46. Song BD, Schmid SL. A molecular motor or a regulator? Dynamin's in a class of its own. Biochemistry 2003; 42: 1369–76.
47. Minshall RD, Sessa WC, Stan RV et al. Caveolin regulation of endothelial function. Am J Physiol Lung Cell Mol Physiol 2003; 285: L1179–L1183.
48. Cao S, Yao J, McCabe TJ et al. Direct interaction between endothelial nitric-oxide synthase and dynamin-2. Implications for nitric-oxide synthase function. J Biol Chem 2001; 276: 14249–56.
49. Cao S, Yao J, Shah V. The proline-rich domain of dynamin-2 is responsible for dynamin-dependent in vitro potentiation of endothelial nitric-oxide synthase activity via selective effects on reductase domain function. J Biol Chem 2003; 278: 5894–901.
50. Chatterjee S, Cao S, Peterson TE et al. Inhibition of GTP-dependent vesicle trafficking impairs internalization of plasmalemmal eNOS and cellular nitric oxide production. J Cell Sci 2003; 116: 3645–55.
51. Sun J, Liao JK. Functional interaction of endothelial nitric oxide synthase with a voltage-dependent anion channel. Proc Natl Acad Sci U S A 2002; 99: 13108–13.
52. Dimmeler S, Fleming I, Fisslthaler B et al. Activation of nitric oxide synthase in endothelial cells by Akt-dependent phosphorylation. Nature 1999; 399: 601–5.
53. Lantin-Hermoso RL, Rosenfeld CR, Yuhanna IS et al. Estrogen acutely stimulates nitric oxide synthase activity in fetal pulmonary artery endothelium. Am J Physiol 1997; 273: L119–L126.
54. Fulton D, Gratton JP, McCabe TJ et al. Regulation of endothelium-derived nitric oxide production by the protein kinase Akt. Nature 1999; 399: 597–601.

55. Kim F, Gallis B, Corson MA. TNF-alpha inhibits flow and insulin signaling leading to NO production in aortic endothelial cells. Am J Physiol Cell Physiol 2001; 280: C1057–C1065.
56. Fleming I, Fisslthaler B, Dimmeler S et al. Phosphorylation of Thr(495) regulates Ca(2+)/calmodulin-dependent endothelial nitric oxide synthase activity. Circ Res 2001; 88: E68–E75.
57. Igarashi J, Bernier SG, Michel T. Sphingosine 1-phosphate and activation of endothelial nitric-oxide synthase. differential regulation of Akt and MAP kinase pathways by EDG and bradykinin receptors in vascular endothelial cells. J Biol Chem 2001; 276: 12420–6.
58. Morales-Ruiz M, Lee MJ, Zollner S et al. Sphingosine 1-phosphate activates Akt, nitric oxide production, and chemotaxis through a Gi protein/phosphoinositide 3-kinase pathway in endothelial cells. J Biol Chem 2001; 276: 19672–7.
59. Thors B, Halldorsson H, Thorgeirsson G. Thrombin and histamine stimulate endothelial nitric-oxide synthase phosphorylation at Ser1177 via an AMPK mediated pathway independent of PI3K-Akt. FEBS Lett 2004; 573: 175–80.
60. Chen ZP, Mitchelhill KI, Michell BJ et al. AMP-activated protein kinase phosphorylation of endothelial NO synthase. FEBS Lett 1999; 443: 285–9.
61. Butt E, Bernhardt M, Smolenski A et al. Endothelial nitric-oxide synthase (type III) is activated and becomes calcium independent upon phosphorylation by cyclic nucleotide-dependent protein kinases. J Biol Chem 2000; 275: 5179–87.
62. Bauer PM, Fulton D, Boo YC et al. Compensatory phosphorylation and protein-protein interactions revealed by loss of function and gain of function mutants of multiple serine phosphorylation sites in endothelial nitric-oxide synthase. J Biol Chem 2003; 278: 14841–9.
63. Lane P, Gross SS. Disabling a C-terminal autoinhibitory control element in endothelial nitric-oxide synthase by phosphorylation provides a molecular explanation for activation of vascular NO synthesis by diverse physiological stimuli. J Biol Chem 2002; 277: 19087–94.
64. Michell BJ, Harris MB, Chen ZP et al. Identification of regulatory sites of phosphorylation of the bovine endothelial nitric-oxide synthase at serine 617 and serine 635. J Biol Chem 2002; 277: 42344–51.
65. Harris MB, Blackstone MA, Sood SG et al. Acute activation and phosphorylation of endothelial nitric oxide synthase by HMG-CoA reductase inhibitors. Am J Physiol Heart Circ Physiol 2004; 287: H560–H566.
66. Gallis B, Corthals GL, Goodlett DR et al. Identification of flow-dependent endothelial nitric-oxide synthase phosphorylation sites by mass spectrometry and regulation of phosphorylation and nitric oxide production by the phosphatidylinositol 3-kinase inhibitor LY294002. J Biol Chem 1999; 274: 30101–8.
67. Kou R, Greif D, Michel T. Dephosphorylation of endothelial nitric-oxide synthase by vascular endothelial growth factor. Implications for the vascular responses to cyclosporin A. J Biol Chem 2002; 277: 29669–73.
68. Lin MI, Fulton D, Babbitt R et al. Phosphorylation of threonine 497 in endothelial nitric-oxide synthase coordinates the coupling of L-arginine metabolism to efficient nitric oxide production. J Biol Chem 2003; 278: 44719–26.
69. Fleming I, Bara AT, Busse R. Calcium signalling and autacoid production in endothelial cells are modulated by changes in tyrosine kinase and phosphatase activity. J Vasc Res 1996; 33: 225–34.
70. Fleming I, Bauersachs J, Fisslthaler B et al. Ca^{2+}-independent activation of the endothelial nitric oxide synthase in response to tyrosine phosphatase inhibitors and fluid shear stress. Circ Res 1998; 82: 686–695.

30

Molecular mechanisms of myocardial remodeling in hypertensive heart disease

Javier Díez

INTRODUCTION

It is now accepted that besides left ventricular hypertrophy (LVH) that characterizes hypertensive heart disease (HHD), changes in the composition of myocardial tissue (i.e. remodeling) develop in the hypertensive heart.[1] Whereas LVH provides the adaptive response of the cardiomyocyte compartment to pressure overload in an attempt to normalize systolic wall stress, myocardial remodeling is mostly the consequence of a number of neurohormonally and cytokine-mediated pathological processes occurring both in the cardiomyocyte and the noncardiomyocyte compartments of the hypertensive heart. Some of these processes are related to the exaggerated loss of cardiomyocytes due to apoptosis and the excessive accumulation of collagen type I and III fibers in the myocardium. This chapter deals with the potential molecular mechanisms involved in both the origin and the consequences of apoptosis and fibrosis in HHD.

APOPTOSIS

Cardiomyocyte apoptosis, as assessed by the TUNEL assay, has been shown to be abnormally stimulated in patients with HHD, no angiographic evidence of coronary artery disease, and normal cardiac function.[2,3] This finding has been confirmed by Koda et al.[4] using a more specific assay (*Taq* assay) to detect apoptotic cell death. In addition, recent findings from our laboratory indicate that cardiomyocyte apoptosis is stimulated in patients with HHD and heart failure.[5] In fact, we found increased TUNEL-positive cardiomyocytes and enhanced active caspase-3 expression in hypertensive failing hearts compared with hypertensive hypertrophied hearts and normotensive hearts.

Origin

Cardiomyocyte apoptosis has been proposed to occur as a result of an imbalance between the factors that induce or suppress apoptosis.[6] Thus, arterial hypertension may represent a condition in which inducers of cardiomyocyte apoptosis predominate over suppressors of cardiomyocyte apoptosis (Figure 30.1).[7]

The pro-apoptotic component

It is now recognized that besides the mechanical factor secondary to hemodynamic overload, a number of systemic and local humoral factors may induce cardiomyocyte apoptosis in HHD. Mechanical overload secondary to aortic banding has been shown to induce cardiomyocyte apoptosis in the rat.[8] Overstretching of isolated papillary muscles in vitro, which mimics an elevation of diastolic stress in vivo, resulted in an increase in cardiomyocyte apoptosis.[9,10] Interestingly, augmented superoxide formation and expression of Fas receptor were observed in this condition. The addition of the nitric oxide (NO)-releasing drug, C87–3754, prevented apoptosis and superoxide anion formation.[9] Therefore, the induction of superoxide seems to be a relevant factor in overstretching-induced cardiomyocyte apoptosis. On the other hand, mechanical stretch causes release of humoral factors from cardiomyocytes that may induce apoptosis in these cells.[11]

Several in vivo observations suggest that effector hormones of the renin-angiotensin-aldosterone system (RAAS) may be involved in cardiomyocyte apoptosis in HHD. First, cardiomyocyte apoptosis increases in angiotensin (Ang) II-infused hypertensive Sprague-Dawley rats and blockade of the Ang II type 1 (AT_1) receptor with losartan prevents this effect despite the persistence of increased blood pressure.[12] Second,

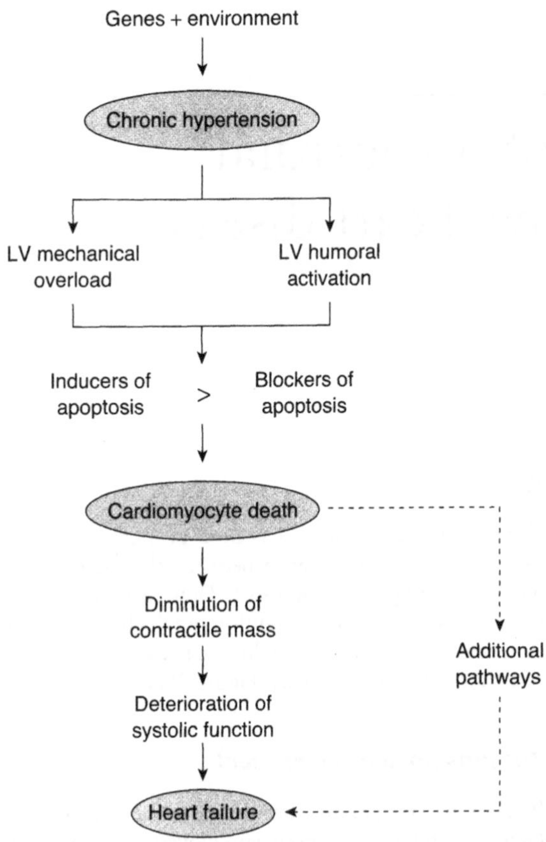

Figure 30.1 Diagram illustrating the cascade of events involved in the origin and consequences of cardiomyocyte apoptosis in hypertensive heart disease. LV, left ventricle; > indicates that the expression and/or activity of inducers of apoptosis predominates over the expression and/or activity of blockers of apoptosis

an association has been found between enhanced cardiomyocyte apoptosis and exaggerated angiotensin converting enzyme (ACE) activity in the hypertrophied left ventricle of spontaneously hypertensive rats (SHR).[13] Third, chronic treatment with losartan at doses that do not normalize blood pressure is associated with reduction of cardiomyocyte apoptosis in both SHR[14] and patients with HHD.[2] Finally, De Angelis et al.[15] have reported that infusion of aldosterone induces ventricular cardiomyocyte apoptosis in the rat.

In vitro studies have shown that Ang II binding to AT_1 receptors triggers apoptosis by a mechanism involving stimulation of p38 MAP kinase activity, activation of p53 protein and subsequent decrease of the Bcl-2 to Bax protein ratio, activation of caspase-3, stimulation of calcium-dependent DNase I, and internucleosomal DNA fragmentation.[16–20] Although Ang II has been shown to induce apoptosis in other cardiovascular cells through stimulation of the AT_2 receptor,[21] recent findings suggest that it is unlikely that this receptor is a strong signal to induce cardiomyocyte apoptosis in vivo. In fact, apoptosis is not increased in the heart of transgenic mice overexpressing AT_2 receptors in the myocardium.[22] In addition, Diep et al. have reported that blockade of AT_1 receptors with losartan is accompanied by normalization of cardiac apoptosis in rats with Ang II-induced hypertension that exhibit increased expression of AT_2 receptors in the heart.[12] Interestingly, cardiomyocyte apoptosis induced by infusion of Ang II is reduced by 50% in hearts of rats pretreated with spironolactone,[15] suggesting that the pro-apoptotic effect of the peptide could be due, at least in part, to aldosterone.

The anti-apoptotic component

Biomechanical stress of the heart that occurs in conditions of pressure overload can also induce survival pathways in the cardiomyocyte.[23,24] The transmembrane signal transducer gp130 molecule has been proposed to exert a survival effect in cardiomyocytes, mediating apoptosis-suppressor signals triggered by members of the interleukin-6 (IL-6) cytokine family, including cardiotrophin-1 (CT-1) and leukemia inhibitory factor (LIF).[25] In support of this, it has been shown that left ventricular gp130 knockout mice develop a rapid dilated cardiomyopathy with massive cardiomyocyte apoptosis in response to mechanical overload.[26] Interestingly, an association of diminished expression of gp130 and LIF proteins with increased cardiomyocyte apoptosis has been found in the heart of SHR.[27] It thus can be hypothesized that inhibition of the gp130 signaling pathway in arterial hypertension decreases the survival capability of cardiomyocytes and makes them more susceptible to apoptotic factors. In accordance with this possibility are findings from our laboratory showing that compared with cardiomyocytes isolated from normotensive Wistar-Kyoto (WKY) rats, cardiomyocytes isolated from SHR exhibit increased susceptibility to the apoptotic effects of angiotensin II.[27]

Consequences

It has been hypothesized that cardiomyocyte apoptosis is one of the mechanisms involved in the loss of contractile mass that facilitates the transition to heart failure in HHD (Figure 30.1).[28,29] In support of this possibility are recent findings from our group showing that increased cardiomyocyte apoptosis is associated with diminished cardiomyocyte density and reduced ejection fraction in patients with HHD and heart failure.[5] In addition, impaired contractile function may reflect not only a decrease in the number of viable, fully functional cardiomyocytes, but also a decline in the function of viable cardiomyocytes, or a combination of these mechanisms. It has been reported recently that caspase-3 cleaves cardiomyocyte myofibrillar proteins, resulting in depression of cardiomyocyte contractile function.[30] In addition, Laugwitz et al.[31] have demonstrated that blockade of caspase-3 activation improves contractility in the failing myocardium. This possibility is of interest, taking into account that overexpression of the active form of caspase-3 has been reported in the myocardium of patients with HHD.[5]

FIBROSIS

The available evidence indicates that myocardial fibrosis due to an exaggerated accumulation of fibrillar collagen types I and III within the myocardial interstitium and surrounding intramural coronary arteries and arterioles is one of the key pathologic features of myocardial remodeling in human HHD. In fact, a number of studies performed in post mortem human hearts[32–34] and endomyocardial human biopsies[35–38] have shown that myocardial collagen volume fraction, a morphometric measure of the amount of tissue collagen, is constantly increased in patients with HHD compared with normotensive controls.

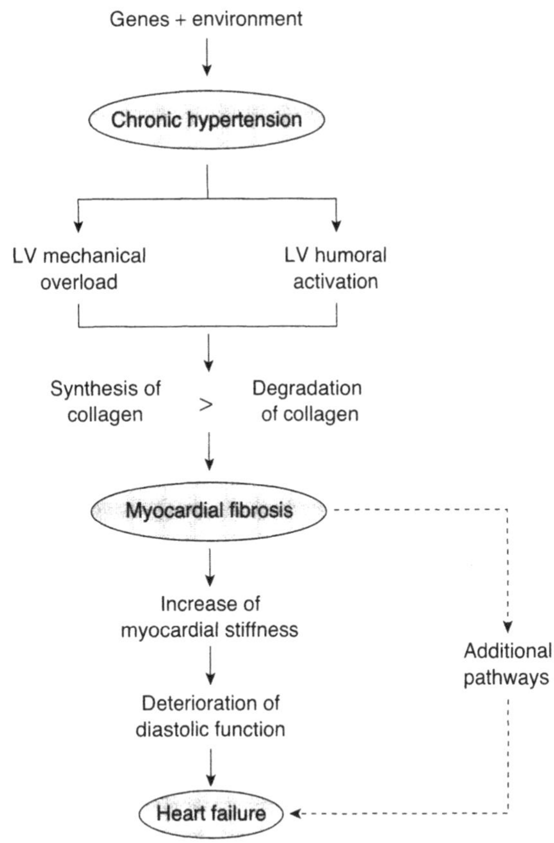

Figure 30.2 Diagram illustrating the cascade of events involved in the origin and consequences of myocardial fibrosis in hypertensive heart disease. LV, left ventricle; > indicates that the synthesis of collagen predominates over its degradation

Origin

It has been proposed that the excess of myocardial collagen seen in HHD is mainly due to the uncoupling between increased synthesis and unchanged or decreased degradation of collagen-type fibers by matrix metalloproteinases (MMPs) (Figure 30.2).[39] Hemodynamic loading and a number of humoral factors may be involved in such an uncoupling.[39]

The hemodynamic component

As shown by in vivo experiments, pressure overload of the left ventricle is associated with increased collagen synthesis and reduced MMP-1 or collagenase activity.[40,41] In addition, in vitro studies have shown that collagen type I synthesis is stimulated and collagenase expression inhibited in cardiac fibroblasts submitted to mechanical load.[40,41] Thus, hemodynamic overload of the left ventricle due to hypertension may contribute to myocardial fibrosis. Several clinical observations support this possibility. Tanaka et al.[32] reported that collagen volume fraction increased from the outer to the inner third of the left ventricular free wall, probably reflecting transmural gradients of wall stress. Rossi[34] found that the extent and severity of myocardial fibrosis paralleled the enlargement of cardiomyocytes. Finally, Querejeta et al.[38] reported that collagen volume fraction correlated with systolic blood pressure and pulse pressure in the myocardium of patients with HHD.

The nonhemodynamic component

Two types of findings suggest that nonhemodynamic factors may also contribute to myocardial fibrosis in human hypertension. First, myocardial fibrosis has been found not only in the left ventricle but also in the right ventricle,[33,42] the interventricular septum,[43] and the left atria[44] of patients with HHD. Second, it has been shown that the ability of antihypertensive treatment to regress fibrosis in hypertensives is independent of its antihypertensive efficacy.[37,45] Thus, fibrosis may be the consequence of the loss of reciprocal regulation that normally exists between profibrotic and antifibrotic humoral factors.[39] Again the RAAS appears to be involved in the development of hypertensive fibrosis.

Pharmacological interventions with ACE inhibitors[36,37] and AT_1 receptor antagonists[45,46] have underscored the importance of circulating or locally produced Ang II in the development of myocardial fibrosis in patients with HHD. This is supported by a number of experimental findings indicating that Ang II exerts multiple profibrotic effects within the heart including induction of fibroblast hyperplasia, activation of collagen biosynthetic pathways and inhibition of collagen degradative pathways.[47] Furthermore, recent data suggest that crosstalk between some factors produced by cardiomyocytes (i.e. osteopontin), macrophages (i.e. plasminogen activator inhibitor-1), and fibroblasts (i.e. transforming growth factor-β_1, connective tissue growth factor) mediates the profibrotic effects of Ang II.[48] Additionally, fibrosis may represent the reparative response to inflammation and oxidative stress induced by Ang II through the interaction with AT_1 receptors located in cells from the cardiac microvasculature.[49,50]

Aldosterone has been shown to stimulate collagen synthesis through the mineralocorticoid receptor in cultured cardiac fibroblasts.[51] In in vivo studies on rats with renovascular hypertension, hyperaldosteronism, or spontaneous hypertension, the aldosterone antagonist spironolactone was able to prevent or reverse the development of myocardial fibrosis even though the drug did not normalize blood pressure.[52–55] Thus, aldosterone may promote myocardial fibrosis, probably through a direct action on cardiac cells mediated by the mineralocorticoid receptor. In addition, increasing evidence suggests that aldosterone may mediate and exacerbate the proinflammatory and profibrotic effects of Ang II on the heart.[56]

Consequences

A linkage between fibrosis and left ventricular dysfunction/failure may be established (Figure 30.2). Initially, fibrosis of the myocardial interstitium compromises the rate of relaxation, diastolic suction and passive stiffness, contributing to impaired diastolic function.[57] In accordance with this, we have shown recently that an association exists between myocardial collagen content and left ventricular chamber stiffness in patients with HHD.[46] A continued accumulation of fibrous tissue further impairs diastolic filling and now compromises transduction of cardiomyocyte contraction into myocardial force development, thus impairing systolic performance.[58] In support of this possibility is the finding that an association exists between severe myocardial fibrosis and deterioration of the ejection fraction in patients with HHD.[59,60]

CONCLUSIONS

Changes in the composition of myocardial tissue develop in HHD leading to structural remodeling of the myocardium. Myocardial remodeling may contribute to the increased risk of developing heart failure in patients with HHD. Remodeling is the result of a number of mechanical, neurohormonal and cytokine-mediated processes occurring both in the cardiomyocyte and the noncardiomyocyte compartments of the heart. Evidence reviewed in this chapter suggests that these processes lead to cardiomyocyte apoptosis and interstitial and perivascular fibrosis in the hypertensive heart. Furthermore, a growing body of data suggests a critical role for Ang II and aldosterone in the mediation of apoptosis and fibrosis. This may provide an explanation for the cardioprotective effects demonstrated in hypertensive patients by pharmacological agents interfering with the RAAS.

REFERENCES

1. Swynghedauw B. Molecular mechanisms of myocardial remodeling. Physiol Rev 1999; 79: 215–62.
2. González A, López B, Ravassa S et al. Stimulation of cardiac apoptosis in essential hypertension: potential role of angiotensin II. Hypertension 2002; 39: 75–80.
3. Yamamoto S, Sawada K, Shimomura H et al. On the nature of cell death during remodeling of hypertrophied human myocardium. J Mol Cell Cardiol 2000; 32: 161–75.
4. Koda M, Takemura G, Kanoh M et al. Myocytes positive for in situ markers for DNA breaks in human hearts which are hypertrophic, but neither failed nor dilated: a manifestation of cardiac hypertrophy rather than failure. J Pathol 2003; 199: 229–36.
5. González A, Fortuño MA, Querejeta R et al. Cardiomyocyte apoptosis in hypertensive cardiomyopathy. Cardiovasc Res 2003; 59: 549–62.
6. Anversa P, Olivetti G, Leri A et al. Myocyte death and ventricular remodeling. Curr Opin Nephrol Hypertens 1997; 6: 169–76.
7. Fortuño MA, Ravassa S, Fortuño A et al. Cardiomyocyte apoptotic cell death in arterial hypertension. Mechanisms and potential management. Hypertension 2001; 38: 1406–12.

8. Teiger E, Than VD, Richard L et al. Apoptosis in pressure overload-induced heart hypertrophy in the rat. J Clin Invest 1996; 97: 2891–7.
9. Cheng W, Li B, Kajstura J, Li P et al. Stretch-induced programmed myocyte cell death. J Clin Invest 1995; 96: 2247–59.
10. Leri A, Claudio PP, Li Q et al. Stretch-mediated release of angiotensin II induces myocyte apoptosis by activating p53 that enhances the local renin-angiotensin system and decreases the Bcl-2-to-Bax protein ratio in the cell. J Clin Invest 1998; 101: 1326–42.
11. Sadoshima J, Izumo S. The cellular and molecular response of cardiac myocytes to mechanical stress. Annu Rev Physiol 1997; 59: 551–71.
12. Diep QN, El Mabrouk M, Yue P et al. Effect of AT(1) receptor blockade on cardiac apoptosis in angiotensin II-induced hypertension. Am J Physiol 2002; 282: H1635–H1641.
13. Díez J, Panizo A, Hernández M et al. Cardiomyocyte apoptosis and cardiac angiotensin-converting enzyme in spontaneously hypertensive rats. Hypertension 1997; 30: 1029–34.
14. Olivetti G, Melissari M, Balbi T et al. Myocyte nuclear and possible cellular hyperplasia contribute to ventricular remodeling in the hypertrophic senescent heart in humans. J Am Coll Cardiol 1994; 24: 140–9.
15. De Angelis N, Fiordaliso F, Latini R et al. Appraisal of the role of angiotensin II and aldosterone in ventricular myocyte apoptosis in adult normotensive rat. J Mol Cell Cardiol 2002; 34: 1655–65.
16. Cheng W, Li B, Kajstura J et al. Stretch-induced programmed myocyte cell death. J Clin Invest 1995; 96: 2247–59.
17. Sharov VG, Todor A, Suzuki G et al. Hypoxia, angiotensin-II, and norepinephrine mediated apoptosis is stimulus specific in canine failed cardiomyocytes: a role for p38 MAPK, Fas-L and cyclin D(1). Eur J Heart Fail 2003; 5: 121–9.
18. Cigola E, Kajstura J, Li B, Meggs LG et al. Angiotensin II activates programmed myocyte cell death in vitro. Exp Cell Res 1997; 231: 363–71.
19. Kajstura J, Cheng W, Sarangarajan R et al. Necrotic and apoptotic myocyte cell death in the aging heart of Fischer 344 rats. Am J Physiol Heart Circ Physiol 1996; 271: H1215–H1228.
20. Ravassa S, Fortuño MA, González A et al. Mechanisms of increased susceptibility to angiotensin II-induced apoptosis in ventricular cardiomyocytes of spontaneously hypertensive rats. Hypertension 2000; 36: 1065–71.
21. Matsubara H. Pathophysiological role of angiotensin II type 2 receptor in cardiovascular and renal diseases. Circ Res 1998; 83: 1182–91.
22. Sugino H, Ozono R, Kurisu S et al. Apoptosis is not increased in myocardium overexpressing type 2 angiotensin II receptor in transgenic mice. Hypertension 2001; 37: 1394–8.
23. Chien K. Stress pathways in heart failure. Cell 1999; 98: 555–8.
24. Hunter J, Chien KR. Signaling pathways for cardiac hypertrophy and failure. N Engl J Med 1999; 341: 1276–83.
25. López N, Diez J, Fortuño MA. Characterization of the protective effects of cardiotrophin-1 against non-ischemic death stimuli in adult cardiomyocytes. Cytokine 2005; 30: 283–92.
26. Sam F, Samyer DB, Chang DL et al. Progressive left ventricular remodeling and apoptosis late after myocardial infarction in mouse heart. Am J Physiol 2000; 279: H422–H428.
27. Ravassa S, Ardanáz N, López B et al. Involvement of cardiotrophin-1 signaling pathway in cardiac apoptosis of spontaneously hypertensive rats. J Hypertens 2002; 20 (Suppl 4): S30.
28. Bing OHL. Hypothesis. Apoptosis may be a mechanism for the transition to heart failure with chronic pressure overload. J Mol Cell Cardiol 1994; 26: 943–8.
29. Fortuño MA, González A, Ravassa S et al. Clinical implications of apoptosis in hypertensive heart disease. Am J Physiol Heart Circ Physiol 2003; 284: H1495–H1506.
30. Communal C, Sumandea M, de Tombe P et al. Functional consequences of caspase activation in cardiac myocytes. Proc Natl Acad Sci U S A 2002; 99: 6252–6.
31. Laugwitz KL, Moretti A, Weig HJ et al. Blocking caspase-activated apoptosis improves contractility in failing myocardium. Hum Gene Ther 2001; 12: 2051–63.
32. Tanaka M, Fujiwara H, Onodera T et al. Quantitative analysis of myocardial fibrosis in normals, hypertensive hearts, and hypertrophic cardiomyopathy. Br Heart J 1986; 55: 575–81.
33. Olivetti G, Melissari M, Balbi T et al. Myocyte cellular hypertrophy is responsible for ventricular remodelling in the hypertrophied heart of middle aged individuals in the absence of cardiac failure. Cardiovasc Res 1994; 28: 1199–208.
34. Rossi MA. Pathologic fibrosis and connective tissue matrix in left ventricular hypertrophy due to chronic arterial hypertension in humans. J Hypertens 1998; 16: 1031–41.
35. Ciulla M, Paliotti R, Hess DB et al. Echocardiographic patterns of myocardial fibrosis in hypertensive patients: Endomyocardial biopsy versus ultrasonic tissue characterization. J Am Soc Echocardiogr 1997; 10: 657–64.
36. Schwartzkopff B, Brehm M, Mundehenke M, Strauer BE. Repair of coronary arterioles after treatment with perindopril in hypertensive heart disease. Hypertension 2000; 36: 220–5.
37. Brilla CG, Funck RC, Rupp RH. Lisinopril-mediated regression of myocardial fibrosis in patients with hypertensive heart disease. Circulation 2000; 102: 1388–93.
38. Querejeta R, Varo N, López B et al. Serum carboxy-terminal propeptide of procollagen type I is a marker of myocardial fibrosis in hypertensive heart disease. Circulation 2000; 101: 1729–35.
39. Weber KT. Fibrosis and hypertensive heart disease. Curr Opin Cardiol 2000; 15: 264–72.
40. Bishop JE, Lindahl G. Regulation of cardiovascular collagen synthesis by mechanical load. Cardiovasc Res 1999; 42: 27–44.
41. López B, González A, Díez J. Role of matrix metalloproteinases in hypertension-associated cardiac fibrosis. Curr Opin Nephrol Hypertens 2004; 13: 197–204.
42. Amanuma S, Sekiguchi M, Ogasawara S et al. Biventricular endomyocardial biopsy findings in essential hypertension of graded severity. Postgrad Med J 1994; 70 (Suppl 1): S67–S71.
43. Pearlman ES, Weber KT, Janicki JS et al. Muscle fiber orientation and connective tissue content in the hypertrophied human heart. Lab Invest 1982; 46: 158–64.
44. Boldt A, Wetzel U, Lauschke J et al. Fibrosis in left atrial tissue of patients with atrial fibrillation with and without underlying mitral valve disease. Heart 2004; 90: 400–5.
45. López B, Querejeta R, Varo N et al. Usefulness of serum carboxy-terminal propeptide of procollagen type I in assessment of the cardioreparative ability of antihypertensive treatment in hypertensive patients. Circulation 2001; 104: 286–91.
46. Díez J, Querejeta R, López B et al. Losartan-dependent regression of myocardial fibrosis is associated with reduction of left ventricular chamber stiffness in hypertensive patients. Circulation 2002; 105: 2512–17.
47. González A, López B, Querejeta R et al. Regulation of myocardial fibrillar collagen by angiotensin II. A role in hypertensive heart disease? J Mol Cell Cardiol 2002; 34: 1585–93.
48. Díez J. Profibrotic effects of angiotensin II in the heart. A matter of mediators. Hypertension 2004; 43: 1164–5.
49. Tokuda K, Kai H, Kuwahara F et al. Pressure-independent effects of angiotensin II on hypertensive myocardial fibrosis. Hypertension 2004; 43: 499–503.

50. Yoshida J, Yamamoto K, Mano T et al. AT1 receptor blocker added to ACE inhibitor provides benefits at advanced stage of hypertensive diastolic failure. Hypertension 2004; 43: 686–91.
51. Brilla CG, Zhou G, Matsubara L et al. Collagen metabolism in cultured adult rat cardiac fibroblasts: response to angiotensin II and aldosterone. J Mol Cell Cardiol 1994; 26: 809–20.
52. Brilla CG, Matsubara LS, Weber KT. Anti-aldosterone treatment and the prevention of myocardial fibrosis in primary and secondary aldosteronism. J Mol Cell Cardiol 1993; 25: 563–75.
53. Brilla CG, Pick R, Tan LB et al. Remodeling of the rat right and left ventricles in experimental hypertension. Circ Res 1990; 67: 1355–64.
54. Brilla CG, Matsubara LS, Weber KT. Antifibrotic effects of spironolactone in preventing myocardial fibrosis in systemic arterial hypertension. Am J Cardiol 1993; 71: 12A–16A.
55. Nicoletti A, Heudes D, Hinglais N et al. Left ventricular fibrosis in renovascular hypertensive rats. Effect of losartan and spironolactone. Hypertension 1995; 26: 101–11.
56. Struthers AD, MacDonald TM. Review of aldosterone- and angiotensin II-induced target organ damage and prevention. Cardiovasc Res 2004; 61: 663–70.
57. Burlew BS, Weber KT. Cardiac fibrosis as a cause of diastolic dysfunction. Herz 2002; 27: 92–8.
58. Burlew BS, Weber KT. Connective tissue and the heart. Functional significance and regulatory mechanisms. Cardiol Clin 2000; 18: 435–42.
59. McLenachan JM, Dargie JH. Ventricular arrhythmias in hypertensive left ventricular hypertrophy. Relation to coronary artery disease, left ventricular dysfunction, and myocardial fibrosis. Am J Hypertens 1990; 3: 735–40.
60. Querejeta R, López B, González A et al. Increased collagen type I synthesis in patients with heart failure of hypertensive origin. Relation to myocardial fibrosis. Circulation 2004; 110: 1263–8.

31

Apoptosis: molecular mechanisms in hypertension

Taben M Hale, David Duguay and Denis deBlois

INTRODUCTION

Apoptosis is a highly regulated form of cell death that acts as the essential counterpart of cell proliferation.[1] Initially described in the context of organ morphogenesis in the invertebrate nematode and mammalian embryo, apoptosis is often referred to as 'programmed cell death'. For instance, an increase in programmed cell death of cardiomyocytes in the right ventricle has been implicated in normal assymetrical postnatal morphogenesis of the cardiac chambers.[2] The identification over the last 15 years of the key genes mediating apoptotic cell death in mammalians has set the stage for a remarkable increase in studies implicating apoptosis in cardiovascular diseases. As discussed below, these include conditions where apoptosis is increased relative to cell replication, such as in cardiomyocyte loss during progression to heart failure, arterial atrophy leading to aneurysm, and capillary rarefaction in hypertension. In contrast, decreased apoptosis relative to cell replication can lead to tissue hyperplasia, as in arterial remodeling in hypertension and atherosclerosis. Finally, enhanced cell turnover due to an increase in both apoptosis and cell proliferation has been proposed as a mechanism leading to premature endothelial cell senescence.

PATHWAYS OF APOPTOSIS

Apoptosis is regulated by a complex interplay of environmental cues that are not specific for apoptosis but are shared with common major signaling pathways for cell growth and differentiation. These include, for instance, cytokines (e.g. Fas, tumor necrosis factor (TNF), interleukin (IL)-6), growth factors (e.g. platelet-derived growth factor (PDGF), insulin-like growth factor (IGF)-1), endocrine mediators (angiotensin (Ang) II, endothelin), reactive oxygen species (ROS, e.g. superoxide, hydrogen peroxide) and specific ($\alpha_v\beta_3$,β_1) integrin engagement with extracellular matrix components.[3,4] Several of these cues promote cell growth by increasing cell survival via the activation of protein kinase pathways such as with PDGF or IGF-1 receptor, ERK-1/2, phosphatidylinositol 3-kinase (PI3K)/Akt pathway or focal adhesion kinase-1 (FAK-1) pathways. The regulation of apoptosis shows a high degree of cell specificity. For instance, AT_1 receptors for Ang II stimulate replication in vascular smooth muscle cells (SMCs) and cardiac fibroblasts, and enhance apoptosis in cardiomyocytes and macrovascular endothelial cells.[5] In addition to target cell type, the effects on cell growth versus apoptosis are also dependent on the type and amount of inducer, e.g. with low versus high levels of ROS having opposite effects.[6]

In contrast to necrotic death – where cells typically swell and show random DNA cleavage and lytic disintegration of cytoplasmic and nuclear membranes, eventually triggering inflammation – apoptotic cells show a characteristic well-ordained sequence of morphological changes.[1,7] These include chromatin condensation and margination in sharply delineated masses at the nuclear envelope, cytoplasmic condensation and rigidification, cell volume shrinkage, as well as budding of nuclear and plasma membranes to produce apoptotic bodies containing closely packed, well-preserved organelles. Figure 31.1 summarizes key intracellular pathways of apoptosis. A specific feature of apoptosis is the activation of calcium-dependent cysteine proteases present as zymogen in all cell types: the caspases.[8] Over the recent 15 years, the identification of the key genes regulating apoptosis in mammalian cells has generated investigative tools and spurred a wealth of studies that have greatly increased our understanding of the role

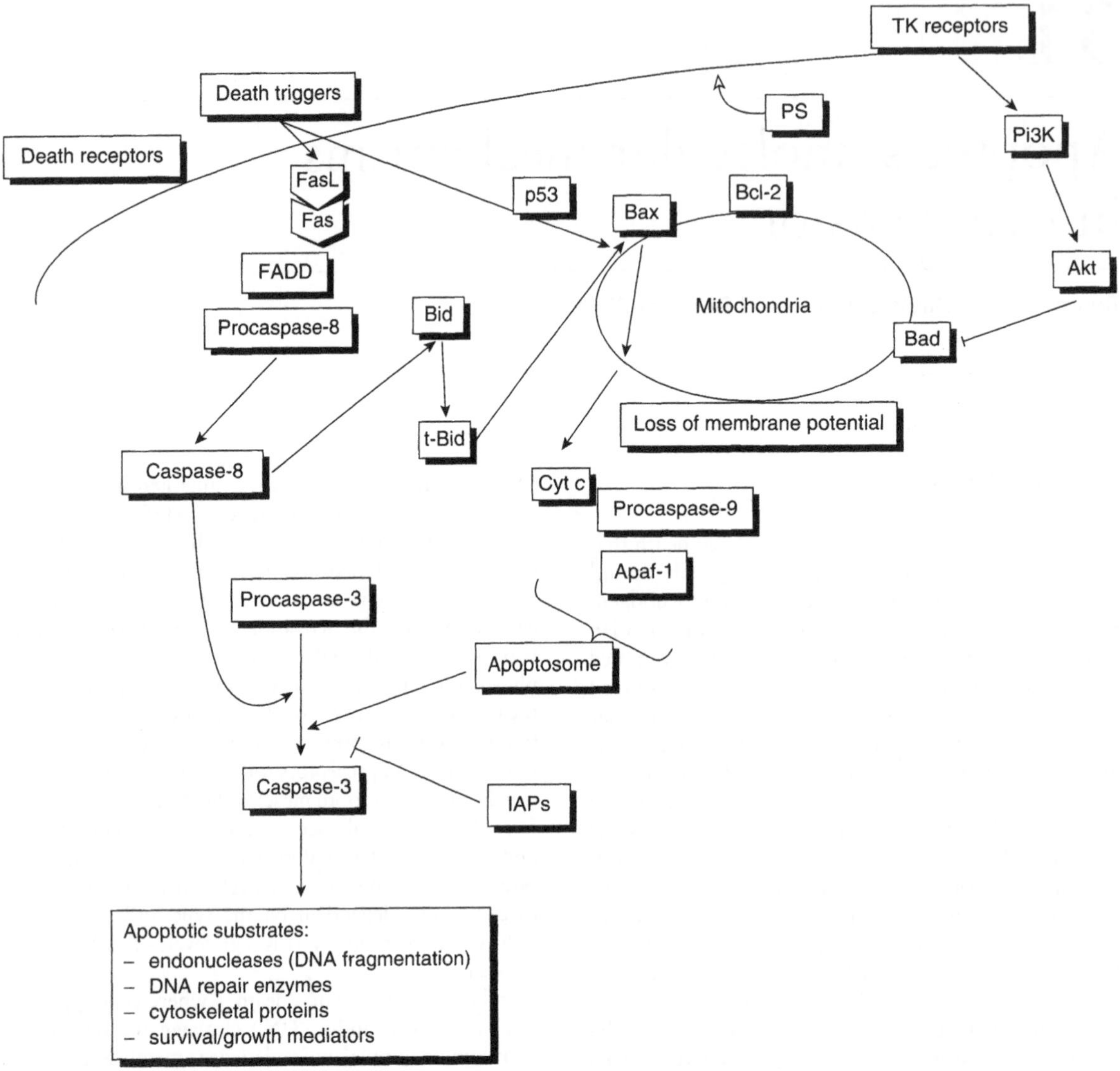

Figure 31.1 Pathways involved in death receptor or mitochondrial-mediated apoptosis. Death receptor (e.g. Fas) stimulation, causes recruitment of fas associated death domain (FADD) and, activation of caspase-8, which then activates the executioner caspases (e.g. caspase-3), responsible for typical apoptotic morphological changes. Activation of the pro-apoptotic factor, Bid (via caspase-8), results in translocation of Bax to the mitochondrial membrane and release of cytochrome c (Cyt c), which then associates with apoptotic protease activating factor-1 (APAF-1) and caspase-9 causing activation of caspase-3. The mitochondrial pathway of apoptosis can be stimulated directly by certain death triggers (e.g. oxidative stress) leading to an upset in the balance between pro-apoptotic (e.g. Bax, Bad) and anti-apoptotic (e.g. Bcl-2) mitochondrial factors, and subsequent Cyt c release. Stimulation of tyrosine kinase (TK) receptors may inhibit apoptosis via phosphatidylinositol 3-kinase (PI3K) and Akt activation. Finally, inhibitors of apoptosis proteins (IAPs) can prevent caspase-3 activation. PS, phosphatidyl serine

of apoptosis in cardiovascular disorders. In addition to morphology, apoptosis is now defined biochemically as 'caspase-dependent cell death'[9] (other types of 'programmed cell death' exist but are much less prevalent[10]).

To date, the caspase family includes 14 members mainly involved in apoptosis initiation (e.g. caspase-8 and -9), execution (e.g. caspase-3) or in cytokine maturation (e.g. caspase-1, also called interleukin-1 converting enzyme). Caspases are activated by homo- or hetero-dimerization followed by limited proteolysis and generation of the active enzyme. Apoptosis can be triggered either by activation of the death receptor superfamily, such as Fas/CD95 or TNF receptor, or by the loss of mitochondrial membrane potential leading to the release of caspase activating factors. The death receptor pathway involves clustering of activated death receptor and the formation of a death-inducing signaling complex (DISC) at the intracellular domain of the receptors. The DISC includes the adaptor molecule Fas-associated death domain (FADD), which recruits several procaspase-8 molecules. Proximity facilitates the mutual cleavage of procaspase-8 molecules, ultimately releasing active caspase-8 into the cytoplasm. The mitochondrial pathway of apoptosis can be triggered by multiple signals including oxidative stress, calcium overload or pro-apoptotic members of the Bcl-2 family of apoptosis regulatory proteins. Loss of mitochondrial membrane potential leads to the release of cyctochrome c. Cytochrome c forms a multimeric complex called the apoptosome, which includes the adaptor molecule Apaf-1, ATP, and procaspase-9.

The death receptor and mitochondrial pathways converge toward the activation of cytoplasmic caspases, among which caspase-3 is the prototypical member, to execute the apoptotic program. The two pathways are also linked and regulated by pro-apoptotic (Bax, Bid) and anti-apoptotic (Bcl-2, Bcl-X_L) members of the Bcl-2 protein family. The balance between anti- and pro-apoptotic Bcl-2 family members is critical to determine if a cell undergoes apoptosis.[11] For instance, the mitochondrial pathway can be activated via caspase-8 cleaveage of cytoplasmic Bid. Following a death signal, Bid and/or Bax can associate with the mitochondria to induce membrane depolarization and formation of the apoptosome complex.[12,13] In contrast, up-regulated expression of Bcl-2 inhibits apoptosis in most models. Caspases further facilitate apoptosis by degrading a wide array of target proteins including DNA repair enzymes such as poly(ADP-ribose) polymerase (PARP), cytoskeletal proteins such as actin and gelosin and important survival/growth mediators such as Bcl-2 and ERK kinase kinase 1. Thus, the death receptor and mitochondrial pathways are not mutually exclusive and show coordinate activation in most cells. Depending on the condition, the mitochondrial pathway may trigger or act as an amplifier of the apoptotic process. The proteolytic activity of caspases results in the activation of specific endonucleases that cut genomic DNA between nucleosomes to generate fragments of approximately 180 base pairs, a hallmark of apoptosis showing up as a DNA ladder following agarose gel electrophoresis. Finally, the control of intracellular K^+ ion appears to play an important role in apoptosis regulation.[14–16] Enhanced K^+ efflux is an essential mediator of not only early apoptotic shrinkage but also downstream caspase activation and DNA fragmentation.[17]

APOPTOSIS IN HYPERTENSION

The initial observation implicating apoptosis in hypertension came from studies in spontaneously hypertensive rats (SHRs), a model of genetically determined hypertension showing aortic, cardiac, and renal hyperplasia, as well as accelerated loss of neuronal cells. Using *in situ* radioactive labeling of internucleosomal DNA fragmentation Hamet et al.[18] reported that apoptosis is enhanced in target organs (aortic SMCs, heart, kidney and brain) of hypertension in young adult rats and mice as compared with normotensive controls. Further studies showed that neonatal cardiac hyperplasia in SHRs is associated with increased DNA replication and reduced apoptosis within 24 hours of birth.[19,20] Moreover, radioactive labeling of genomic DNA in utero revealed a 50% decrease in the half-life of DNA in the kidney, heart and thoracic aorta in pre-hypertensive SHRs as compared with Wistar-Kyto (WKY) rats, suggesting increased cell turnover in this model of hypertension.[21,22] The Ang II pathway has been implicated in these differences in cell turnover.[21,23] As shown in Table 31.1,[24–63] current evidence indicates that apoptosis is differentially regulated in a wide variety of tissues (cardiovascular and non-cardiovascular) in SHRs relative to normotensive WKY rats. Most, although not all, of these differences remain after blood pressure reduction or when cells are cultured in vitro. Together these data implicate both hemodynamic and non-hemodynamic (genetic, humoral) components in apoptosis regulation in SHRs. It is important to note however, that SMCs and cardiomyocytes cultured from SHRs show enhanced susceptibility to apoptosis induction in response to serum withdrawal or stimulation of the cyclic AMP pathway.[18,42,64–70] Alterations in apoptosis regulation are not specific to the SHR model, since aortic SMCs from DOCA-salt rats also show increased DNA laddering, caspase-3 activation and Bax to Bcl-2 protein ratio.[31] Paradoxically, Ang II infusion in rats enhanced SMC apoptosis with caspase-3 activation and increased Bax to Bcl-2 protein ratio.[71] Other studies showed that Ang II infusion induces SMC DNA replication.[72] Consistent with this, previous studies in c-myc transfected SMCs suggested that proliferating cells are at higher risk of undergoing apoptosis.[73]

Table 31.1 Differential apoptosis in spontaneously hypertensive rats (SHRs) relative to normotensive rats

Organ/cell type	*Change in SHRs vs normotensive rats*	*Detection method*	*Comment/suggested role*	*References*
Vascular				
Endothelial cells	↑	Ethidium bromide staining, caspase-3 expression	Capillary rarefaction, prevented by adrenalectomy	24–27
	↓ (mesenteric vessels)	TUNEL and DNA laddering	1–2-week-old SHR, role in increasing media-to-lumen ratio	28
	No difference (aorta)	TUNEL and morphology	4–12-week-old SHR	29
SMCs	↑ (mesenteric vessels)	TUNEL and morphology	4–12-week-old SHR, role in maintenance of eutrophic remodeling	29
	↓ (intra-myocardial arteries)	Bax and Bcl-2 protein expression	36-week-old SHR Normalization by ACE inhibitor Role in hypertrophic remodeling	30
	↑ (aorta)	DNA fragmentation, TUNEL, caspase-3, increased Bax to Bcl-2 protein ratio, reduced cell number	Young adult SHR Induction with ACE inhibitor, ARB, CCB and ET_A endothelin receptor blockade	31,32 33–36
Adventitial fibroblasts	↓ (mesenteric vessels)	TUNEL and DNA laddering	1–2-week-old SHR, role in increasing adventitial mass	28
Cardiac				
Whole heart	↓	DNA fragmentation, TUNEL, morphology	1–2-week-old SHR Establishment of hypertophy/ hyperplasia	20
Whole heart	↑		4–24-week-old SHR	18, 37, 38
Cardiomyocytes	↑	TUNEL, annexin V binding, caspase-3 cleavage, increased Bax to Bcl-2 protein ratio	Transition from compensated hypertrophy to heart failure Prevented By ACE inhibitors, ARB, CCB and vasopeptidase inhibitors	39 40–42 43
Fibroblasts	↑	TUNEL, DNA fragmentation, caspase-3 cleavage, increased Bax to Bcl-2 protein ratio	Transient induction with ACE inhibitor, ARB, CCB Reversal of fibroblast hyperplasia	44, 45
Renal				
Kidney	↓		1–2-week-old SHR Establishment of hypertophy/ hyperplasia	20
	↑		4–24-week-old SHRs In the inner cortex and medulla	18
Mesangial cells	↑	TUNEL, propidium iodide staining, increased Bax to Bcl-2 protein ratio	In response to serum deprivation in cultured cells	46

Table 31.1 *(Continued)*

Organ/cell type	*Change in SHRs vs normotensive rats*	*Detection method*	*Comment/suggested role*	*References*
Glomerular cells	↑	Caspase-3 expression	Prevented by omapatrilat Bradykinin was implicated	47
Tubular epithelial and interstitial cells	↑	TUNEL, increased Bax to Bcl-X_L protein ratio	SHR with 5/6 renal mass reduction, attenuated by renin-angiotensin system inhibitors	48
Brain				
Brain	↑		In the cortex, striatum, hippocampus and thalamus	18
	↑ (frontal and occipital cortex)	TUNEL	24-week-old SHR	49
	↑ (CA_1 and dentate gyrus in hippocampus)	TUNEL	In 24-week-old SHR Linked to a decrease in white and gray matter volume	50
Neurons	↑ (retinal ganglionic neurons and photoreceptors)	TUNEL	Attenuated by blood pressure lowering No change in other retinal cells populations	51
Other				
Hepatocytes	↓	TUNEL	Following CCL_4 in vivo Suggested as an anti-apoptotic effect of the sympathetic nervous system that promotes liver fibrosis	52
Instestinal cells	↑ (cells of the jejunal crypt)	Morphology	Increased sensibility to radiation Prevented by reserpine (sympathetic dysfunction)	53
Osteocytes	↑	Morphology and TUNEL	During development of femoral head osteonecrosis	54
Prostate cells	↑ (prostate epithelium or no change)	TUNEL, caspase-3 and -8 expression	SHR is a prostatic hyperplasia model Proliferation is more increased than apoptosis	55–58
Immune system				
Lymphocytes	↑ (thymus)		8-week-old SHR	59
Thymocytes	↑	TUNEL, propidium iodide staining, DNA fragmentation	Decrease in number of CD8+ cells in thymus and peripheral T cells DNA fragmentation in thymus prevented by adrenalectomy	60–63

TUNEL, terminal transferase dUTP, nick and labeling; ACE, angiotensin converting enzyme; ARB, AT_1 receptor blocker for angiotensin II; CCB, calcium channel blocker.

Increased telomerase activity has been implicated in vascular SMC (VSMC) growth.[74,75] Telomerase activity is enhanced in aortic VSMCs from SHRs between the age of 2 and 12 weeks,[70] a period of active vascular remodeling. Disruption of telomerase activity in normotensive VSMCs induces cell growth arrest.[74] In contrast, it induces apoptosis in SHR VSMCs, a response that can be prevented by overexpression of p53.[70] Thus, not only do SHR VSMCs express increased telomerase activity, but they appear to be more dependent on it for their survival, compared with VSMCs isolated from normotensive animals. The in vivo significance of these observations remains unclear, although 'premature cell senescence' can result from enhanced activation of growth pathways,[76] as seen in hypertensive cells.[77] Increased pulse pressure in hypertension is associated with reduced telomere length, suggestive of accelerated cardiovascular aging.[78,79] Telomerase activity is increasingly being implicated in cell growth and inhibition of apoptosis.[80] In SHR the increase in both growth and apoptosis in SMCs may contribute to the increased cell turnover.[21] As an alternate mechanism, it should be noted that oxidative stress has also been demonstrated to shorten telomere length.

SMC apoptosis in hypertension

Vascular remodeling can occur as a normal adaptive response to long-term changes in arterial pressure or blood flow, a pathologic result of vessel injury, progression of vascular disease, or as a result of pharmacological intervention. For example, in hypertension vessels undergo structural changes that result in an increase in vascular mass characterized by increases in cell number (hyperplasia), cell size (cellular hypertrophy), or both. Whether these changes occur prior to or as a result of elevation in blood pressure is a widely debated issue. Regardless, evidence has accumulated to show that dysregulation of the balance between VSMC growth and death is critical in the development of vascular hypertrophy. Several proteins known to be involved in cell growth and death have been shown to be expressed at different levels when comparing arteries from normotensive and hypertensive rats. These altered expression levels can suggest the mechanism by which the past growth occurred (e.g. ↑mitogen-activated protein kinase (MAPK)),[81] or counter-regulatory mechanisms that may control further proliferation (e.g. ↑peroxisome proliferator-activated receptor (PPAR)).[82]

While the mechanisms involved in structural modification of vessels have not been fully elucidated, apoptosis has been shown to play a role with impact varying with disease, drug treatment, and vessel type. VSMC apoptosis in resistance arteries has been shown to occur in vivo during development of hypertension[29]and as a result of changes in blood flow.[83] For example, apoptosis was significantly increased in mesenteric small resistance arteries of SHRs vs WKY rats after 8 and 12 weeks of age, a time when blood pressure is rising, media to lumen ratio is increased, and hypertension is being established.[29] Vascular remodeling due to long-term changes in blood flow has been demonstrated experimentally in carotid and mesenteric arteries. In the studies with mesenteric arteries, ligation of one artery results in reduction of flow downstream, and a redirection of blood to an adjacent artery thereby exposing it to a sudden increase in flow. Apoptosis has been shown to be evident in both low flow and high flow arteries during the respective reduction and increase in medial size.[83] Similar studies in the carotid arteries demonstrate increases in apoptosis resulting from significant decreases in blood flow.[84]

Changes in wall stress and stretch have been shown to modulate cell survival both in vivo and in vitro. While the mechanisms mediating these changes have not been fully elucidated, integrin signaling,[85] ROSs,[86] nitric oxide (NO),[86] and stimulation of AT_2 and ET_B receptors[86,87] have been proposed to be involved. The stimuli for vascular remodeling are equally diverse. Vessels must maintain the ability to change their structure in order to maintain perfusion to vital organs as well as minimize large variations in wall stress. Indeed, increases in wall stress and circumferential stretch of VSMCs can stimulate vascular remodeling, although the mechanisms have not been fully elucidated. Proposed mechanisms have involved changes in integrin signaling and receptor populations. Stretch-induced signaling through β_1 integrin has been demonstrated to increase activation of p38 MAPK to directly phosphorylate p53.[85] Further studies revealed that stretch could directly trigger the TNF receptor pathway, even in the absence of ligand. Stretch of VSMCs led to increased association of TNF receptor 1 with TRAF-2, resulting in sustained JNK and p38 activation and apoptosis.[88] In addition, endothelin has also been proposed to play a role in stretch-induced apoptosis.[87] Endothelin-1 (ET-1), acting on ET_A receptor is a potent vasoconstrictor and mitogen for VSMCs.[89] In contrast, stimulation of ET_B receptors on VSMCs has been shown to promote relaxation and apoptosis.[87] Stretch causes endothelial cells to increase production of ET-1, and smooth muscle cells to shift their receptor population from predominantly ET_A to ET_B. This results in direct stimulation of the ET_B receptor, resulting in VSMC apoptosis.[87] This effect has further been shown in an ex vivo model, where perfusion pressure was increased in isolated rat carotid arteries. As with increased stretch in cultured cells, increases in perfusion pressure resulted in significant ET_B-mediated apoptosis of VSMCs.[90]

Ang II also plays an important role in both physiological and pathophysiological vascular remodeling. Like ET-1, Ang II is a potent vasoconstrictor and mitogen. These primary effects are mediated through the AT_1 receptor located on the SMC.[91] Stimulation of the AT_2 receptor, however, leads to SMC relaxation, growth inhibition and apoptosis.[36,91] In addition, experimental studies using AT_1 receptor blockers (ARBs) in hypertensive rats have demonstrated AT_2 receptor-mediated apoptosis.[36] While blockade of AT_2 receptors under normal conditions does not impact on VSMC survival, during AT_1 antagonism there is a marked increase in apoptosis. It is therefore suggested that blocking the AT_1 receptor allows for unopposed stimulation of AT_2 receptors by Ang II. While the exact signaling pathway remains unknown, the down-regulation of Bax and sequential activation of caspases-3 and -9 have been shown.[35] Furthermore, caspase inhibition using the pan-caspase inhibitor Z-VAD resulted in a marked attenuation of the regression of vascular hypertrophy and SMC apoptosis, suggesting that apoptosis is an obligatory step in losartan (AT_1 antagonist)-induced vascular remodeling.[35]

One of the mechanisms by which Ang II stimulates VSMC growth is via generation of ROS. It, along with other factors involved in cellular growth/death responses, including (but not limited to) TNF, PDGF, Ox-LDL, high glucose, and vascular endothelial growth factor (VEGF) generate ROS such as H_2O_2, superoxide and peroxynitrite.[6] ROS are increased in arteries of SHR vs WKY rats,[92] as well as in atherosclerotic lesions.[6] Downstream mediators are also diverse with targets that include ERK, SAPK, NFκB, caspases, and Akt kinase. While it was long understood that ROS were involved in vascular pathologies, recent evidence has suggested that these species may also play a role in normal vascular physiology. In fact, there is now a growing understanding that ROS can participate in growth, survival and death responses in VSMCs. The ultimate effect is highly context-dependent, with the species and amount of oxidant produced, and the local milieu playing critical roles.[6]

In addition to Ang II antagonists, other antihypertensive agents, including angiotensin converting enzyme (ACE) inhibitors and calcium channel blockers, have also been shown to induce apoptosis in SHR aortic SMCs.[33] While the exact mechanisms involved in this process have not been fully elucidated, it has been determined that in each case, there is a 30% reduction in cell number. Importantly, treatment with the vasodilator hydralazine does not result in aortic SMC apoptosis or regression of hypertrophy, despite similar reduction in blood pressure.[33] More recently the cholesterol-lowering drugs that inhibit the enzyme HMG coA-reductase, commonly known as 'statins', have also been shown to induce apoptosis in hypertensive arteries.[93,94] The current state of knowledge suggests that this apoptosis occurs via the mitochondrial pathway. During exposure to statins, in the VSMC there is a decrease in Bcl-2 levels, no change in Bax, and caspase-9 activation.[93] Further, these agents have been shown to sensitize human cultured SMCs to FAS and cytokine-induced apoptosis.[94] Therefore, not only are these agents able to induce apoptosis directly, but they also cause the cells to be more susceptible to cell death. Whether these findings can be replicated in vivo is the focus of ongoing experiments.

Recently, the PPARs have been shown to also play a role in vascular remodeling. Much of the early work on this receptor system focused on metabolism, diabetes, and atherosclerosis. The findings that came from the atherosclerosis work led to the investigation of these receptors in other vascular growth disorders, including hypertension. PPARα and PPARγ have both been shown to have a significantly higher expression in aorta and mesenteric arteries of adult SHRs relative to age-matched WKY rats.[82] Given that stimulation of these receptors on VSMCs induces apoptosis, the current hypothesis is that this increased expression may serve as a counter-regulatory mechanism to limit the hyperplasia seen in hypertensive vessels. PPARγ-induced apoptosis appears to occur in part, through transforming growth factor (TGF)-β1-mediated nuclear recruitment of phosphorylated SMAD-2,[95] while PPARα mediates this effect, in part through a p38 MAPK pathway and through alterations of the mitochondrial membrane potential leading to cytochrome c release.[96]

While VSMC turnover is a rare event in fully developed arteries, it remains an option for at least some cells. Traditionally evidence of apoptosis has been considered an area of concern and associated with vascular disease and pathology. However, we have since learned that this is an important mechanism by which vessels can adapt their structure to maintain appropriate perfusion. Furthermore, apoptosis has also been shown to play a role in the secondary benefits associated with certain pharmacotherapies.

The role of apoptosis in the different modes of (hypertrophic, eutrophic, atrophic) arterial remodeling in hypertension remains unclear. SMC apoptosis has been implicated in the development of saccular cerebral aneurysm both in rodent models[97] and in humans, where it is associated with activation of the c-JNK/c-Jun pathway,[98] vessel rupture and stroke.[99] In human essential hypertension, SMC hyperplasia is observed in large arteries, whereas small resistance vessels are mainly characterized by inward eutrophic remodeling.[29,86,100] Remodeling of resistance arteries with antihypertensive drug treatment involves outward remodeling and decrease in the wall to lumen ratio. Because apoptosis induction by therapeutic drugs appears to occur selectively in large rather than small arteries, its role is probably more important in controlling vascular compliance and atherosclerotic progression than in systemic blood pressure regulation.

Therapeutic apoptosis in pulmonary hypertension

As the first study showing that neointimal hyperplasia could be reversible by apoptosis induction, Pollman et al. showed that antisense oligonucleotides targeting the anti-apoptotic gene bcl-x_L resulted in vascular lesion regression by inducing SMC apoptosis in rabbit carotid arteries with an established intimal lesion several weeks after ballon injury.[101] SMCs found in the intima are phenotypically distinct from medial SMCs in terms of extracellular matrix production and proliferation.[102] The sensitivity to basal or drug-induced apoptosis is enhanced in intimal SMC in vitro[103] and in vivo,[104] a feature that is associated with the up-regulation of apoptotic genes.[101,105–109] The field of pulmonary hypertension has been among the most active in documenting the potential therapeutic role of apoptosis induction to control intimal hyperplasia. The monocrotaline-injected rat is a well-characterized model of pulmonary hypertension showing a marked increase in pulmonary artery pressure (due to endothelial injury, intimal hyperplasia and stenosis of peripheral pulmonary vessels), right ventricular hypertrophy and ultimately death within weeks. Candidate approaches currently being evaluated and showing the ability to induce intimal SMC apoptosis in pulmonary hypertension include phosphiodiesterase 5 inhibition (e.g. with sildenafil),[110] statins,[68,111] Rho-kinase inhibition,[112] and elastase inhibition.[113] In the latter study, complete reversal of fatal pulmonary hypertension was attained with a serine elastase inhibitor acting via a decrease in tenascin and other matrix components interacting with the $\alpha_v\beta_3$ integrin pathway. Additional candidate pathways for intimal SMC apoptosis induction in pulmonary hypertension include inactivation of survivin[114] and activation of the bone morphogenetic protein type II receptor/smad-1 pathway.[115] It remains unclear whether endothelin antagonists, a current therapy of pulmonary hypertension, induce SMC apoptosis to regress SMC hyperplasia in pulmonary arteries.[116]

Apoptosis in vascular endothelial cells

Capillary formation by angiogenesis is an important determinant of the balance between tissue perfusion and ischemia. Capillary rarefaction is commonly observed in hypertensive organs, suggesting reduced endothelial cell survival.[117] Enhanced endothelial apoptosis contributing to capillary rarefaction has been reported in SHRs, glucocorticoid-mediated hypertension in rats, renal hypertension in rats, and peripheral skeletal muscle (after experimental heart failure) in rabbits.[24,59,118,119]

Current evidence suggests that endothelial apoptosis is regulated differently in capillaries versus larger vessels. Notably, AT_1 receptors for Ang II inhibit caspase-3 activation and apoptosis in microvascular endothelial cells deprived of serum in vitro or in a murine model of retinal vascular regression.[120] AT_1 receptor-mediated survival is attributed to the stimulation of the PI3K/Akt pathway, epidermal growth factor receptor transactivation and up-regulation of survivin but not activation of ERK1/2 or ROS. In mouse models of angiogenesis induced by peripheral artery ligation, AT_1 receptors stimulate angiogenesis via the VEGF/endothelial nitric oxide synthase (eNOS) pathway whereas AT_2 receptors suppress angiogenesis by inducing endothelial apoptosis.[121,122] Interestingly, aldosterone stimulates angiogenesis in part via the inhibition of AT_2 receptor expression.[123] In contrast, stimulation of macrovascular endothelial cells with Ang II induces apoptosis via the activation of AT_1 and AT_2 receptors, the MAP kinase phosphatase-3-dependent dephosphorylation of ERK1/2, leading to the degradation of Bcl-2.[124,125] Inducers of endothelial apoptosis also include ROS, in part due to Ang II stimulation of NADPH oxidase in hypertension.[126] It should be emphasized, however, that ROS can increase endothelial cell survival at low doses.[6] Notably, exposure to low concentrations of H_2O_2 provides protection via induction of the intracellular redox regulator thioredoxin-1.[127] A similar dose-dependent regulation of apoptosis has also been described for statins in angiogenesis.[128] Cytokines such as TNF are also important regulators of endothelial inflammation and apoptosis.[129,130] Notably, TNF was implicated in the pro-apoptotic effect of serum from heart failure patients in cultured human endothelial cells.[131]

Ang II-induced endothelial cell apoptosis is attenuated by NO.[125] Inhibitors of endothelial apoptosis also include laminar fluid shear stress, endothelin ET_B receptors acting via the ERK1/2 pathway,[132,133] NF-κB[134] and NO-induced telomerase activation.[135] Thus, therapies likely to reduce endothelial apoptosis in hypertension include drugs with the potential to reduce vascular inflammation and increase NO bioavailability, such as inhibitors of the renin-angiotensin system (RAS) and calcium channel blockers. The inhibition of endothelial apoptosis may impact favorably on vascular hyperplasia, as suggested by the observation that endothelial cells undergoing apoptosis release a paracrine anti-apoptotic factor for SMCs, acting via ERK1/2 phosphorylation, decreased expression of p53 and increased expression of the anti-apoptotic factor Bcl-x_L in SMCs.[135] This factor was identified as the C-terminal fragment of perlecan domain V.[135]

Apoptosis in the heart

The heart is a complex organ where terminally differentiated cardiomyocytes contribute to >70% of organ mass but only about 30% of cell number. In addition to neurons, the non-cardiomyocyte population includes proliferation-competent cells such as fibroblasts (mainly), vascular cells, and immune cells. The population dynamics for these cell types is regulated in a cell type-specific manner developmentally, during disease and therapy. Following the postnatal period of proliferation, cardiomyocyte or cardiac neuron numbers do not change significantly unless cell loss occurs. A large body of experimental and clinical evidence accumulated over the last 10 years indicates that apoptosis contributes to cardiac damage via the loss of cardiomyocytes or neurons leading to heart failure and cardiac conduction system disorders.[136–139] Some[64] but not all[40,41] studies have documented cardiomyocyte apoptosis in young hypertensive SHRs, an increase that is concomitant with the development of fibroblast hyperplasia.[64] All studies, however, concur in finding an increased cardiac susceptibility to apoptosis as evidenced by an increase Bax to Bcl-2 protein ratio that is not associated with changes in p53 expression levels.[41] The compensated left ventricle of 30-week-old SHRs shows increased cardiomyocyte apoptosis,[39,40] a feature that is reduced by prophylactic treatment with ACE inhibitors or ARBs over 14 weeks.[39–41] In this case, apoptosis inhibition correlates with ventricular ACE inhibition but not blood pressure reduction.[40] Consistent with this, Ang II stimulates apoptosis in cultured cardiomyocytes via AT_1 receptor activation.[42,140,141] Some[42] but not all[140] studies show a pro-apoptotic effect of Ang II AT_2 receptors in cultured cardiomyocytes. When cardiomyocytes from SHRs and normotensive WKY rats are compared in culture, the apoptotic effect of Ang II is greater in SHR than WKY cells.[42] Moreover, cardiomyocytes from SHRs but not WKY rats show AT_2 receptor-mediated apoptosis in vitro.[42] Treatment with a vasopeptidase inhibitor mimicked the protective effect of an AT_1 blocker against remodeling and cardiomyocyte apoptosis in SHRs fed a high salt diet.[142] In long-term studies, the lifespan of stroke-prone SHRs is normalized from 15–18 months to 30 months, either by early-onset treatment (in 1-month-old rats) or late-onset treatment (in 15-month-old rats) with an ACE inhibitor.[143,144]

Non-genetic models of hypertension clearly demonstrate that increased mechanical load induces cardiomyocyte apoptosis. Cardiac pressure overload following aortic coarctation induces a rapid increase in cardiomyocyte apoptosis preceding the development of left ventricular hypertrophy. Under pressure overload, AT_1 receptors recruit the p53 pathway to increase cardiomyocyte apoptosis.[140] In turn, p53 activates the RAS and Ang II production in cardiomyocytes, leading to AT_1-dependent apoptosis.[141] The results of the Randomized Aldactone Evaluation Study (RALES) trial have generated renewed interest in aldosterone and its specific contribution to cardiovascular diseases.[145] Aldosterone stimulates cardiomyocyte apoptosis both in vivo and in cultured cells to a similar extent as Ang II.[146] The occurrence of clinical data underlining the therapeutic potential of aldosterone antagonists, before an established pathophysiological explanation was available, is reminiscent of the rise of ACE inhibitors and beta-blockers in heart failure treatment. Indeed the control of heart failure with beta-blockers is also associated with the inhibition of cardiomyocyte apoptosis.[147] Consistent with this, beta-adrenergic receptor activation enhances apoptosis in cultured cardiomyocytes, via the cAMP/proteine kinase A pathway.[148] Overall the inhibition of cardiomyocyte apoptosis now represents one of the principal reasons for improved clinical outlook in heart failure with these inhibitors. ROS are a class of mediators for which experimental evidence awaits confirmation from direct therapeutic intervention in the clinic.[149] In a dog model of dilated cardiomyopathy induced by ventricular pacing, apoptosis of cardiomyocytes, fibroblasts, and endothelial cells precedes and correlates over time with ventricular decompensation, suggesting that oxidative stress and levels of anti-oxidant defenses may be critical for the regulation of apoptosis in the overloaded heart.[150]

Since cardiomyocytes undergoing hypertrophy are at greater risk of undergoing apoptosis, a key question is to unravel the mechanisms involved in determining the ultimate fate of these cells. Pro-apoptotic pathways include apoptosis signal-regulating kinase-1 and TGF kinase-1, upstream of p38 and JNK MAP kinases.[151,152] Two different isoforms of the MAP kinase p38 show different effects in response to mechanical stress, with p38α promoting p53 activation, Bax expression and activation of the mitochondrial pathway of apoptosis, while p38β promotes hypertrophy.[153] Also, JNK kinase activation alone results in hypertrophy whereas co-activation of JNK and p38 MAP kinases triggers apoptosis. Another pathway of heart failure involves TNF-α.[154] These pro-apoptotic pathways are counterbalanced by the Raf-1 kinase pathway,[155] as well as ligands of the gp130 receptor, including IL-6 and leukemia inhibitor factor, which recruit the JAK/STAT signaling pathway to increase expression of embryonic genes and pro-survival factors (see elsewhere for review[156]). Evidence of apoptosis in the human hypertensive heart remains scarce. A small study showed an increased number of TUNEL-positive cardiomyocytes and non-cardiomyocytes in right septal endomyocardial biopsies obtained from 28 hypertensive patients.[69] At 12 months post-randomization for treatment, losartan reduced the number of TUNEL-positive cardiomyocytes and non-cardiomyocytes while no effect was detected for amlodipine.

The suggestion that increased cardiomyocyte apoptosis participates in the etiology of heart failure[138] probably contributed to the negative view of apoptosis prevalent in the field of cardiovascular diseases. However, the up-regulation of apoptosis in certain cardiovascular cells may contribute to the beneficial action of antihypertensive drugs on cardiovascular structure.[31–33,36,45,157] As an explanation for this apparent discrepancy, the same stimulus, e.g. Ang II acting via AT_1 receptors, can stimulate proliferation in fibroblasts and promote apoptosis in cardiomyocytes.[158–160] Consistent with this pattern of response, fibroblasts undergo apoptosis in SHRs treated with ACE inhibition or AT_1 receptor blockade.[44] In contrast, blood pressure reduction with hydralazine does not induce cardiac apoptosis.[45] It is proposed that inhibitors of the RAS in SHRs increase apoptosis transiently and selectively in cardiac fibroblasts early during drug treatment, while they prevent the progressive deletion of cardiomyocytes during long-term therapy. Another example of cell-specific regulation of apoptosis is beta-adrenergic signaling, which stimulates apoptosis in cardiomyocytes (via the cAMP pathway)[148,161,162] and proliferation in cardiac fibroblasts (via the phosphatidylinositol 3-kinase/Akt pathway).[163,164] As in vascular cells, ROS induce either apoptosis or hypertrophy in cardiac cells in a dose-dependent manner.[165,166] The enhanced apoptosis in all cardiac cells seen in human hypertensive subjects[69] or animal models of heart failure,[150] and its attenuation by therapy, may involve the modulation of cardiac inflammation and oxidative stress. In summary, the regulation of cardiac apoptosis during disease development and therapy is regulated in a time-dependent and cell-specific manner. Whether induction of fibroblast apoptosis is relevant to anti-fibrotic effects of therapeutic drugs remains to be determined.

Apoptosis in the kidney

Hypertension is the second most frequent cause of end-stage renal disease (ESRD), surpassed only by diabetes. It is also a consequence of ESRD, further increasing the rate of renal function loss. Hypertensive nephropathy is characterized by glomerular sclerosis, interstitial fibrosis and tubular atrophy, leading to progressive nephron loss. Apoptosis is increased in the kidney glomerular and tubular compartments in various settings of experimental hypertension,[48,167–170] as is susceptibility to apoptosis in cells from those compartments when compared with a normotensive control.[46–48] Renal apoptosis can be beneficial through deletion of excess resident cells and leukocytes near inflammation sites, but can also contribute to the pathology indirectly by eliminating already injured cells or directly by depletion of glomerular and tubular cells.[170,171] A reduced rate of interstitial cell apoptosis (fibroblasts) may promote renal fibrosis, while increased apoptosis in glomerular capillary endothelial cells may lead to microvascular rarefaction.

In humans, apoptosis is observed in the glomeruli of patients with various pathologic conditions,[172–174] including glomerular sclerosis,[174] and in tubulo-interstitial cells of diabetic kidney.[175] Data on the regulation of renal apoptosis in hypertensive patients are very scarce. Reduced kidney weight and tubular atrophy observed in hypertensive nephropathy, as well as apoptosis in similar nephropathies and experimental models, suggest a role for apoptosis in the progression towards ESRD in hypertensive patients. Ang II-mediated generation of ROS and increased expression of TGF-β, via both AT_1 and AT_2, followed by p38MAPK activation and binding of Fas ligand to Fas, appear to be major pathways of renal apoptosis induction. Damage to the visceral glomerular epithelial cell layer (podocytes) is implicated in numerous renal diseases progressing to ESRD:[176] podocytes represent the last barrier before denudation of the glomerular basal membrane, they have a critical role in maintaining the structure and function of the glomerular filter and their injury is associated with proteinuria.[177] Podocytopenia, due to both detachment and apoptosis followed by a lack of proliferation, is observed in nephropathies associated with glomerular hypertension and contributes to development of glomerulosclerosis.[177] Proteinuria can then promote the secretion of cytokines (e.g. TGF-β), thus contributing to progression of the disease by stimulation of fibrosis and apoptosis in the tubulo-interstitium.[178] Apoptosis is also observed in mesangial cells,[179–181] where accumulation of a matrix of altered quality (e.g. collagen I and fibronectin found in sclerotic glomeruli, as opposed to collagen IV and laminin in normal glomeruli) could reduce their survival.[182,183] Finally, apoptosis is observed in glomerular endothelial cells, playing a role in glomerulosclerosis progression[184,185] and also in the tubulo-interstitium compartment, after the development of fibrosis, and contributing to tubular atrophy.[186,187]

Antihypertensive agents prevent renal apoptosis (podocytes, mesangial and tubular cells) in experimental models of hypertension,[48,180,186,188–191] slowing the progression of renal disease. Interestingly, with the same reduction of blood pressure, hydralazine only partially prevents tubulo-interstitial apoptosis following Ang II infusion, while the AT_1 antagonist losartan prevents it completely.[192] Renal apoptosis prevention by RAS inhibitors can thus be partially dissociated from their blood pressure-lowering action,[193] an effect that could be related to the reduction of renal apoptosis following activation of the kallikrein-kinin system[194] or to the reduction of TGF-β activity.[167] By inhibiting glomerular apoptosis, calcium channel blockers and beta-blockers prevent glomerular injuries in a rat model of severe hypertensive nephrosclerosis,[180,195–197] whereas the pathology was exacerbated by a diuretic.[198] However, new therapies are needed as ESRD continues to increase in the hypertensive population. It is proposed that a targeted inhibition of renal apoptosis, mainly in podocytes, could further reduce progression to ESRD. Activation of IGF-1,[199] nephrin (via VEGF),[200] and the heme oxygenase system,[186,192] as well as inhibition of TGF-β-mediated deleterious renal effects with tranilast[166] represent interesting novel strategies.

CONCLUSION

In summary, apoptosis is a prevalent determinant of cell fate in all target organs of hypertension. Although in many conditions the clinical relevance of apoptosis remains to be established, experimental evidence supporting a causal pathophysiological role is growing, particularly in the progression to heart failure. However, apoptosis, like cell replication, is neither good nor bad but rather context-dependent. Because it is a gene-regulated rather than a chaotic mode of cell death, apoptosis is intrinsically amenable to therapeutic intervention: it may be up- or down-regulated during therapy depending on the cell type. As an important corollary, the development of cardiovascular hyperplasia, with its negative impact on morbidity and mortality, can no longer be considered as an irreversible process. These considerations form the basis for the suggestion that apoptosis will become a major therapeutic target in the near future.

ACKNOWLEDGMENTS

The work was supported in part by a grant from the Canadian Institutes of Health Research (CIHR–45452). D. Duguay holds a Canada Graduate Scholarship-CIHR doctoral Award T.M. Hale holds a CHS-CIHR postdoctoral fellowship.

REFERENCES

1. Majno G, Joris I. Apoptosis, oncosis and necrosis. An overview of cell death. Am J Pathol 1995; 146: 3–15.
2. Kajstura J, Mansukhani M, Cheng W et al. Programmed cell death and expression of the protooncogene bcl-2 in myocytes during postnatal maturation of the heart. Exp Cell Res 1995; 219: 110–21.
3. Green DR, Kroemer G. The pathophysiology of mitochondrial cell death. Science 2004; 305: 626–9.
4. Johnson GL, Lapadat R. Mitogen-activated protein kinase pathways mediated by ERK, JNK, and p38 protein kinases. Science 2002; 298: 1911–12.
5. deBlois D, Orlov SN, Hamet P. Apoptosis in cardiovascular remodeling – effect of medication. Cardiovasc Drugs Ther 2001; 15: 539–45.
6. Irani K. Oxidant signaling in vascular cell growth, death, and survival: a review of the roles of reactive oxygen species in smooth muscle and endothelial cell mitogenic and apoptotic signaling. Circ Res 2000; 87: 179–83.
7. Kerr JF, Wyllie AH, Currie AR. Apoptosis: a basic biological phenomenon with wide-ranging implications in tissue kinetics. Br J Cancer 1972; 26: 239–57.
8. Hengartner MO. The biochemistry of apoptosis. Nature 2000; 407: 770–6.

9. Schwartz SM. Cell death and the caspase cascade. Circulation 1998; 97: 227–9.
10. Kitanaka C, Kuchino Y. Caspase-independent programmed cell death with necrotic morphology. Cell Death Differ 1999; 6: 508–15.
11. Mallat Z, Tedgui A. Apoptosis in the vasculature: mechanisms and functional importance. Br J Pharmacol 2000; 130: 947–62.
12. Silke J, Vaux DL. Cell death: shadow baxing. Curr Biol 1998; 8: R528–R531.
13. Wolter KG, Hsu YT, Smith CL et al. Movement of Bax from the cytosol to mitochondria during apoptosis. J Cell Biol 1997; 139: 1281–92.
14. Taurin S, Seyrantepe V, Orlov SN et al. Proteome analysis and functional expression identify mortalin as an antiapoptotic gene induced by elevation of [Na+]i/[K+]i ratio in cultured vascular smooth muscle cells. Circ Res 2002; 91: 915–22.
15. Orlov SN, Pchejetski D, Taurin S et al. Apoptosis in serum-deprived vascular smooth muscle cells: evidence for cell volume-independent mechanism. Apoptosis 2004; 9: 55–66.
16. Orlov SN, Thorin-Trescases N, Pchejetski D et al. Na+/K+ pump and endothelial cell survival: [Na+]i/[K+]i-independent necrosis triggered by ouabain, and protection against apoptosis mediated by elevation of [Na+]i. Pflugers Arch 2004; 448: 335–45.
17. Remillard CV, Yuan JX. Activation of K+ channels: an essential pathway in programmed cell death. Am J Physiol Lung Cell Mol Physiol 2004; 286: L49–L67.
18. Hamet P, Richard L, Dam TV et al. Apoptosis in target organs of hypertension. Hypertension 1995; 26: 642–8.
19. Walter SV, Hamet P. Enhanced DNA synthesis in heart and kidney of newborn spontaneously hypertensive rats. Hypertension 1986; 8: 520–5.
20. Moreau P, Tea BS, Dam TV et al. Altered balance between cell replication and apoptosis in hearts and kidneys of newborn SHR. Hypertension 1997; 30: 720–4.
21. Thorin-Trescases N, deBlois D, Hamet P. Evidence of an altered in vivo vascular cell turnover in spontaneously hypertensive rats and its modulation by long-term antihypertensive treatment. J Cardiovasc Pharmacol 2001; 38: 764–74.
22. Hamet P, Thorin-Trescases N, Moreau P et al. Workshop: excess growth and apoptosis: is hypertension a case of accelerated aging of cardiovascular cells? Hypertension 2001; 37: 760–6.
23. Choi JH, Yoo KH, Cheon HW et al. Angiotensin converting enzyme inhibition decreases cell turnover in the neonatal rat heart. Pediatr Res 2002; 52: 325–32.
24. Gobe G, Browning J, Howard T et al. Apoptosis occurs in endothelial cells during hypertension-induced microvascular rarefaction. J Struct Biol 1997; 118: 63–72.
25. Greene AS. Life and death in the microcirculation: a role for angiotensin II. Microcirculation 1998; 5: 101–7.
26. Lim HH, DeLano FA, Schmid-Schonbein GW. Life and death cell labeling in the microcirculation of the spontaneously hypertensive rat. J Vasc Res 2001; 38: 228–36.
27. Wu CH, Chi JC, Jerng JS et al. Transendothelial macromolecular transport in the aorta of spontaneously hypertensive rats. Hypertension 1990; 16: 154–61.
28. Dickhout JG, Lee RM. Apoptosis in the muscular arteries from young spontaneously hypertensive rats. J Hypertens 1999; 17: 1413–19.
29. Rizzoni D, Rodella L, Porteri E et al. Time course of apoptosis in small resistance arteries of spontaneously hypertensive rats. J Hypertens 2000; 18: 885–91.
30. Diez J, Panizo A, Hernandez M et al. Is the regulation of apoptosis altered in smooth muscle cells of adult spontaneously hypertensive rats? Hypertension 1997; 29: 776–80.
31. Sharifi AM, Schiffrin EL. Apoptosis in aorta of deoxycorticosterone acetate-salt hypertensive rats: effect of endothelin receptor antagonism. J Hypertens 1997; 15: 1441–8.
32. Sharifi AM, Schiffrin EL. Apoptosis in vasculature of spontaneously hypertensive rats: effect of an angiotensin converting enzyme inhibitor and a calcium channel antagonist. Am J Hypertens 1998; 11: 1108–16.
33. deBlois D, Tea BS, Dam TV et al. Smooth muscle cell apoptosis during vascular regression in spontaneously hypertensive rats. Hypertension 1997; 29 (1pt1): 340–9.
34. Duguay D, Sarkissian SD, Kouz R et al. Kinin B2 receptor is not involved in enalapril-induced apoptosis and regression of hypertrophy in spontaneously hypertensive rat aorta: possible role of B1 receptor. Br J Pharmacol 2004; 141: 728–36.
35. Marchand EL, Der SS, Hamet P et al. Caspase-dependent cell death mediates the early phase of aortic hypertrophy regression in losartan-treated spontaneously hypertensive rats. Circ Res 2003; 92: 777–84.
36. Tea BS, Der Sarkissian S, Touyz RM et al. Proapoptotic and growth-inhibitory role of angiotensin II type 2 receptor in vascular smooth muscle cells of spontaneously hypertensive rats in vivo. Hypertension 2000; 35: 1069–73.
37. Li W, Sun N, Liu W et al. Influence of Valsartan on myocardial apoptosis in spontaneously hypertensive rats. Chin Med J (Engl) 2002; 115: 364–6.
38. Peng L, Bradeley C, Liu J. [Investigation of inhibitory effect of ramipril on apoptosis in spontaneously hypertensive rats.] Hua Xi Yi Ke Da Xue Xue Bao 1999; 30: 40–3 (in Chinese).
39. Li Z, Bing OH, Long X et al. Increased cardiomyocyte apoptosis during the transition to heart failure in the spontaneously hypertensive rat. Am J Physiol 1997; 272: H2313-H2319.
40. Diez J, Panizo A, Hernandez M et al. Cardiomyocyte apoptosis and cardiac angiotensin-converting enzyme in spontaneously hypertensive rats. Hypertension 1997; 30: 1029–34.
41. Fortuno MA, Ravassa S, Etayo JC et al. Overexpression of Bax protein and enhanced apoptosis in the left ventricle of spontaneously hypertensive rats: effects of AT1 blockade with losartan. Hypertension 1998; 32: 280–6.
42. Ravassa S, Fortuno MA, Gonzalez A et al. Mechanisms of increased susceptibility to angiotensin II-induced apoptosis in ventricular cardiomyocytes of spontaneously hypertensive rats. Hypertension 2000; 36: 1065–71.
43. Yu G, Liang X, Xie X et al. Diverse effects of chronic treatment with losartan, fosinopril, and amlodipine on apoptosis, angiotensin II in the left ventricle of hypertensive rats. Int J Cardiol 2001; 81: 123–9.
44. Der Sarkissian S, Marchand EL, Duguay D et al. Reversal of interstitial fibroblast hyperplasia via apoptosis in hypertensive rat heart with valsartan or enalapril. Cardiovasc Res 2003; 57: 775–83.
45. Tea BS, Dam TV, Moreau P et al. Apoptosis during regression of cardiac hypertrophy in spontaneously hypertensive rats: temporal regulation and spatial heterogeneity. Hypertension 1999; 34: 229–35.
46. Rodriguez-Lopez AM, Flores O, Martinez-Salgado C et al. Increased apoptosis susceptibility in mesangial cells from spontaneously hypertensive rats. Microvasc Res 2000; 59: 80–7.
47. Zhou X, Ono H, Ono Y et al. Renoprotective effects of omapatrilat are mediated partially by bradykinin. Am J Nephrol 2003; 23: 214–21.
48. Soto K, Gomez-Garre D, Largo R et al. Tight blood pressure control decreases apoptosis during renal damage. Kidney Int 2004; 65: 811–22.
49. Mignini F, Vitaioli L, Sabbatini M et al. The cerebral cortex of spontaneously hypertensive rats: a quantitative microanatomical study. Clin Exp Hypertens 2004; 26: 287–303.

50. Sabbatini M, Strocchi P, Vitaioli L et al. The hippocampus in spontaneously hypertensive rats: a quantitative microanatomical study. Neuroscience 2000; 100: 251–8.
51. Sabbatini M, Strocchi P, Vitaioli L et al. Changes of retinal neurons and glial fibrillary acid protein immunoreactive astrocytes in spontaneously hypertensive rats. J Hypertens 2001; 19: 1861–9.
52. Hamasaki K, Nakashima M, Naito S et al. The sympathetic nervous system promotes carbon tetrachloride-induced liver cirrhosis in rats by suppressing apoptosis and enhancing the growth kinetics of regenerating hepatocytes. J Gastroenterol 2001; 36: 111–20.
53. Matsuu M, Shichijo K, Nakamura Y et al. The role of the sympathetic nervous system in radiation-induced apoptosis in jejunal crypt cells of spontaneously hypertensive rats. J Radiat Res (Tokyo) 2000; 41: 55–65.
54. Shibahara M, Nishida K, Asahara H et al. Increased osteocyte apoptosis during the development of femoral head osteonecrosis in spontaneously hypertensive rats. Acta Med Okayama 2000; 54: 67–74.
55. Lujan M, Ferruelo A, Paez A et al. Prostate apoptosis after doxazosin treatment in the spontaneous hypertensive rat model. BJU Int 2004; 93: 410–14.
56. Matityahou A, Rosenzweig N, Golomb E. Rapid proliferation of prostatic epithelial cells in spontaneously hypertensive rats: a model of spontaneous hypertension and prostate hyperplasia. J Androl 2003; 24: 263–9.
57. Yamashita M, Zhang X, Shiraishi T et al. Determination of percent area density of epithelial and stromal components in development of prostatic hyperplasia in spontaneously hypertensive rats. Urology 2003; 61: 484–9.
58. Zhang X, Na Y, Guo Y. Biologic feature of prostatic hyperplasia developed in spontaneously hypertensive rats. Urology 2004; 63: 983–8.
59. Suematsu M, Suzuki H, DeLano FA et al. The inflammatory aspect of the microcirculation in hypertension: oxidative stress, leukocytes/endothelial interaction, apoptosis. Microcirculation 2002; 9: 259–76.
60. Fannon LD, Braylan RC, Phillips MI. Alterations of lymphocyte populations during development in the spontaneously hypertensive rat. J Hypertens 1992; 10: 629–34.
61. Takeichi N, Suzuki K, Okayasu T et al. Immunological depression in spontaneously hypertensive rats. Clin Exp Immunol 1980; 40: 120–6.
62. Suzuki H, DeLano FA, Jamshidi N et al. Enhanced DNA fragmentation in the thymus of spontaneously hypertensive rats. Am J Physiol 1999; 276: H2135–H2140.
63. Zhao XS, Tian DZ, Ding YJ et al. Effect of cathepsin B on thymocyte apoptosis in spontaneously hypertensive rats. Acta Pharmacol Sin 2001; 22: 26–31.
64. Liu JJ, Peng L, Bradley CJ et al. Increased apoptosis in the heart of genetic hypertension, associated with increased fibroblasts. Cardiovasc Res 2000; 45: 729–35.
65. Klett CP, Palmer A, Gallagher AM et al. Differences in cultured cardiac fibroblast populations isolated from SHR and WKY rats. Clin Exp Pharmacol Physiol Suppl 1995; 22: S265–S267.
66. Touyz RM, Fareh J, Thibault G et al. Intracellular Ca2+ modulation by angiotensin II and endothelin-1 in cardiomyocytes and fibroblasts from hypertrophied hearts of spontaneously hypertensive rats. Hypertension 1996; 28: 797–805.
67. Ragolia L, Palaia T, Paric E et al. Prostaglandin D2 synthase inhibits the exaggerated growth phenotype of spontaneously hypertensive rat vascular smooth muscle cells. J Biol Chem 2003; 278: 22175–81.
68. Fouty BW, Rodman DM. Mevastatin can cause G1 arrest and induce apoptosis in pulmonary artery smooth muscle cells through a p27Kip1-independent pathway. Circ Res 2003; 92: 501–9.
69. Gonzalez A, Lopez B, Ravassa S et al. Stimulation of cardiac apoptosis in essential hypertension: potential role of angiotensin II. Hypertension 2002; 39: 75–80.
70. Cao Y, Li H, Mu FT et al. Telomerase activation causes vascular smooth muscle cell proliferation in genetic hypertension. FASEB J 2002; 16: 96–8.
71. Diep QN, Li JS, Schiffrin EL. In vivo study of AT(1) and AT(2) angiotensin receptors in apoptosis in rat blood vessels. Hypertension 1999; 34: 617–24.
72. Daemen MJAP, Lombardi DM, Bosman FT et al. Angiotensin II induces smooth muscle cell proliferation in the normal and injured arterial wall. Circ Res 1991; 68: 450–6.
73. Bennett MR, Evan GI, Newby AC. Deregulated expression of the c-myc oncogene abolishes inhibition of proliferation of rat vascular smooth muscle cells by serum reduction, interferon-gamma, heparin, and cyclic nucleotide analogues and induces apoptosis. Circ Res 1994; 74: 525–36.
74. Minamino T, Kourembanas S. Mechanisms of telomerase induction during vascular smooth muscle cell proliferation. Circ Res 2001; 89: 237–43.
75. Liu JP. Studies of the molecular mechanisms in the regulation of telomerase activity. FASEB J 1999; 13: 2091–104.
76. Lloyd AC. Limits to lifespan. Nat Cell Biol 2002; 4: E25–E27.
77. Touyz RM, El Mabrouk M, He G et al. Mitogen-activated protein/extracellular signal-regulated kinase inhibition attenuates angiotensin II-mediated signaling and contraction in spontaneously hypertensive rat vascular smooth muscle cells. Circ Res 1999; 84: 505–15.
78. Aviv A. Chronology versus biology: telomeres, essential hypertension, and vascular aging. Hypertension 2002; 40: 229–32.
79. Jeanclos E, Schork NJ, Kyvik KO et al. Telomere length inversely correlates with pulse pressure and is highly familial. Hypertension 2000; 36: 195–200.
80. Serrano AL, Andres V. Telomeres and cardiovascular disease: does size matter? Circ Res 2004; 94: 575–84.
81. Kim S, Murakami T, Izumi Y et al. Extracellular signal-regulated kinase and c-Jun NH2-terminal kinase activities are continuously and differentially increased in aorta of hypertensive rats. Biochem Biophys Res Commun 1997; 236: 199–204.
82. Diep QN, Schiffrin EL. Increased expression of peroxisome proliferator-activated receptor-alpha and -gamma in blood vessels of spontaneously hypertensive rats. Hypertension 2001; 38: 249–54.
83. Buus CL, Pourageaud F, Fazzi GE et al. Smooth muscle cell changes during flow-related remodeling of rat mesenteric resistance arteries. Circ Res 2001; 89: 180–6.
84. Cho A, Mitchell L, Koopmans D et al. Effects of changes in blood flow rate on cell death and cell proliferation in carotid arteries of immature rabbits. Circ Res 1997; 81: 328–37.
85. Wernig F, Mayr M, Xu Q. Mechanical stretch-induced apoptosis in smooth muscle cells is mediated by {beta} 1-integrin signaling pathways. Hypertension 2003; 41: 903–11.
86. Intengan HD, Schiffrin EL. Vascular remodeling in hypertension: roles of apoptosis, inflammation, and fibrosis. Hypertension 2001; 38: 581–7.
87. Cattaruzza M, Dimigen C, Ehrenreich H et al. Stretch-induced endothelin B receptor-mediated apoptosis in vascular smooth muscle cells. FASEB J 2000; 14: 991–8.
88. Sotoudeh M, Li YS, Yajima N et al. Induction of apoptosis in vascular smooth muscle cells by mechanical stretch. Am J Physiol – Heart Circ Physiol 2002; 282: H1709–H1716.

89. Masaki T, Miwa S, Sawamura T et al. Subcellular mechanisms of endothelin action in vascular system. Eur J Pharmacol 1999; 375: 133–8.
90. Lauth M, Berger MM, Cattaruzza M et al. Elevated perfusion pressure upregulates endothelin-1 and endothelin B receptor expression in the rabbit carotid artery. Hypertension 2000; 35: 648–54.
91. Touyz RM, Berry C. Recent advances in angiotensin II signaling. Braz J Med Biol Res 2002; 35: 1001–15.
92. Taniyama Y, Griendling KK. Reactive oxygen species in the vasculature: molecular and cellular mechanisms. Hypertension 2003; 42: 1075–81.
93. Blanco-Colio LM, Villa A, Ortego M et al. 3-Hydroxy-3-methyl-glutaryl coenzyme A reductase inhibitors, atorvastatin and simvastatin, induce apoptosis of vascular smooth muscle cells by downregulation of Bcl-2 expression and Rho A prenylation. Atherosclerosis 2002; 161: 17–26.
94. Knapp AC, Huang J, Starling G et al. Inhibitors of HMG-CoA reductase sensitize human smooth muscle cells to Fas-ligand and cytokine-induced cell death. Atherosclerosis 2000; 152: 217–27.
95. Redondo S, Ruiz E, Santos-Gallego CG et al. Pioglitazone induces vascular smooth muscle cell apoptosis through a peroxisome proliferator-activated receptor-gamma, transforming growth factor-beta 1, and a Smad2-dependent mechanism. Diabetes 2005; 54: 811–17.
96. Diep QN, Touyz RM, Schiffrin EL. Docosahexaenoic acid, a peroxisome proliferator-activated receptor-alpha ligand, induces apoptosis in vascular smooth muscle cells by stimulation of p38 mitogen-activated protein kinase. Hypertension 2000; 36: 851–55.
97. Kondo S, Hashimoto N, Kikuchi H et al. Apoptosis of medial smooth muscle cells in the development of saccular cerebral aneurysms in rats [see comments]. Stroke 1998; 29: 181–18.
98. Takagi Y, Ishikawa M, Nozaki K et al. Increased expression of phosphorylated c-Jun amino-terminal kinase and phosphorylated c-Jun in human cerebral aneurysms: role of the c-Jun amino-terminal kinase/c-Jun pathway in apoptosis of vascular walls. Neurosurgery 2002; 51: 997–1002.
99. Frosen J, Piippo A, Paetau A et al. Remodeling of saccular cerebral artery aneurysm wall is associated with rupture: histological analysis of 24 unruptured and 42 ruptured cases. Stroke 2004; 35: 2287–93.
100. Mulvany MJ. Small artery remodeling and significance in the development of hypertension. News Physiol Sci 2002; 17: 105–09.
101. Pollman MJ, Hall JL, Mann MJ et al. Inhibition of neointimal cell bcl-x expression induces apoptosis and regression of vascular disease. Nat Med 1998; 4: 222–7.
102. Schwartz SM, deBlois D, O'Brien ER. The intima. Soil for atherosclerosis and restenosis. Circ Res 1995; 77: 445–65.
103. Bennett MR, Evan GI, Schwartz SM. Apoptosis of human vascular smooth muscle cells derived from normal vessels and coronary atherosclerotic plaques. J Clin Invest 1995; 95: 2266–74.
104. Walsh K, Smith RC, Kim HS. Vascular cell apoptosis in remodeling, restenosis, and plaque rupture. Circ Res 2000; 87: 184–8.
105. Izumi Y, Kim S, Yoshiyama M et al. Activation of apoptosis signal-regulating kinase 1 in injured artery and its critical role in neointimal hyperplasia. Circulation 2003; 108: 2812–18.
106. Sata M, Tanaka K, Ishizaka N et al. Absence of p53 leads to accelerated neointimal hyperplasia after vascular injury. Arterioscl Thromb Vasc Biol 2003; 23: 1548–52.
107. Blanc-Brude OP, Yu J, Simosa H et al. Inhibitor of apoptosis protein survivin regulates vascular injury. Nat Med 2002; 8: 987–94.
108. Yoshimura S, Morishita R, Hayashi K et al. Inhibition of intimal hyperplasia after balloon injury in rat carotid artery model using cis-element 'decoy' of nuclear factor-kappaB binding site as a novel molecular strategy. Gene Ther 2001; 8: 1635–42.
109. Cai W, Devaux B, Schaper W et al. The role of Fas/APO 1 and apoptosis in the development of human atherosclerotic lesions. Atherosclerosis 1997; 131: 177–86.
110. Wharton J, Strange JW, Moller GM et al. Anti-proliferative effects of phosphodiesterase type 5 inhibition in human pulmonary artery cells. Am J Respir Crit Care Med 2005; 172: 105–13.
111. Nishimura T, Vaszar LT, Faul JL et al. Simvastatin rescues rats from fatal pulmonary hypertension by inducing apoptosis of neointimal smooth muscle cells. Circulation 2003; 108: 1640–5.
112. Abe K, Shimokawa H, Morikawa K et al. Long-term treatment with a Rho-kinase inhibitor improves monocrotaline-induced fatal pulmonary hypertension in rats. Circ Res 2004; 94: 385–93.
113. Cowan KN, Heilbut A, Humpl T et al. Complete reversal of fatal pulmonary hypertension in rats by a serine elastase inhibitor. Nat Med 2000; 6: 698–702.
114. McMurtry MS, Archer SL, Altieri DC et al. Gene therapy targeting survivin selectively induces pulmonary vascular apoptosis and reverses pulmonary arterial hypertension. J Clin Invest 2005; 115: 1479–91.
115. Zhang S, Fantozzi I, Tigno DD et al. Bone morphogenetic proteins induce apoptosis in human pulmonary vascular smooth muscle cells. Am J Physiol Lung Cell Mol Physiol 2003; 285: L740–L754.
116. Barton M, Kiowski W. The therapeutic potential of endothelin receptor antagonists in cardiovascular disease. Curr Hypertens Rep 2001; 3: 322–30.
117. Kiefer FN, Neysari S, Humar R et al. Hypertension and angiogenesis. Curr Pharm Des 2003; 9: 1733–44.
118. Vega F, Panizo A, Pardo-Mindan J et al. Susceptibility to apoptosis measured by MYC, BCL-2, and BAX expression in arterioles and capillaries of adult spontaneously hypertensive rats. Am J Hypertens 1999; 12: 815–20.
119. Nusz DJ, White DC, Dai Q et al. Vascular rarefaction in peripheral skeletal muscle after experimental heart failure. Am J Physiol Heart Circ Physiol 2003; 285: H1554–H1562.
120. Ohashi H, Takagi H, Oh H et al. Phosphatidylinositol 3-kinase/Akt regulates angiotensin II-induced inhibition of apoptosis in microvascular endothelial cells by governing survivin expression and suppression of caspase-3 activity. Circ Res 2004; 94: 785–93.
121. Silvestre JS, Tamarat R, Senbonmatsu et al. Antiangiogenic effect of angiotensin II type 2 receptor in ischemia-induced angiogenesis in mise hindlimb. Circ Res 2002; 90: 1072–9.
122. Benndorf R, Boger RH, Ergun S et al. Angiotensin II type 2 receptor inhibits vascular endothelial growth factor-induced migration and in vitro tube formation of human endothelial cells. Circ Res 2003; 93: 438–47.
123. Michel F, Ambroisine ML, Duriez M et al. Aldosterone enhances ischemia-induced neovascularization through angiotensin II-dependent pathway. Circulation 2004; 109: 1933–7.
124. Rossig L, Hermann C, Haendeler J et al. Angiotensin II-induced upregulation of MAP kinase phosphatase-3 mRNA levels mediates endothelial cell apoptosis. Basic Res Cardiol 2002; 97: 1–8.
125. Dimmeler S, Rippmann V, Weiland U et al. Angiotensin II induces apoptosis of human endothelial cells. Protective effect of nitric oxide. Circ Res 1997; 81: 970–6.

126. Li JM, Shah AM. Endothelial cell superoxide generation: regulation and relevance for cardiovascular pathophysiology. Am J Physiol Regul Integr Comp Physiol 2004; 287: R1014–R1030.
127. Haendeler J, Tischler V, Hoffmann J et al. Low doses of reactive oxygen species protect endothelial cells from apoptosis by increasing thioredoxin-1 expression. FEBS Lett 2004; 577: 427–33.
128. Weis M, Heeschen C, Glassford AJ et al. Statins have biphasic effects on angiogenesis. Circulation 2002; 105: 739–45.
129. Barinaga M. Life-death balance within the cell. Science 1996; 274: 724.
130. Van Antwerp DJ, Martin SJ, Kafri T et al. Suppression of TNF-alpha-induced apoptosis by NF-kappaB. Science 1996; 274: 787–9.
131. Rossig L, Haendeler J, Mallat Z et al. Congestive heart failure induces endothelial cell apoptosis: protective role of carvedilol. J Am Coll Cardiol 2000; 36: 2081–9.
132. Shichiri M, Yokokura M, Marumo F et al. Endothelin-1 inhibits apoptosis of vascular smooth muscle cells induced by nitric oxide and serum deprivation via MAP kinase pathway. Arterioscl Thromb Vasc Biol 2000; 20: 989–97.
133. Shichiri M, Kato H, Marumo F et al. Endothelin-1 as an autocrine/paracrine apoptosis survival factor for endothelial cells. [Published erratum appears Hypertension 1998; 31: 723.] Hypertension 1997; 30: 1198–203.
134. Scatena M, Almeida M, Chaisson ML et al. NF-kappaB mediates alphavbeta3 integrin-induced endothelial cell survival. J Cell Biol 1998; 141: 1083–93.
135. Raymond MA, Desormeaux A, Laplante P et al. Apoptosis of endothelial cells triggers a caspase-dependent anti-apoptotic paracrine loop active on vascular smooth muscle cells. FASEB J 2004; 18: 705–7.
136. Teiger E, Dam TV, Richard L et al. Apoptosis in pressure overload-induced heart hypertrophy in the rat. J Clin Invest 1996; 97: 2891–7.
137. Haunstetter A, Izumo S. Apoptosis: basic mechanisms and implications for cardiovascular disease. Circ Res 1998; 82: 1111–29.
138. Anversa P, Olivetti G, Leri A et al. Myocyte cell death and ventricular remodeling. Curr Opin Nephrol Hypertens 1997; 6: 169–76.
139. James TN. Normal and abnormal consequences of apoptosis in the human heart. Annu Rev Physiol 1998; 60: 309–25.
140. Leri A, Claudio PP, Li Q et al. Stretch-mediated release of angiotensin II induces myocyte apoptosis by activating p53 that enhances the local renin-angiotensin system and decreases the Bcl-2-to-Bax protein ratio in the cell. J Clin Invest 1998; 101: 1326–42.
141. Leri A, Fiordaliso F, Setoguchi M et al. Inhibition of p53 function prevents renin-angiotensin system activation and stretch-mediated myocyte apoptosis. Am J Pathol 2000; 157: 843–57.
142. Groholm T, Finckenberg P, Palojoki E et al. Cardioprotective effects of vasopeptidase inhibition vs angiotensin type 1-receptor blockade in spontaneously hypertensive rats on a high salt diet. Hypertens Res 2004; 27: 609–18.
143. Linz W, Wohlfart P, Schoelkens BA et al. Late treatment with ramipril increases survival in old spontaneously hypertensive rats. Hypertension 1999; 34: 291–5.
144. Linz W, Jessen T, Becker RH et al. Long-term ACE inhibition doubles lifespan of hypertensive rats. Circulation 1997; 96: 3164–72.
145. Pitt B. Effect of aldosterone blockade in patients with systolic left ventricular dysfunction: implications of the RALES and EPHESUS studies. Mol Cell Endocrinol 2004; 217: 53–8.
146. De Angelis N, Fiordaliso F, Latini R et al. Appraisal of the role of angiotensin II and aldosterone in ventricular myocyte apoptosis in adult normotensive rat. J Mol Cell Cardiol 2002; 34: 1655–65.
147. Sabbah HN, Sharov VG, Gupta RC et al. Chronic therapy with metoprolol attenuates cardiomyocyte apoptosis in dogs with heart failure. J Am Coll Cardiol 2000; 36: 1698–705.
148. Iwai-Kanai E, Hasegawa K, Araki M et al. Alpha- and beta-adrenergic pathways differentially regulate cell type-specific apoptosis in rat cardiac myocytes. Circulation 1999; 100: 305–11.
149. Ferrari R, Guardigli G, Mele D et al. Oxidative stress during myocardial ischaemia and heart failure. Curr Pharm Des 2004; 10: 1699–711.
150. Cesselli D, Jakoniuk I, Barlucchi L et al. Oxidative stress-mediated cardiac cell death is a major determinant of ventricular dysfunction and failure in dog dilated cardiomyopathy. Circ Res 2001; 89: 279–86.
151. Izumiya Y, Kim S, Izumi Y et al. Apoptosis signal-regulating kinase 1 plays a pivotal role in angiotensin II-induced cardiac hypertrophy and remodeling. Circ Res 2003; 93: 874–83.
152. Zhang D, Gaussin V, Taffet GE et al. TAK1 is activated in the myocardium after pressure overload and is sufficient to provoke heart failure in transgenic mice. Nat Med 2000; 6: 556–63.
153. Wang Y, Huang S, Sah VP et al. Cardiac muscle cell hypertrophy and apoptosis induced by distinct members of the p38 mitogen-activated protein kinase family. J Biol Chem 1998; 273: 2161–8.
154. Ananthakrishnan R, Moe GW, Goldenthal MJ et al. Akt signaling pathway in pacing-induced heart failure. Mol Cell Biochem 2005; 268: 103–10.
155. Harris IS, Zhang S, Treskov I et al. Raf-1 kinase is required for cardiac hypertrophy and cardiomyocyte survival in response to pressure overload. Circulation 2004; 110: 718–23.
156. Fortuno MA, Gonzalez A, Ravassa S et al. Clinical implications of apoptosis in hypertensive heart disease. Am J Physiol Heart Circ Physiol 2003; 284: H1495–H1506.
157. Lemay J, Hamet P, deBlois D. Losartan-induced apoptosis as a novel mechanism for the prevention of vascular lesion formation after vascular injury. Journal of Renin-Angiotensin-Aldosterone System 2000; 1: 39–42.
158. Sadoshima J, Izumo S. Molecular characterization of angiotensin II-induced hypertrophy of cardiac myocytes and hyperplasia of cardiac fibroblasts. Critical role of the AT1 receptor subtype. Circ Res 1993; 73: 413–23.
159. Horiuchi M, Akishita M, Dzau VJ. Molecular and cellular mechanism of angiotensin II-mediated apoptosis. Endocr Res 1998; 24: 307–14.
160. Opie LH, Sack MN. Enhanced angiotensin II activity in heart failure: reevaluation of the counterregulatory hypothesis of receptor subtypes. Circ Res 2001; 88: 654–8.
161. Communal C, Singh K, Pimentel DR et al. Norepinephrine stimulates apoptosis in adult rat ventricular myocytes by activation of the beta-adrenergic pathway. Circulation 1998; 98: 1329–34.
162. Shizukuda Y, Buttrick PM, Geenen DL et al. Beta-adrenergic stimulation causes cardiocyte apoptosis: influence of tachycardia and hypertrophy. Am J Physiol 1998; 275 (3 Pt 2): H961–H968.
163. Colombo F, Noel J, Mayers P et al. Beta-adrenergic stimulation of rat cardiac fibroblasts promotes protein synthesis via the activation of phosphatidylinositol 3-kinase. J Mol Cell Cardiol 2001; 33: 1091–106.
164. Colombo F, Gosselin H, El Helou V et al. Beta-adrenergic receptor-mediated DNA synthesis in neonatal rat cardiac fibroblasts proceeds via a phosphatidylinositol 3-kinase dependent pathway refractory to the antiproliferative action of cyclic AMP. J Cell Physiol 2003; 195: 322–30.

165. Li PF, Dietz R, von Harsdorf R. Superoxide induces apoptosis in cardiomyocytes, but proliferation and expression of transforming growth factor-beta1 in cardiac fibroblasts. FEBS Lett 1999; 448: 206–10.
166. Kwon SH, Pimentel DR, Remondino A et al. H_2O_2 regulates cardiac myocyte phenotype via concentration-dependent activation of distinct kinase pathways. J Mol Cell Cardiol 2003; 35: 615–21.
167. Kelly DJ, Zhang Y, Gow R et al. Tranilast attenuates structural and functional aspects of renal injury in the remnant kidney model. J Am Soc Nephrol 2004; 15: 2619–29.
168. Kobayashi S, Moriya H, Nakabayashi I et al. Angiotensin II and IGF-I may interact to regulate tubulointerstitial cell kinetics and phenotypic changes in hypertensive rats. Hypertens Res 2002; 25: 257–69.
169. Ono H, Ono Y, Takanohashi A et al. Apoptosis and glomerular injury after prolonged nitric oxide synthase inhibition in spontaneously hypertensive rats. Hypertension 2001; 38: 1300–6.
170. Ying WZ, Wang PX, Sanders PW. Induction of apoptosis during development of hypertensive nephrosclerosis. Kidney Int 2000; 58: 2007–17.
171. Ortiz A, Lorz C, Justo P et al. Contribution of apoptotic cell death to renal injury. J Cell Mol Med 2001; 5: 18–32.
172. Savill J, Mooney A, Hughes J. Apoptosis and renal scarring. Kidney Int Suppl 1996; 54: S14–S17.
173. Thomas SE, Andoh TF, Pichler RH et al. Accelerated apoptosis characterizes cyclosporine-associated interstitial fibrosis. Kidney Int 1998; 53: 897–908.
174. Sugiyama H, Kashihara N, Makino H et al. Apoptosis in glomerular sclerosis. Kidney Int 1996; 49: 103–11.
175. Kumar D, Robertson S, Burns KD. Evidence of apoptosis in human diabetic kidney. Mol Cell Biochem 2004; 259: 67–70.
176. Kriz W, LeHir M. Pathways to nephron loss starting from glomerular diseases – insights from animal models. Kidney Int 2005; 67: 404–19.
177. Mundel P, Shankland SJ. Podocyte biology and response to injury. J Am Soc Nephrol 2002; 13: 3005–15.
178. Topaloglu R. Progression to renal failure. Turk J Pediatr 2005; 47 (Suppl): 3–8.
179. Okado T, Terada Y, Tanaka H et al. Smad7 mediates transforming growth factor-beta-induced apoptosis in mesangial cells. Kidney Int 2002; 62: 1178–86.
180. Ono H, Saitoh M, Ono Y et al. Imidapril improves L-NAME-exacerbated nephrosclerosis with TGF-beta 1 inhibition in spontaneously hypertensive rats. J Hypertens 2004; 22: 1389–95.
181. Singhal PC, Gibbons N, Franki N et al. Simulated glomerular hypertension promotes mesangial cell apoptosis and expression of cathepsin-B and SGP-2. J Investig Med 1998; 46: 42–50.
182. Mooney A, Jackson K, Bacon R et al. Type IV collagen and laminin regulate glomerular mesangial cell susceptibility to apoptosis via beta(1) integrin-mediated survival signals. Am J Pathol 1999; 155: 599–606.
183. Singhal PC, Franki N, Kumari S et al. Extracellular matrix modulates mesangial cell apoptosis and mRNA expression of cathepsin-B and tissue transglutaminase. J Cell Biochem 1998; 68: 22–30.
184. Kitamura H, Shimizu A, Masuda Y et al. Apoptosis in glomerular endothelial cells during the development of glomerulosclerosis in the remnant-kidney model. Exp Nephrol 1998; 6: 328–36.
185. Yamanaka N, Shimizu A. Role of glomerular endothelial damage in progressive renal disease. Kidney Blood Press Res 1999; 22: 13–20.
186. Bhaskaran M, Reddy K, Radhakrishanan N et al. Angiotensin II induces apoptosis in renal proximal tubular cells. Am J Physiol Renal Physiol 2003; 284: F955–F965.
187. Quiroz Y, Bravo J, Herrera-Acosta J et al. Apoptosis and NFkappaB activation are simultaneously induced in renal tubulointerstitium in experimental hypertension. Kidney Int Suppl 2003; S27–S32.
188. Ding G, Reddy K, Kapasi AA et al. Angiotensin II induces apoptosis in rat glomerular epithelial cells. Am J Physiol Renal Physiol 2002; 283: F173–F180.
189. Durvasula RV, Petermann AT, Hiromura K et al. Activation of a local tissue angiotensin system in podocytes by mechanical strain. Kidney Int 2004; 65: 30–9.
190. Lodha S, Dani D, Mehta R et al. Angiotensin II-induced mesangial cell apoptosis: role of oxidative stress. Mol Med 2002; 8: 830–40.
191. Wolf G, Chen S, Ziyadeh FN. From the periphery of the glomerular capillary wall toward the center of disease: podocyte injury comes of age in diabetic nephropathy. Diabetes 2005; 54: 1626–34.
192. Aizawa T, Ishizaka N, Kurokawa K et al. Different effects of angiotensin II and catecholamine on renal cell apoptosis and proliferation in rats. Kidney Int 2001; 59: 645–53.
193. Kriz W. Podocytes as a target for treatment with ACE inhibitors and/or angiotensin-receptor blockers. Kidney Int 2004; 65: 333–4.
194. Chao J, Chao L. Kallikrein-kinin in stroke, cardiovascular and renal disease. Exp Physiol 2005; 90: 291–8.
195. Inada H, Ono H, Minami J et al. Nipradilol prevents L-NAME-exacerbated nephrosclerosis with decreasing of caspase-3 expression in SHR. Hypertens Res 2002; 25: 433–40.
196. Watanabe S, Ono H, Ishimitsu T et al. Calcium antagonist inhibits glomerular cell apoptosis and injuries of L-NAME exacerbated nephrosclerosis in SHR. Hypertens Res 2000; 23: 683–91.
197. Zhou X, Ono H, Ono Y et al. N- and L-type calcium channel antagonist improves glomerular dynamics, reverses severe nephrosclerosis, and inhibits apoptosis and proliferation in an l-NAME/SHR model. J Hypertens 2002; 20: 993–1000.
198. Ono Y, Ono H, Frohlich ED. Hydrochlorothiazide exacerbates nitric oxide-blockade nephrosclerosis with glomerular hypertension in spontaneously hypertensive rats. J Hypertens 1996; 14: 823–8.
199. Bridgewater DJ, Ho J, Sauro V et al. Insulin-like growth factors inhibit podocyte apoptosis through the PI3 kinase pathway. Kidney Int 2005; 67: 1308–14.
200. Foster RR, Saleem MA, Mathieson PW et al. Vascular endothelial growth factor and nephrin interact and reduce apoptosis in human podocytes. Am J Physiol Renal Physiol 2005; 288: F48–F57.

32

Na,K-ATPase inhibitors in hypertension

John M Hamlyn

INTRODUCTION

In the USA, hypertension affects over 60 million adults and, depending on diagnostic criteria, the risk of developing hypertension for otherwise normotensive adults aged 55 years has been estimated as 60–90%. Much has been learned about the epidemiology and treatment of hypertension and many mechanisms involved in blood pressure control have been identified; yet there is little or no compelling evidence that abnormalities in one or more of the currently identified mechanisms can explain a significant portion of essential hypertension. This chapter presents a brief overview of the sodium pump-sodium calcium exchange-hypertension hypothesis and recent developments that now suggest that the linked functions of a circulating cardiac glycoside steroid and two membrane transporters participate in the etiology of salt-sensitive essential hypertension.

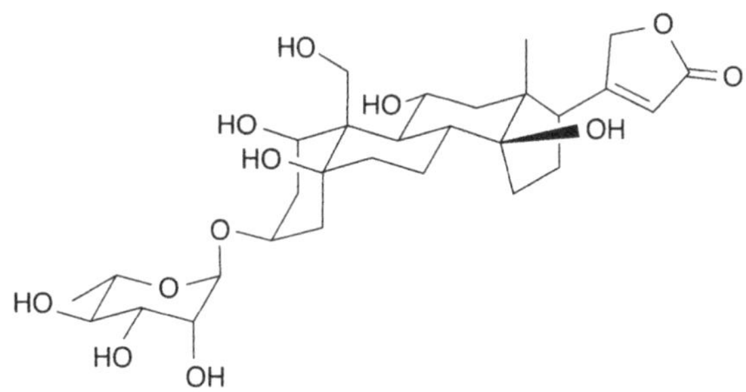

Figure 32.1 The structure of ouabain. Note the β oriented hydroxyl groups at positions 5 and 14, the 3-0 linked sugar L-rhamnose, and the β oriented lactone ring at position 19. These features contribute critically to the ability of ouabain to inhibit the sodium-potassium pump with high affinity, whereas only some of the aforementioned features influence its hypertensinogenic activity

THE SODIUM POTASSIUM PUMP (NA PUMP)

Most mammalian cells use plasma membrane Na pumps to maintain low intracellular sodium and high cell potassium concentrations. The pump couples the free energy from ATP hydrolysis to ion translocation. Normally, three sodium ions are pumped out of the cell in exchange for two entering potassium ions and the transported ions move against their respective electrochemical gradients. The Na pump is comprised of α and β subunits and a third (γ) subunit of low molecular weight is present in the kidney. The α subunit exists in four isoforms (1–4) encoded by four chromosomally dispersed genes and directly mediates ion movement, ATP hydrolysis, and the binding of cardiac glycosides[1] (Figure 32.1) and their signaling effects.[2] The α-4 subunit is expressed in sperm and is unlikely to have any role in cardiovascular regulation and α-1 is expressed by most mammalian cells and has a housekeeping function. The α-2 and α-3 isoforms are co-expressed with α-1 primarily in muscle (including arterial myocytes) and nerve, respectively. The α-3 isoform is relevant to a number of neurological disorders while the peripheral α-2 isoform is likely to be relevant to long-term cardiovascular function in adult mammals.

THE NA PUMP IN HYPERTENSION

A link between diminished Na pump activity and experimental hypertension was proposed by Haddy and colleagues in 1976.[3] The first comprehensive and compelling mechanism linking humoral Na pump inhibitors with arterial Na pump activity, cellular calcium metabolism and hypertension was proposed a year later by Blaustein.[4] The Blaustein hypothesis was extraordinarily specific; it proposed distinct roles for three molecular entities that together elevated both the cytoplasmic calcium concentration and the tone of arterial myocytes in a manner predicted to cause hypertension. The components of this molecular trinity included: 1) a circulating material that, analogous to ouabain, depressed active Na extrusion; 2) a vascular myocyte ouabain-sensitive Na pump; 3) a membrane transport system that specifically exchanged sodium for calcium ions and that translated the effects of reduced Na pump activity into changes in arterial diameter via calcium ions. Figure 32.2 includes the key molecular elements of the original 1977 hypothesis and the role of recently described pharmacological agents. At the time of the hypothesis the evidence for the humoral factor was sparse; the chemical nature would remain unknown for another 15 years. In addition, the existence of a vascular sodium calcium exchanger was in doubt[5] and there was evidence that clinically relevant Na pump inhibitors actually lowered blood pressure in some patients with essential hypertension.[6] These apparently insurmountable problems now have solutions.

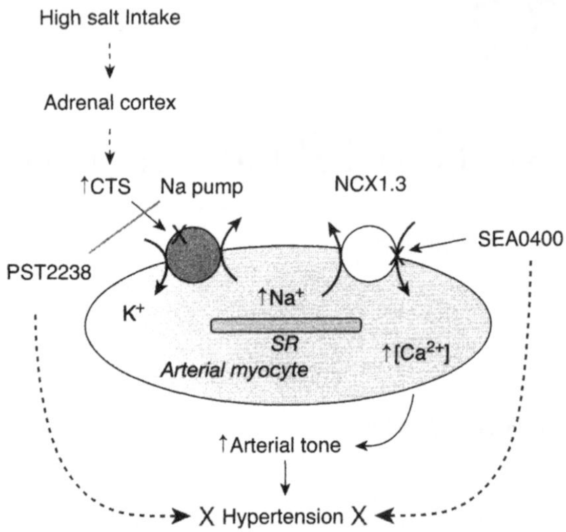

Figure 32.2 Mechanism of the long-term increase in vascular tone in salt-sensitive hypertension. Chronic high salt intake stimulates an increase in circulating cardiotonic steroids secreted by the adrenal gland. Inhibition of the α-2 isoform of the Na pump leads to an increase in sub-plasmalemmal sodium (Na^+) concentration, stimulates the reverse mode NCX-1.3-mediated influx of calcium ions (Ca^{2+}) and thereby elevates arterial tone and blood pressure. NCX1.3, vascular myocyte form of the sodium calcium exchanger; SEA0400, a selective inhibitor of NCX1.3 that blocks Ca^{2+} entry; PST2238, a synthetic furane analog of digitoxigenin that antagonizes the interaction of ouabain with the Na pumps

The primary evidence initially linking Na pump inhibitors with high blood pressure was the depression of active sodium transport that occurred when boiled plasma supernatants from animals with hypertension were applied to isolated vascular preparations. Typically, the plasma from rats with sodium- and volume-sensitive forms of hypertension depressed Na pump-mediated Rb (rubidium) fluxes.[3] Usually, the depression of the ion flux was modest (10–25%), and this now seems compatible with the ratio (4:1) of the ouabain-sensitive α-2 and ouabain-insensitive α-1 Na pump isoforms in rat conduit arteries.[7] Subsequent measurements of Na pump inhibitors used commercial antibodies raised against digoxin because they often cross-reacted with unknown materials ('false positives') in the circulation of individuals with no known intake of digitalis.[8] In general, higher levels of digoxin-like immunoreactivity did not appear to be linked with hypertension unless renal failure was co-present,[9] whereas ouabain immunocross-reactive materials were correlated with blood pressure in patients with aldosterone-secreting tumors.[10–12] Later assay methods led to more reliable estimates in the circulation and tissues[10–16] and in 1991 endogenous ouabain (EO) was identified as the first link in the chain that links Na pump activity with hypertension.[17]

Two in vivo tissue targets have been suggested for EO. Circulating EO may enter the central nervous system and thereby increase peripheral sympathetic nerve activity and blood pressure.[18] In contrast, the Blaustein hypothesis envisages that vascular myocytes are the primary target for EO. There is evidence for a role for both targets, although recent work appears to favor a vascular mechanism. In vascular myocytes, the membrane distribution of the highly ouabain-sensitive α-2 isoform (originally suggested to be α-3) is clustered in microdomains where the underlying endoplasmic reticulum approaches the plasmalemma.[7] Inhibition of the ouabain-sensitive α-2 Na pumps affects myocyte calcium homeostasis.[19] As ouabain failed to induce hypertension in transgenic animals in which the α-2 isoform of the Na pump was rendered ouabain-insensitive,[20] the α-2 isoform of the Na pump is a critical link between ouabain and hypertension. High ouabain sensitivity is thus a crucial property of α-2 and it is of interest that the long-term hemodynamic consequences (i.e. hypertension) of reduced α-2 expression are the same as those induced by low dose ouabain.[21]

Because the pituitary hormone ACTH is a powerful stimulus for the adrenocortical secretion of corticosteroids and EO in rats, cattle and humans,[22–25] it is of great interest that ACTH induces hypertension in animals with ouabain-sensitive α-2 Na pump isoforms (i.e. the wild-type) but not in their ouabain-insensitive α-2 counterparts (J.B. Lingrel, personal communication). As the classical adrenocortical steroids do not interact with the ouabain binding site, the induction and maintenance of ACTH hypertension apparently depends critically upon Na pump inhibitors that originate from the adrenal cortex.

THE ROLE OF SODIUM CALCIUM EXCHANGE (NCX) IN HYPERTENSION

The phenomenon of sodium calcium exchange was described in 1969.[26] Subsequently, the exchanger was cloned[27] and is a family of three genes (NCX1–3). Each gene is expressed in a tissue-specific manner with alternative splicing variants. Vascular smooth muscle expresses the NCX1 isoform[28] with specific splice variants (e.g. NCX1.3 and NCX1.7) that are highly sensitive to the inhibitor SEA0400.[29] Recently, a series of seminal observations were made concerning the critical role of the vascular NCX1 in virtually all forms of salt-dependent hypertension[30] and the mechanism by which ouabain elevates arterial tone. The selective NCX1 inhibitor, SEA0400, was an effective antihypertensive in salt- and ouabain-dependent forms of hypertension. This showed that the 'reverse' mode of NCX1 operated in vascular myocytes in vivo to deliver the calcium that elevated the blood pressure. Further, the antihypertensive specificity of SEA0400 in vivo was proven by the absence of cardiovascular effects in transgenic animals in which the otherwise normal NCX1 bore a mutation that prevented drug binding to the transporter. In addition, in NCX1 heterozygote animals in which the vascular expression of NCX1 was genetically reduced, blood pressure remained normal and was salt-insensitive. In contrast, salt sensitivity and hypertension occurred in the NCX1 overexpressors. Collectively, these observations leave little doubt concerning the key role of the vascular form of NCX1 as a primary calcium influx pathway in salt-sensitive and ouabain-dependent hypertension.

MULTIPLE Na PUMP INHIBITORS?

The search for Na pump inhibitors revealed four specific inhibitors in the human circulation.[31] To date, only the most biologically active of the circulating materials (i.e. EO) has been identified[14,17] and this same material has been isolated from brain and the adrenal glands.[32–34] The nature of the three unidentified materials in human plasma remains unknown; they may represent biosynthetic intermediates in the EO pathway that have biological activity and that are secreted by the adrenal gland. Steroids that resemble digoxin, proscillaridin, bufalin, resibufagenin, telocinobufagin, and marinobufagenin have also been described in mammalian tissues.[34–41] The origin of some of these materials and their relationship to the above-mentioned circulating materials is not clear. One of the latter materials has also been linked with sodium-sensitive experimental hypertension, essential hypertension, and heart failure.[29,40,41]

ELEVATED EO IN HYPERTENSION

Increased plasma EO was observed in ~55% of patients with adrenocortical tumors causing aldosterone excess[42] and circulating EO is also elevated in states of sustained positive sodium balance including congestive heart failure[43] and chronic renal failure.[44] Circulating levels of EO are increased 30–200% in many forms of hypertension including essential hypertension.[10–12,42,44–48] Analysis of the distribution of plasma EO in essential hypertension showed that between ~45 and 50% of untreated patients exhibited elevated circulating levels. Multiple regression analyses revealed significant relationships among blood pressure, body mass index, age, and EO, whereas these parameters were not associated with plasma renin activity or aldosterone.[42,47,48] A relationship between plasma EO and peripheral vascular resistance across many different pathological and physiological conditions is evident, suggesting that the primary long-term action of EO is to raise the effective filling pressure of the circulation. Hence, the mechanisms that underlie the elevated EO in essential hypertension and its long-term pressor actions are of considerable medical significance.

DOES ELEVATED EO CAUSE HYPERTENSION?

The prolonged peripheral administration of ouabain induces sustained hypertension in the rat.[18,49,50] Typically, a prehypertensive period lasting 1–2 weeks is followed by the development of a normal renin form of hypertension characterized by increased total peripheral resistance (TPR).[49] Maneuvers that increase sodium retention, such as the surgical reduction of renal mass, augment the hypertensinogenic effect of ouabain in the rat[50] and co-administration of subpressor amounts of aldosterone and digoxin induce sustained hypertension in sheep;[51] similar results occur in rats given mineralocorticoids with ouabain.[52] The amplification of the hypertensinogenic impact of exogenous Na pump inhibitors probably results from the combination of increased actual volume in a circulation where the effective filling pressure is already raised by a vasoconstrictor mechanism.

The steady-state circulating concentrations of ouabain needed to raise blood pressure in rats are remarkably low – ranging between 1 and 5 nmoles/L[49] and similar to the plasma levels of EO measured in some patients with essential hypertension with the same assay.[42] The hypertension is fully reversible. Across the inbred Dahl rat strains, the circulating levels of EO are correlated with blood pressure.[53] In Dahl SS/jr, plasma EO is elevated and does not change with a high salt intake whereas Dahl SR/jr rats are resistant to EO and ouabain. Dahl SS/jr rats with active immunity against ouabain develop lower blood pressures when salt-fed,[54] while immunization was less effective in preventing reduced renal mass/saline hypertension.[55]

In normal and hypertensive humans, the acute administration of cardiac glycosides evokes transient increases of blood pressure and augments the pressor response to vasoactive agents.[56–59] In patients with compromised short-term cardiovascular reflexes, acute administration of ouabain raises blood pressure dramatically.[59–61] The effects of prolonged administration of ouabain in humans are not described but it may be inappropriate to assume that the same conclusions from the experience with digitalis glycosides apply. For example, the prolonged use of digitalis glycosides does not induce sustained hypertension in man or in various animals,[6,42] and digitalis preparations normalize blood pressure in rats with ouabain-induced hypertension[62] and in certain patients with essential hypertension.[6] Moreover, the synthetic furane ring aglycone analog of digitoxin, PST2238, which was developed as a receptor antagonist of ouabain, lowers blood pressure in ouabain-induced hypertension[63] and in a large portion of patients with essential hypertension (P. Ferrari, personal communication). Similarly, the reduction of EO in humans with digoxin antibody fragments (that bind ouabain and EO with moderate affinity[64]) lowers blood pressure in hypertensive rats and eclamptic women.[65–69] Conversely, hypersecretion of EO by adrenocortical tumors is invariably associated with hypertension,[11,12,42,45,70] which can be corrected by either surgery or therapy. Collectively, these studies imply that there is a direct and meaningful relationship between circulating EO and blood pressure in humans and also that the cardiovascular actions of digitalis glycosides and its analogs are diametrically opposite to ouabain and EO.

SUMMARY

The etiology of salt-sensitive hypertension appears to involve a molecular trinity comprised of EO, and specific vascular isoforms of the Na pump and the sodium calcium exchanger. The coordinated function of this molecular trinity has long-term direct effects on vascular tone and peripheral resistance and will likely be a fruitful target for novel therapeutic agents.

ACKNOWLEDGMENTS

This work was supported in part by NIH Award HL075584.

REFERENCES

1. Blanco G, Mercer RW. Isozymes of the Na-K-ATPase: heterogeneity in structure, diversity in function. Am J Physiol 1998; 275 (5 Pt 2): F633–F650.
2. Xie Z, Askari A. Na^+/K^+-ATPase as a signal transducer. Eur J Biochem 2002; 269: 2434–9.
3. Haddy FJ, Overbeck H. The role of humoral agents in volume expanded hypertension. Life Sci 1976; 19: 935–48.
4. Blaustein MP. Sodium ions, calcium ions, blood pressure regulation, and hypertension: a reassessment and a hypothesis. Am J Physiol 1977; 232: C165–C173.
5. Mulvany MJ, Aalkjaer C, Jensen PE. Sodium-calcium exchange in vascular smooth muscle. Ann N Y Acad Sci 1991; 639: 498–504.
6. Abarquez RF. Digitalis in the treatment of hypertension, a preliminary report. Acta Med Philipp 1967; 3: 161–70.
7. Juhaszova M, Blaustein MP. Na^+ pump low and high ouabain affinity alpha subunit isoforms are differently distributed in cells. Proc Natl Acad Sci U S A 1997; 94: 1800–5.
8. Gruber KA, Whitaker JM, Buckalew VM Jr. Endogenous digitalis-like substance in plasma of volume-expanded dogs. Nature 1980; 287: 743–5.
9. Tzou MC, Reuning RH, Sams RA. Quantitation of interference in digoxin immunoassay in renal, hepatic, and diabetic disease. Clin Pharmacol Ther 1997; 61: 429–41.
10. Masugi F, Ogihara T, Hasegawa T et al. Ouabain and non-ouabain-like factors in plasma of patients with essential hypertension. Clin Exp Hypertens 1987; A9: 1233–42.
11. Masugi F, Ogihara T, Hasegawa T et al. Normalization of high plasma level of ouabain-like immunoreactivity in primary aldosteronism after removal of adrenals. J Hum Hypertens 1988; 2: 409–20.
12. Masugi F, Ogihara T, Hasegawa T et al. Circulating factor with ouabain-like immunoreactivity in patients with primary aldosteronism. Biochem Biophys Res Commun 1986; 135: 41–5.

13. Hamlyn JM, Ringel R, Schaeffer J et al. A circulating inhibitor of $(Na^{+}+K^{+})$ATPase associated with essential hypertension. Nature 1982; 300: 650–2.
14. Hamlyn JM, Harris DW, Ludens JH. Digitalis-like activity in human plasma: purification, affinity and mechanism. J Biol Chem 1989; 264: 7395–404.
15. Goto A, Yamada K, Ishii M et al. Digitalis-like activity in human plasma: relation to blood pressure and sodium balance. Am J Med 1990; 89: 420–6.
16. Goto A, Yamada K, Yagi N et al. Digoxin-like immunoreactivity: is it still worth measuring? Life Sci 1991; 49: 1667–78.
17. Hamlyn JM, Blaustein MP, Bova S et al. Identification and characterization of a ouabain-like compound from human plasma. Proc Natl Acad Sci U S A 1991; 88: 6259–63.
18. Huang BS, Huang X, Harmsen E et al. Chronic versus peripheral ouabain, BP and sympathetic activity in rats. Hypertension 1994; 23 (Pt 2): 1087–90.
19. Golovina VA, Song H, James PF et al. Na^{+} pump α2-subunit expression modulates Ca^{2+} signaling. Am J Physiol Cell Physiol 2003; 284: C475–C486.
20. Dostanic I, Paul RJ, Lorenz JN et al. The α2-isoform of Na-K-ATPase mediates ouabain-induced hypertension in mice and increased vascular contractility in vitro. Am J Physiol Heart Circ Physiol 2005; 288: H477–H485.
21. Zhang J, Chen L, Lee MY et al. Reduced expression of Na pumps with α-2 but not α-1 subunits increases myogenic tone and blood pressure. FASEB J 19: abstract 914.16.
22. Goto A, Yamada K, Hazama H et al. Ouabainlike compound in hypertension associated with ectopic corticotrophin syndrome. Hypertension 1996; 28: 421–5.
23. Yamada K, Goto A, Omata M. Adrenocorticotropin-induced hypertension in rats: role of ouabain-like compound. Am J Hypertens 1997; 10 (4 Pt 1): 403–8.
24. Laredo J, Hamilton BP, Hamlyn JM. Ouabain is secreted by bovine adrenocortical cells. Endocrinology 1994; 135: 794–7.
25. Sophocleous A, Elmatzoglou I, Souvatzoglou A. Circulating endogenous digitalis-like factor(s) (EDLF) in man is derived from the adrenals and its secretion is ACTH-dependent. J Endocrinol Invest 2003; 26: 668–74.
26. Baker PF, Blaustein MP, Hodgkin AL et al. The influence of calcium on sodium efflux in squid axons. J Physiol 1969; 200: 431–58.
27. Komuro I, Wenninger KE, Philipson KD et al. Molecular cloning and characterization of the human cardiac Na^{+}/Ca^{2+} exchanger cDNA. Proc Natl Acad Sci U S A 1992; 89: 4769–73.
28. Nakasaki Y, Iwamoto T, Hanada H et al. Cloning of the rat aortic smooth muscle Na^{+}/Ca^{2+} exchanger and tissue-specific expression of isoforms. J Biochem (Tokyo) 1993; 114: 528–34.
29. Iwamoto T, Kita S, Uehara A et al. Molecular determinants of Na^{+}/Ca^{2+} exchange (NCX1) inhibition by SEA0400. J Biol Chem 2004; 279: 7544–53.
30. Iwamoto T, Kita S, Zhang J et al. Salt-sensitive hypertension is triggered by Ca^{2+} entry via Na^{+}/Ca^{2+} exchanger type-1 in vascular smooth muscle. Nat Med 2004; 10: 1193–9.
31. Harris DW, Clark MA, Fisher JF et al. Development of an immunoassay for endogenous digitalis-like factor. Hypertension 1991; 17: 936–43.
32. Kawamura A, Guo J, Itagaki Y et al. On the structure of endogenous ouabain. Proc Natl Acad Sci U S A 1999; 96: 6654–9.
33. Tymiak AA, Norman JA, Bolgar M et al. Physicochemical characterization of a ouabain isomer isolated from bovine hypothalamus. Proc Natl Acad Sci U S A 1993; 90: 8189–93.
34. Schneider R, Wray V, Nimtz M et al. Bovine adrenals contain, in addition to ouabain, a second inhibitor of the sodium pump. J Biol Chem 1998; 273: 784–92.
35. Qazzaz HM, Cao Z, Bolanowski DD et al. De novo biosynthesis and radiolabeling of mammalian digitalis-like factors. Clin Chem 2004; 50: 612–20.
36. Lichtstein D, Kachalsky S, Deutsch J. Identification of a ouabain-like compound in toad skin and plasma as a bufodieneolide derivative. Life Sci 1986; 38: 1261–70.
37. Lichtstein D, Gati I, Samuelov S et al. Identification of digitalis-like compounds in human cataractous lenses. Eur J Biochem 1993; 216: 261–8.
38. Komiyama Y, Dong XH, Nishimura N et al. A novel endogenous digitalis, telocinobufagin, exhibits elevated plasma levels in patients with terminal renal failure. Clin Biochem 2005; 38: 36–45.
39. Fedorova OV, Kolodkin NI, Agalakova NI et al. Antibody to marinobufagenin lowers blood pressure in pregnant rats on a high NaCl intake. J Hypertens 2005; 23: 835–42.
40. Bagrov AY, Fedorova OV, Dmitrieva RI et al. Characterization of a urinary bufodienolide Na+,K+-ATPase inhibitor in patients after acute myocardial infarction. Hypertension 1998; 31: 1097–103.
41. Fedorova OV, Talan MI, Agalakova NI et al. Endogenous ligand of alpha(1) sodium pump, marinobufagenin, is a novel mediator of sodium chloride-dependent hypertension. Circulation 2002; 105: 1122–7.
42. Rossi GP, Manunta P, Hamlyn JM et al. Endogenous ouabain in primary aldosteronism and essential hypertension: relationship with plasma renin, aldosterone and blood pressure. J Hypertens 1995; 13: 1181–91.
43. Gottlieb SS, Rogowski AC, Weinberg M et al. Elevated concentrations of endogenous ouabain in patients with congestive heart failure. Circulation 1992; 86: 420–5.
44. Schaeffer JS, Talartschik J, Koch KM et al. Increased plasma levels of ouabain-like compound in dialysis patients: relationship with interdialytic volume changes. J Am Soc Nephrol 1991; 2: 348 (abstract 34P).
45. Manunta P, Evans G, Hamilton BP et al. A new syndrome with elevated plasma ouabain and hypertension secondary to an adrenocortical tumor. J Hypertens 1992; 10: S27 (abstract P36).
46. Goto A, Yamada K, Yagi N et al. Novel concepts on the roles of ouabain-like compound (OLC) in hypertension. J Hypertens 1992; 10 (Suppl 4): S50 (abstract P52).
47. Manunta P, Stella P, Rivera R et al. Left ventricular mass, stroke volume, and ouabain-like factor in essential hypertension. Hypertension 1999; 34: 450–6.
48. Pierdomenico SD, Bucci A, Manunta P et al. Endogenous ouabain and hemodynamic and left ventricular geometric patterns in essential hypertension. Am J Hypertens 2001; 14: 44–50.
49. Manunta P, Rogowski AC, Hamilton BP, Hamlyn JM. Ouabain-induced hypertension in the rat: relationships among circulating and tissue ouabain and blood pressure. J Hypertens 1994; 12: 549–60.
50. Yuan C, Manunta P, Hamlyn JM et al. Chronic ouabain administration produces hypertension in rats. Hypertension 1993; 22: 178–87.
51. Spence CD, Coghlan JP, Whitworth JA et al. Digoxin administration enhances the pressor response to aldosterone administration in conscious sheep. Clin Exp Pharmacol Physiol 1989 16: 211–22.
52. Sekihara H, Yazaki Y, Kojima T. Ouabain as an amplifier of mineralocorticoid-induced hypertension. Endocrinology 1992; 131: 3077–82.
53. Lighthall GK, Manunta P, Hamlyn JM. Increased circulating ouabain in Dahl SS/JR rats. J Hypertens 1994; 12: S158 (abstract 870).
54. Gomez-Sanchez EP, Gomez-Sanchez CE, Fort C. Immunization of Dahl SS/jr rats with an ouabain conjugate mitigates hypertension. Am J Hypertens 1994; 7: 591–6.

55. Yamada K, Goto A, Nagoshi H et al. Participation of ouabainlike compound in reduced renal mass-saline hypertension. Hypertension 1994; 23 (Suppl I): I-110–13.
56. Pidgeon GB, Richards AM, Nicholls MG et al. Acute effects of intravenous ouabain in healthy volunteers. Clin Sci 1994; 86: 391–7.
57. Cappuccio FP, Markandu ND, Sagnella GA et al. The effect of oral digoxin on sodium excretion, renin-angiotensin-aldosterone system and blood pressure in normotensive subjects. Postgrad Med J 1986; 62: 265–8.
58. Guthrie GP Jr. Effects of digoxin on responsiveness to the pressor actions of angiotensin and norepinephrine in man. J Clin Endocrinol Metab 1984; 58: 76–80.
59. Mason DT, Braunwald E. Studies on digitalis. X. Effects of ouabain on forearm vascular resistance and venous tone in normal subjects and in patients in heart failure. J Clin Invest 1964; 43: 532–43.
60. Kumar R, Yankopoulos NA, Abelman WH. Ouabain-induced hypertension in a patient with decompensated hypertensive heart disease. Chest 1973; 63: 105–7.
61. Ross J, Waldhausen JA, Braunwald E. Studies on digitalis I: direct effects on peripheral vascular resistance. J Clin Invest 1960; 39: 930–8.
62. Manunta P, Rogowski AC, Hamilton BP, Hamlyn JM. Chronic reversible hypertension in rats induced by ouabain but not digoxin. Hypertension 1992; 20: 404 (abstract 30).
63. Ferrari P, Torielli L, Ferrandi M et al. PST2238: a new antihypertensive compound that antagonizes the long-term pressor effect of ouabain. J Pharmacol Exp Ther 1998; 285: 83–94.
64. Pullen MA, Brooks DP, Edwards RM. Characterization of the neutralizing activity of digoxin-specific Fab toward ouabain-like steroids. J Pharmacol Exp Ther 2004; 310: 319–25.
65. Goodlin RC. Antidigoxin antibodies in eclampsia. N Engl J Med 1988; 318: 518–19.
66. Kunes J, Stolba P, Pohlova I et al. The importance of endogenous digoxin-like factors in rats with various forms of experimental hypertension. Clin Exp Hypertens 1985; 7: 707–20.
67. Huang CT, Smith RM. Lowering of blood pressure in chronic aortic coarctate hypertensive rats with digoxin antiserum. Life Sci 1984; 35: 115–18.
68. Mann JFE, Miemitz R, Ganten U et al. Haemodynamic effects of intact digoxin antibody and its Fab fragments in experimental hypertension. J Hypertension 1987; 5: 543–9.
69. Balzan S, Montali U, Biver P et al. Digoxin-binding antibodies reverse the effect of endogenous digitalis-like compounds on Na,K-ATPase in erythrocytes. J Hypertens 1991; 9 (Suppl 6): S304–S305.
70. Komiyama Y, Nishimura N, Munakata M et al. Increases in plasma ouabainlike immunoreactivity during surgical extirpation of pheochromocytoma. Hypertens Res 1999; 22: 135–9.

33

Oxidative events in cell and vascular biology

David G Harrison and Sergey Dikalov

INTRODUCTION

The earth formed approximately 4.5 billion years ago and unicellular organisms, which received their nutrients from surrounding media, appeared approximately one billion years later.[1] It has been estimated that the earth was anoxic for at least 2 billion years. Around 2.3 billion years ago, there was a sudden increase in oxygen in the oceans and atmosphere. It is thought that the first photosynthetic organisms, cyanobacteria, were responsible for this 'great oxidation event'; however, there was also depletion of other gases, such as methane and hydrogen, which permitted oxygen to accumulate.[2] The appearance of oxygen on the surface of the earth subsequently triggered the development of complex multicellular organisms that could utilize oxygen.[3] The symbiotic relationship that subsequently evolved between plants and animals served both kingdoms well in the ensuing millions of years; however, a very complex biology arose as a result of this dependence on oxygen. Prokaryotic and eukaryotic cells adapted small molecules as antioxidants and developed enzymes that produce, scavenge and utilize reactive oxygen species (ROS) and other enzymes that can repair oxidative damage. Interestingly, some of these enzymes are highly preserved from bacteria to man, supporting the concept that the co-existence with oxygen metabolites has been essential for millions of years. Further and not well understood, eukaryotic cells have begun to use ROS and their targets as signaling molecules. This latter phenomenon has radically changed our view and treatment of oxidative injury, because we now realize that removal of all oxygen metabolites could have untoward effects.

REACTIVE OXYGEN SPECIES

The term reactive oxygen species has been adapted to refer to oxygen metabolites likely to participate in oxidation/reduction reactions. Some ROS, illustrated in Table 33.1, possess unpaired electrons in their outer electronic orbital and are therefore free radicals, while others do not contain unpaired electrons; however, they are prone to accept or donate electrons and are therefore 'reactive'.

Table 33.1 Reactive oxygen species

Oxygen radicals		*Oxygen species*	
$^•OH$	hydroxyl	ONOOH	peroxynitrous acid
R-O$^•$	alkoxyl	$ONOO^-$	peroxynitrite
Aryl-O$^•$	phenoxyl	$Fe^{IV}=O$	ferryl
R-OO$^•$	peroxyl	$^1O_2$	singlet oxygen
$HO_2^•$	hydroperoxyl	HOCl	hypochloric acid
$O_2^{•-}$	superoxide	LOOH	lipid peroxide
$NO^•$	nitric oxide	H_2O_2	hydrogen peroxide

Reactivity is decreasing from the top to the bottom of the table.

According to quantum chemistry, electrons are located on atomic orbitals (s, p, d...) with distinct energy levels, such that the electrons can absorb or release a discrete quantum of energy. In compound molecules, there are respective molecular orbitals (σ, π, δ...).[4] The majority of radicals relevant to cell biology contain unpaired electrons in their σ or π orbitals. Sigma orbitals have their major electron density on the axis connecting two atoms, while π orbitals have most of their electron density adjacent to the bond axis and not localized to one atom, but are distributed throughout the molecule (Figure 33.1). Because of this, free radicals containing an uncoupled electron on the σ orbital will gain substantial energy by acquiring an additional electron in that σ orbital. This makes oxygen- and carbon-centered radicals, like hydroxyl ($^•OH$), alkoxyl (R-O$^•$) and alkyl (R$^•$) radicals, very reactive and capable of causing lipid and

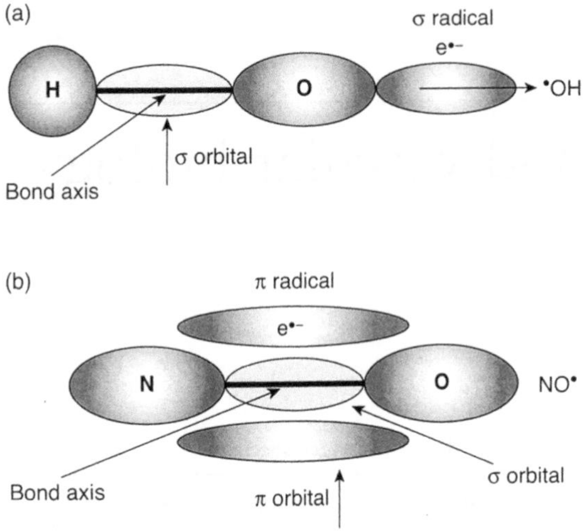

Figure 33.1 Comparison of pi and sigma radicals. Note locations of the σ and π orbitals. (a) A schematic diagram of the hydroxyl radical. The location of the σ radical is along the bond axis. (b) A schematic diagram of nitric oxide (NO) with its unpaired electron in the π orbital, which is delocalized

protein damage. Due to this property, the oxygen-centered σ radicals $^{\bullet}OH$ and R-O• react with numerous targets and there are not antioxidants that specifically target them. Thus, carbon-centered (R-C•), sulfur-centered (R-S•) and nitrogen-centered (R-N•) σ radicals can be scavenged by antioxidants such as glutathione and ascorbate, although these reactions are not specific.

In contrast, superoxide and nitric oxide are π radicals. Likewise, many antioxidants like ascorbate, α-tocopherol, uric acid and flavanoids donate an electron to scavenge radicals and in this process are left with an unpaired electron in their π orbital. This unpaired electron in the π orbital is distributed throughout the molecule rather than being restricted to a single atom (Figure 33.1). In this case the electron is delocalized. This reduces its reactivity and prevents the antioxidant radical from being pro-oxidant.

Thus, the reactivity of radicals depends not only on their core structure, but also on the nature of their unpaired electron(s). Radicals with unpaired electrons in the σ orbital (•OH, RO•, L•) are more reactive than those with electrons in the π orbital ($O_2^{\bullet-}$, NO•). When the unpaired electron is distributed throughout the molecule on the π orbital (delocalized), the radical is relatively less reactive. This is the case for the ascorbyl (vitamin C) radical, the phenoxy- (vitamin E) semiquinone radical, and the cation radical of compound I, which exists in

Table 33.2 Redox couples and the respective one electron reduction potentials

Couple	*E° (mV)*
$^{\bullet}OH/H_2O$	2310
RO•/ROH (aliphatic alkoxyl)	1600
$ONOO^-/NO_2^{\bullet}$	1400
$NO^+/NO^{\bullet}$	1210
$HO_2^{\bullet}/H_2O_2$	1060
ROO•/ROOH	1000
$NO_2^{\bullet}/NO_2^-$	990
HRP-II/HRP	970
$O_2^{\bullet-}/H_2O_2$	940
$RS^{\bullet}/RS^-$ (cysteine)	920
$^1O_2/O_2^{\bullet-}$	650
L•/L-H (polyunsaturated fatty acid)	600
$HU^{\bullet-}/UH_2$ (urate)	590
α-Tocopheroxyl/α-tocopherol	500
Trolox C (TO•/TO-H)	480
$H_2O_2/^{\bullet}OH$	320
Ascorbate•/ascorbate	282
$O_2/O_2^{\bullet-}$	–160
RSSR/RSSR•	–1500
$CO_2/CO_2^{\bullet}$	–1800

From Buettner et al., Arch Biochem Biophys 1993;[5] used with permission from Dr Buettner and Elsevier Science.

activated forms of myeloperoxidase and cytochrome P-450.

Buettner and colleagues have presented and popularized the concept of a 'pecking' order of ROS, which refers to the fact that these possess different one electron reduction potentials.[5] Table 33.2 provides reduction potentials for a variety of biologically relevant ROS. The arrangement is such that the strongest oxidizing agents are at the top, and the strongest reducing agents at the bottom. Thus, any molecule above will oxidize any molecule below it, and alternatively, molecules below will reduce those above. The likelihood that a reaction between two different molecules will occur depends on how widely separated the two respective redox potentials are and the relative concentrations of the two. Thus, even if two molecules have relatively similar redox potentials, if one is present in large excess it can oxidize or reduce another in much lower concentration. Some of the more biologically relevant ROS will be discussed later.

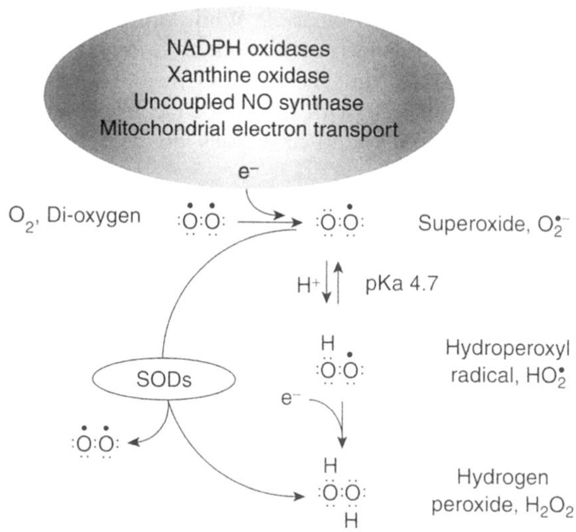

Figure 33.2 Lewis dot diagrams showing sequential reduction of oxygen. A one electron oxidation of oxygen leads to formation of superoxide, which is in equilibrium with the hydroperoxyl radical, although this equilibrium at a physiological pH favors superoxide. The one electron oxidation of hydroperoxyl leads to formation of hydrogen peroxide (H_2O_2). Superoxide dismutases (SODs) utilize two molecules of superoxide to form H_2O_2 and oxygen

Molecular oxygen

Oxygen (O_2) is generally not considered a ROS; however, it possesses two electrons which are unpaired (Figure 33.2), resulting in it being a di-radical. Because of this, oxygen is a mild oxidizing agent. In biology, oxygen readily combines with heme iron in the ferrous (Fe^{2+}) state.

Superoxide ($O_2^{\bullet-}$)

The properties of $O_2^{\bullet-}$ have been extensively reviewed.[6] The one electron reduction of oxygen leads to formation of superoxide. In biological solutions, superoxide exists in equilibrium (pKa 4.7) with the hydroperoxy radical, ($HO_2^{\bullet}$, Figure 33.2). At physiological pH, this equilibrium highly favors the deprotonated form; however, because the hydroperoxy radical is uncharged, it can enter lipid bilayers and can cross cell membranes.

Superoxide can be stored as its salt form (KO_2) and, in fact, $O_2^{\bullet-}$ can be generated in the laboratory by dissolving KO_2 in aqueous solution at physiological pH. Superoxide is also stable in highly alkaline solutions (pH > 14). Its intracellular concentration is minimized by superoxide dismutase (SOD) spontaneous dismutation and its reactivity with other molecules, and its intracellular lifetime has been estimated to be as low as 1 millisecond.

As is evident from its position in the pecking order (Table 33.2), $O_2^{\bullet-}$ is generally an oxidant, but can reduce some molecules. In fact, the classical assay for detection of $O_2^{\bullet-}$ is reduction of cytochrome c. An important reaction of $O_2^{\bullet-}$ is its oxidation of NO. This is covered in the section below on peroxynitrite. In the mitochondria $O_2^{\bullet-}$ can react with the FeS clusters in aconitase leading to release of Fe^{2+} and inactivation of this enzyme. This can lead to loss of energy production and the liberation of iron can cause further radical-mediated damage.[7]

Superoxide is a progenitor of many other ROS. In some cases, it has been difficult to precisely separate an action of $O_2^{\bullet-}$ *per se* vs an effect of an oxidant derived from $O_2^{\bullet-}$. For example, systems that generate $O_2^{\bullet-}$ do not initiate lipid oxidation unless they are in the presence of metals, or if $O_2^{\bullet-}$ is converted to hydrogen peroxide (H_2O_2) in the presence of a peroxidase.[8]

An acceptable approach to implicating $O_2^{\bullet-}$ in a biological process is to show that its effect is diminished or removed by treatment with SOD. This is discussed more completely in the section below on SODs.

Nitric oxide and related compounds

Nitric oxide (NO) is more properly considered a reactive nitrogen species (RNS); however, it is highly reactive with other ROS and plays a crucial role in vascular biology and hypertension. Nitrogen is somewhat unique in that it contains five electrons in its outer valance shell, and therefore, can exist in states ranging from +5 to −3, leading to formation of many different molecules (Table 33.3).[9] NO contains its unpaired electron in the π orbital and is therefore a π radical, and as discussed below, can react rapidly with $O_2^{\bullet-}$.

In mammalian cells, NO is synthesized by one of three isoforms of NO synthase (NOS).[10] In vascular cells, endothelial cells express eNOS or NOS III. The neuronal isoform, nNOS or NOS I has been found in vascular smooth muscle cells and seems to blunt constrictor responses.[11,12] The inducible NOS, iNOS or NOS II, is not normally present, but can be induced by cytokines and bacterial endotoxin and is largely responsible for the hemodynamic consequences of septic shock.[13]

All three isoforms of NOS have reductase domains, which contain binding sites for NADPH and the flavins FAD and FMN. Electrons are shuttled from NADPH to the flavins where they are stored in a p450 reductase-like fashion. Upon calmodulin binding, electrons are then transferred to a heme group in the

Table 33.3 Various oxides of nitrogen

Oxide	*Nitrogen species*	*Properties*
N_2O	Nitrous oxide	Anesthetic
HNO	Nitroxyl	Product of Angell's salt
$N{=}O^{\bullet}$	Nitric oxide	Radical gas, signalling molecule
HONO	Nitrous acid	Product of acidified NO
NO^+	Nitrosonium cation	Nitrosating agent
RS-NO	Nitrosothiol	NO donor/nitrosating agent
$NO_2^{\bullet}$	Nitrogen dioxide radical	Nitrosating agent
NO_2^-	Nitrite	Oxidation product of NO
NO_3^-	Nitrate	Oxidation product of NO

oxygenase domain. Near the heme group are binding sites for tetrahydrobiopterin (BH_4) and L-arginine. BH_4 plays a critical role in allowing transfer of electrons to the guanidino-nitrogens of L-arginine, one of which is ultimately oxidized to NO, forming citrulline as a byproduct.[10]

NO can also be formed non-enzymatically. An often-used trick in the laboratory is to acidify nitrite leading to formation HONO, which via a series of reactions can yield NO and nitrosating molecules (reactions 1–3):

$$NO_2^- + H^+ \leftrightarrow HONO \text{ (reaction 1)}$$

$$HONO + HONO \rightarrow H_2O + N_2O_3\ (NO^+ - NO_2^-) \text{ (reaction 2)}$$

$$N_2O_3 \leftrightarrow NO^{\bullet} + {}^{\bullet}NO_2 \text{ (reaction 3)}$$

There is evidence that these reactions can occur in vivo. In the setting of severe myocardial ischemia, where profound acidosis occurs, NO formation from nitrite has been detected.[14] A potentially very important non-enzymatic mechanism for formation of NO from nitrite involves a reaction with deoxyhemoglobin. In hypoxic regions of the circulation where deoxyhemoglobin is formed, this can serve a physiological role to promote NO formation and vasodilatation.[15]

The best characterized and understood signaling events mediated by NO are due to its reaction with Fe^{2+} in heme centers. In the vessel, the reaction of NO with the heme center of guanylate cyclase leads to a conformational change in the enzyme such that it becomes catalytically active and converts GTP to cyclic GMP, which in turn activates cGMP-dependent protein kinase or G-kinase.[16] While other pathways have been proposed,[17] activation of G-kinase is the principal mechanism whereby NO mediates vasodilatation. In keeping with this, mice lacking G-kinase are hypertensive and their vessels do not dilate in response to NO.[18,19]

Another target of NO is mitochondrial cytochrome c oxidase or complex IV, which also contains a heme group. The reaction of NO with cytochrome c oxidase can inhibit electron transfer and oxygen utilization by the mitochondrial electron transport chain. Like binding to guanylate cyclase, cytochrome c oxidase is exquisitely sensitive to NO and this binding is reversible.[20] Loss of NO can contribute to enhanced myocardial oxygen consumption in conditions such as heart failure.[21]

The end oxidation products of NO in solution are nitrate (NO_3^-) and nitrite (NO_2^-). In physiological buffers, the ratio of these is approximately one to one; however, in the presence of oxyhemoglobin and other heme groups, NO and nitrite are rapidly converted to nitrate. Both nitrate and nitrite are devoid of vasodilator activity. At physiological pH, very high concentrations of nitrite (100 μmoles/L) can result in nanomolar levels of NO that can produce vasodilatation. Organic nitrates like nitroglycerin, isosorbide mononitrate and isosorbide dinitrate are commonly employed as vasodilators; however, their conversion to NO or a related compound is enzymatically mediated in vascular cells. Recently aldehyde dehydrogenase has been shown to mediate some of this enzymatic activity.[22]

S-Nitrosothiols (RS-N=O) have been detected in the plasma and cells although their mechanism of formation is unclear. A commonly held misconception stated in the literature is that NO will readily react with thiols to form S-nitrosothiols.[23] This reaction is impossible. To form nitrosothiols, SH groups must be exposed to nitrosating agents such as the nitrogen dioxide radical ($NO_2^{\bullet}$), another nitrosothiol, or N_2O_3 as the source of nitrosonium cation (NO^+).[23] The latter does not exist in solution, but is transferred from one molecule to another. It is also possible for NO to react with a thiyl radical ($R\text{-}S^{\bullet}$) to form a nitrosothiol (reactions 4–5).

$$NO + NO_2 \rightarrow N_2O_3;\ ONONO \leftrightarrow NO^+NO_2^-;$$
$$RSH + N_2O_3 \rightarrow HNO_2 + RSNO \text{ (reaction 4)}$$

$$\text{II. } RSH + NO_2 \rightarrow HNO_2 + RS^{\bullet};$$
$$RS^{\bullet} + NO^{\bullet} \rightarrow RSNO \text{ (reaction 5)}$$

Nitrosothiols have been implicated in some of the biological activity of NO, although their role is debated. For example, in classical bioassay experiments, the biological activity of the endothelium-derived relaxing factor

(EDRF) is more closely mimicked by S-nitrosocysteine than by authentic nitric oxide.[24] It has been proposed that NO binding to cysteine 93 of the beta chain of hemoglobin can modulate oxygen release from the heme group, and that in fact, NO might switch from the cysteine to the heme group in hemoglobin to modulate the conformation of hemoglobin.[25] This remains extremely controversial.[26–30] S-Nitrosoalbumin and S-nitrosohemoglobin have also been proposed to serve as circulating sources of NO that can promote vasodilatation at sites remote from its production.[31]

S-Nitrosothiols can be cleaved homolytically, to yield NO and a thiyl radical (R-S•),[32] and can also undergo heterolytic scission to yield R-S⁻ and the nitrosonium cation (NO^+).[33] As mentioned above, NO^+ is very reactive, and does not exist in solution, but readily reacts via an intramolecular transfer mechanism with another R-SH group. This represents a mechanism whereby NO could be shuttled from one molecule to another, and in fact, from one site in the cell to another. The homolytic cleavage of S-nitrosothiols is likely very important in signaling. When two different S-nitrosothiols are present, this can lead to formation of two thiyl radicals that can readily react with one another to form a mixed disulfide. The attachment of small thiols to cysteine residues of larger proteins, known as thiolation, likely occurs via such mechanisms. Glutathionylation is one such thiolation reaction, which imparts signaling properties (discussed below).

Hydrogen peroxide (H_2O_2)

A body of recent literature has shown that H_2O_2 not only modulates intracellular redox status, but also acts as a signaling molecule. H_2O_2 is uncharged and relatively long-lived, the intracellular lifetime being approximately 1 second. Because of this, H_2O_2 can readily cross cell membranes, and is therefore likely to participate in intracellular cell signaling.[34,35]

H_2O_2 is formed by dismutation of $O_2^{\bullet-}$ or by a one electron reduction of $O_2^{\bullet-}$ (Figure 33.2). Some enzymes such as NOX4, xanthine oxidase and glucose oxidase perform two electron reductions or at least sequential one electron reductions of oxygen such that H_2O_2 is the predominant ROS that they form.[36]

H_2O_2 is a mild oxidizing agent on its own, but participates in redox reactions in mammalian cells in manners beyond its direct oxidizing effects. A major role of H_2O_2 is to serve as a co-substrate for myeloperoxidase and the related enzyme eosinophil peroxidase.[37] H_2O_2 has no direct reaction with NO; however, it has recently been demonstrated that H_2O_2 reacts with the heme center of myeloperoxidase to produce Fe^{44}, which in turn can

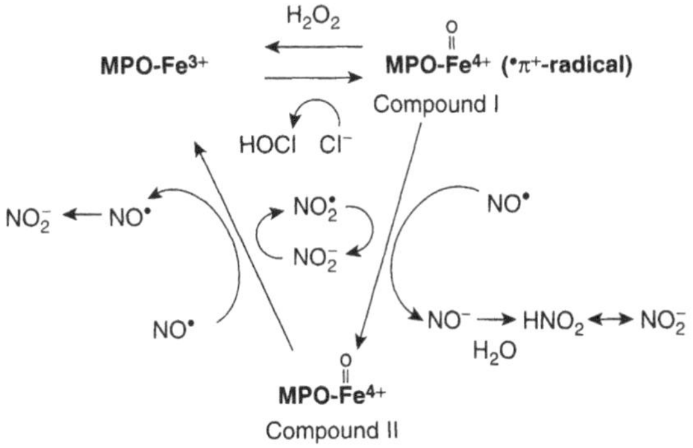

Figure 33.3 Reactions of myeloperoxidase (MPO) with nitric oxide (NO). The iron catalytic center of MPO exists in the ferric state (Fe^{3+}) at baseline. Upon reaction with H_2O_2, the Fe is oxidized to Fe^{4+}, which is a π radical, also referred to as compound I. In this process, halide anions like bromide and chloride are used to form hypochlorous and hypobromic acid. Compound I can oxidize NO to nitrite and can further oxidize nitrite to the nitrogen dioxide radical, and in extracting an electron from either NO or nitrite, is converted to compound II. Compound II can also oxidize another molecule of NO to nitrite. Thus, MPO can consume NO and form nitrogen dioxide, which is a strong nitrosating agent. (Adapted from Abu-Soud and Hazen[38] and used with permission from Dr Hazen and the publisher.)

oxidize NO to NO_2^- and to further oxidize NO_2^- to the nitrogen dioxide radical ($NO_2^{\bullet}$) (Figure 33.3).[38] This is discussed in greater detail below.

Hydroxyl radical (HO•)

The σ radical hydroxyl is extraordinarily oxidizing, its extraction of an electron from virtually any other target leading to formation of water. An enormous literature has arisen regarding the formation of hydroxyl from the combinations of the Haber Weiss reaction (reaction 6) and Fenton chemistry (reactions 7–8). These reactions have been reviewed in detail elsewhere[39] and will only be briefly described here.

$$O_2^{\bullet-} + H_2O_2 \rightarrow O_2 + OH^- + OH \text{ (reaction 6)}$$

The Haber Weiss reaction (reaction 6) is unfavorable in aqueous solutions, but it can be sustained by a metal catalyst such as iron via the Fenton reaction:

$$Fe^{3+} + O_2^{\bullet-} \rightarrow Fe^{2+} + O_2 \text{ (reaction 7)}$$

$$Fe2^{+} + H_2O_2 \rightarrow Fe^{3+} + OH^- + OH \text{ (reaction 8)}$$

These observations have emphasized the role of iron and, in particular, free or catalytically active iron in the formation of the hydroxyl radical in biological systems. Other transition metals can replace Fe^{3+}, but in vivo, only copper and iron are usually sufficiently high to be relevant. Related to this issue, there is debate about how likely reaction 7 is in vivo. It has been argued that $O_2^{\bullet -}$ is more likely to provide ferrous iron by oxidizing [4Fe-4S] clusters in enzymes like aconitase and fumarase.[40] Free iron and iron overload have been implicated in a wide variety of diseases, including neurodegenerative diseases,[41,42] atherosclerosis,[43] and hypertension;[44] and hydroxyl generation by Fenton/Haber Weiss-like reactions are often implicated. With the discovery of peroxynitrite and the observation that peroxynitrite could leave behind hydroxyl-like footprints, debate has arisen about how likely hydroxyl is to be formed in vivo by the Fenton/Haber Weiss-like reactions.[45]

In vivo, one of the markers of oxidative stress is 8-hydroxy-2′-deoxyguanosine, which is formed by the reaction of hydroxyl-like species with guanasine residues in DNA.[46] The presence of 8-hydroxy-2′-deoxyguanosine has been used to support the concept that hydroxyl is produced in nuclei of cells. There are, however, other ROS that can lead to formation of 8-OH-deoxyguanosine. As discussed below, peroxynitrite can exhibit hydroxyl-like activity, perhaps by releasing hydroxyl, and has been shown to form 8-OH-deoxyguanosine.

Because of its high level of reactivity, there is really no specific scavenger of hydroxyl. The free hydroxyl radical reacts instantly at a diffusion-limited rate with any nearby organic molecule. Its intracellular lifetime has been estimated to be less than 10^{-9} seconds.[47]

Peroxynitrite anion ($OONO^-$)

The reaction of $O_2^{\bullet -}$ with NO leads to formation of the peroxynitrite anion. This reaction is one of the fastest in biology, and is essentially diffusion-limited.[48,49] This reaction leads to inactivation of NO and is thought to account for reduced ‘bioavailability’ of NO in a variety of common diseases.[50]

At physiological pHs, peroxynitrite is readily protonated (pKa 6.8) to form peroxynitrous acid (HONOO), which has been proposed to produce the nitrogen dioxide and hydroxyl radicals via HO-ONO homolysis.

$$ONOO + H+ \rightarrow HONOO \text{ (reaction 9)}$$

$$HONOO \rightarrow OH^{\bullet} + NO_2^{\bullet} \text{ (reaction 10)}$$

Whether or not this reaction actually occurs in vivo has been debated,[51] but many of the biological consequences of peroxynitrite can be explained by both nitrosation reactions and hydroxylation-like reactions.[52] Related to nitrosation reactions, nitrotyrosine has been considered a marker of peroxynitrite formation, although there are other more likely mechanisms for its formation in vivo, described below.

The reactivity of peroxynitrite is influenced by carbon dioxide, which is ubiquitous in vivo and in most physiological buffers. The reaction of peroxynitrite with CO_2 leads to formation of the nitrosocarbonate anion $ONOOCOO^-$.[53] This has been reported to both enhance,[54] and to reduce[55] the reactivity of peroxynitrite, and its ultimate effect seems to depend on the environment in which it is formed. In lipid-rich environments, such as membrane bilayers, the nitrosocarbonate anion can at least theoretically produce the nitrosating radical $NO_2^{\bullet}$ and the carbonate radical CO_3. In aqueous solutions, alternate pathways have been proposed that could lead to peroxynitrite scavenging by CO_2.[53] These scavenging reactions with $CO_2^{\bullet}$ are not so avid as to prevent oxidation of thiols in the cytoplasm.

Lipid radicals

Long chain polyunsaturated fatty acids (PUFAs) are prone to oxidation because of the presence of bis-allylic carbons, situated between carbons with double bonds. The energy needed to break the bond between such a carbon and one of its hydrogen atoms (dissociation energy) is lower than any other carbon-hydrogen bonds in the PUFA (Figure 33.4).[56] The result of this is that these hydrogens are particularly prone to abstraction. Indeed, the likelihood that a fatty acid will undergo oxidation has been shown to be dependent on its content of bis-allylic hydrogens and the degree of oxidation of any PUFA is often normalized to the number of these hydrogens. Oxidation of fatty acids occurs via a series of reactions illustrated in Figure 33.5. These involve: 1) extraction by an oxidant of a bys-allylic hydrogen, leaving behind an unpaired electron on the previous bis-allylic carbon (a carbon-centered radical). 2) Rearrangement of double bonds shifting the carbon-centered radical and attachment of an oxygen molecule, yielding a lipid peroxy radical. 3) Reaction of the peroxy radical can react with another lipid to yield a peroxide and another carbon-centered radical (reactions 11–13).

$$LH + R^{\bullet} - \rightarrow L^{\bullet} + RH \text{ (reaction 11)}$$

$$L^{\bullet} + O_2 - \rightarrow LOO^{\bullet} \text{ (reaction 12)}$$

$$LOO^{\bullet} + LH - \rightarrow L^{\bullet} + LOOH \text{ (reaction 13)}$$

As is apparent, this subsequent formation of another carbon-centered radical begins an oxidation

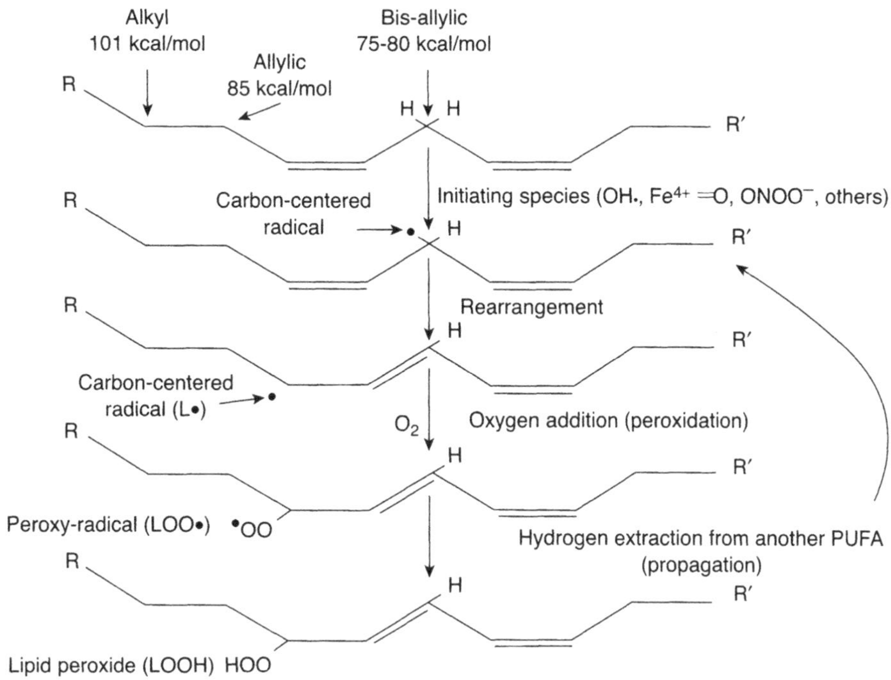

Figure 33.4 Mechanisms of lipid peroxidation: a polyunsaturated fatty acid (PUFA) with two double bonds separated by a bis-allylic carbon. The dissociation energies for hydrogen abstraction at various carbons (bis-allylic, allylic and alkyl) are shown. Reaction of the PUFA with an initiating oxidant leads to hydrogen abstraction, preferably from the bis-allylic carbon, leading to formation of a carbon-centered radical. This is followed by rearrangement of double bonds, addition of oxygen and formation of a peroxy-radical. The lipid peroxy-radical readily abstracts a hydrogen from another PUFA, forming another carbon-centered lipid radical, leading to a radical-chain reaction and propagation of oxidation

chain reaction that can continue unabated unless a chain-breaking antioxidant is introduced. Such chain-breaking antioxidants have been considered to include compounds like tocopherol, probucol, and flavanoids. Surprisingly, upon hydrogen donation (its method of radical scavenging), tocopherol forms the tocopheroxyl radical, which may paradoxically enhance lipid oxidation, depending on the rate of radical flux, the presence of co-antioxidants and other factors.[57]

Nitric oxide can also serve as a chain-breaking antioxidant by reacting with lipid peroxy and alkoxy radicals, forming LOONO and LONO.[58] Both of these latter species have been detected in human atherosclerotic lesions, reflecting the potential importance of NO as an inhibitor of lipid peroxidation.

Extensive oxidation of polyunsaturated fatty acids can lead to bond breaks in the carbon backbone, yielding fragments that are three to nine carbons in length.[59] These carbon fragments are often referred to as reactive carbonyls, a term that refers to compounds that contain an oxygen double bonded to a carbon group: a ketone if the oxygen is bonded to a carbon flanked by other carbons, and a reactive aldehyde if the oxygen is bound to a terminal carbon. These include compounds such as malondialdehyde (Figure 33.5), and glyoxyl. One of the most commonly produced of the reactive aldehydes is hydroxynonenol (Figure 33.5). Many of these reactive aldehydes are effectively ROS, in that they are electrophillic and can abstract electrons from a variety of targets. Moreover, these molecules are stable, and can traverse cell membranes to oxidize targets in adjacent cells. One of the carbon derivatives of lipid oxidation is ethane, which can be detected in exhaled breath and has been used as a marker of oxidative stress in human studies. The reaction of these with proteins is discussed below in the section on protein oxidation.

The 8-F_2 isoprostanes are non-enzymatic products of lipid oxidation. These can be detected by either gas chromatography/mass spectrometry or liquid chromatography/mass spectrometry in urine and plasma and such assays have been employed to quantify levels

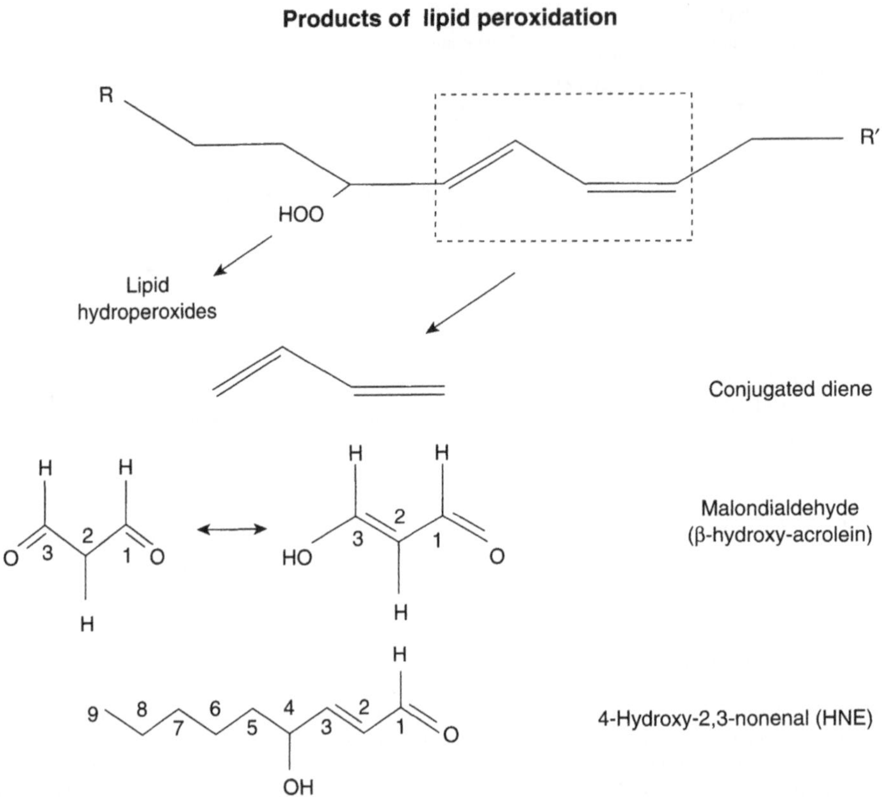

Figure 33.5 Formation of carbonyl groups. Extensive oxidation of polyunsaturated fatty acids leads to breaks in the carbon backbone and release of carbonyls

of oxidative stress in vivo.[60] Urinary and plasma 8-F_2 isoprostanes are elevated in a variety of human pathophysiological processes, including atherosclerosis, diabetes, cancer, and lung disease.[61,62] The 8-F_2 isoprostanes can produce vasoconstriction both by direct activation of the thromboxane receptor and by stimulating release of cyclooxygenase products.[63]

There are also important enzymatic sources of fatty acid oxidation. These include cyclooxygenases, the cytochrome p450 reductases and the lipoxygenases, which respectively form prostaglandins, epoxides and hydroperoxy (HPODE) and hydrodecanoeic acid (HODE). These have been covered extensively in other reviews and will not be discussed further here except to emphasize that these oxidized lipid intermediates have extremely important signaling properties that control numerous cellular events and physiological functions.

Lipid peroxides can activate gene transcription. One of their principal targets is the transcription factor NFκB, which when activated can promote transcription of a variety of pro-inflammatory molecules like MCP1 and VCAM1, leading to macrophage recruitment and infiltration into the vessel wall.[64,65] These molecular events are some of the earliest events in atherosclerotic lesion development.

TARGETS OF OXIDATION

Virtually all components of the cells, including lipids, thiols, proteins, and DNA can be modified by ROS. Lipid oxidation is discussed in the preceding section.

Thiols

Thiols (RSH) readily react with peroxynitrite (ONOOH), nitrogen dioxide ($^{\bullet}NO_2$), the phenoxyl radical of vitamin E, and both carbon and oxygen radicals. Because of this, thiols are both important endogenous antioxidants and also targets for oxidative modification. The major intracellular small molecule

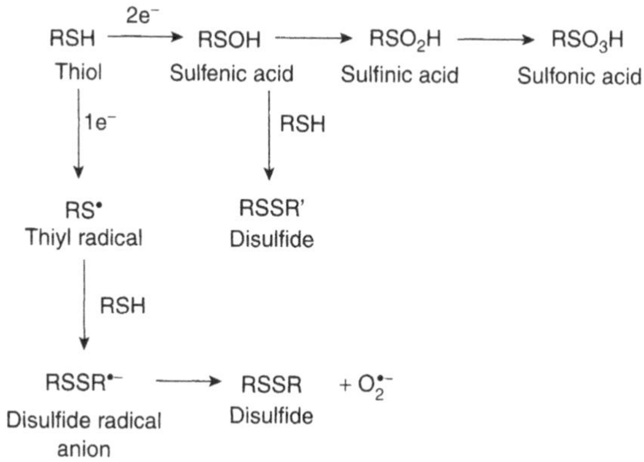

Figure 33.6 Products of thiol (sulfhydryl) oxidation. These reactions can occur with small molecule thiols such as cysteine and glutathione, or can occur with thiol-containing amino acids in proteins

antioxidant is glutathione, a tripeptide composed of glycine, cysteine and glutamine, which is synthesized by the sequential actions of the enzymes gamma-glutamyl cysteine synthetase and glutathione synthetase.[66] Via this pathway, cysteine is rapidly converted to GSH when taken up by cells. N-Acetylcysteine, which is used both experimentally and therapeutically as an antioxidant, functions largely to bolster intracellular levels of glutathione. In the cell, GSH is present in concentrations approaching 10 mM, while the oxidized form of glutathione (GSSG) is maintained at levels that are 1–2% of this, largely because GSSG is rapidly reduced to GSH by glutathione reductase and is also transported from the cell.

The oxidation of thiols in proteins leads to a myriad of products (Figure 33.6) that represent important post-translational modifications that can alter protein and enzyme function. Recently, Xu and Chance have used radiolysis to oxidize protein thiols and have analyzed the products of these reactions using X-ray crystallography.[67] Radiolysis of cysteine led to formation of cysteine sulfonic acid and cystine as the major products. Radiolysis of cystine led to oxidative opening of the disulfide bond and generation of cysteine sulfonic acid and sulfinic acid; however, the rate of this reaction was significantly less than that for cysteine. Radiolysis of methionine predominantly led to formation of methionine sulfoxide (M–S=O), which could be further oxidized to methionine sulfone.

In the above study, radiolysis, which generates hydroxyl radical, was used. In vivo, more commonly encountered oxidants have differing effects on protein methionine residues. Methionine residues in proteins are relatively resistant to oxidation by H_2O_2, but can be oxidized by stronger oxidants, such as HOCl, forming sulfoxides. Recently, oxidation of methionine 116 in cathepsin G by HOCl has been shown to cause release of a peptide from the protein and loss of its catalytic activity, thus protecting native proteins from degradation by this protease.[68] Likewise, oxidation of methionine in calmodulin decreases its binding activity – a phenomenon that could have important implications for activation of NOS.[69]

An important modification of protein thiols is formation of mixed disulfides, in particular, the attachment of a protein thiol with glutathione (glutathionylation). This can occur via the reaction of two nitrosothiols, by oxidation of one thiol to a sulfoxide, which will react with another thiol, or by the reaction of two thiyl radicals.[70–74] This post-translational modification can alter protein function, and therefore, can serve as a signaling mechanism in a manner similar to serine or tyrosine phosphorylation. As examples, the mitochondrial complex 1 is glutathionylated, leading to increased superoxide production from this site.[73] S-Glutathionylation of actin has been reported to affect actin filament formation.[75] Likewise, glutathionylation of the NFκB subunit p50 inhibits its DNA binding.[76] Numerous other examples of protein modification by glutathionylation have been documented, although the in vivo significance of many of these has not been well established. The enzyme glutaredoxin reduces mixed disulfides, and in particular, reduces glutathionylated proteins.[77] In this fashion, glutaredoxin reverses the signaling events caused by glutathionylation in a manner similar to how phosphatases reverse protein phosphorylation signaling.

Proteins

Proteins can directly react with oxidants, particularly on lysine, arginine and proline residues (Figure 33.7). This reaction can break the five-membered ring of proline and cause alterations in the side chain structures of arginine and lysine residues, leading to the formation of semialdehydes. One such is prevalent in Apo(B)-100 in human atherosclerotic lesions.[78]

As discussed above, extensive peroxidation of thiols leads to breaks in the carbon backbone, leading to formation of protein carbonyls such as 4-hydroxy-2-nonenol (HNE, Figure 33.5). HNE and other reactive aldehydes can react with the lysine, histadine and cysteine residues in proteins leading to adducts, which can alter protein confirmation, enzyme function and target proteins for rapid degradation.[79] HNE-modified proteins have been identified in numerous human pathologies, including Alzheimer's disease,[80] rheumatoid

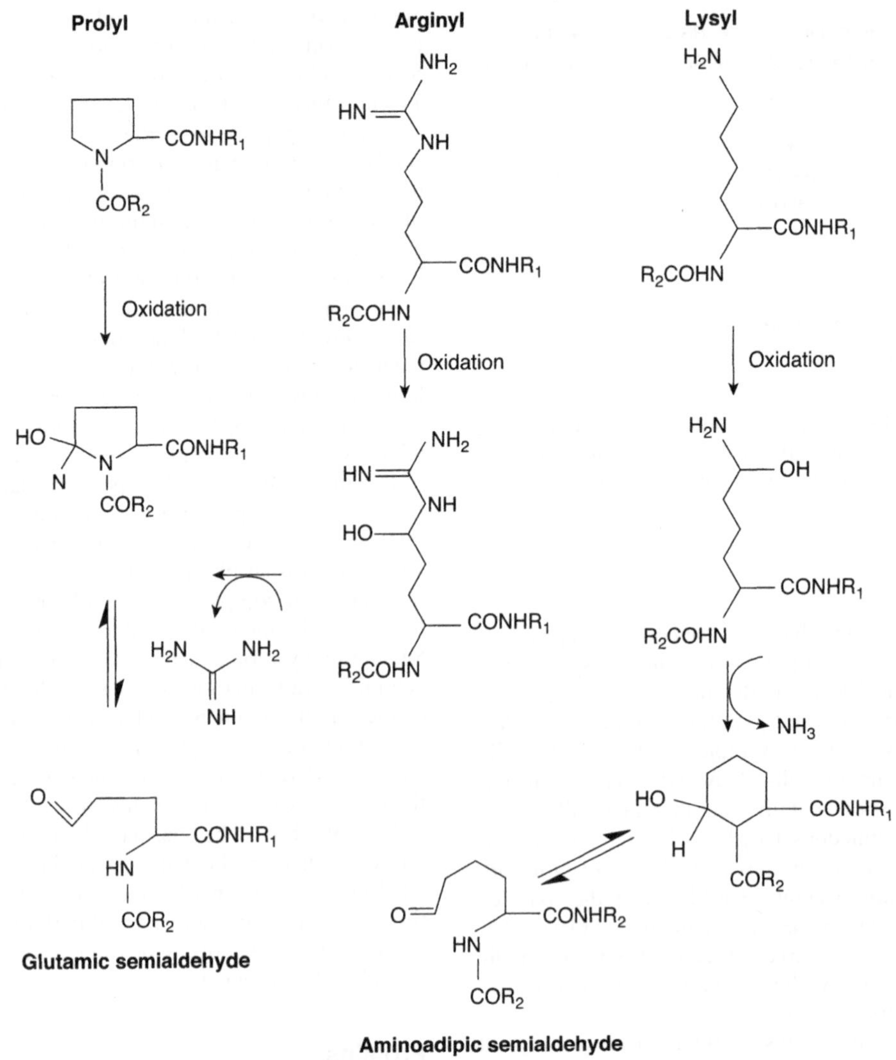

Figure 33.7 Effect of oxidation of amino acid residues in proteins. In particular, proline, lysine and arginine residues are prone to oxidation with dramatic changes in structure

arthritis,[81] and aging.[82] HNE-modified proteins are markedly increased in both experimental and human atherosclerotic lesions. While HNE and other reactive aldehydes have been shown to have various effects on cell signaling, most of their effects are likely non-specific. HNE is converted to non-reactive products by a variety of enzymes, including aldose and aldehyde reductases.

The oxidative modification of proteins can also affect prosthetic groups such as flavins, BH_4 and [4Fe-4S] clusters. A particular event relevant to vascular biology and hypertension is the oxidation of BH_4.[83,84] In particular, peroxynitrite oxidizes BH_4 to the $BH_3^{\bullet}$ radical. This radical can be reduced back to BH_4 by physiologic levels of ascorbate. Likewise, uric acid prevents oxidation of BH_4 by scavenging peroxynitrite.[85] These interactions have been shown to be important for function of the endothelial cell NO synthase as discussed below.

DNA

DNA oxidation has been reviewed in detail previously.[86] All four bases of DNA and the deoxyribose moiety can be oxidatively modified; however, the oxidation of guanosine to 8-hydroxyguanosine (8-OH guanosine) seems most prevalent and best characterized. The oxidation of guanosine to 8-OH-guanosine most often leads to an effective G→T substitution, although oxidation of DNA can lead to conformational changes, changes in transcription factor binding, promoter activity and epigenetic regulation. For nuclear DNA, there are a number of DNA repair mechanisms, which minimize the effect of DNA oxidation. These DNA repair mechanisms are much less effective in the mitochondria and mitochondrial DNA seems more susceptible to oxidative damage than nuclear DNA.[87] This can lead to deletions of mitochondrial DNA, miscoding of mitochondrial proteins and increased electron leak from alterations in the mitochondrial electron transport chain.[88] In this regard, mitochondrial oxidative stress can beget increased mitochondrial dysfunction. Deletions of mitochondrial DNA have been observed in humans with cardiomyopathy and in atherosclerotic lesions.[89] Interestingly, mice heterozygotic for the mitochondrial SOD (MnSOD or SOD2) have mitochondrial DNA deletions and increased atherosclerosis when crossed with Apo(E)-deficient mice.

MAMMALIAN ENZYMES CAPABLE OF GENERATING ROS – RELEVANCE TO VASCULAR BIOLOGY

While there are numerous enzyme systems that produce ROS in mammalian cells, five enzyme systems seem to predominate, particularly in vascular cells, renal cells and cells of the central nervous system. These include the NADPH oxidases, xanthine oxidase, uncoupled NO synthase, mitochondrial sources and myeloperoxidase. A recurring theme is that there appears to be substantial interplay between these sources, such that activation of one can lead to activation of the others (Figure 33.8). This can lead to feed-forward processes, which further augment ROS production and oxidant stress. These interactions will be discussed in depth below.

NADPH oxidases

The NADPH oxidase was first identified in phagocytic cells and is responsible for the respiratory burst that these cells exhibit when activated. It is now clear that many cells contain variations of the NADPH oxidase and that these are a major source of ROS in non-phagocytic cells. There are important differences between the phagocytic and non-phagocytic NADPH oxidases. The phagocytic oxidases produce high levels of $O_2^{\bullet-}$ upon stimulation. In contrast, the non-phagocytic oxidases produce ROS constantly at much lower levels.

The Nox proteins are the catalytic subunits of these enzymes, and vary in terms of their mode of activation and need for co-factor activation.[90] Nox1 was first identified in colon carcinoma cells, but is also present at low levels in vascular cells. Nox2, previously known as gp91phox, is the large catalytic subunit of the phagocyte cytochrome b558. It is also expressed in endothelial and adventitial cells and in the vascular smooth muscle cells of smaller vessels.[91–94] Nox3 is present in the hair cells of the inner ear, and plays an important role in development of these cells. Because of this, mice lacking Nox3 have difficulty with balance. Nox4 is constitutively expressed and constitutively active in vascular smooth muscle and endothelial cells.[95,96] In the absence of other stimuli, Nox4 is expressed at the highest level in vascular cells. Nox5 is unique in that it contains EF-hand domains which convey calcium sensitivity.

A variety of pathological stimuli, such as angiotensin (Ang) II, stretch, endothelin-1, thrombin, and catecholamines acutely activate the NADPH oxidases in both vascular smooth muscle and endothelial cells. The biochemical pathway leading to activation of the NADPH oxidase in response to Ang II involves activation of the tyrosine kinase c-Src, transactivation of the EGF receptor and ultimate activation and translocation of the small g protein Rac-1 (Figure 33.8).[97] Phosphorylation and translocation of the cytoplasmic component $p47^{phox}$ is also a critical step.[98] Activation of Nox1 and Nox2 also require translocation of cytoplasmic subunits, including $p47^{phox}$ or analogs of $p47^{phox}$ and p67phox termed NoxO1 and NoxA.[99,100] In the case of Nox5, calcium binding to the EF-hand domains in the C-terminus leads to a conformational change, such that the C-terminus associates with the catalytic N-terminus. In this fashion, the C-terminal domain seems to substitute for the cytoplasmic subunits used by the other Nox isoforms and Nox5 does not seem to require cytosolic subunits for full activation.

It seems that all the Nox enzymes require $p22^{phox}$, which functions as a docking protein for other subunits and stabilizes the Nox proteins.[101] The phagocytic NADPH oxidase requires activated Rac-2, while the non-phagocytic oxidases require Rac1. These small G proteins are critical for activation, and require the isoprenoid geranylgeranyl pyrophosphate (GGPP) for membrane attachment. The HMG-CoA reductase inhibitors reduce cellular production of GGPP, and

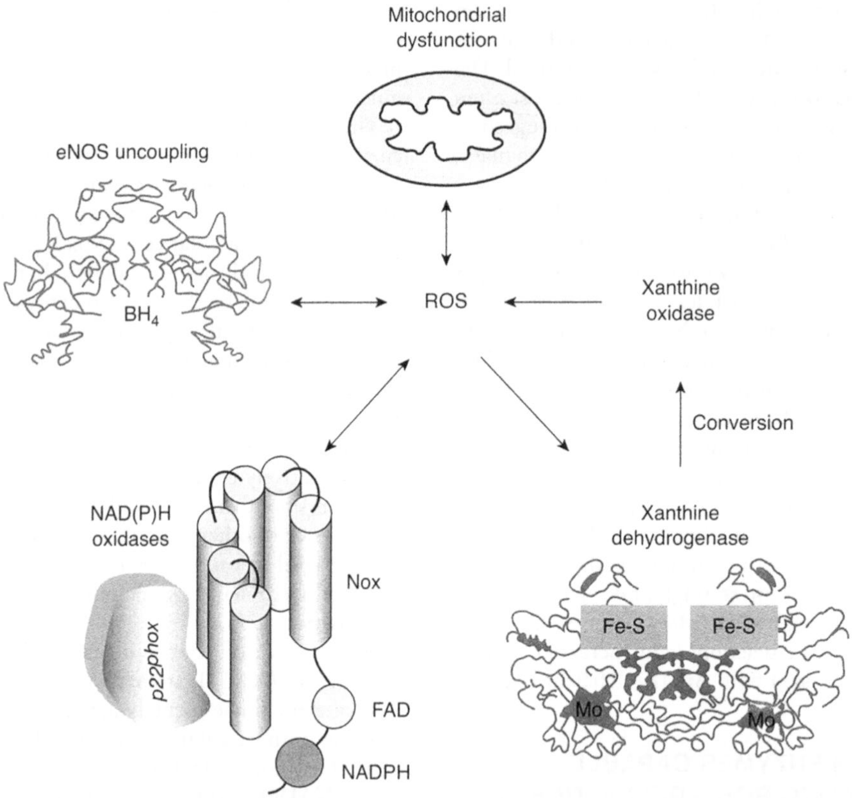

Figure 33.8 Interaction of various sources of reactive oxygen species (ROS). The production of ROS from any one source can lead to activation of the NADPH oxidase or conversion of xanthine dehydrogenase to xanthine oxidase. ROS such as peroxynitrite can lead to oxidation of tetrahydrobiopterin and uncoupling of the endothelial nitric oxide synthase such that this enzyme begins to produce superoxide. Finally, ROS can lead to DNA damage in the mitochondria promoting mitochondrial ROS production

via this mechanism reduce NADPH oxidase activity in vascular cells.

Interestingly, pathophysiological stimuli such as Ang II, hypercholesterolemia, growth factors and serum can also increase expression of several of the NADPH oxidase subunits, including $p22^{phox}$, Nox1 and Nox4, further promoting an increase in ROS production.[90] The biochemical pathways regulating expression of these subunits have not been elucidated. An increase in $p22^{phox}$ could lead to stabilization of various Nox proteins via protein/protein interactions, resulting in coordinated up-regulation of several different oxidase subunits. In keeping with this concept, we recently created a mouse with targeted over-expression of $p22^{phox}$ in the smooth muscle and have found that these animals have a striking up-regulation of Nox1.[102] Recent data indicate that within the same cell, different Nox isoforms can have very different functions. This is likely related to the subcellular location. For example, in vascular smooth muscle cells, Nox1 is localized to caveoli and focal adhesion contacts and seems to play a role in proliferation. In contrast, Nox4 is localized to the actin cytoskeleton and seems to play a role in cellular differentiation. This concept is in keeping with the idea presented above that oxidative stress can affect function in localized compartments of the cell.

Of interest, the vascular NADPH oxidase can be activated by both H_2O_2 and lipid peroxides. Thus, production of ROS via either the NADPH oxidase or other enzymes can stimulate production of other ROS in a feed-forward fashion (Figure 33.7).

Xanthine oxidase

Another source of ROS in mammalian cells is xanthine oxidoreductase (XOR). XOR exists in two forms, as xanthine dehydrogenase (XDH), and xanthine oxidase

(XO).[103] XDH utilizes NAD^+ to receive electrons from hypoxanthine and xanthine yielding NADH and uric acid. In contrast, XO utilizes oxygen as an electron acceptor from these same substrates to form $O_2^{\bullet-}$ and H_2O_2.

The ratio of XO to XDH in the cell is therefore critical to determine the amount of ROS produced by these enzymes. Conversion of XDH to XO is stimulated by inflammatory cytokines like TNF-α, and also by oxidation of critical cysteine residues by oxidants such as peroxynitrite.[104,105] Recently, we have shown in bovine and mouse aortic endothelial cells that the relative levels of XO and XDH are markedly altered by the presence of a functioning NADPH oxidase, such that in cells with an absence of the NADPH oxidase, the levels of XO are extremely low.[106,107] Activation of the NADPH oxidase by either angiotensin or mechanical forces leads to an increase in intracellular calcium that activates degradation of XDH.[108] Thus, this pathway represents a second instance in which cellular production of ROS from the NADPH oxidase further begets ROS production.

In human endothelial cells, there is debate as to whether XDH is expressed under normal conditions. We have been unable to detect XDH protein in cultured human umbilical endothelial cells or in human aortic endothelial cells, and immunohistochemical studies of normal human tissues have failed to demonstrate XDH in endothelial cells or other cardiovascular tissues.[107] In contrast, it is clear that XO can produce ROS and affect endothelial function in humans in the setting of pathology.[109–112] This might be due to stimulation of XDH expression by inflammatory cytokines or other stimuli in these conditions. For example, Sohn et al. demonstrated that hypoxia induces activity of XO in human umbilical vein endothelial cells.[113]

There is evidence that XO present in endothelial cells originates from other organs and that the enzyme is probably taken up via heparin binding sites.[109,114,115] Interestingly, XO can masquerade as an NADH oxidase, particularly when deprived of molybdenum. In this form, the enzyme can use NADH as an electron donor to produce $O_2^{\bullet-}$. This enzyme activity is not inhibited by allopurinol or oxypurinol.

Recent studies have demonstrated that ROS produced by XO contribute to endothelial dysfunction in humans. Landmesser et al. showed that XO activity correlates inversely with endothelial function in patients with heart failure and in subjects with atherosclerosis.[109,116] Furthermore, the improvement in flow-mediated vasodilatation caused by intra-arterial infusion of vitamin C was directly correlated with levels of vascular bound XO.

Uncoupled eNOS

A third major contributor to vascular ROS generation is uncoupled endothelial NO synthase (eNOS). The normal product of this enzyme is NO; however, in the absence of either L-arginine or BH_4, the NO synthases are incapable of transferring electrons to L-arginine, and begin to use oxygen as a substrate for $O_2^{\bullet-}$ formation.[117]

Uncoupling of eNOS has been demonstrated in various pathophysiological conditions including diabetes, chronic exposure to Ang II,[118] hypercholesterolemia,[119] and hypertension (Figure 33.9).[120] In DOCA-salt hypertension, oxidation of BH_4 occurs as a result of ROS (in particular peroxynitrite) produced by the NADPH oxidase. Oral treatment of mice that have DOCA-salt hypertension with BH_4 're-couples' eNOS, leading to increased vascular NO production, decreased $O_2^{\bullet-}$ production and lowering of blood pressure.[120]

Recent studies have demonstrated that BH_4 is particularly susceptible to oxidation when compared with other endogenous antioxidants such as urate, ascorbate, cysteine, and glutathione.[85] Studies in vitro and in cultured cells suggest an important interaction between these various endogenous antioxidants and BH_4 and the ability of these to maintain eNOS catalysis. According to these studies, urate serves as a critical scavenger of peroxynitrite. The resultant urate radical is recycled to urate by ascorbate. The immediate reaction of BH_4 with peroxynitrite leads to formation of the $BH_3^{\bullet}$ radical. The $BH_3^{\bullet}$ radical is transient and within several seconds degrades to BH_2, which cannot be reduced to BH_4 by ascorbate. Thus, in this pathway, BH_2 represents a terminal oxidation product, although extensive oxidation of BH_4 likely leads to breaks in the pterin ring. Importantly, ascorbate plays a critical role in that it converts the $BH_3^{\bullet}$ radical back to BH_4 (Figure 33.10). In this manner, ascorbate serves to sustain eNOS enzyme activity and endothelial cell BH_4 levels.[85,121,122]

Related to the above situation, eNOS is subject to regulation by H_2O_2, which both acutely activates the enzyme, and over the longer term, increases its expression.[34,123] Thus increased expression of eNOS in the setting of oxidant stress leads to a situation in which high levels of the uncoupled enzyme generate even greater amounts of $O_2^{\bullet-}$. It should be stressed that it is unlikely that all eNOS becomes uncoupled, such that some of the enzyme continues to produce NO, leading to a condition favoring production of peroxynitrite.

Mitochondrial electron transport

In many organs and tissues, the mitochondrial electron transport chain is thought to represent the predominant

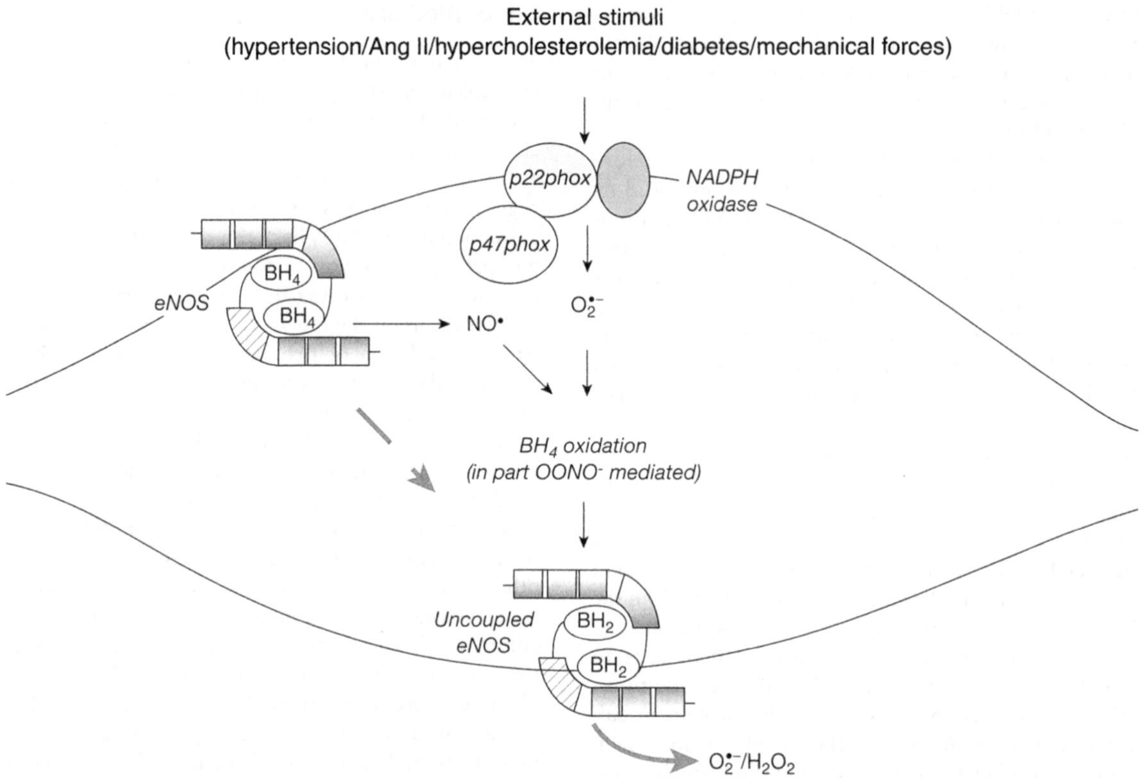

Figure 33.9 Uncoupling of the endothelial nitric oxide synthase (eNOS) by oxidation of tetrahydrobiopterin (BH_4). Oxidation of BH_4 leads to formation of dihydrobiopterin (BH_2) and other oxidized species. In the absence of BH_4, eNOS produces $O_2^{\bullet-}$ rather than NO. (Reproduced with permission from Landmesser et al. J Clin Invest 2003; 111: 1201–9.[83])

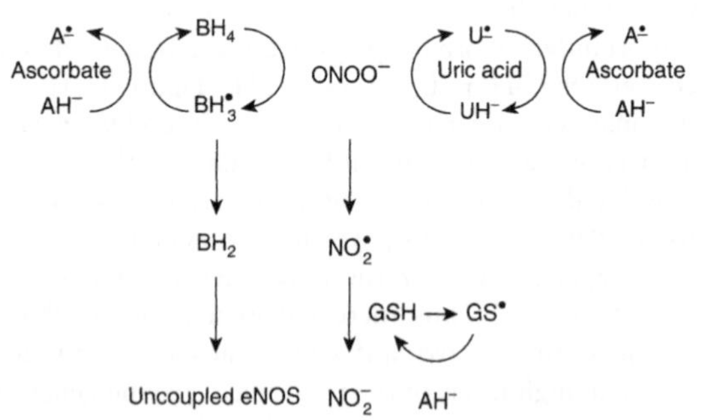

Figure 33.10 Oxidation pathway of tetrahydrobiopterin (BH_4) and roles of endogenous antioxidants. BH_4 is oxidized by peroxynitrite ($ONOO^-$) to the $BH_3^{\bullet}$ radical, which can be recycled to BH_4 by ascorbate. The $BH_3^{\bullet}$ radical is metastable, and degrades to BH_4 in the absence of ascorbate. Uric acid can scavenge $ONOO^-$ and the urate radical can be regenerated to uric acid by ascorbate. (Reproduced with permission from Kuzkaya et al. J Biol Chem 2003; 278: 22546–54.[85])

source of $O_2^{\bullet-}$ and consequently H_2O_2. While most of the oxygen entering the respiratory chain is reduced to H_2O, it has been estimated that between 1 and 4% of the oxygen is incompletely reduced and forms O_2. While this is probably a high approximation, it is clear that the mitochondrial respiratory chain represents a substantial source of cellular superoxide and H_2O_2. This 'electron leak' occurs mainly at two sites in the respiratory chain, complex I and complex III.

In the vessel wall, the precise contribution of mitochondria to the total ROS production remains unclear. This is in part because pharmacological agents have been used to inhibit the various complexes and these have not been well characterized. As with all pharmacologic inhibitors, their non-specific effects are unknown. Furthermore, some agents have been reported to have varying effects. For example, rotenone has been used to both stimulate and inhibit radical production by the mitochondria. Furthermore, inhibition of mitochondrial function alters many other aspects of cell metabolism, making interpretation of these interventions difficult. Nevertheless, there is ample evidence that mitochondria play an important role in vascular ROS production. Stimuli such as high glucose, cyclical strain, leptin, and cigarette smoking have been shown to damage aortic mitochondrial DNA and alter mitochondrial enzyme activity. The precise mechanisms whereby such extracellular signals could alter mitochondrial function have not been precisely defined.

Defects in mitochondrial DNA can be inherited or can develop as a result of disease, and markedly augment ROS production by these organelles. Interestingly, exposure of endothelial or vascular smooth muscle cells to exogenous peroxynitrite or H_2O_2 leads to mitochondrial DNA damage. This represents yet another mechanism whereby the oxidant stress could beget further oxidant stress.

Myeloperoxidase (MPO)

Recent evidence has implicated MPO as playing a central role in vascular pathology, lipid peroxidation, and atherosclerosis. MPO participates in a number of oxidative reactions that have relevance to vascular biology. Most notably, MPO utilizes H_2O_2 as a co-substrate to form the chlorinating species HOCl. HOCl is the predominant oxidant formed by neutrophils and is essential for bactericidal function. Likewise, the reaction of activated MPO with NO (discussed above in the discussion regarding H_2O_2) not only consumes NO, but also forms nitrosating species that readily react with various targets. In particular, the reaction of $NO_2^{\bullet}$ with tyrosine leads to formation of nitrotyrosine, previously thought to be predominantly caused by reactions of peroxynitrite with tyrosine. Likewise, HOCl and HOBr can react with tyrosines to form chloro- and bromotyrosines. These have been recently used as markers of inflammation and oxidative stress and are elevated in the plasma of subjects with coronary artery disease.[124] HOCl and nitrosating species formed by MPO react with low-density lipoprotein (LDL) to form particles that are avidly taken up by macrophage scavenger receptors. Moreover, MPO is present in human high density lipoprotein (HDL), and humans with cardiovascular disease (CVD) have increased contents of chloro- and nitro-tyrosines in ApoA1, the atheroprotective protein of the HDL particle. Moreover, oxidatively modified ApoA1 has been found to be dysfunctional in terms of promoting cholesterol ester efflux from macrophage-like cells.[125]

MPO is produced by neutrophils, monocytes, and tissue macrophages and is secreted by these cells upon their activation. While MPO is not usually present in vascular cells, once released by inflammatory cells in the vessel wall it can be taken up via pinocytotic mechanisms into endothelial cells. Thus, although endothelial cells do not normally produce MPO, they can acquire this protein in inflammatory conditions. When present in vascular cells, MPO and its product HOCl can contribute to endothelial dysfunction both via oxidation of NO and also by chlorinating L-arginine, the substrate for NOS, as discussed earlier. The loss of NO production can promote many aspects of atherosclerotic lesion formation, including platelet deposition and adhesion molecule expression. HOCl has also been shown to activate matrix metalloproteinases and to cause endothelial cell apoptosis, events which would clearly predispose to atherosclerosis. By reducing the vasodilatation caused by endothelium-derived NO, MPO might also contribute to hypertension.

NON-ENZYMATIC SOURCES OF ROS (EXPERIMENTAL CONSIDERATIONS)

ROS can form non-enzymatically, especially via reactions with transition metals. In fact, the enzymatic and the non-enzymatic formation of radicals are similar in that most enzymes that form ROS utilize a transition metal (iron, copper, molybdenum, manganese) at their catalytic site.

The classic non-enzymatic formation of radicals is the Haber-Weiss reaction or Fenton reaction, which was discussed in detail in the earlier section on the hydroxyl radical. Likely more important is the direct reaction of Fe^{2+} with dioxygen, leading to FeO_2 and FeO_4, which then generate Fe^{3+} and $O_2^{\bullet-}$. This reaction can occur in the absence of preformed H_2O_2 and can be catalyzed by reducing agents which convert ferric iron to ferrous iron.[126]

Despite the fact that iron-binding proteins both in the cell and in extracellular fluids minimize the levels of free iron, there is an abundance of evidence that catalytically active iron exists in vivo and contributes to disease. Iron-mediated oxidation reactions occur in proteins, perhaps because certain proteins bind iron at specific sites where these oxidation footprints have been observed. Thus, certain proteins chelate iron and likely do not negate its redox activity. This leads to iron-mediated oxidative modifications of proteins at certain 'hot spots'. Interestingly, Duffy and co-workers have shown that infusion of the iron chelator deferoxamine improved endothelium-dependent vasodilatation in a group of subjects with coronary artery disease, strongly implicating free iron as a source of radicals in the clinical setting.[127]

In a small study of patients on dialysis, it has recently been found that subjects with increased carotid intimal medial thickness were more likely to have received intravenous iron therapy and had higher plasma levels of ferritin than those without increased carotid thickness.[128] There are also studies which tend to refute the role of iron in atherosclerosis. Injections of iron dextran in cholesterol-fed rabbits to produce iron overload surprisingly reduced aortic arch lesion formation, but this was confounded by the fact that this treatment concomitantly reduced plasma cholesterol levels.[129] Treatment of Apo(E)-deficient mice with oral iron also was found to decrease atherosclerosis.[130] Interestingly, in the Health Professionals Follow-up Study of more than 38 000 men, the lifetime history of blood donation had no relationship to the incidence of myocardial infarction or fatal coronary heart disease, although it was correlated strongly with serum ferritin levels.[131]

Whatever their importance is in vivo, reactions with iron and other transition metals can be a major source of experimental error. Even the most fastidiously prepared buffers, made with the highest grade chemicals are contaminated in this way, and major efforts should be made to eliminate this contamination when performing studies of isolated tissues, membranes and enzyme systems. In our experience, if this is not done, fully one-half of the $O_2^{\bullet -}$ formed in a study of isolated tissue homogenates can be attributed to artifact due to these reactions. These can be eliminated by treating buffers for several hours with chelex and using diethylenetriamine-penta-acetic acid (DTPA) in near millimolar concentrations. Experiments with the buffer as a background also provide valuable controls to assure that the major amount of contaminating metals have been removed.

ANTIOXIDANT ENZYMES

Superoxide dismutases

The SODs are a family of metalloenzymes that catalyze the dismutation of $O_2^{\bullet -}$ to oxygen and $H_2O_2^{\bullet}$.[132] The catalytic mechanism of SOD scavenging of $O_2^{\bullet -}$ consists of two consecutive reactions: oxidation of the first molecule of $O_2^{\bullet -}$ to oxygen and reduction of the second molecule of $O_2^{\bullet -}$ to $H_2O_2^{\bullet}$. As an example for the copper-containing SODs, the reaction with $O_2^{\bullet -}$ proceeds as illustrated in reactions 14–16:

$$O_2^{\bullet -} + Cu^{2+}SOD \rightarrow O_2 + Cu^{+}SOD \text{ (reaction 14)}$$

$$O_2^{\bullet -} + Cu^{+}SOD \rightarrow H_2O_2 + Cu^{2+}SOD \text{ (reaction 15)}$$

$$\text{Composite: } 2\ O_2^{\bullet -} + 2\ H^{+} \rightarrow H_2O_2 + O_2 \text{ (reaction 16)}$$

The last reaction occurs even in the absence of SOD, but SOD accelerates it by 1000-fold, minimizing the concentration of available superoxide.

Mammalian cells contain three major SOD isoforms.[133] In most mammalian cells, the predominant form of SOD is the cytoplasmic Cu/Zn SOD (SOD1). The manganese SOD (MnSOD or SOD2) is transcribed in the nucleus and translated in the cytoplasm, but has a sequence which targets it to the mitochondria.[133] At this site, MnSOD protects against mitochondrial DNA damage. MnSOD knockout animals are not viable, and die of a cardiomyopathy within 10 days of birth and have a deficiency of several mitochondrial enzymes, likely due to oxidative damage to the genes encoding them.[134] The extracellular SOD, SOD3, is secreted from cells and is bound by heparin sulfates. In vessels, expression of SOD3 is particularly high, representing 30–50% of the total SOD activity.[135] Recently, it has been recognized that fibulin-5 also plays a major role in binding of SOD3 to the extracellular matrix.[136]

The copper and zinc containing SODs (SOD1 and SOD3) play a major role in modulation of vascular tone. Pharmacological inhibition of these enzymes with diethyl-dihydrocarbonate (DETC) results in a situation in which NO is produced, but is oxidatively inactivated by superoxide before or while leaving the endothelial cell.[137] Likewise, feeding rats a copper-deficient diet leads to an alteration of endothelium-dependent vasodilatation.[138] In keeping with this, SOD1-deficient mice are viable, but have altered vascular reactivity.[139] Because of its location, SOD3 likely protects NO from oxidative degradation as it diffuses from the endothelium to adjacent vascular smooth muscle cells. In keeping with this, mice lacking SOD3 have impaired endothelium-dependent vasodilatation and are predisposed to hypertension.[140]

There is an interesting chemistry that occurs at the copper center of the copper-containing SODs. As is apparent in reactions 14–16, the copper in SOD1 and SOD3 undergoes an initial reduction and then re-oxidation. Exposure of Cu^{+} to H_2O_2, particularly in the presence of bicarbonate, leads to formation of a Cu^{2+}-OH species, which in the absence of any intervention leads to oxidation of nearby histidines that coordinate the copper.[141] This ultimately can inactivate the enzyme, unless a small molecule anionic antioxidant, such as urate, tocopherol or nitrate is present to reduce the Cu-OH. In vitro studies have indicated that the small molecule most effective in protecting the copper-containing SODs in physiological concentrations is uric acid. In keeping with this, recent studies have indicated that both SOD1 and SOD3 are partially inactivated in vessels of Apo(E)-deficient mice. In these mice, vascular production of H_2O_2 is increased, and treatment with oxonic acid, which increases serum uric acid levels, restores activity of SOD1 and SOD3.[142]

An acceptable approach to implicating $O_2^{\bullet-}$ in a biological process is to show that its effect is diminished or removed by treatment with SOD. Because the SODs are large proteins, they do not enter cells and when given intravenously, they are rapidly eliminated from the circulation. For this reason, a variety of modifications of SODs have been made to permit effective membrane targeting and to increase cellular uptake. These include attachment of polyethylene glycol,[143] incorporation of SOD into liposomes,[144,145] and creation of recombinant forms of SOD containing heparin binding sites.[146] It should be stressed that even when these forms of SOD are used, several hours of incubation are required to allow intracellular entry of the molecule. SOD mimetics such as metal-based porphyrinic compounds have been employed; however, these have other effects beyond simply scavenging $O_2^{\bullet-}$, and thus, must be used with caution as specific probes for $O_2^{\bullet-}$.[147,148]

Catalase and glutathione peroxidase

In eukaryotic cells, catalase and gluthatione peroxidase (GPx) are the major scavengers of the H_2O_2. Catalase converts H_2O_2 to water and oxygen via a series of reactions (17–20).

$$H_2O_2 + \text{catalase} \rightarrow H_2O + \text{compound I (reaction 17)}$$

$$\text{Compound I} + H_2O_2 \rightarrow \text{catalase} + H_2O + O_2 \text{ (reaction 18)}$$

$$\text{Composite: } 2\ H_2O_2 \rightarrow 2\ H_2O + O_2 \text{ (reaction 19)}$$

$$\text{Peroxidative activity: compound I} + \text{NADPH} \rightarrow \text{NADP} + \text{compound II (reaction 20)}$$

Formation of compound I in the reaction of catalase heme with H_2O_2 is fast ($k \sim 10^7\ M^{-1}s^{-1}$), but the second peroxidative reaction proceeds relatively slowly ($k \sim 10^2\ M^{-1}s^{-1}$).

An acceptable approach to implicating H_2O_2 in a biological process is to show that its effect is eliminated by catalase when used in reasonable concentrations. In very high concentrations (> 1000 U/ml), catalase can scavenge NO and this should be taken into consideration in systems where both NO and H_2O_2 could have an effect.[149]

The glutathione peroxidases are a group of selenoproteins that utilize H_2O_2 and reduced glutathione as co-substrates leading to formation of water and oxidized glutathione (GSSG).[150] Via this reaction, H_2O_2 plays a crucial role in regulation of the redox status of glutathione, importantly modulating the GSH/GSSG ratio. Glutathione peroxidase can also decompose a number of organic hydroperoxides (ROOH) via similar reactions (reactions 21–24).[151]

$$H_2O_2 + \text{GPx-Se-H} \rightarrow H_2O + \text{GPx-Se-OH (reaction 21)}$$

$$\text{GPx-Se-OH} + \text{GSH} \rightarrow H_2O + \text{GPx-Se-SG (reaction 22)}$$

$$\text{GPx-Se-SG} + \text{GSH} \rightarrow \text{GSSG} + \text{GPx-Se-H (reaction 23)}$$

$$\text{Composite: } 2\ \text{GSH} + H_2O_2 \rightarrow 2\ H_2O + \text{GSSG (reaction 24)}$$

There are four known glutathione peroxidases, and these vary depending on their reactivity and cellular distribution. The phospholipid hydroperoxide glutathione peroxidase (Gpx4) utilizes lipid hydroperoxides in a fashion similar to the reactions above for H_2O_2.[152] Ebselen is a selenium-containing compound that is an effective glutathione peroxidase mimetic. It not only scavenges hydrogen and lipid peroxides, but also peroxynitrite.[153]

Thioredoxin

Thioredoxin (Trx) is a small (Mr 12 000) multifunctional ubiquitous protein characterized by having a redox-active disulfide/dithiol within the conserved active site sequence.[154] Oxidized thioredoxin ($Trx\text{-}S_2$) has a disulfide, and reduced thioredoxin [$Trx\text{-}(SH)_2$] a dithiol. Thioredoxin specifically reduces disulfide bonds in a variety of target proteins. The NADPH-dependent thioredoxin reductase in turn reduces $Trx\text{-}S_2$ to $Trx\text{-}(SH)_2$ (reactions 25–26).

$$Trx\text{-}(SH)_2 + \text{protein-}S_2 \rightarrow Trx\text{-}S_2 + \text{protein-}(SH)_2 \text{ (reaction 25)}$$

$$Trx\text{-}S_2 + \text{NADPH} \rightarrow Trx\text{-}(SH)_2 + \text{NADP}^+ \text{ (reaction 26)}$$

Thioredoxin plays an important role in regulation of gene expression by modulating DNA binding of transcription factors such as Ref1, NFκB and AP1.[155] Thioredoxin also binds to the MAP3 kinase apoptosis signaling kinase-1 (ASK1), which inhibits the ability of ASK1 to activate JNK and p38 MAP kinases, which in turn stimulate adhesion molecules like VCAM1.[156] Oxidation of thioredoxin prevents its binding to ASK1 and promotes this inflammatory pathway. Thioredoxin is also bound by the thioredoxin interacting protein (Txnip), which also prevents its binding to ASK1.[156] These interactions between ASK1, Txnip, thioredoxin and the oxidized state of thioredoxin are illustrated in Figure 33.11.

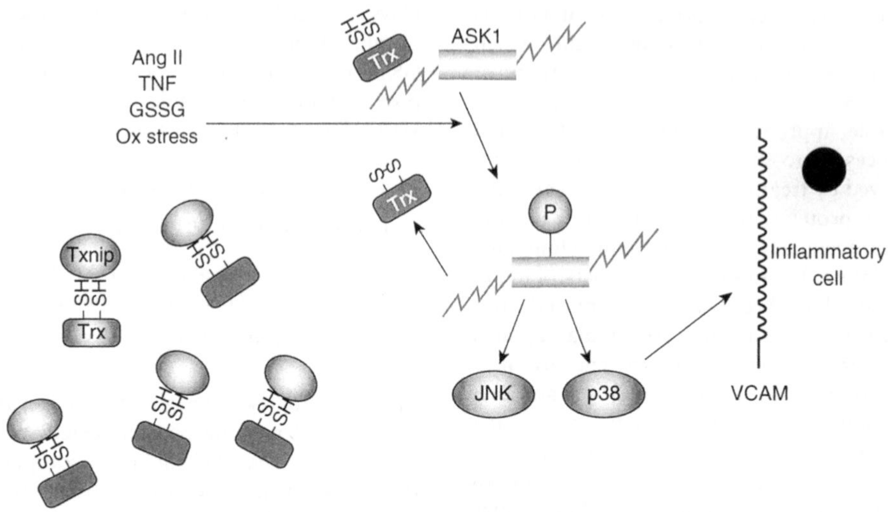

Figure 33.11 Role of thioredoxin (Trx) in modulation of the apoptosis signaling kinase 1 (ASK1). Trx binds ASK1 and inhibits its activation. Several stimuli, including angiotensin II (Ang II), cytokines, oxidative (ox stress) stress and oxidized glutathione (GSSG) can lead to oxidation of the critical cysteine thiols of thioredoxin, leading to its dissociation from ASK1. ASK1 can then be activated by phosphorylation, leading to downstream oxidation of MAP kinases p38 and jun-terminal kinase (JNK), which can then stimulate adhesion molecule expression such as the vascular cell adhesion molecule (VCAM). The thioredoxin interacting protein (Txnip) can bind thioredoxin and inhibit its interaction with ASK1

PEROXIREDOXINS

The peroxiredoxins are a family of six related homodimeric proteins that are expressed at high levels in eukaryotic cells.[157–160] These are peroxidases that have a major role in removing hydroperoxides including H_2O_2 and are differentially distributed in the cell.[160] Peroxiredoxins I and II are located in the cytoplasm. Peroxiredoxin III is targeted to the mitochondria, and peroxiredoxin IV is secreted from the cell. Like thioredoxin, peroxiredoxins I through V have two cysteines. Upon reaction with H_2O_2, one of the cysteines forms sulfenic acid, which then reacts with the adjacent cysteine to form a disulfide (see Figure 33.6 for an example of this reaction).[159] This disulfide is then reduced by thioredoxin. Peroxiredoxin V has been shown to reduce peroxynitrite via a nucleophilic attack on the OO bond with a very high rate constant.[161] Overexpression of wild-type peroxiredoxin II has been shown to inhibit peroxide levels in response to TNF-α, while overexpression of a dominant negative peroxiredoxin II enhanced intracellular peroxide levels in cell culture.[162] Likewise, adenoviral overexpression of peroxiredoxin VI has been shown to protect against hyperoxic lung injury.[163] The role of the peroxiredoxins in modulating oxidant stress in the cardiovascular system is likely important, but has not been well defined.

Normal functions of ROS – signaling properties

The bulk of research before the mid-1990s was performed with the view that ROS were simply injurious byproducts formed by pathologically altered metabolic pathways. While this is true for some ROS, it has become clear that these molecules have important signaling functions.

Of particular interest, H_2O_2 has been implicated in a variety of signaling processes. The mechanisms involved in these signaling events are varied. An important reaction is oxidation of critical cysteines to sulfenic acids, which in turn can serve as precursors to sulfonic acid and/or disulfide formation (Figure 33.6). Disulfide formation can further lead to glutathionylation and protein crossbridging. These modifications can alter the function of a number of enzymes, including protein tyrosine phosphatases, glyceraldehyde-3-phosphate dehydrogenase, and peroxiredoxin. The effect of H_2O_2 on tyrosine phosphatases has been studied in depth. It is now clear that growth factors stimulate cellular H_2O_2 production, which in turn leads to oxidation of critical cysteines of protein tyrosine phosphatases to sulfenic acid, inhibition of tyrosine phosphatase activity, sustained tyrosine phosphorylation, and subsequently, cell proliferation.[164–167] In contrast, reducing agents and thioredoxin have been shown to inhibit cell growth by converting these sulfenic groups to reduced thiols and thereby inhibiting tyrosine phosphatases.[165,167] An important concept is that H_2O_2 seems to have different roles on cell growth depending on its concentration. In low concentrations, H_2O_2 stimulates vascular smooth muscle proliferation and hypertrophy, while at high concentrations it stimulates apoptosis.[168]

H_2O_2 has effects on vasomotion, and has been shown to be a potent stimulus for eNOS activation and over the long term increases eNOS mRNA and protein expression.[34,123] It has recently been recognized that H_2O_2 is very likely one of the endothelium-derived hyperpolarizing factors but it can also activate guanylate cyclase, thereby promoting vasodilatation.[169,170]

The notion that ROS can modulate signaling events under normal circumstances represents a paradigm shift in our understanding of these molecules, and prompts reconsideration of the use of various antioxidant agents that can remove these molecules, thus altering potentially important signaling processes.

A related action of ROS is that they may stimulate compensatory signaling events. For example, mice that have targeted overexpression of $p22^{phox}$ in the smooth muscle have a lifelong increase in vascular $O_2^{\bullet-}$ and H_2O_2 production. Recent studies have shown that these animals have a seemingly compensatory increase in eNOS and ecSOD expression, and that their vessels produce sevenfold more NO than vessels of control animals in response to calcium ionophore stimulation. H_2O_2 seems to mediate these responses because crossing these animals with catalase overexpressing mice negated these compensatory mechanisms.[102,171] In view of this, removal of H_2O_2 without inhibiting the source of ROS could be deleterious.

THE CONCEPT OF OXIDATIVE STRESS AND CLOSING COMMENTS

The term oxidative stress was first introduced by Sies to refer to a condition in which the balance between cellular oxidants and antioxidants is altered, favoring the former.[172] It has become apparent that this condition only applies to the most extreme states and that within the cell there are numerous compartments and targets of ROS which can be modified without a change in the overall cellular redox state. An important concept is that within localized compartments of the cell, specific molecules exist that have reduction potentials such that electron transfer flows from one to the next in an organized fashion. Perturbations of this normal circuitry can lead to disturbed redox signaling such that the 'correct' redox product is not formed and an incorrect product is formed. In the mitochondria, for example, electrons normally flow from NADH sequentially to complex I through complex IV, leading to formation of water, ATP and NAD^+. When electrons begin to 'leak' from this normal flow, they can lead to formation of $O_2^{\bullet-}$ and ultimately cause oxidative damage to DNA in a localized area. This can happen without greatly changing the redox status of the cytoplasm. Likewise, the NOS enzyme, present in the cytoplasm and membranes, normally transfers electrons from NADPH to flavins in the reductase domain to a heme group and ultimately to L-arginine. In pathological states, this electron flow can be disrupted, leading to formation of superoxide and other ROS and ultimately to oxidation of target molecules. Changes in the oxidation state of thiols can independently occur in the nucleus, cytoplasm, mitochondria and even in tiny subcellular spaces such as caveoli. Oxidative and nitrosative modifications of proteins can change enzyme function, protein localization, and protein/protein interaction. Very specific targets such as these could markedly alter cell function with altering the overall redox status. In keeping with this, numerous ROS-generating enzymes have specialized subcellular locations, and their activation has very different consequences on cell function. For example, in vascular smooth muscle cells, Nox1 is localized to caveoli while Nox4 is associated with the cell cytoskeleton.[96]

These considerations confound the use of antioxidants in treatment of various diseases. An ideal antioxidant would have a redox potential that would redirect electron flow from a pathological target to its correct downstream target, would reduce an oxidized protein to its correct native state or would remove a nitrogroup from a modified protein, while having no other effects. Unfortunately, this is almost impossible. It is, therefore, not surprising that several recent clinical trials have failed to show any benefit of antioxidant vitamins or of antioxidant vitamin cocktails, and in some cases, antioxidants have proven harmful.[173]

Likewise, the subcellular location of redox reactions makes the use of plasma and urinary biomarkers to detect overall oxidative stress difficult. In some cases, these assays have provided valuable information; however, it is unlikely that subtle degrees of oxidation will be reflected by such global markers.

Consequently, it remains extremely important that we continue to refine our methods of detecting ROS, and in particular, molecular targets that have been modified by oxidative and nitrosative reactions. In this regard, proteomic and metabolomic approaches will likely become increasing valuable experimental and clinical tools. Methods of detecting specific protein or small molecule modifications that are specific to certain pathways are promising in this regard. For example, oxidatively modified tyrosines have proven useful in identifying subjects with active coronary artery disease and have responded to therapeutic interventions.[174,175] Likewise, an oxidized pro-domain of matrix metalloproteinase-7 has been reported to be released upon exposure to $HOCl^-$.[176] In addition, we need to continue to advance our understanding of the basic mechanisms underlying oxidative events and develop therapies directed to normalize these in pathological conditions. For example, in the case of eNOS uncoupling, treatment with BH_4 has proven effective.[83] This corrects electron flow through the eNOS enzyme without actually scavenging radicals. Likewise, specific inhibitors of enzymes that produce ROS may be more effective than scavenging radicals after they have been formed. To accomplish this; however, it is essential that we precisely identify the source of ROS in various pathological conditions and develop specific inhibitors of these enzymes.

REFERENCES

1. Raven JA, Johnston AM, Kubler JE et al. Seaweeds in cold seas: evolution and carbon acquisition. Ann Bot (Lond) 2002; 90: 525–36.
2. Kerr RA. Earth science. The story of O_2. Science 2005; 308: 1730–2.
3. Hedges SB, Blair JE, Venturi ML et al. A molecular timescale of eukaryote evolution and the rise of complex multicellular life. BMC Evol Biol 2004; 4: 2.
4. Wong Y. Atomic orbitals version 1.0. Workbook edition. Sudbury, MA: Jones & Bartlett Publishers, 1997.
5. Buettner GR. The pecking order of free radicals and antioxidants: lipid peroxidation, alpha-tocopherol, and ascorbate. Arch Biochem Biophys 1993; 300: 535–43.
6. Afanas Ev IB. Superoxide ion chemistry and biological implications. Boca Raton: CRC Press, 1989.
7. Gardner PR. Superoxide-driven aconitase FE-S center cycling. Biosci Rep 1997; 17: 33–42.
8. Chisolm GM 3rd, Hazen SL, Fox PL et al. The oxidation of lipoproteins by monocytes-macrophages. Biochemical and biological mechanisms. J Biol Chem 1999; 274: 25959–62.
9. Harrison DG, Bates JN. The nitrovasodilators. New ideas about old drugs. Circulation 1993; 87: 1461–7.
10. Stuehr DJ. Mammalian nitric oxide synthases. Biochim Biophys Acta 1999; 1411: 217–30.
11. Boulanger CM, Heymes C, Benessiano J et al. Neuronal nitric oxide synthase is expressed in rat vascular smooth muscle cells: activation by angiotensin II in hypertension. Circ Res 1998; 83: 1271–8.
12. Brophy CM, Knoepp L, Xin J et al. Functional expression of NOS 1 in vascular smooth muscle. Am J Physiol Heart Circ Physiol 2000; 278: H991–H997.
13. Stoclet JC, Muller B, Gyorgy K et al. The inducible nitric oxide synthase in vascular and cardiac tissue. Eur J Pharmacol 1999; 375: 139–55.
14. Zweier JL, Wang P, Samouilov A et al. Enzyme-independent formation of nitric oxide in biological tissues. Nat Med 1995; 1: 804–9.
15. Cosby K, Partovi KS, Crawford JH et al. Nitrite reduction to nitric oxide by deoxyhemoglobin vasodilates the human circulation. Nat Med 2003; 9: 1498–505.
16. Murad F, Waldman S, Molina C et al. Regulation and role of guanylate cyclase-cyclic GMP in vascular relaxation. Prog Clin Biol Res 1987; 249: 65–76.
17. Adachi T, Weisbrod RM, Pimentel DR et al. S-Glutathiolation by peroxynitrite activates SERCA during arterial relaxation by nitric oxide. Nat Med 2004; 10: 1200–7.
18. Feil R, Lohmann SM, de Jonge H et al. Cyclic GMP-dependent protein kinases and the cardiovascular system: insights from genetically modified mice. Circ Res 2003; 93: 907–16.
19. Pfeifer A, Klatt P, Massberg S et al. Defective smooth muscle regulation in cGMP kinase I-deficient mice. EMBO J 1998; 17: 3045–51.
20. Moncada S. Nitric oxide and cell respiration: physiology and pathology. Verh K Acad Geneeskd Belg 2000; 62: 171–9; discussion 179–81.
21. Trochu JN, Bouhour JB, Kaley G et al. Role of endothelium-derived nitric oxide in the regulation of cardiac oxygen metabolism: implications in health and disease. Circ Res 2000; 87: 1108–17.
22. Chen Z, Zhang J, Stamler JS. Identification of the enzymatic mechanism of nitroglycerin bioactivation. Proc Natl Acad Sci U S A 2002; 99: 8306–11.
23. Stamler JS, Jaraki O, Osborne J et al. Nitric oxide circulates in mammalian plasma primarily as an S-nitroso adduct of serum albumin. Proc Natl Acad Sci U S A 1992; 89: 7674–7.
24. Myers PR, Minor RL Jr, Guerra R Jr et al. Vasorelaxant properties of the endothelium-derived relaxing factor more closely resemble S-nitrosocysteine than nitric oxide. Nature 1990; 345: 161–3.
25. Gow AJ, Stamler JS. Reactions between nitric oxide and haemoglobin under physiological conditions. Nature 1998; 391: 169–73.
26. Jaszewski AR, Fann YC, Chen YR et al. EPR spectroscopy studies on the structural transition of nitrosyl hemoglobin in the arterial-venous cycle of DEANO-treated rats as it relates to the proposed nitrosyl hemoglobin/nitrosothiol hemoglobin exchange. Free Radic Biol Med 2003; 35: 444–51.
27. Gladwin MT, Schechter AN. NO contest: nitrite versus S-nitroso-hemoglobin. Circ Res 2004; 94: 851–5.
28. Patel RP, Hogg N, Spencer NY et al. Biochemical characterization of human S-nitrosohemoglobin. Effects on oxygen binding and transnitrosation. J Biol Chem 1999; 274: 15487–92.
29. Patel RP. Biochemical aspects of the reaction of hemoglobin and NO: implications for Hb-based blood substitutes. Free Radic Biol Med 2000; 28: 1518–25.
30. Crawford JH, White CR, Patel RP. Vasoactivity of S-nitrosohemoglobin: role of oxygen, heme, and NO oxidation states. Blood 2003; 101: 4408–15.
31. Foster MW, Pawloski JR, Singel DJ et al. Role of circulating S-nitrosothiols in control of blood pressure. Hypertension 2005; 45: 15–17.
32. Grossi L, Montevecchi PC. A kinetic study of S-nitrosothiol decomposition. Chemistry 2002; 8: 380–7.
33. Tsikas D, Sandmann J, Rossa S et al. Investigations of S-transnitrosylation reactions between low- and high-molecular-weight S-nitroso compounds and their thiols by high-performance liquid chromatography and gas chromatography-mass spectrometry. Anal Biochem 1999; 270: 231–41.
34. Cai H, Davis ME, Drummond GR et al. Induction of endothelial NO synthase by hydrogen peroxide via a

Ca(2+)/calmodulin-dependent protein kinase II/janus kinase 2-dependent pathway. Arterioscler Thromb Vasc Biol 2001; 21: 1571–6.
35. Inoue N, Ramasamy S, Fukai T et al. Shear stress modulates expression of Cu/Zn superoxide dismutase in human aortic endothelial cells. Circ Res 1996; 79: 32–7.
36. Yamazaki I. One-electron and two-electron transfer mechanisms in enzymic oxidation-reduction reactions. Adv Biophys 1971; 2: 33–76.
37. Klebanoff SJ. Myeloperoxidase: friend and foe. J Leukoc Biol 2005; 77: 598–625.
38. Abu-Soud HM, Hazen SL. Nitric oxide is a physiological substrate for mammalian peroxidases. J Biol Chem 2000; 275: 37524–32.
39. Kehrer JP. The Haber-Weiss reaction and mechanisms of toxicity. Toxicology 2000; 149: 43–50.
40. Liochev SI, Fridovich I. The relative importance of HO• and ONOO- in mediating the toxicity of O•. Free Radic Biol Med 1999; 26: 777–8.
41. Youdim MB, Ben-Shachar D, Riederer P. The possible role of iron in the etiopathology of Parkinson's disease. Mov Disord 1993; 8: 1–12.
42. Jellinger KA. The role of iron in neurodegeneration: prospects for pharmacotherapy of Parkinson's disease. Drugs Aging 1999; 14: 115–40.
43. Qayyum R, Schulman P. Iron and atherosclerosis. Clin Cardiol 2005; 28: 119–22.
44. Saito K, Ishizaka N, Aizawa T et al. Role of aberrant iron homeostasis in the upregulation of transforming growth factor-beta1 in the kidney of angiotensin II-induced hypertensive rats. Hypertens Res 2004; 27: 599–607.
45. Koppenol WH. The basic chemistry of nitrogen monoxide and peroxynitrite. Free Radic Biol Med 1998; 25: 385–91.
46. Floyd RA, Carney JM. Free radical damage to protein and DNA: mechanisms involved and relevant observations on brain undergoing oxidative stress. Ann Neurol 1992; 32 (Suppl): S22–S27.
47. Finkelstein E, Rosen GM, Rauckman EJ. Spin trapping of superoxide and hydroxyl radical: practical aspects. Arch Biochem Biophys 1980; 200: 1–16.
48. Jourd'heuil D, Miranda KM, Kim SM et al. The oxidative and nitrosative chemistry of the nitric oxide/superoxide reaction in the presence of bicarbonate. Arch Biochem Biophys 1999; 365: 92–100.
49. Beckman JS, Koppenol WH. Nitric oxide, superoxide, and peroxynitrite: the good, the bad, and ugly. Am J Physiol 1996; 271: C1424–C1437.
50. Harrison DG. Cellular and molecular mechanisms of endothelial cell dysfunction. J Clin Invest 1997; 100: 2153–7.
51. Kissner R, Nauser T, Kurz C et al. Peroxynitrous acid – where is the hydroxyl radical? IUBMB Life 2003; 55: 567–72.
52. Koppenol WH. The basic chemistry of nitrogen monoxide and peroxynitrite. Free Radic Biol Med 1998; 25: 385–91.
53. Vesela A, Wilhelm J. The role of carbon dioxide in free radical reactions of the organism. Physiol Res 2002; 51: 335–9.
54. Yermilov V, Yoshie Y, Rubio J et al. Effects of carbon dioxide/bicarbonate on induction of DNA single-strand breaks and formation of 8-nitroguanine, 8-oxoguanine and base-propenal mediated by peroxynitrite. FEBS Lett 1996; 399: 67–70.
55. Padmaja S, Squadrito GL, Lemercier JN et al. Peroxynitrite-mediated oxidation of D,L-selenomethionine: kinetics, mechanism and the role of carbon dioxide. Free Radic Biol Med 1997; 23: 917–26.
56. Wagner BA, Buettner GR, Burns CP. Free radical-mediated lipid peroxidation in cells: oxidizability is a function of cell lipid bis-allylic hydrogen content. Biochemistry 1994; 33: 4449–53.
57. Thomas SR, Davies MJ, Stocker R. Oxidation and antioxidation of human low-density lipoprotein and plasma exposed to 3-morpholinosydnonimine and reagent peroxynitrite. Chem Res Toxicol 1998; 11: 484–94.
58. O'Donnell VB, Chumley PH, Hogg N et al. Nitric oxide inhibition of lipid peroxidation: kinetics of reaction with lipid peroxyl radicals and comparison with alpha-tocopherol. Biochemistry 1997; 36: 15216–23.
59. Uchida K. Role of reactive aldehyde in cardiovascular diseases. Free Radic Biol Med 2000; 28: 1685–96.
60. Liu TZ, Stern A, Morrow JD. The isoprostanes: unique bioactive products of lipid peroxidation. An overview. J Biomed Sci 1998; 5: 415–20.
61. Morrow JD. Quantification of isoprostanes as indices of oxidant stress and the risk of atherosclerosis in humans. Arterioscler Thromb Vasc Biol 2005; 25: 279–86.
62. Mayne ST. Antioxidant nutrients and chronic disease: use of biomarkers of exposure and oxidative stress status in epidemiologic research. J Nutr 2003; 133 (Suppl 3): 933S–940S.
63. Cracowski JL, Devillier P, Durand T et al. Vascular biology of the isoprostanes. J Vasc Res 2001; 38: 93–103.
64. Dwarakanath RS, Sahar S, Reddy MA et al. Regulation of monocyte chemoattractant protein-1 by the oxidized lipid, 13-hydroperoxyoctadecadienoic acid, in vascular smooth muscle cells via nuclear factor-kappa B (NF-kappa B). J Mol Cell Cardiol 2004; 36: 585–95.
65. Natarajan R, Reddy MA, Malik KU et al. Signaling mechanisms of nuclear factor-kappab-mediated activation of inflammatory genes by 13-hydroperoxyoctadecadienoic acid in cultured vascular smooth muscle cells. Arterioscler Thromb Vasc Biol 2001; 21: 1408–13.
66. Dickinson D, Forman H. Glutathione in defense and signaling: lessons from a small thiol. Ann N Y Acad Sci 2002; 973: 488–504.
67. Xu G, Chance MR. Radiolytic modification of sulfur-containing amino acid residues in model peptides: fundamental studies for protein footprinting. Anal Chem 2005; 77: 2437–49.
68. Shao B, Belaaouaj A, Verlinde CL et al. Methionine sulfoxide and proteolytic cleavage contribute to the inactivation of cathepsin G by hypochlorous acid: an oxidative mechanism for regulation of serine proteinases by myeloperoxidase. J Biol Chem 2005; 280: 29311–21.
69. Gao J, Yin DH, Yao Y et al. Loss of conformational stability in calmodulin upon methionine oxidation. Biophys J 1998; 74: 1115–34.
70. Mohr S, Hallak H, de Boitte A et al. Nitric oxide-induced S-glutathionylation and inactivation of glyceraldehyde-3-phosphate dehydrogenase. J Biol Chem 1999; 274: 9427–30.
71. O'Brian CA, Chu F. Post-translational disulfide modifications in cell signaling – role of inter-protein, intra-protein, S-glutathionyl, and S-cysteaminyl disulfide modifications in signal transmission. Free Radic Res 2005; 39: 471–80.
72. Ghezzi P. Regulation of protein function by glutathionylation. Free Radic Res 2005; 39: 573–80.
73. Hurd TR, Costa NJ, Dahm CC et al. Glutathionylation of mitochondrial proteins. Antioxid Redox Signal 2005; 7: 999–1010.
74. Fratelli M, Gianazza E, Ghezzi P. Redox proteomics: identification and functional role of glutathionylated proteins. Expert Rev Proteomics 2004; 1: 365–76.
75. Dalle-Donne I, Rossi R, Giustarini D et al. Actin S-glutathionylation: evidence against a thiol-disulphide exchange mechanism. Free Radic Biol Med 2003; 35: 1185–93.
76. Pineda-Molina E, Klatt P, Vazquez J et al. Glutathionylation of the p50 subunit of NF-kappaB: a mechanism for redox-induced inhibition of DNA binding. Biochemistry 2001; 40: 14134–42.

77. Shelton MD, Chock PB, Mieyal JJ. Glutaredoxin: role in reversible protein s-glutathionylation and regulation of redox signal transduction and protein translocation. Antioxid Redox Signal 2005; 7: 348–66.
78. Pietzsch J, Julius U. Different susceptibility to oxidation of proline and arginine residues of apolipoprotein B-100 among subspecies of low density lipoproteins. FEBS Lett 2001; 491: 123–6.
79. Zhang WH, Liu J, Xu G et al. Model studies on protein side chain modification by 4-oxo-2-nonenal. Chem Res Toxicol 2003; 16: 512–23.
80. Takeda A, Smith MA, Avila J et al. In Alzheimer's disease, heme oxygenase is coincident with Alz50, an epitope of tau induced by 4-hydroxy-2-nonenal modification. J Neurochem 2000; 75: 1234–41.
81. Selley ML, Bourne DJ, Bartlett MR et al. Occurrence of (E)-4-hydroxy-2-nonenal in plasma and synovial fluid of patients with rheumatoid arthritis and osteoarthritis. Ann Rheum Dis 1992; 51: 481–4.
82. Poon HF, Calabrese V, Scapagnini G et al. Free radicals and brain aging. Clin Geriatr Med 2004; 20: 329–59.
83. Landmesser U, Dikalov S, Price S et al. Oxidation of tetrahydrobiopterin leads to uncoupling of endothelial cell nitric oxide synthase in hypertension: role of the NADPH-oxidase. J Clin Invest 2003; 111: 1201–9.
84. Laursen JB, Somers M, Kurz S et al. Endothelial regulation of vasomotion in apoE-deficient mice: implications for interactions between peroxynitrite and tetrahydrobiopterin. Circulation 2001; 103: 1282–8.
85. Kuzkaya N, Weissmann N, Harrison DG et al. Interactions of peroxynitrite, tetrahydrobiopterin, ascorbic acid, and thiols: implications for uncoupling endothelial nitric-oxide synthase. J Biol Chem 2003; 278: 22546–54.
86. Cooke M, MD E, Dizdaroglu M et al. Oxidative DNA damage: mechanisms, mutation, and disease. FASEB J 2003; 17: 1195–214.
87. Richter C. Oxidative damage to mitochondrial DNA and its relationship to ageing. Int J Biochem Cell Biol 1995; 27: 647–53.
88. Ballinger SW, Patterson C, Yan CN et al. Hydrogen peroxide- and peroxynitrite-induced mitochondrial DNA damage and dysfunction in vascular endothelial and smooth muscle cells. Circ Res 2000; 86: 960–6.
89. Ballinger SW, Patterson C, Knight-Lozano CA et al. Mitochondrial integrity and function in atherogenesis. Circulation 2002; 106: 544–9.
90. Lassegue B, Clempus RE. Vascular NAD(P)H oxidases: specific features, expression, and regulation. Am J Physiol Regul Integr Comp Physiol 2003; 285: R277–R297.
91. Gorlach A, Brandes RP, Nguyen K et al. A gp91phox containing NADPH oxidase selectively expressed in endothelial cells is a major source of oxygen radical generation in the arterial wall. Circ Res 2000; 87: 26–32.
92. Jones SA, O'Donnell VB, Wood JD et al. Expression of phagocyte NADPH oxidase components in human endothelial cells. Am J Physiol 1996; 271: H1626–H1634.
93. Touyz RM, Chen X, Tabet F et al. Expression of a functionally active gp91phox-containing neutrophil-type NAD(P)H oxidase in smooth muscle cells from human resistance arteries: regulation by angiotensin II. Circ Res 2002; 90: 1205–13.
94. Wang HD, Pagano PJ, Du Y et al. Superoxide anion from the adventitia of the rat thoracic aorta inactivates nitric oxide. Circ Res 1998; 82: 810–18.
95. Ago T, Kitazono T, Ooboshi H et al. Nox4 as the major catalytic component of an endothelial NAD(P)H oxidase. Circulation 2004; 109: 227–33.
96. Hilenski LL, Clempus RE, Quinn MT et al. Distinct subcellular localizations of Nox1 and Nox4 in vascular smooth muscle cells. Arterioscler Thromb Vasc Biol 2004; 24: 677–83.
97. Seshiah PN, Weber DS, Rocic P et al. Angiotensin II stimulation of NAD(P)H oxidase activity: upstream mediators. Circ Res 2002; 91: 406–13.
98. Touyz RM, Yao G, Schiffrin EL. c-Src induces phosphorylation and translocation of p47phox: role in superoxide generation by angiotensin II in human vascular smooth muscle cells. Arterioscler Thromb Vasc Biol 2003; 23: 981–7.
99. Takeya R, Ueno N, Kami K et al. Novel human homologues of p47phox and p67phox participate in activation of superoxide-producing NADPH oxidases. J Biol Chem 2003; 278: 25234–46.
100. Banfi B, Clark RA, Steger K et al. Two novel proteins activate superoxide generation by the NADPH oxidase NOX1. J Biol Chem 2003; 278: 3510–13.
101. Ambasta RK, Kumar P, Griendling KK et al. Direct interaction of the novel Nox proteins with p22phox is required for the formation of a functionally active NADPH oxidase. J Biol Chem 2004; 279: 45935–41.
102. Laude K, Cai H, Fink B et al. Hemodynamic and biochemical adaptations to vascular smooth muscle overexpression of p22phox in mice. Am J Physiol Heart Circ Physiol 2005; 288: H7–H12.
103. Harrison R. Structure and function of xanthine oxidoreductase: where are we now? Free Radic Biol Med 2002; 33: 774–97.
104. Sakuma S, Fujimoto Y, Sakamoto Y et al. Peroxynitrite induces the conversion of xanthine dehydrogenase to oxidase in rabbit liver. Biochem Biophys Res Commun 1997; 230: 476–9.
105. Friedl HP, Till GO, Ryan US et al. Mediator-induced activation of xanthine oxidase in endothelial cells. FASEB J 1989; 3: 2512–18.
106. McNally JS, Davis ME, Giddens DP et al. Role of xanthine oxidoreductase and NAD(P)H oxidase in endothelial superoxide production in response to oscillatory shear stress. Am J Physiol Heart Circ Physiol 2003; 285: H2290–H2297.
107. Linder N, Rapola J, Raivio KO. Cellular expression of xanthine oxidoreductase protein in normal human tissues. Lab Invest 1999; 79: 967–74.
108. McNally JS, Saxena A, Cai H et al. Regulation of xanthine oxidoreductase protein expression by hydrogen peroxide and calcium. Arterioscler Thromb Vasc Biol 2005; 25: 1623–8.
109. Spiekermann S, Landmesser U, Dikalov S et al. Electron spin resonance characterization of vascular xanthine and NAD(P)H oxidase activity in patients with coronary artery disease: relation to endothelium-dependent vasodilation. Circulation 2003; 107: 1383–9.
110. Guthikonda S, Sinkey C, Barenz T et al. Xanthine oxidase inhibition reverses endothelial dysfunction in heavy smokers. Circulation 2003; 107: 416–21.
111. Cardillo C, Kilcoyne CM, Cannon RO 3rd et al. Xanthine oxidase inhibition with oxypurinol improves endothelial vasodilator function in hypercholesterolemic but not in hypertensive patients. Hypertension 1997; 30: 57–63.
112. Farquharson CA, Butler R, Hill A et al. Allopurinol improves endothelial dysfunction in chronic heart failure. Circulation 2002; 106: 221–6.
113. Sohn HY, Krotz F, Gloe T et al. Differential regulation of xanthine and NAD(P)H oxidase by hypoxia in human umbilical vein endothelial cells. Role of nitric oxide and adenosine. Cardiovasc Res 2003; 58: 638–46.
114. Fukushima T, Adachi T, Hirano K. The heparin-binding site of human xanthine oxidase. Biol Pharm Bull 1995; 18: 156–8.
115. Houston M, Estevez A, Chumley P et al. Binding of xanthine oxidase to vascular endothelium. Kinetic characterization and

oxidative impairment of nitric oxide-dependent signaling. J Biol Chem 1999; 274: 4985–94.
116. Landmesser U, Spiekermann S, Dikalov S et al. Vascular oxidative stress and endothelial dysfunction in patients with chronic heart failure: role of xanthine-oxidase and extracellular superoxide dismutase. Circulation 2002; 106: 3073–8.
117. Vasquez-Vivar J, Kalyanaraman B, Martasek P et al. Superoxide generation by endothelial nitric oxide synthase: the influence of cofactors. Proc Natl Acad Sci U S A 1998; 95: 9220–5.
118. Hink U, Li H, Mollnau H et al. Mechanisms underlying endothelial dysfunction in diabetes mellitus. Circ Res 2001; 88: E14–E22.
119. Stroes E, Kastelein J, Cosentino F et al. Tetrahydrobiopterin restores endothelial function in hypercholesterolemia. J Clin Invest 1997; 99: 41–6.
120. Landmesser U, Dikalov S, Price SR et al. Oxidation of tetrahydrobiopterin leads to uncoupling of endothelial cell nitric oxide synthase in hypertension. J Clin Invest 2003; 111: 1201–9.
121. Heller R, Unbehaun A, Schellenberg B et al. L-ascorbic acid potentiates endothelial nitric oxide synthesis via a chemical stabilization of tetrahydrobiopterin. J Biol Chem 2001; 276: 40–7.
122. Huang A, Vita JA, Venema RC et al. Ascorbic acid enhances endothelial nitric-oxide synthase activity by increasing intracellular tetrahydrobiopterin. J Biol Chem 2000; 275: 17399–406.
123. Drummond GR, Cai H, Davis ME et al. Transcriptional and posttranscriptional regulation of endothelial nitric oxide synthase expression by hydrogen peroxide. Circ Res 2000; 86: 347–54.
124. Zhang R, Brennan ML, Fu X et al. Association between myeloperoxidase levels and risk of coronary artery disease. JAMA 2001; 286: 2136–42.
125. Zheng L, Nukuna B, Brennan ML et al. Apolipoprotein A-I is a selective target for myeloperoxidase-catalyzed oxidation and functional impairment in subjects with cardiovascular disease. J Clin Invest 2004; 114: 529–41.
126. Qian SY, Buettner GR. Iron and dioxygen chemistry is an important route to initiation of biological free radical oxidations: an electron paramagnetic resonance spin trapping study. Free Radic Biol Med 1999; 26: 1447–56.
127. Duffy SJ, Biegelsen ES, Holbrook M et al. Iron chelation improves endothelial function in patients with coronary artery disease. Circulation 2001; 103: 2799–804.
128. Reis KA, Guz G, Ozdemir H et al. Intravenous iron therapy as a possible risk factor for atherosclerosis in end-stage renal disease. Int Heart J 2005; 46: 255–64.
129. Dabbagh AJ, Shwaery GT, Keaney JF Jr et al. Effect of iron overload and iron deficiency on atherosclerosis in the hypercholesterolemic rabbit. Arterioscler Thromb Vasc Biol 1997; 17: 2638–45.
130. Kirk EA, Heinecke JW, LeBoeuf RC. Iron overload diminishes atherosclerosis in apoE-deficient mice. J Clin Invest 2001; 107: 1545–53.
131. Ascherio A, Rimm EB, Giovannucci E et al. Blood donations and risk of coronary heart disease in men. Circulation 2001; 103: 52–7.
132. Beyer W, Imlay J, Fridovich I. Superoxide dismutases. Prog Nucleic Acid Res Mol Biol 1991; 40: 221–53.
133. Zelko IN, Mariani TJ, Folz RJ. Superoxide dismutase multigene family: a comparison of the CuZn-SOD (SOD1), Mn-SOD (SOD2), and EC-SOD (SOD3) gene structures, evolution, and expression. Free Radic Biol Med 2002; 33: 337–49.
134. Li Y, Huang TT, Carlson EJ et al. Dilated cardiomyopathy and neonatal lethality in mutant mice lacking manganese superoxide dismutase. Nat Genet 1995; 11: 376–81.
135. Fukai T, Folz RJ, Landmesser U et al. Extracellular superoxide dismutase and cardiovascular disease. Cardiovasc Res 2002; 55: 239–49.
136. Nguyen AD, Itoh S, Jeney V et al. Fibulin-5 is a novel binding protein for extracellular superoxide dismutase. Circ Res 2004; 95: 1067–74.
137. Mugge A, Elwell JH, Peterson TE et al. Release of intact endothelium-derived relaxing factor depends on endothelial superoxide dismutase activity. Am J Physiol 1991; 260: C219–C225.
138. Alvarez B, Demicheli V, Duran R et al. Inactivation of human Cu,Zn superoxide dismutase by peroxynitrite and formation of histidinyl radical. Free Radic Biol Med 2004; 37: 813–22.
139. Didion SP, Ryan MJ, Didion LA et al. Increased superoxide and vascular dysfunction in CuZnSOD-deficient mice. Circ Res 2002; 91: 938–44.
140. Jung O, Marklund SL, Geiger H et al. Extracellular superoxide dismutase is a major determinant of nitric oxide bioavailability: in vivo and ex vivo evidence from ecSOD-deficient mice. Circ Res 2003; 93: 622–9.
141. Goss SP, Singh RJ, Kalyanaraman B. Bicarbonate enhances the peroxidase activity of Cu,Zn-superoxide dismutase. Role of carbonate anion radical. J Biol Chem 1999; 274: 28233–9.
142. Hink H, Santanam N, Dikalov S et al. Peroxidase properties of the extracellular superoxide dismutase: role of uric acid in modulating in vivo activity. Arterioscler, Thromb Vasc Biol 2002; 22: 1402–8.
143. Tamura Y, Chi LG, Driscoll EM Jr et al. Superoxide dismutase conjugated to polyethylene glycol provides sustained protection against myocardial ischemia/reperfusion injury in canine heart. Circ Res 1988; 63: 944–59.
144. Munzel T, Sayegh H, Freeman BA et al. Evidence for enhanced vascular superoxide anion production in nitrate tolerance. A novel mechanism underlying tolerance and cross-tolerance. J Clin Invest 1995; 95: 187–94.
145. Laursen JB, Rajagopalan S, Galis Z et al. Role of superoxide in angiotensin II-induced but not catecholamine-induced hypertension. Circulation 1997; 95: 588–93.
146. Inoue M, Watanabe N, Utsumi T et al. Targeting SOD by gene and protein engineering and inhibition of free radical injury. Free Radic Res Commun 1991; 12–13 (Pt 1): 391–9.
147. Perez MJ, Cederbaum AI. Antioxidant and pro-oxidant effects of a manganese porphyrin complex against CYP2E1-dependent toxicity. Free Radic Biol Med 2002; 33: 111–27.
148. Ross AD, Sheng H, Warner DS et al. Hemodynamic effects of metalloporphyrin catalytic antioxidants: structure-activity relationships and species specificity. Free Radic Biol Med 2002; 33: 1657–69.
149. Brunelli L, Yermilov V, Beckman JS. Modulation of catalase peroxidatic and catalatic activity by nitric oxide. Free Radic Biol Med 2001; 30: 709–14.
150. Brigelius-Flohe R. Tissue-specific functions of individual glutathione peroxidases. Free Radic Biol Med 1999; 27: 951–65.
151. Aumann KD, Bedorf N, Brigelius-Flohe R et al. Glutathione peroxidase revisited – simulation of the catalytic cycle by computer-assisted molecular modelling. Biomed Environ Sci 1997; 10: 136–55.
152. Schuckelt R, Brigelius-Flohe R, Maiorino M et al. Phospholipid hydroperoxide glutathione peroxidase is a selenoenzyme distinct from the classical glutathione peroxidase as evident from cDNA and amino acid sequencing. Free Radic Res Commun 1991; 14: 343–61.
153. Cotgreave IA, Duddy SK, Kass GE et al. Studies on the anti-inflammatory activity of ebselen. Ebselen interferes with granulocyte oxidative burst by dual inhibition of NADPH oxidase and protein kinase C? Biochem Pharmacol 1989; 38: 649–56.
154. Watson WH, Yang X, Choi YE et al. Thioredoxin and its role in toxicology. Toxicol Sci 2004; 78: 3–14.

155. Lean J, Kirstein B, Urry Z et al. Thioredoxin-1 mediates osteoclast stimulation by reactive oxygen species. Biochem Biophys Res Commun 2004; 321: 845–50.
156. Yamawaki H, Pan S, Lee RT, Berk BC. Fluid shear stress inhibits vascular inflammation by decreasing thioredoxin-interacting protein in endothelial cells. J Clin Invest 2005; 115: 733–8.
157. Flohe L, Budde H, Hofmann B. Peroxiredoxins in antioxidant defense and redox regulation. Biofactors 2003; 19: 3–10.
158. Hofmann B, Hecht HJ, Flohe L. Peroxiredoxins. Biol Chem 2002; 383: 347–64.
159. Wood ZA, Schroder E, Robin Harris J et al. Structure, mechanism and regulation of peroxiredoxins. Trends Biochem Sci 2003; 28: 32–40.
160. Rhee SG, Chae HZ, Kim K. Peroxiredoxins: a historical overview and speculative preview of novel mechanisms and emerging concepts in cell signaling. Free Radic Biol Med 2005; 38: 1543–52.
161. Dubuisson M, Vander Stricht D, Clippe A et al. Human peroxiredoxin 5 is a peroxynitrite reductase. FEBS Lett 2004; 571: 161–5.
162. Kang SW, Chang TS, Lee TH et al. Cytosolic peroxiredoxin attenuates the activation of Jnk and p38 but potentiates that of Erk in Hela cells stimulated with tumor necrosis factor-alpha. J Biol Chem 2004; 279: 2535–43.
163. Wang Y, Manevich Y, Feinstein SI et al. Adenovirus-mediated transfer of the 1-cys peroxiredoxin gene to mouse lung protects against hyperoxic injury. Am J Physiol Lung Cell Mol Physiol 2004; 286: L1188–L1193.
164. Denu JM, Tanner KG. Specific and reversible inactivation of protein tyrosine phosphatases by hydrogen peroxide: evidence for a sulfenic acid intermediate and implications for redox regulation. Biochemistry 1998; 37: 5633–42.
165. Lee SR, Kwon KS, Kim SR et al. Reversible inactivation of protein-tyrosine phosphatase 1B in A431 cells stimulated with epidermal growth factor. J Biol Chem 1998; 273: 15366–72.
166. Salmeen A, Andersen JN, Myers MP et al. Redox regulation of protein tyrosine phosphatase 1B involves a sulphenyl-amide intermediate. Nature 2003; 423: 769–73.
167. Denu JM, Tanner KG. Redox regulation of protein tyrosine phosphatases by hydrogen peroxide: detecting sulfenic acid intermediates and examining reversible inactivation. Methods Enzymol 2002; 348: 297–305.
168. Griendling KK, Harrison DG. Dual role of reactive oxygen species in vascular growth. Circ Res 1999; 85: 562–3.
169. Matoba T, Shimokawa H, Kubota H et al. Hydrogen peroxide is an endothelium-derived hyperpolarizing factor in human mesenteric arteries. Biochem Biophys Res Commun 2002; 290: 909–13.
170. Burke TM, Wolin MS. Hydrogen peroxide elicits pulmonary arterial relaxation and guanylate cyclase activation. Am J Physiol 1987; 252: H721–H732.
171. Weber DS, Rocic P, Mellis AM et al. Angiotensin II-induced hypertrophy is potentiated in mice overexpressing p22phox in vascular smooth muscle. Am J Physiol Heart Circ Physiol 2005; 288: H37–H42.
172. Cadenas E, Wefers H, Muller A et al. Active oxygen metabolites and their action in the hepatocyte. Studies on chemiluminescence responses and alkane production. Agents Actions Suppl 1982; 11: 203–16.
173. Kritharides L, Stocker R. The use of antioxidant supplements in coronary heart disease. Atherosclerosis 2002; 164: 211–19.
174. Shishehbor MH, Aviles RJ, Brennan ML et al. Association of nitrotyrosine levels with cardiovascular disease and modulation by statin therapy. JAMA 2003; 289: 1675–80.
175. Shishehbor MH, Brennan ML, Aviles RJ et al. Statins promote potent systemic antioxidant effects through specific inflammatory pathways. Circulation 2003; 108: 426–31.
176. Fu X, Kassim SY, Parks WC et al. Hypochlorous acid generated by myeloperoxidase modifies adjacent tryptophan and glycine residues in the catalytic domain of matrix metalloproteinase-7 (matrilysin): an oxidative mechanism for restraining proteolytic activity during inflammation. J Biol Chem 2003; 278: 28403–9.

34

Oxidative stress in hypertension

Rhian M Touyz

INTRODUCTION

Reactive oxygen species (ROS) and reactive nitrogen (RNS) species are highly reactive byproducts of O_2 metabolism that play an important physiological role in vascular biology and a pathophysiological role in hypertensive vascular disease.[1,2] Normally the rate of ROS production is balanced by the rate of elimination. However, an imbalance between ROS production and the ability to defend against them by antioxidants results in increased bioavailability of ROS leading to oxidative excess.[2,3] The pathogenic outcome of oxidative stress is oxidative damage, a major cause of vascular, renal, and cardiac injury in cardiovascular disease, including hypertension. Among the major ROS important in these processes are superoxide anion ($\bullet O_2^-$), hydrogen peroxide (H_2O_2), hydroxyl radical ($\bullet OH$), and the RNS, nitric oxide (NO) and peroxynitrite ($ONOO^-$). Under physiological conditions, ROS/RNS are produced in a controlled manner at low concentrations and function as signaling molecules to maintain vascular integrity by regulating vascular smooth muscle cell contraction-relaxation, vascular smooth muscle cell growth, and endothelial function.[4,5] Under pathological conditions increased ROS production leads to endothelial dysfunction, increased contractility, vascular smooth muscle cell growth and apoptosis, monocyte migration, lipid peroxidation, inflammation and increased deposition of extracellular matrix proteins, major processes contributing to vascular injury in hypertension.[6,7]

Myriad experimental studies together with clinical investigations provide compelling evidence that oxidative stress is involved in the pathogenesis of cardiovascular diseases, including atherosclerosis, diabetes, cardiac failure, and hypertension. In experimental models of hypertension, production of cardiac, renal, neural and vascular ROS is increased.[8–10] Mouse models deficient in ROS-generating oxidases have lower blood pressure compared with wild-type counterparts and angiotensin (Ang) II infusion in these mice fails to induce hypertension.[11] In human hypertension, plasma and urine levels of thiobarbituric acid-reactive substances (TBARS) and 8-epi-isoprostane, markers of systemic oxidative stress, are elevated.[12,13] Treatment with antioxidants or superoxide dismutase (SOD) mimetics improves vascular function and structure and reduces blood pressure in experimental and human hypertension.[14–16] Many of the adverse consequences of hypertension on endothelial function may be reversed by intra-arterial infusion of antioxidants, such as vitamin C.[17] Furthermore, in cultured vascular smooth muscle cells (VSMCs) and isolated arteries from hypertensive rats and humans, production of ROS is enhanced and antioxidant capacity is reduced.[18,19] Hence, evidence at multiple levels supports a role for oxidative excess in the pathogenesis of hypertension.

The cardiovascular, renal and central nervous systems, all important in the development of hypertension, are major targets for oxidative damage by ROS.[8,20,21] The present chapter highlights recent developments relating to vascular ROS in hypertension and considers the significance of oxidative stress in clinical hypertension. In addition, strategies to reduce oxidative stress as potential therapeutic agents in the management of hypertension are discussed.

PRO-OXIDANT AND ANTIOXIDANT SYSTEMS IN THE VASCULATURE

ROS can be produced from multiple sources in the vessel wall, including leakage from the mitochondrial electron transport chain, small molecules, enzymes, including cyclooxygenase, lipoxygenase, heme oxygenase, cytochrome p450 monooxygenase, xanthine oxidase,

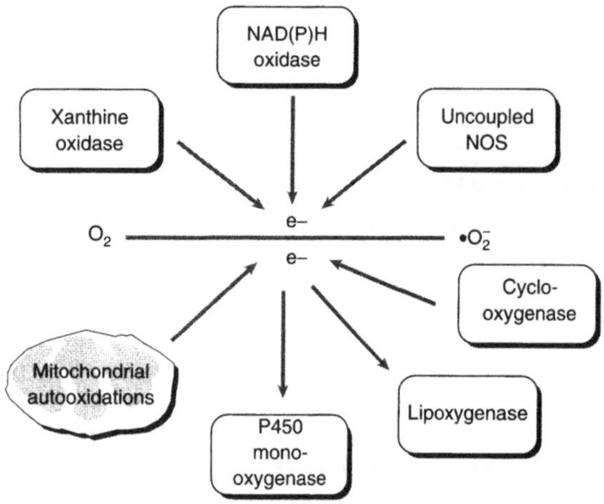

Figure 34.1 Multiple enzymes contribute to vascular superoxide ($•O_2^-$) generation, of which non-phagocytic nicotinamide adenine dinucleotide phosphate (NAD(P)H) oxidase, is the major source

and NAD(P)H (nicotinamide adenine dinucleotide phosphate, reduced form) oxidase[22–24] (Figure 34.1). However, only a few $•O_2^-$ generating enzymes have been implicated in vascular disease, including xanthine oxidase, which oxidizes xanthine and hypoxanthine to form $•O_2^-$, H_2O_2 and uric acid, cytochrome p450, and NAD(P)H oxidase.[25,26] In addition it is becoming increasingly evident that $•O_2^-$ can be generated by nitric oxide synthase (NOS) when it is deprived of its critical cofactor tetrahydrobiopterin (BH_4) or its substrate L-arginine.[27] NOS uncoupling is usually associated with endothelial dysfunction and states of oxidative stress.[28,29]

Of the many enzymatic sources of ROS, NAD(P)H oxidase appears to be of major importance in the vasculature (Figure 34.2). NAD(P)H oxidase, a multi-subunit enzyme[30] catalyzes the production of $•O_2^-$ by the one electron reduction of oxygen using NAD(P)H as the electron donor: $2O_2 + NAD(P)H \rightarrow 2O_2^- + NAD(P)H + H^+$. The prototypical NAD(P)H oxidase is that found in phagocytes[31] and comprises five components (phox for PHagocyte OXidase): p47phox, p67phox, p40phox, p22phox, and gp91phox.[31,32] In unstimulated cells, p40phox, p47phox, and p67phox exist in the cytosol, whereas p22phox and gp91phox are located in the membranes, where they occur as a heterodimeric flavoprotein, cytochrome b558. Upon cell stimulation, p47phox becomes phosphorylated, the cytosolic subunits form a complex, which migrates to the membrane where it associates with cytochrome b558 to assemble the active oxidase, which now transfers electrons from the substrate to O_2 leading to $•O_2^-$ generation.[33]

Non-phagocytic NAD(P)H oxidase is the primary source of $•O_2^-$ in the vasculature[30,34–36] and is functionally active in all layers of the vessel wall, in the endothelium,[11,37] the media,[38] the adventitia,[39] and in cultured VSMCs.[40,41] Unlike phagocytic NAD(P)H oxidase, which is activated only upon stimulation and which generates $•O_2^-$ in a burst-like manner extracellularly, vascular oxidases are constitutively active, produce $•O_2^-$ intracellularly in a slow and sustained fashion and act as intracellular signaling molecules.[30] All of the phagocytic NAD(P)H oxidase subunits are expressed, to varying degrees, in vascular cells.[30] Recent studies demonstrated that the newly discovered gp91phox homologues, nox1 and nox4, are also found in the vasculature.[41–46] Nox1 mRNA is expressed in rat aortic VSMCs and may be a substitute for gp91phox in these cells.[41] Although initial studies suggested that nox1 is a subunit-independent low capacity $•O_2^-$-generating enzyme involved in the regulation of mitogenesis, recent data indicate that nox1 requires p47phox and p67phox and that it is regulated by NoxO1 (Nox organizer 1) and NoxA1 (Nox activator 1).[44] The exact role of NoxO1 and NoxA1 in vascular cells is currently unknown. Nox1 may be important in pathological processes as it is significantly up-regulated in vascular injury.[44] Nox4 appears to be abundantly expressed in all vascular cell types[44] and may play an important role in constitutive production of $•O_2^-$ in differentiating cells. The exact role of gp91phox homologs in vascular biology awaits further clarification.

Activity of vascular NAD(P)H oxidase and expression of oxidase subunits are regulated by cytokines, growth factors and vasoactive agents.[47–50] Of particular significance, with respect to hypertension, is angiotensin II (Ang II).[18,32,39] Ang II induces activation of NAD(P)H oxidase, increases expression of NAD(P)H oxidase subunits and stimulates ROS production in cultured VSMCs and intact arteries.[18,32,39] Mechanisms linking Ang II to the enzyme and upstream signaling molecules modulating NAD(P)H oxidase in vascular cells have not been fully elucidated, but PLD, PKC, c-Src, PI3K, and Rac may be important.[6,18,40,51–54] Platelet-derived growth factor (PDGF), endothelin-1, transforming growth factor-β (TGF-β), tumour necrosis factor (TNF)-α and thrombin as well as mechanical factors, such as stretch, pulsatile strain, and shear stress stimulate NAD(P)H oxidase activation.[55–58] Increasing levels of catalase or the antioxidant glutathione prevent agonist-induced ROS generation.[59,60]

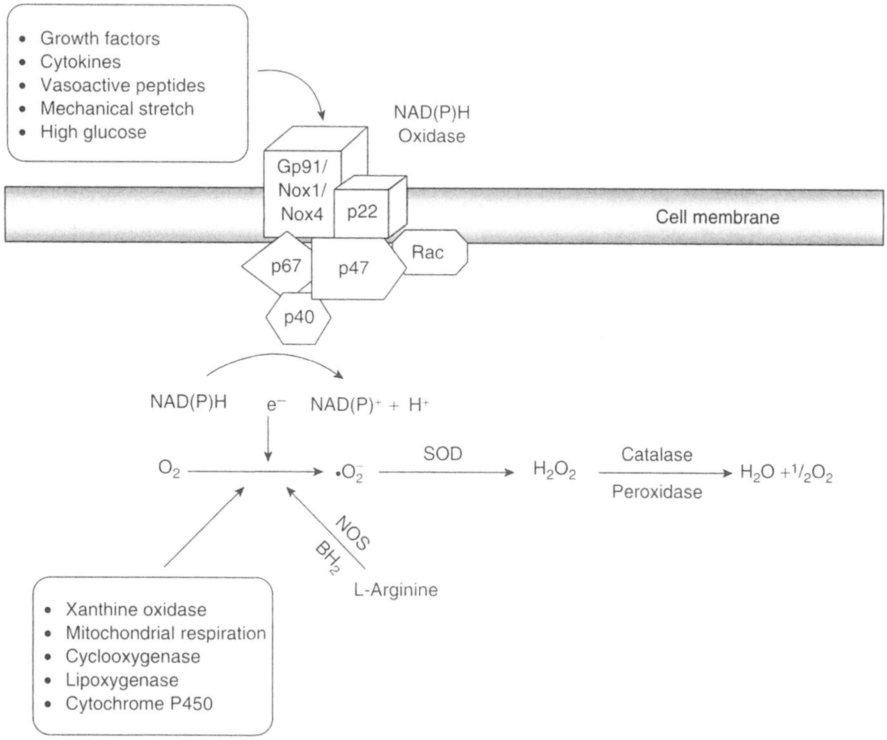

Figure 34.2 Non-phagocytic NADPH oxidase, a multi-subunit enzyme, catalyzes the production of $•O_2^-$ by the one electron reduction of oxygen using NAD(P)H as the electron donor. Multiple factors, including humoral and physical factors, influence activity of vascular NADPH oxidase. Antioxidant enzymes, such as superoxide dismutase (SOD), catalase and peroxidase, maintain cellular redox status

It should be stressed that in addition to vascular NAD(P)H oxidase, phagocytic NADPH oxidase contributes to oxidative stress in the vascular system, since peripheral polymorphonuclear leukocytes can infiltrate cardiovascular tissues in pathological processes.[61,62] This is evidenced by findings of enhanced phagocytic NADPH oxidase-dependent $•O_2^-$ generation in hypertensive patients.[63]

Under certain conditions, such as substrate (arginine) or cofactor BH_4 deficiency, nitric oxide synthase (NOS) can produce $•O_2^-$.[64] These findings have led to the concept of 'NOS uncoupling', where activity of the enzyme for NO production is decreased in association with an increase in NOS-dependent $•O_2^-$ formation. All NOS isoforms require BH_4 for NOS homodimerization and for electron transfer during arginine oxidation. Decreased bioavailability of BH_4 or oxidation of BH_4 to produce cofactor-inactive pterins results in BH_4-deficient NOS, which catalyzes $•O_2^-$ and H_2O_2 formation. Vascular $•O_2^-$ production appears to be partially mediated by BH_4-dependent eNOS uncoupling in various vascular pathologies, including atherosclerosis, diabetes, hyperhomocystinemia, and hypertension.[65–68] This is further supported in human studies where increased endothelial $•O_2^-$ production in vessels from diabetic and hypertensive patients is inhibited by sepiapterin, precursor of BH_4.[69,70] The relative importance of NOS- versus NAD(P)H oxidase-mediated $•O_2^-$ generation in hypertension probably relates to the magnitude of endothelial dysfunction, since most conditions in which $•O_2^-$ is derived from NOS are associated with marked endothelial dysfunction.

Major antioxidant enzymes in the vessel wall include SOD (copper/zinc SOD (SOD1), mitochondrial MnSOD (SOD2), and extracellular SOD (SOD3)), catalase and glutathione peroxidase, whereas non-enzymatic sources include small molecules and vitamins.[71] The concentration of SOD in the extracellular fluid is lower than in the intracellular fluid, which enables $•O_2^-$ to survive longer and to travel further once it gains access to the extracellular space. Arteries contain large amounts of extracellular SOD in the interstitium, suggesting an important role for this SOD isoform within the vessel wall.[72,73] SOD converts $\bullet O_2^-$ to H_2O_2, which is hydrolyzed by catalase and glutathione peroxidase to H_2O and O_2. Glutathione peroxidase is the major enzyme protecting the cell membrane against lipid peroxidation, since reduced glutathione (GSH) donates protons to membrane lipids maintaining them in a reduced state. In addition to endogenous enzyme antioxidants, numerous non-enzymatic antioxidants are found in biological systems. Scavenging antioxidants include water-soluble ascorbic acid (vitamin C), lipid-soluble α-tocopherol (vitamin E), flavonoids, carotenoids, bilirubin, and thiols.[74] Decreased bioavailability of antioxidants results in accumulation of oxygen intermediates and consequent oxidative excess. Based on this paradigm it has been suggested that antioxidant supplementation may have beneficial therapeutic effects in reducing oxidative stress in diseases.

ROLE OF ROS IN VASCULAR (PATHO)PHYSIOLOGY

Molecular processes underlying ROS-induced vascular changes involve activation of redox-sensitive signaling pathways. Superoxide anion and H_2O_2 stimulate MAP kinases, tyrosine kinases and transcription factors (NFκB, AP-1, and HIF-1) and inactivate protein tyrosine phosphatases.[75] ROS also increase $[Ca^{2+}]_i$ and up-regulate proto-oncogene and proinflammatory gene expression.[76,77] These processes occur through oxidative modification of proteins by altering important amino acid residues, by inducing protein dimerization, and by interacting with metal complexes such as Fe-S moieties.[75,77,78] Changes in intracellular redox state through thioredoxin and glutathione systems may also influence signaling events.

In hypertension, oxidative stress promotes vascular smooth muscle cell proliferation and hypertrophy, collagen deposition, inflammation and alterations in activity of matrix metalloproteinases (MMPs), which lead to thickening of the vascular media and arterial remodeling (Figure 34.3). Superoxide anion and H_2O_2 stimulate growth factor-like cellular responses, such as intracellular alkalinization, MAP kinase phosphorylation, and tyrosine kinase activation. H_2O_2 induces vascular smooth muscle cell DNA synthesis, increases expression of proto-oncogenes and promotes cell growth.[75–79] During vascular damage in hypertension when oxidative stress is increased redox-sensitive growth actions may lead to accelerated proliferation and hypertrophy, further contributing to vascular injury and structural changes.[80,81] Enhanced activation of NAD(P)H oxidase and up-regulation of NAD(P)H oxidase subunits seems to be critically involved in redox-mediated vascular remodeling in hypertension. This has recently been confirmed in transgenic mice overexpressing vascular p22phox.[82] In these mice, p22phox overexpression is associated with increased generation of ROS and vascular hypertrophy.[82] ROS also influence vascular structure by increasing deposition of extracellular matrix proteins, such as collagen and fibronectin. Superoxide anion and H_2O_2 modulate activity of vascular MMP2 and MMP9, which promote degradation of basement membrane and elastin respectively.[83]

Redox-sensitive inflammatory processes, including expression of proinflammatory molecules, such as vascular cell adhesion molecule-1 (VCAM-1), intercellular adhesion molecule-1 (ICAM-1), interleukins, and monocyte chemotactic protein-1 (MCP-1), as well as redox-regulated lipid peroxidation and cell migration also contribute to vascular remodeling in hypertension.[84,85]

Impaired endothelium-mediated vasodilatation and endothelial dysfunction have been linked to decreased NO bioavailability. This may be secondary to decreased NO synthesis and/or increased degradation of NO because of its interaction with $\bullet O_2^-$ to form $ONOO^-$.[86,87] Peroxynitrite is a weak vasodilator compared with NO and has pro-inflammatory potential. Decreased NO is associated with reduced vasodilation, platelet aggregation and leukocyte adhesion to the vascular wall. In addition NO reduction leads to increased endothelial permeability, extravasation of plasma proteins and other macromolecules, and consequent recruitment of phagocytic cells and inflammatory proteins, which further impair endothelial function and aggravate vascular damage.[88,89]

ROS IN HYPERTENSION

A plethora of experimental and clinical data implicates oxidative excess as being pathophysiologically important in hypertension. This is evidenced by findings that oxidative stress is increased in hypertension and that treatment with antioxidants or agents that inhibit NAD(P)H oxidase-driven generation of ROS reduces, and may even prevent, blood pressure elevation.

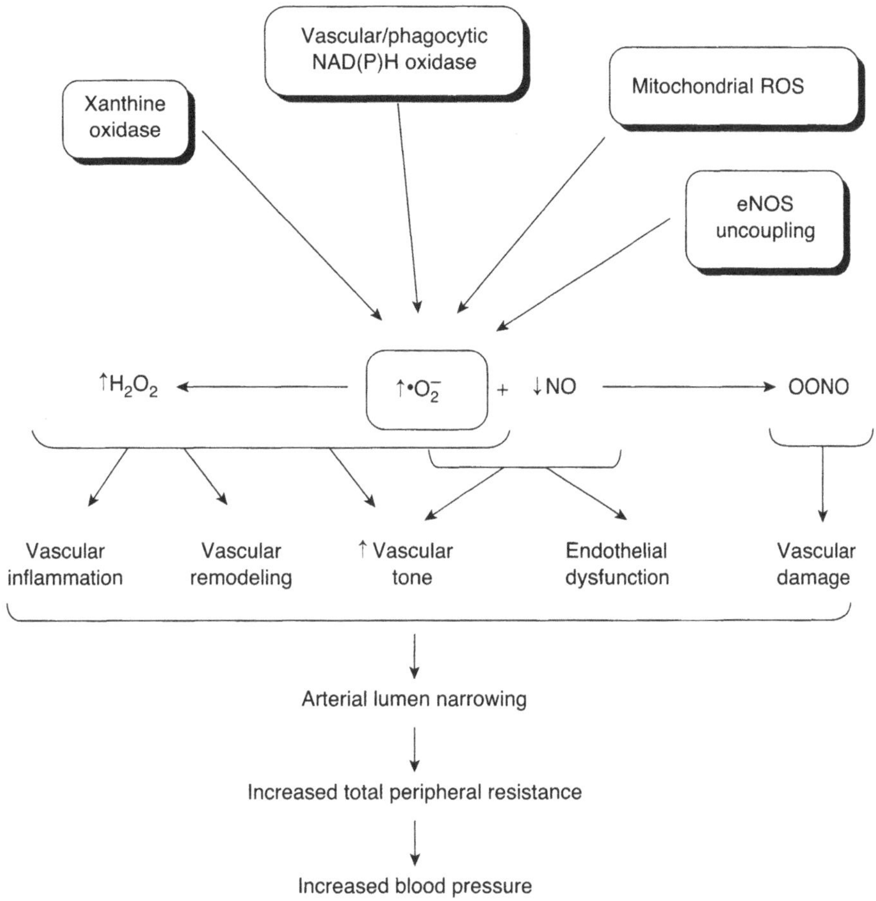

Figure 34.3 Possible role of reactive oxygen species (ROS) in the pathogenesis of hypertension. Production of vascular ROS leads to activation of multiple redox-dependent signaling pathways. These events contribute to vascular inflammation, growth, altered contraction/dilation (vascular tone) and endothelial dysfunction, which lead to vascular remodeling, arterial narrowing, increased peripheral resistance and consequently to increased blood pressure

Oxidative stress in genetic models of hypertension

Genetically hypertensive rats, such as spontaneously hypertensive rats (SHRs) and stroke-prone SHRs (SHRSP), which develop hypertension spontaneously, exhibit enhanced NAD(P)H oxidase-mediated •O_2^- generation in resistance arteries (mesenteric), conduit vessels (aorta), and kidneys.[90,91] These processes are associated with increased expression of NAD(P)H oxidase subunits, particularly p22phox and p47phox, and increased activity of the enzyme.[30,92] In many cases this up-regulation of NAD(P)H oxidase occurs primarily in vascular smooth muscle and adventitia rather than in the endothelium, where eNOS uncoupling may be more important.[93] 8-Hydroxy-2′-deoxyguanosine, a marker for oxidative stress-induced DNA damage, and protein carbonylation, a marker for oxidation status of proteins are enhanced in aorta, heart, and kidney, whereas endogenous antioxidants, including glutathione peroxidase and thioredoxin, are markedly suppressed in SHR and SHRSP compared with normotensive Wistar Kyoto (WKY) rats.[94,95] Male SHRs have higher vascular •O_2^- concentration than female counterparts, a phenomenon that has been linked to up-regulation of AT_1 receptors in male SHR arteries.[96]

Several polymorphisms in the promoter region of the p22phox gene have been identified in SHR, which could contribute to enhanced NAD(P)H oxidase activity.[97] These findings may have clinical relevance since an association between a p22phox gene polymorphism and NAD(P)H oxidase-mediated $\cdot O_2^-$ production in the vascular wall of patients with atherosclerosis and hypertension has been described.[98,99] Increased expression of p47phox has been demonstrated in the renal vasculature, macula densa, and distal nephron from young SHRs, suggesting that up-regulation of renal NAD(P)H oxidase precedes development of hypertension.[100] The importance of p47phox was demonstrated in p47phox–/– mice, which failed to develop hypertension in response to Ang II infusion.[101] Diminished NO bioavailability as a consequence of enhanced vascular $\cdot O_2^-$ generation may also contribute to oxidative stress in SHR and SHRSP. Treatment with antioxidant vitamins, NAD(P)H oxidase inhibitors, SOD mimetics, BH_4, and AT_1 receptor blockers decreases vascular $\cdot O_2^-$ production and attenuates, to varying degrees, the increase in blood pressure in these genetic models of hypertension.[102–104] Lifelong treatment with antioxidants can even prevent development of hypertension in SHR.[105]

Dominiczak and colleagues have taken advantage of rat strains with genetic hypertension to search for candidate genes implicated in oxidative stress associated with hypertension.[106] Using a congenic strain derived from SHRSP and WKY rats combined with gene expression profiling, the gene for glutathione S-transferase (Gstm1), an antioxidant enzyme, was identified as a candidate gene for hypertension.[107] Expression of Gstm1 was reduced in prehypertensive (5 week) and adult (15 week) animals and could indicate attenuated antioxidant capacity in these rats.[107,108] This gene is considered a putative positional and physiological candidate and its pathophysiological role in hypertension is likely to involve defense against oxidative stress.

Oxidative stress and experimentally induced hypertension

Oxidative excess has been demonstrated in many models of experimental hypertension, including Ang II-induced hypertension,[109–111] Dahl salt-sensitive hypertension,[112] lead-induced hypertension,[113] obesity-associated hypertension,[114] mineralocorticoid hypertension,[115] aldosterone-provoked hypertension,[116] 2-kidney, 1-clip hypertension,[117] and in models of postmenopausal hypertension.[118] Vascular and renal oxidative stress is evident in the prehypertensive phase in SHR, SHRSP and Ren-2 transgenic rats, indicating that ROS may be causally linked to the development of hypertension.[107,108,119,120] Enhanced activation of vascular and renal NAD(P)H oxidase and xanthine oxidase and uncoupling of eNOS have been implicated in enhanced $\cdot O_2^-$ generation in experimental hypertension.[121–123] Recent evidence indicates that mitochondrial sources may also contribute to oxidative excess in cardiovascular disease.[124] Inhibition of ROS production with apocynin (NADPH oxidase inhibitor), allopurinol (xanthine oxidase inhibitor), quercetin (dietary flavonoid) and scavenging of free radicals with antioxidants or SOD mimetics, such as Tempol, reduces oxidative stress, decreases blood pressure and prevents development of hypertension in most models of experimental hypertension.[125–128] These antihypertensive actions have been attributed to improved endothelial function, regression of cardiovascular remodeling, improved renal function and reduced vascular, cardiac and renal inflammation. On the other hand, deliberately increasing levels of oxidative stress by glutathione depletion leads to hypertension.[129] Of importance, norepinephrine-induced hypertension is not associated with enhanced vascular oxidative stress and SOD does not decrease blood pressure in this model.[109,130] These findings, together with the fact that increased oxidative stress precedes development of hypertension, suggest that blood pressure itself is not the primary cause of oxidative excess in hypertension and that not all forms of hypertension are redox-sensitive. However, it is possible that hypertension promotes generation of ROS, which would further amplify the oxidative stress–hypertension interaction. Kim and Vaziri demonstrated that induction of hypertension in normotensive rats causes a spontaneous increase in ROS generation in circulating and splenic leukocytes, thereby contributing to oxidative stress, inflammation, and cardiovascular and renal complications in hypertensive animals.[131]

Oxidative stress in human hypertension

Clinical studies have demonstrated that production of reactive oxygen species is increased whereas levels/activity of antioxidant systems are decreased in hypertensive patients.[132–135] This may be due to increased formation of reactive oxygen species and/or to decreased activity/levels of endogenous antioxidants.[14–17] Oxidative excess has been shown in patients with essential hypertension, salt-sensitive hypertension, renovascular hypertension, malignant hypertension, and in preeclampsia.[85,136–139] Most of these findings are based on elevated levels of lipid peroxidation byproducts, including plasma and urine TBARS, malondialdehyde and 8-epi-isoprostanes.[140,141]

Increased plasma, platelet and leukocyte $\bullet O_2^-$ and H_2O_2 concentrations have been demonstrated in hypertensive patients.[142,143] Studies in cultured vascular smooth muscle cells derived from resistance arteries of hypertensive patients revealed enhanced formation of ROS.[144] Accumulation of ROS byproducts from oxidized genomic and mitochondrial DNA has also been shown in hypertensive individuals. Increased levels/activity of vascular NAD(P)H oxidase have been implicated as the primary source of excess $\bullet O_2^-$ in essential hypertension.[135] Polymorphonuclear leukocytes, resident macrophages and platelets, rich $\bullet O_2^-$ sources, further participate in cardiovascular and renal oxidative stress and inflammation in hypertensive patients.[145,146]

Activation of the renin-angiotensin system (RAS) has been proposed as a major mediator of NAD(P)H oxidase activation and ROS production in human hypertension.[19,132,144] Ang II is a potent stimulator of NAD(P)H oxidase and up-regulates expression of NAD(P)H oxidase subunits in human vascular smooth muscle cells, fibroblasts and endothelial cells.[147,148] In addition to its interactions with NAD(P)H oxidase, Ang II induces LOX-1 expression, the human endothelial receptor for oxidized LDL.[149] Because of this interaction between Ang II and $\bullet O_2^-$-generating systems, it is not surprising that some of the therapeutic blood pressure-lowering actions of angiotensin converting enzyme (ACE) inhibitors and AT_1 receptor blockers may be mediated by inhibiting NAD(P)H oxidase activity and reducing ROS production.[150]

Polymorphisms in the p22phox gene have been suggested to play a role in altered NAD(P)H oxidase-generated $\bullet O_2^-$ production in human cardiovascular disease.[151] In particular the -930(A/G) polymorphism in the p22(phox) promoter may be a novel genetic marker associated with hypertension.[99] A single nucleotide polymorphism in the p22phox gene has been linked to altered arterial compliance.[152] However, to confirm that these polymorphisms are indeed markers for hypertension, studies in large populations are necessary.

Although experimental evidence and clinical studies provide compelling evidence that oxidative stress is important in the pathophysiology of hypertension, not all human hypertension is redox-dependent. In never-treated mild to moderate hypertension lipid peroxidation is not increased.[153] In some studies AT_1 receptor blockade did not improve endothelial function and $\bullet O_2^-$ production was unaltered in hypertensive subjects.[154] Furthermore many large clinical trials on antioxidants failed to demonstrate beneficial therapeutic effects on blood pressure and cardiovascular outcomes.[155–157] Reasons for these discrepancies probably relate to the heterogeneous nature of hypertension and to the complexities of redox biology in the cardiovascular system.

STRATEGIES TO REDUCE OXIDATIVE STRESS IN HUMAN HYPERTENSION

Since ROS appear to be important in hypertension and other cardiovascular diseases, there has been considerable interest in developing strategies to reduce oxidative stress. Therapeutic approaches that have been considered include mechanisms to increase antioxidant bioavailability through diet or supplementation and/or to reduce generation of ROS by decreasing activity of $\bullet O_2^-$-generating enzymes and by increasing levels of BH_4 (Box 34.1). Gene therapy approaches for cardiovascular disease are also under development.

Antioxidants

The potential value of antioxidants in treating conditions associated with oxidative stress, such as hypertension, is suggested by experimental data.[10–16] This is further supported by observational and epidemiological data in humans.[158–161] Evidence from prospective studies suggests that a high intake of antioxidant vitamins is protective for hypertension and cardiovascular disease. Numerous animal studies support this thesis as do a number of short-term functional studies in humans.[161–163] However, many of these studies used supra-physiological concentrations of vitamins. Despite convincing evidence demonstrating beneficial cardiovascular effects of antioxidants, randomized clinical trials have produced contrasting results.[155–157] Of the larger trials, only two studies, the Cambridge Heart Antioxidant Study (CHAOS)[164] and the Anti-oxidant Supplementation in Atherosclerosis Prevention Study (ASAP)[165] demonstrated positive effects. Most trials, including the Alpha Tocopherol, Beta-Carotene Cancer Prevention Study (ATBC), the GISSI-Prevenzione trial, the Heart Outcomes Prevention Evaluation (HOPE) study, the HOPE-TOO, the MRC/BHF Heart Protection Study and the Primary Prevention Project (PPP),[166–170] failed to show any significant benefit on cardiovascular outcomes. Thus, the overall results of clinical trials have been disappointing given the consistent and promising findings from experimental investigations, epidemiological data and human studies.

Possible reasons why primary and secondary prevention trials of antioxidant protocols have provided such negative results may relate to inappropriate choice of antioxidants, insufficient dosing regimens or durations of antioxidant therapy, harmful interactions between

Box 34.1 Strategies to reduce oxidative stress in hypertension

Antioxidants/radical scavengers

Vitamins C, E
Beta carotene
Complex Q
Quercitin
Polyphenols
Flavonoids
Thiol-containing compounds (lipoic acid, N-acetylcysteine)
Edaravone (3-methyl-1-phenyl-2-pyrazolin 5-one)
Tempol (SOD mimetic)

NAD(P)H oxidase inhibitors

DPI
Apocynin
S17834 (benzo(b)pyran-4-one)
Gp91ds-tat

Xanthine oxidase inhibitors

Allopurinol
Febuxostat (TMX-67, nonpurine selective inhibitor)

Conventional drugs

3-Hydroxy-3-methylglutaryl-CoA (statins)
Ca^{2+} channel blockers
ACE inhibitors
AT_1 receptor blockers
Beta-blockers

antioxidant agents, and cellular compartmentalization of antioxidants. Moreover in large clinical trials, patients had significant cardiovascular disease, in which case damaging effects of oxidative stress may be irreversible. Also, most of the enrolled patients were taking aspirin prophylactically. Since aspirin has intrinsic antioxidant properties[171,172] additional antioxidant therapy with vitamin C or vitamin E may be ineffective. Finally, in patients studied in whom negative results were obtained, it was never proven that these subjects did in fact have increased oxidative stress. In fact, negative results of clinical trials should be interpreted with caution in the absence of verification that antioxidant therapy successfully reduces vascular oxidative stress.

Based on the current data, it is recommended that the general population should consume a balanced diet with emphasis on antioxidant-rich fruits and vegetables and whole grains. This recommendation, which is consistent with the dietary guidelines of the American Heart Association[173] and the recommendations of the Canadian Hypertension Education Program (CHEP),[174] considers the role of the total diet in influencing disease risk, and is supported by findings from the Dietary Approaches to Stop Hypertension (DASH) study.[175] It is likely that dietary antioxidant vitamins act in synergy with other antioxidants, such as flavonoids and other phenolic compounds, to provide a better antioxidant environment than that achieved with vitamin supplementation alone.[176]

Pharmacological/molecular inhibition of NAD(P)H oxidase

Since NAD(P)H oxidase is considered the major source of $\bullet O_2^-$ in the cardiovascular system, this enzyme has been considered an important target to reduce oxidative stress. Several pharmacological and molecular approaches directly targeting NAD(P)H oxidase have been proposed. Diphenyleneiodinium is a non-specific inhibitor of flavin-containing enzymes that effectively blocks activation of NAD(P)H oxidase.[176] Apocynin, a methoxy-substituted carbechol, acts by inhibiting translocation and assembly of p47phox:p67phox to the membrane complex.[177,178] Apocynin inhibits NAD(P)H-driven generation of $\bullet O_2^-$ in rat, mouse, and human vascular tissue, increases NO production, improves endothelial function, and lowers blood pressure.[179] S17834, a benzo(b)pyran-4-one, has recently been shown to inhibit NAD(P)H oxidase activity, reduce formation of ROS and attenuate atherosclerosis in apolipoprotein E-deficient mice.[180] Although these pharmacological agents are effective in reducing NAD (P)H-driven $\bullet O_2^-$ formation, they need to be administered in high doses and effects are not vascular-specific, which makes their clinical use questionable. Pagano and colleagues used another approach to target NAD(P)H oxidase by designing a chimeric peptide (gp91ds-tat) that inhibits p47phox association with gp91phox, thereby reducing functional assembly of the oxidase complex.[181] gp91ds-tat infusion inhibits $\bullet O_2^-$ formation and attenuates blood pressure elevation in experimental models of hypertension. Another strategy that has been shown to be effective in oxidative stress-related hypertension in animals is BH_4, which prevents NOS uncoupling and decreases NOS-generated ROS. Use of such strategies in humans still needs to be explored.

Increasing evidence indicates that some of the beneficial actions of classical antihypertensive agents such as β-adrenergic blockers, ACE inhibitors, AT_1

receptor antagonists and Ca^{2+} channel blockers may be mediated, in part, by decreasing vascular oxidative stress. 3-Hydroxy-3-methylglutaryl-CoA reductase inhibitors (statins) have also been shown to have NAD(P)H oxidase inhibitory effects.[182–185] Oxidative stress-lowering actions of these drugs have been attributed to direct inhibition of NAD(P)H oxidase activity, as shown for AT_1 receptor blockers, and to intrinsic antioxidant properties of the agents. The role of antihypertensive drugs as modulators of vascular oxidative stress is currently an active area of research.

Reduction of oxidative stress by gene transfer strategies

Studies aimed at overexpression of antioxidant genes, including eNOS, nNOS, extracellular SOD, glutathione peroxidase and catalase demonstrated, for the most part, improved endothelial and vascular function in various animal models.[176,186] However, in many of these studies gene transfer was not tissue-specific. Enormous effort is now being focused on methodologies to direct viral vectors to defined vascular cells and regions.[186,187] This would allow better control over transgene expression, use of lower vector doses and an improved safety profile of these agents. Such strategies to up-regulate antioxidant systems and/or to down-regulate $\cdot O_2^-$-generating systems may provide additional therapeutic options in the treatment of hypertension and other cardiovascular diseases.

CONCLUSIONS

ROS are produced in the cardiovascular system in a controlled and tightly regulated manner. Superoxide and H_2O_2 have important signaling properties, mainly through oxidative modification of proteins and activation of transcription factors that maintain vascular, cardiac and renal function and structure. In hypertension, dysregulation of enzymes such as NAD(P)H oxidase, NOS, xanthine oxidase, mitochondrial enzymes or SOD that generate $\cdot O_2^-$, H_2O_2 and $\cdot OH$, altered thioredoxin and glutathione systems or reduced scavenging by antioxidants, results in increased formation of ROS, which has damaging actions on the vasculature. ROS in hypertension contribute to vascular injury by promoting vascular smooth muscle cell growth, extracellular matrix protein deposition, activation of MMPs, inflammation, endothelial dysfunction, and increased vascular tone. In experimental hypertension oxidative stress is increased and antioxidant levels/activity are decreased. Clinical data suggest that hypertensive patients, especially those with severe hypertension, salt-sensitive hypertension, and renovascular hypertension, exhibit oxidative excess. Although inconclusive at present, treatment strategies to alter ROS bioavailability by decreasing production and/or by increasing radical scavenging, may regress vascular remodeling, prevent further vascular injury and reduce blood pressure and associated target organ damage in hypertensive patients. The potential of SOD mimetics, NAD(P)H oxidase inhibitors and gene transfer strategies to enhance NO and antioxidant bioactivity may provide additional and improved therapeutic options in the management of hypertension and other cardiovascular diseases.

ACKNOWLEDGMENTS

Studies performed by the author were supported by grants 57786 and 44018 and a grant to the Multidisciplinary Research Group on Hypertension, all from the Canadian Institutes of Health Research.

REFERENCES

1. Zalba G, San Jose G, Moreno MU et al. Oxidative stress in arterial hypertension: role of NAD(P)H oxidase. Hypertension 2001; 38: 1395–9.
2. Landmesser U, Harrison DG. Oxidative stress and vascular damage in hypertension. Coron Artery Dis 2001; 12: 455–61.
3. Griendling KK, Sorescu D, Lassegue B, Ushio-Fukai M. Modulation of protein kinase activity and gene expression by reactive oxygen species and their role in vascular physiology and pathophysiology. Arterioscler Thromb Vasc Biol 2000; 20: 2175–83.
4. Cosentino F, Sill JC, Katusic ZS. Role of superoxide anions in the mediation of endothelium-dependent contractions. Hypertension 1994; 23: 229–35.
5. Rao GN, Berk BC. Active oxygen species stimulate vascular smooth muscle cell growth and proto-oncogene expression. Circ Res 1992; 70: 593–9.
6. Touyz RM, Schiffrin EL. Ang II-stimulated superoxide production is mediated via phospholipase D in human vascular smooth muscle cells. Hypertension 1999; 34 (4 Pt 2): 976–82.
7. Chin JH, Azhar S, Hoffman BB. Inactivation of endothelium derived relaxing factor by oxidized lipoproteins. J Clin Invest 1992; 89: 10–18.
8. Zimmerman MC, Lazartigues E, Lang JA et al. Superoxide mediates the actions of angiotensin II in the central nervous system. Circ Res 2002; 91: 1038–45.
9. Kerr S, Brosnan J, McIntyre M, Reid JL, Dominiczak AF, Hamilton CA. Superoxide anion production is increased in a model of genetic hypertension. Role of endothelium. Hypertension 1999; 33: 1353–8.
10. Chen X, Touyz RM, Park JB, Schiffrin EL. Antioxidant effects of vitamins C and E are associated with altered activation of vascular NAD(P)H oxidase and superoxide dismutase in stroke-prone SHR. Hypertension 2001; 38: 606–11.

11. Li JM, Shah AM. Mechanism of endothelial cell NADPH oxidase activation by angiotensin II. Role of the p47phox subunit. J Biol Chem 2003; 278: 12094–100.
12. Quinones-Galvan A, Pucciarelli A, Fratta-Pasini A et al. Effective blood pressure treatment improves LDL-cholesterol susceptibility to oxidation in patients with essential hypertension. J Intern Med 2001; 250: 322–6.
13. Napoli C, Sica V, de Nigris F et al. Sulfhydryl angiotensin-converting enzyme inhibition induces sustained reduction of systemic oxidative stress and improves the nitric oxide pathway in patients with essential hypertension. Am Heart J 2004; 148: 172–6.
14. Hoagland KM, Maier KG, Roman RJ. Contributions of 20-HETE to the antihypertensive effects of Tempol in Dahl salt-sensitive rats. Hypertension 2003; 41 (3 Pt 2): 697–702.
15. Sharma RC, Hodis HN, Mack WJ. Probucol suppresses oxidant stress in hypertensive arteries. Immunohistochemical evidence. Am J Hypertens 1996; 9: 577–90.
16. Schnackenberg CG, Welch W, Wilcox CS. Normalization of blood pressure and renal vascular resistance in SHR with a membrane-permeable superoxide dismutase mimetic. Role of nitric oxide. Hypertension 1999; 32: 59–64.
17. Taddei S, Virdis A, Ghiadoni L, Magagna A, Salvetti A. Vitamin C improves endothelium-dependent vasodilation by restoring nitric oxide activity in essential hypertension. Circulation 1998; 97: 2222–9.
18. Cruzado MC, Risler NR, Miatello RM, Yao G, Schiffrin EL, Touyz RM. Vascular smooth muscle cell NAD(P)H oxidase activity during the development of hypertension: effect of angiotensin II and role of insulinlike growth factor-1 receptor transactivation. Am J Hypertens 2005; 18: 81–7.
19. Berry C, Hamilton CA, Brosnan MJ et al. Investigation into the sources of superoxide in human blood vessels: angiotensin II increases superoxide production in human internal mammary arteries. Circulation 2000; 101: 2206–12.
20. Cantor EJ, Mancini EV, Seth R, Yao XH, Netticadan T. Oxidative stress and heart disease: cardiac dysfunction, nutrition, and gene therapy. Curr Hypertens Rep 2003; 5: 215–20.
21. Wilcox CS. Reactive oxygen species: roles in blood pressure and kidney function. Curr Hypertens Rep 2002; 4: 160–6.
22. Touyz RM, Yao G, Viel E, Amiri F, Schiffrin EL. Angiotensin II and endothelin-1 regulate MAP kinases through different redox-dependent mechanisms in human vascular smooth muscle cells. J Hypertens 2004; 22: 1141–9.
23. Wang D, Hope S, Du Y. Paracrine role of adventitial superoxide anion in a model of genetic hypertension. Role of endothelium. Hypertension 1999; 33: 1353–8.
24. Jones A, O'Donnell VB, Wood JD. Expression of phagocyte NADPH oxidase components in human endothelial cells. Am J Physiol 1996; 271 (4 pt 2): H1626–H1634.
25. Abe J-I, Berk BC. Reactive oxygen species of signal transduction in cardiovascular disease. Trends Cardiovasc Med 1998; 8: 59–64.
26. Rajagopalan S, Kurz S, Munzel T. Angiotensin II mediated hypertension in the rat increases vascular superoxide production via membrane NADH/NADPH oxidase activation: contribution to alterations of vasomotor tone. J Clin Invest 1996; 97: 1916–23.
27. Milstien S, Katusic Z. Oxidation of tetrahydrobiopterin by peroxynitrite: implications for vascular endothelial function. Biochem Biophys Res Commun 1999; 263: 681–4.
28. Cosentino F, Barker JE, Brand MP et al. Reactive oxygen species mediate endothelium-dependent relaxations in tetrahydrobiopterin-deficient mice. Arterioscler Thromb Vasc Biol 2001; 21: 496–502.
29. Landmesser U, Dikalov S, Price SR et al. Oxidation of tetrahydrobiopterin leads to uncoupling of endothelial cell nitric oxide synthase in hypertension. J Clin Invest 2003; 111: 1201–9.
30. Lassegue B, Clempus RE. Vascular NAD(P)H oxidases: specific features, expression, and regulation. Am J Physiol Regul Integr Comp Physiol 2003; 285: R277–R297.
31. Babior BM, Lambeth JD, Nauseef W. The neutrophil NADPH oxidase. Arch Biochem Biophys 2002; 397: 342–4.
32. Griendling KK, Sorescu D, Ushio-Fukai M. NAD(P)H oxidase: role in cardiovascular biology and disease. Circ Res 2000; 86: 494–501.
33. Touyz RM, Yao G, Schiffrin EL. c-Src induces phosphorylation and translocation of p47phox: role in superoxide generation by angiotensin II in human vascular smooth muscle cells. Arterioscler Thromb Vasc Biol 2003; 23: 981–7.
34. Touyz RM, Chen X, He G, Quinn MT, Schiffrin EL. Expression of a gp91phox-containing leukocyte-type NADPH oxidase in human vascular smooth muscle cells – modulation by Ang II. Circ Res 2002; 90: 1205–13.
35. Bendall JK, Cave AC, Heymes C, Gall N, Shah AM. Pivotal role of a gp91(phox)-containing NADPH oxidase in angiotensin II-induced cardiac hypertrophy in mice. Circulation 2002; 105: 293–6.
36. Cai H, Harrison DG. Endothelial dysfunction in cardiovascular diseases: the role of oxidant stress. Circ Res 2000; 87: 840–4.
37. Muzaffar S, Jeremy JY, Angelini GD, Stuart-Smith K, Shukla N. Role of the endothelium and nitric oxide synthases in modulating superoxide formation induced by endotoxin and cytokines in porcine pulmonary arteries. Thorax 2003; 58: 598–604.
38. Rey FE, Pagano PJ. The reactive adventitia: fibroblast oxidase in vascular function. Arterioscler Thromb Vasc Biol 2002; 22: 1962–71.
39. Griendling KK, Minieri CA, Ollerenshaw JD, Alexander RW. Angiotensin II stimulates NADH and NADPH oxidase activity in cultured vascular smooth muscle cells. Circ Res 1994; 74: 1141–8.
40. Seshiah PN, Weber DS, Rocic P, Valppu L, Taniyama Y, Griendling KK. Angiotensin II stimulation of NAD(P)H oxidase activity. Upstream mediators. Circ Res 2002; 91: 406–13.
41. Suh YA, Arnold RS, Lassegue B. Cell transformation by the superoxide-generating Mox-1. Nature 1999; 410: 79–82.
42. Lassegue B, Sorescu D, Szocs K et al. Novel gp91(phox) homologues in vascular smooth muscle cells: nox1 mediates angiotensin II-induced superoxide formation and redox-sensitive signaling pathways. Circ Res 2001; 88: 888–94.
43. Banfi B, Clark RA, Steger K, Krause K-H. Two novel proteins activate superoxide generation by the NADPH oxidase Nox1. J Biol Chem 2003; 278: 3510–13.
44. Wingler K, Wunsch S, Kreutz R, Rothermund L, Paul M, Schmidt HH. Upregulation of the vascular NAD(P)H-oxidase isoforms Nox1 and Nox4 by the renin-angiotensin system in vitro and in vivo. Free Radic Biol Med 2001; 31: 1456–64.
45. Leusen JHW, Verhoeven AJ, Roos D. Interactions between the components of the human NADPH oxidase: a review about the intrigues in the phox family. Front Biosci 1996; 1: 72–90.
46. Ellmark SH, Dusting GJ, Fui MN, Guzzo-Pernell N, Drummond GR. The contribution of Nox4 to NADPH oxidase activity in mouse vascular smooth muscle. Cardiovasc Res 2005; 65: 495–504.
47. Callera GE, Touyz RM, Tostes RC et al. Aldosterone activates vascular p38MAP kinase and NADPH oxidase via c-Src. Hypertension 2005; 45: 773–9.
48. Guzik TJ, Sadowski J, Kapelak B et al. Systemic regulation of vascular NAD(P)H oxidase activity and nox isoform expression in human arteries and veins. Arterioscler Thromb Vasc Biol 2004; 24: 1614–20.

49. Touyz RM, Yao G, Schiffrin EL. Role of the actin cytoskeleton in angiotensin II signaling in human vascular smooth muscle cells. Can J Physiol Pharmacol 2005; 83: 91–7.
50. Li JM, Fan LM, Christie MR, Shah AM. Acute tumor necrosis factor alpha signaling via NADPH oxidase in microvascular endothelial cells: role of p47phox phosphorylation and binding to TRAF4. Mol Cell Biol 2005; 25: 2320–30.
51. Fan CY, Katsuyama M, Yabe-Nishimura C. PKC-delta mediates up-regulation of NOX1, a catalytic subunit of NADPH oxidase, via transactivation of the EGF receptor: possible involvement of PKCdelta in vascular hypertrophy. Biochem J 2005; 390 (Pt 3): 761–7.
52. Reinehr R, Becker S, Eberle A, Grether-Beck S, Haussinger D. Involvement of NADPH oxidase isoforms and SRC family kinases in CD95-dependent hepatocyte apoptosis. J Biol Chem 2005; 280: 27179–94.
53. Touyz RM, Yao G, Quinn MT, Pagano PJ, Schiffrin EL. p47phox associates with the cytoskeleton through cortactin in human vascular smooth muscle cells: role in NAD(P)H oxidase regulation by angiotensin II. Arterioscler Thromb Vasc Biol 2005; 25: 512–18.
54. Yamamori T, Inanami O, Nagahata H, Kuwabara M. Phosphoinositide 3-kinase regulates the phosphorylation of NADPH oxidase component p47(phox) by controlling cPKC/PKCdelta but not Akt. Biochem Biophys Res Commun 2004; 316: 720–30.
55. Grote K, Flach I, Luchtefeld M et al. Mechanical stretch enhances mRNA expression and proenzyme release of matrix metalloproteinase-2 (MMP-2) via NAD(P)H oxidase-derived reactive oxygen species. Circ Res 2003; 92: e80–e86.
56. De Keulenaer GW, Alexander RW, Ushio-Fukai M, Ishizaka N, Griendling KK. Tumour necrosis factor alpha activates a p22phox-based NADH oxidase in vascular smooth muscle. Biochem J 1998; 329: 653–7.
57. Gorlach A, Diebold I, Schini-Kerth VB et al. Thrombin activates the hypoxia-inducible factor-1 signaling pathway in vascular smooth muscle cells: Role of the p22(phox)-containing NADPH oxidase. Circ Res 2001; 89: 47–54.
58. Ghosh M, Wang HD, McNeill JR. Role of oxidative stress and nitric oxide in regulation of spontaneous tone in aorta of DOCA-salt hypertensive rats. Br J Pharmacol 2004; 141: 562–73.
59. Tian N, Thrasher KD, Gundy PD, Hughson MD, Manning RD. Antioxidant treatment prevents renal damage and dysfunction and reduces arterial pressure in salt-sensitive hypertension. Hypertension 2005; 45: 934–40.
60. Zhang Y, Handy DE, Loscalzo J. Adenosine-dependent induction of glutathione peroxidase 1 in human primary endothelial cells and protection against oxidative stress. Circ Res 2005; 96: 831–7.
61. Stralin P, Karlsson K, Johannson BO, Marklund SL. The interstitium of the human arterial wall contains very large amounts of extracellular superoxide dismutase. Arterioscler Thromb Vasc Biol 1995; 15: 2032–6.
62. Sela S, Mazor R, Amsalam M, Yagil C, Yagil Y, Kristal B. Primed polymorphonuclear leukocytes, oxidative stress, and inflammation antecede hypertension in the Sabra rat. Hypertension 2004; 44: 764–9.
63. Fortuno A, Olivan S, Beloqui O et al. Association of increased phagocytic NADPH oxidase-dependent superoxide production with diminished nitric oxide generation in essential hypertension. J Hypertens 2004; 22: 2169–75.
64. Witteveen CF, Giovanelli J, Kaufman S. Reactivity of tetrahydrobiopterin bound to nitric-oxide synthase. J Biol Chem 1999; 274: 29755–62.
65. Wang CH, Li SH, Weisel RD et al. Tetrahydrobiopterin deficiency exaggerates intimal hyperplasia after vascular injury. Am J Physiol Regul Integr Comp Physiol 2005; 289: R299–304.
66. Vasquez-Vivar J, Duquaine D, Whitsett J, Kalyanaraman B, Rajagopalan S. Altered tetrahydrobiopterin metabolism in atherosclerosis: implications for use of oxidized tetrahydrobiopterin analogues and thiol antioxidants. Arterioscler Thromb Vasc Biol 2002; 22: 1655–61.
67. Satoh M, Fujimoto S, Haruna Y et al. NAD(P)H oxidase and uncoupled nitric oxide synthase are major sources of glomerular superoxide in rats with experimental diabetic nephropathy. Am J Physiol Renal Physiol 2005; 288: F1144–F1452.
68. Virdis A, Iglarz M, Neves MF et al. Effect of hyperhomocystinemia and hypertension on endothelial function in methylenetetrahydrofolate reductase-deficient mice. Arterioscler Thromb Vasc Biol 2003; 23: 1352–7.
69. Guzik TJ, Mussa S, Gastaldi D et al. Mechanisms of increased vascular superoxide production in human diabetes mellitus: role of NAD(P)H oxidase and endothelial nitric oxide synthase. Circulation 2002; 105: 1656–62.
70. Higashi Y, Sasaki S, Nakagawa K et al. Tetrahydrobiopterin enhances forearm vascular response to acetylcholine in both normotensive and hypertensive individuals. Am J Hypertens 2002; 15: 326–32.
71. McIntyre M, Bohr DF, Dominiczak AF. Endothelial function in hypertension. The role of superoxide anion. Hypertension 1999; 34: 539–45.
72. Sekiguchi F, Yanamoto A, Sunano S. Superoxide dismutase reduces the impairment of endothelium-dependent relaxation in the spontaneously hypertensive rat aorta. J Smooth Muscle Res 2004; 40: 65–74.
73. Jung O, Marklund SL, Geiger H, Pedrazzini T, Busse R, Brandes RP. Extracellular superoxide dismutase is a major determinant of nitric oxide bioavailability: in vivo and ex vivo evidence from ecSOD-deficient mice. Circ Res 2003; 93: 622–9.
74. Yeum KJ, Russell RM, Krinsky NI, Aldini G. Biomarkers of antioxidant capacity in the hydrophilic and lipophilic compartments of human plasma. Arch Biochem Biophys 2004; 430: 97–103.
75. Finkel T. Oxygen radicals and signaling. Curr Opin Cell Biol 1998; 10: 248–53.
76. Tabet F, Savoia C, Schiffrin EL, Touyz RM. Differential calcium regulation by hydrogen peroxide and superoxide in vascular smooth muscle cells from spontaneously hypertensive rats. J Cardiovasc Pharmacol 2004; 44: 200–8.
77. Haddad JJ. Antioxidant and prooxidant mechanisms in the regulation of redox(y)-sensitive transcription factors. Cell Signal 2002; 14: 879–97.
78. Droge W. Free radicals in the physiological control of cell function. Physiol Rev 2001; 82: 47–95.
79. Turpaev KT. Reactive oxygen species and regulation of gene expression. Biochemistry 2002; 67: 281–92.
80. Suematsu M, Suzuki H, Delano FA, Schmid-Schonbein GW. The inflammatory aspect of the microcirculation in hypertension: oxidative stress, leukocytes/endothelial interaction, apoptosis. Microcirculation 2002; 9: 259–76.
81. Luft FC. Mechanisms and cardiovascular damage in hypertension. Hypertension 2001; 37: 594–8.
82. Weber DS, Rocic P, Mellis AM et al. Angiotensin II-induced hypertrophy is potentiated in mice overexpressing p22phox in vascular smooth muscle. Am J Physiol 2005; 1: H37–H42.
83. Rajagopalan S, Meng XP, Ramasamy S, Harrison DG, Galis ZS. Reactive oxygen species produced by macrophage-derived foam cells regulate the activity of vascular matrix metalloproteinases in vitro. J Clin Invest 1996; 98: 2572–9.

84. Virdis A, Schiffrin EL. Vascular inflammation: a role in vascular disease in hypertension? Curr Opin Nephrol Hypertens 2003; 12: 181–7.
85. Kristal B, Shurta-Swirrski R, Chezar J. Participation of peripheral polymorphonuclear leukocytes in the oxidative stress and inflammation in patients with essential hypertension. Am J Hypertens 1998; 11: 921–8.
86. List BM, Klosch B, Volker C et al. Characterization of bovine endothelial nitric oxide synthase as a homodimer with down-regulated uncoupled NADPH oxidase activity: tetrahydrobiopterin binding kinetics and role of haem in dimerization. Biochem J 1997; 323 (Pt 1): 159–65.
87. Somers MJ, Harrison DG. Reactive oxygen species and the control of vasomotor tone. Curr Hypertens Rep 1999; 1: 102–8.
88. Szabo C. Multiple pathways of peroxynitrite cytotoxicity. Toxicol Lett 2003; 140: 105–12.
89. Alexander RW. Hypertension and the pathogenesis of atherosclerosis. Oxidative stress and the mediation of arterial inflammatory response: a new perspective. Hypertension 1995; 25: 155–61.
90. Touyz RM, Schiffrin EL. Reactive oxygen species in vascular biology: implications in hypertension. Histochem Cell Biol 2004; 122: 339–52.
91. Park JB, Touyz RM, Chen X, Schiffrin EL. Chronic treatment with a superoxide dismutase mimetic prevents vascular remodeling and progression of hypertension in salt-loaded stroke-prone spontaneously hypertensive rats. Am J Hypertens 2002; 15 (1 Pt 1): 78–84.
92. Chabrashvili T, Tojo A, Onozato ML et al. Expression and cellular localization of classic NADPH oxidase subunits in the spontaneously hypertensive rat kidney. Hypertension 2002; 39: 269–74.
93. Li J-M, Shah AM. Endothelial cell superoxide generation: regulation and relevance for cardiovascular pathophysiology. Am J Physiol 2004; 287: 1014–30.
94. Tanito M, Nakamura H, Kwon YW et al. Enhanced oxidative stress and impaired thioredoxin expression in spontaneously hypertensive rats. Antioxid Redox Signal 2004; 6: 89–97.
95. Kumar U, Chen J, Sapoznikhov V, Canteros G, White BH, Sidhu A. Overexpression of inducible nitric oxide synthase in the kidney of the spontaneously hypertensive rat. Clin Exp Hypertens 2005; 27: 17–31.
96. Silva-Antonialli MM, Tostes RC, Fernandes L et al. A lower ratio of AT1/AT2 receptors of angiotensin II is found in female than in male spontaneously hypertensive rats. Cardiovasc Res 2004; 62: 587–93.
97. Zalba G, San Jose G, Beaumont FJ, Fortuno MA, Fortuno A, Diez J. Polymorphisms and promoter overactivity of the p22 (phox) gene in vascular smooth muscle cells from spontaneously hypertensive rats. Circ Res 2001; 88: 217–22.
98. Guzik TJ, West NE, Black E et al. Functional effect of the C242T polymorphism in the NAD(P)H oxidase p22phox gene on vascular superoxide production in atherosclerosis. Circulation 2000; 102: 1744–7.
99. San Jose G, Moreno MU, Olivan S et al. Functional effect of the p22phox-930A/G polymorphism on p22phox expression and NADPH oxidase activity in hypertension. Hypertension 2004; 44: 163–9.
100. Paravicini TM, Chrissobolis S, Drummond GR, Sobey CG. Increased NADPH-oxidase activity and Nox4 expression during chronic hypertension is associated with enhanced cerebral vasodilatation to NADPH in vivo. Stroke 2004; 35: 584–9.
101. Landmesser U, Cai H, Dikalov S et al. Role of p47(phox) in vascular oxidative stress and hypertension caused by angiotensin II. Hypertension 2002; 40: 511–15.
102. Hong HJ, Hsiao G, Cheng TH, Yen MH. Supplemention with tetrahydrobiopterin suppresses the development of hypertension in spontaneously hypertensive rats. Hypertension 2001; 38: 1044–8.
103. Brosnan MJ, Hamilton CA, Graham D, Lygate CA, Jardine E, Dominiczak AF. Irbesartan lowers superoxide levels and increases nitric oxide bioavailability in blood vessels from spontaneously hypertensive stroke-prone rats. J Hypertens 2002; 20: 281–6.
104. Rodriguez-Iturbe B, Zhan CD, Quiroz Y, Sindhu RK, Vaziri ND. Antioxidant-rich diet relieves hypertension and reduces renal immune infiltration in spontaneously hypertensive rats. Hypertension 2003; 41: 341–6.
105. Ratnayake WM, Plouffe L, Hollywood R et al. Influence of sources of dietary oils on the life span of stroke-prone spontaneously hypertensive rats. Lipids 2000; 35: 409–20.
106. Dominiczak AF, Graham D, McBride MW et al. Cardiovascular genomics and oxidative stress. Hypertension 2005; 45: 636–42.
107. McBride MW, Farr JF, Graham D et al. Microarray analysis of rat chromosome 2 congenic strains. Hypertension 2003; 41: 847–53.
108. McBride MW, Miller WH, Brosnan MJ et al. Identification of Gstm1 differential expression by microarray profiling in rat chromosome 2 congenic strains during the development of hypertension. Hypertension 2004; 44: 510 (abstract).
109. Laursen JB, Rajagopalan S, Galis Z, Tarpey M, Freeman BA, Harrison DG. Role of superoxide in angiotensin II-induced but not catecholamine-induced hypertension. Circulation 1997; 95: 588–93.
110. Virdis A, Fritsch Neves M, Amiri F, Viel E, Touyz RM, Schiffrin EL. Spironolactone improves angiotensin-induced vascular changes and oxidative stress. Hypertension 2002; 40: 504–10.
111. Reckelhoff JF, Romero JC. Role of oxidative stress in angiotensin-induced hypertension. Am J Physiol Regul Integr Comp Physiol 2003; 284: R893–R912.
112. Tojo A, Onozato ML, Kobayashi N, Goto A, Matsuoka H, Fujita T. Angiotensin II and oxidative stress in Dahl Salt-sensitive rat with heart failure. Hypertension 2002; 40: 834–9.
113. Ding Y, Gonick HC, Vaziri ND, Liang K, Wei L. Lead-induced hypertension. III. Increased hydroxyl radical production. Am J Hypertens 2001; 14: 169–73.
114. Dobrian AD, Davies MJ, Schriver SD, Lauterio TJ, Prewitt RL. Oxidative stress in a rat model of obesity-induced hypertension. Hypertension 2001; 37: 554–60.
115. Wu R, Millette E, Wu L, de Champlain J. Enhanced superoxide anion formation in vascular tissues from spontaneously hypertensive and desoxycorticosterone acetate-salt hypertensive rats. J Hypertens 2001; 19: 741–8.
116. Iglarz M, Touyz RM, Viel EC, Amiri F, Schiffrin EL. Involvement of oxidative stress in the profibrotic action of aldosterone. Interaction wtih the renin-angiotension system. Am J Hypertens 2004; 17: 597–603.
117. Welch WJ, Mendonca M, Aslam S, Wilcox CS. Roles of oxidative stress and AT1 receptors in renal hemodynamics and oxygenation in the postclipped 2K,1C kidney. Hypertension 2003; 41 (3 Pt 2): 692–6.
118. Javeshghani D, Touyz RM, Sairam MR, Virdis A, Neves MF, Schiffrin EL. Attenuated responses to angiotensin II in follitropin receptor knockout mice, a model of menopause-associated hypertension. Hypertension 2003; 42: 761–7.
119. Vaneckova I, Kramer HJ, Novotna J et al. Roles of nitric oxide and oxidative stress in the regulation of blood pressure and renal function in prehypertensive Ren-2 transgenic rats. Kidney Blood Press Res 2005; 28: 117–26.

120. Nabha L, Garbern JC, Buller CL, Charpie JR. Vascular oxidative stress precedes high blood pressure in spontaneously hypertensive rats. Clin Exp Hypertens 2005; 27: 71–82.
121. Wallwork CJ, Parks DA, Schmid-Schonbein GW. Xanthine oxidase activity in the dexamethasone-induced hypertensive rat. Microvasc Res 2003; 66: 30–7.
122. Touyz RM. Oxidative stress and vascular damage in hypertension. Curr Hypertens Rep 2000; 2: 98–105.
123. Schnackenberg CS. Oxygen radicals in cardiovascular-renal disease. Curr Opin Pharmacol 2002; 2: 121–5.
124. Kimura S, Zhang GX, Nishiyama A et al. Mitochondria-derived reactive oxygen species and vascular MAP kinases: comparison of angiotensin II and diazoxide. Hypertension 2005; 45: 438–44.
125. Park JB, Touyz RM, Chen X, Schiffrin EL. Chronic treatment with a superoxide dismutase mimetic prevents vascular remodeling and progression of hypertension in salt-loaded stroke-prone spontaneously hypertensive rats. Am J Hypertens 2002; 15: 78–84.
126. Frenoux JM, Noirot B, Prost ED et al. Very high alpha-tocopherol diet diminishes oxidative stress and hypercoagulation in hypertensive rats but not in normotensive rats. Med Sci Monit 2002; 8: BR401–BR407.
127. Girouard H, Chulak C, LeJossec M, Lamontagne D, De Champlain J. Chronic antioxidant treatment improves sympathetic function and beta-adrenergic pathway in the SHR. J Hypertens 2003; 21: 179–88.
128. Garcia-Saura MF, Galisteo M, Villar IC et al. Effects of chronic quercetin treatment in experimental renovascular hypertension. Mol Cell Biochem 2005; 270: 147–55.
129. Vaziri ND, Wang XQ, Oveisi F, Rad B. Induction of oxidative stress by glutathione depletion causes severe hypertension in normal rats. Hypertension 2000; 36: 142–6.
130. Aizawa T, Ishizaka N, Usui S, Ohashi N, Ohno M, Nagai R. Angiotensin II and catecholamines increase plasma levels of 8-epi-prostaglandin F(2alpha) with different pressor dependencies in rats. Hypertension 2002; 39: 149–54.
131. Kim CH, Vaziri ND. Hypertension promotes integrin expression and reactive oxygen species generation by circulating leukocytes. Kidney Int 2005; 67: 1462–70.
132. Hamilton CA, Brosnan MJ, McIntyre M, Graham D, Dominiczak AF. Superoxide excess in hypertension and aging: a common cause of endothelial dysfunction. Hypertension 2001; 37: 529–34.
133. Minuz P, Patrignani P, Gaino S et al. Increased oxidative stress and platelet activation in patients with hypertension and renovascular disease. Circulation 2002; 106: 2800–5.
134. Sagar S, Kallo IJ, Kaul N, Ganguly NK, Sharma BK. Oxygen free radicals in essential hypertension. Mol Cell Biochem 1992; 111: 103–8.
135. Redon J, Oliva MR, Tormos C et al. Anti-oxidant activities and oxidative stress by-products in human hypertension. Hypertension 2003; 41: 1096–101.
136. Lip GY, Edmunds E, Nuttall SL, Landray MJ, Blann AD, Beevers DG. Oxidative stress in malignant and non-malignant phase hypertension. J Hum Hypertens 2002; 16: 333–6.
137. Lee VM, Quinn PA, Jennings SC, Ng LL. Neutrophil activation and production of reactive oxygen species in pre-eclampsia. J Hypertens 2003; 21: 395–402.
138. Parslow RA, Sachdev P, Salonikas C, Lux O, Jorm AF, Naidoo D. Associations between plasma antioxidants and hypertension in a community-based sample of 415 Australians aged 60–64. J Hum Hypertens 2005; 19: 219–26.
139. Ward NC, Hodgson JM, Puddey IB, Mori TA, Beilin LJ, Croft KD. Oxidative stress in human hypertension: association with antihypertensive treatment, gender, nutrition, and lifestyle. Free Radic Biol Med 2004; 36: 226–32.
140. Stojiljkovic MP, Lopes HF, Zhang D, Morrow JD, Goodfriend TL, Egan BM. Increasing plasma fatty acids elevates F2-isoprostanes in humans: implications for the cardiovascular risk factor cluster. J Hypertens 2002; 20: 1215–21.
141. Murphey LJ, Morrow JD, Sawathiparnich P, Williams GH, Vaughan DE, Brown NJ. Acute angiotensin II increases plasma F2-isoprostanes in salt-replete human hypertensives. Free Radic Biol Med 2003; 35: 711–18.
142. Mehta JL, Lopez LM, Chen L, Cox OE. Alterations in nitric oxide synthase activity, superoxide anion generation and platelet aggregation in systemic hypertension and effects of celiprolol. Am J Cardiol 1994; 74: 901–5.
143. Lacy F, O'Connor DT, Schmid-Schonbein GW. Plasma hydrogen peroxide production in hypertensives and normotensive subjects at genetic risk of hypertension. J Hypertens 1998; 16: 291–303.
144. Touyz RM, Schiffrin EL. Increased generation of superoxide by angiotensin II in smooth muscle cells from resistance arteries of hypertensive patients: role of phospholipase D-dependent NAD(P)H oxidase-sensitive pathways. J Hypertens 2001; 19: 1245–54.
145. Germano G, Sanguigni V, Pignatelli P et al. Enhanced platelet release of superoxide anion in systemic hypertension: role of AT1 receptors. J Hypertens 2004; 22: 1151–6.
146. Minuz P, Patrignani P, Gaino S et al. Determinants of platelet activation in human essential hypertension. Hypertension 2004; 43: 64–70.
147. Rueckschloss U, Quinn MT, Holtz J, Morawietz H. Dose-dependent regulation of NAD(P)H oxidase expression by angiotensin II in human endothelial cells: protective effect of angiotensin II type 1 receptor blockade in patients with coronary artery disease. Arterioscler Thromb Vasc Biol 2002; 22: 1845–51.
148. Dechend R, Viedt C, Muller DN et al. AT1 receptor agonistic antibodies from preeclamptic patients stimulate NADPH oxidase. Circulation 2003; 107: 1632–9.
149. Limor R, Kaplan M, Sawamura T et al. Angiotensin II increases the expression of lectin-like oxidized low-density lipoprotein receptor-1 in human vascular smooth muscle cells via a lipoxygenase-dependent pathway. Am J Hypertens 2005; 18: 299–307.
150. Welch WJ, Wilcox CS. AT1 receptor antagonist combats oxidative stress and restores nitric oxide signaling in the SHR. Kidney Int 2001; 59: 1257–63.
151. Schachinger V, Britten MB, Dimmeler S, Zeiher AM. NADH/NADPH oxidase p22phox gene polymorphism is associated with improved coronary endothelial vasodilator function. Eur Heart J 2001; 22: 96–101.
152. Drummond RS, Brosnan MJ, Tan C. A single nucleotide polymorphism in the p22phox gene affects arterial compliance. Hypertension 2003; 42: 393–4.
153. Cracowski JL, Baguet JP, Ormezzano O et al. Lipid peroxidation is not increased in patients with untreated mild-to-moderate hypertension. Hypertension 2003; 41: 286–8.
154. Ghiadoni L, Magagna A, Versari D et al. Different effect of antihypertensive drugs on conduit artery endothelial function. Hypertension 2003; 41: 1281–6.
155. Jialal I, Devaraj S. Anti-oxidants and atherosclerosis: don't throw out the baby with the bath water. Circulation 2003; 107: 926–8.
156. Abrescia P, Golino P. Free radicals and antioxidants in cardiovascular diseases. Expert Rev Cardiovasc Ther 2005; 3: 159–71.
157. Vivekananthan DP, Penn MS, Sapp SK, Hsu A, Topol EJ. Use of antioxidant vitamins for the prevention of cardiovascular disease: meta-analysis of randomised trials. Lancet 2003; 361: 2017–23.
158. Digiesi D, Lenuzza M, Digiese G. Prospects for the use of antioxidant therapy in hypertension. Ann Ital Med Int 2001; 16: 93–100.

159. Stampfer MJ, Hennekens CH, Manson JE, Colditz GA, Rosner B, Willett WC. Vitamin E consumption and the risk of coronary heart disease in women. N Engl J Med 1993; 328: 1444–9.
160. Khaw K-T, Bingham S, Welch A et al. Relation between plasma ascorbic acid and mortality in men and women in EPIC-Norfolk prospective study: a prospective population study. Lancet 2001; 357: 657–63.
161. Duffy SJ, Gokce N, Holbrook M et al. Treatment of hypertension with ascorbic acid. Lancet 1999; 354: 2048–9.
162. Galley HF, Thornton J, Howdle PD, Walker BE, Webster NR. Combination oral antioxidant supplementation reduces blood pressure. Clin Sci (Lond) 1997; 92: 361–5.
163. Fotheby MD, Williams JC, Forster LA, Craner P, Ferns GA. Effect of vitamin C on ambulatory blood pressure and plasma lipids in older patients. J Hypertens 2000; 18: 411–15.
164. Stephens NG, Parsons A, Schofield PM, Kelly F, Cheeseman K, Mitchinson MJ. Randomised controlled trial of vitamin E in patients with coronary disease: Cambridge Heart Antioxidant Study (CHAOS). Lancet 1996; 347: 781–6.
165. Salonen RM, Nyyssonen K, Kaikkomen J. Six year effect of combined vitamin C and E supplementation on atherosclerotic progression: the Antioxidant Supplementation in Atherosclerosis Prevention (ASAP) Study. Circulation 2003; 107: 947–953.
166. GISSI-Prevenzione Investigators. Dietary supplementation with n-3 polyunsaturated fatty acids and vitamin E after myocardial infarction: results of the GISSI-Prevenzione trial. Gruppo Italiano per lo Studio della Sopravvivenza nell'Infarto miocardico. Lancet 1999; 354: 447–55.
167. MRC/BHF Heart protection study of antioxidant vitamin supplementation in 20 536 high-risk individuals: a randomized placebo-controlled trial. Lancet 2002; 360: 23–33.
168. de Gaetano G. Collaborative Group of the Primary Prevention Project. Low-dose aspirin and vitamin E in people at cardiovascular risk: a randomised trial in general practice. Collaborative Group of the Primary Prevention Project. Lancet 2001; 357: 89–95.
169. HOPE Investigators. Vitamin E supplementation and cardiovascular events in high risk patients. N Engl J Med 2000; 342: 154–60.
170. The HOPE-TOO Trial Investigators. Effects of long-term vitamin E supplementation on cardiovascular events and cancer. A randomized controlled trial. JAMA 2005; 293: 1338–47.
171. Wu R, Lamontagne D, de Champlain J. Antioxidative properties of acetylsalicylic acid on vascular tissues from normotensive and spontaneously hypertensive rats. Circulation 2002; 105: 387–92.
172. Dragomir E, Manduteanu I, Voinea M, Costache G, Manea A, Simionescu M. Aspirin rectifies calcium homeostasis, decreases reactive oxygen species, and increases NO production in high glucose-exposed human endothelial cells. J Diabetic Complications 2004; 18: 289–99.
173. Tribble DL. AHA Science Advisory. Antioxidant consumption and risk of coronary heart disease: emphasis on vitamin C, vitamin E and β-carotene. A statement for the healthcare professionals from the American Heart Association. Circulation 1999; 99: 591–5.
174. Touyz RM, Campbell N, Logan A, Gledhill N, Petrella R, Padwal R. Canadian Hypertension Education Program. The 2004 Canadian recommendations for the management of hypertension: Part III – Lifestyle modifications to prevent and control hypertension. Can J Cardiol 2004; 20: 55–9.
175. Sacks FM, Svetkey LP, Vollmer WM et al. DASH-Sodium Collaborative Research Group. Effects on blood pressure of reduced dietary sodium and the Dietary Approaches to Stop Hypertension (DASH) diet. DASH-Sodium Collaborative Research Group. N Engl J Med 2001; 344: 3–10.
176. Hamilton CA, Miller WH, Al-Benna S et al. Strategies to reduce oxidative stress in cardiovascular disease. Clin Sci 2004; 106: 219–34.
177. Stolk J, Hiltermann TJ, Dijkman JH, Verhoeven AJ. Characteristics of the inhibition of NADPH oxidase activation in neutrophils by apocynin, a methoxy-substituted catechol. Am J Respir Cell Mol Biol 1994; 11: 95–102.
178. Van den Worm E, Beukelman CJ, Van den Berg AJ, Kroes BH, Labadie RP, Van Dijk H. Effects of methoxylation of apocynin and analogs on the inhibition of reactive oxygen species production by stimulated human neutrophils. Eur J Pharmacol 2001; 433: 225–30.
179. Virdis A, Neves MF, Amiri F, Touyz RM, Schiffrin EL. Role of NAD(P)H oxidase on vascular alterations in angiotensin II-infused mice. J Hypertens 2004; 22: 535–42.
180. Cayatte AJ, Rupin A, Oliver-Krasinski J. S17834, a new inhibitor of cell adhesion and atherosclerosis that targets NADPH oxidase. Arterioscler Thromb Vasc Biol 2001; 21: 1577–84.
181. Rey FE, Kiarash CA, Quinn MT, Pagano PJ. Novel competitive inhibitor of NAD(P)H oxidase assembly attenuates vascular O_2^- and systolic blood pressure in mice. Circ Res 2001; 89: 408–14.
182. Muda P, Kampus P, Zilmer M et al. Effect of antihypertensive treatment with candesartan or amlodipine on glutathione and its redox status, homocysteine and vitamin concentrations in patients with essential hypertension. J Hypertens 2005; 23: 105–12.
183. Ghiadoni L, Virdis A, Magagna A, Taddei S, Salvetti A. Effect of the angiotensin II type I receptor blocker candesartan on endothelial function in patients with essential hypertension. Hypertension 2000; 35: 501–6.
184. Takayama T, Wada A, Tsutamoto T et al. Contribution of vascular NAD(P)H oxidase to endothelial dysfunction in heart failure and the therapeutic effects of HMG-CoA reductase inhibitor. Circ J 2004; 68: 1067–75.
185. Schiffrin EL, Touyz RM. Multiple actions of angiotensin II in hypertension: benefits of AT1 receptor blockade. J Am Coll Cardiol 2003; 42: 911–13.
186. Liu J, Ormsby A, Oja-Tebbe N, Pagano PJ. Gene transfer of NAD(P)H oxidase inhibitor to the vascular adventitia attenuates medial smooth muscle hypertrophy. Circ Res 2004; 95: 587–94.
187. Katusic ZS, Caplice NM, Nath KA. Nitric oxide synthase gene transfer as a tool to study biology of endothelial cells. Arterioscler Thromb Vasc Biol 2003; 23: 1990–4.

35

Inflammation, cardiovascular disease, and hypertension: molecular mechanisms

Tetsuya Matoba and Bradford C Berk

INFLAMMATION, HYPERTENSION AND CARDIOVASCULAR EVENTS

Inflammatory events in hypertension have been proposed for many years. Recent data suggest that inflammation causes vascular oxidative stress through stimulation of reactive oxygen species (ROS) production by leukocytes and vascular wall cells. The increased ROS change protein function and gene expression leading to activation of other inflammatory events including adhesion molecule and cytokine expression, recruitment and activation of leukocytes and vascular cells. Inflammation also causes endothelial dysfunction through either direct interaction between inflammatory cytokines and endothelial cells, or indirectly through increased oxidative stress. Finally changes in vascular wall structure and function ensue mediated by vascular smooth muscle cell (VSMC) proliferation establishing hypertension and augmenting cardiovascular disease (Figure 35.1).

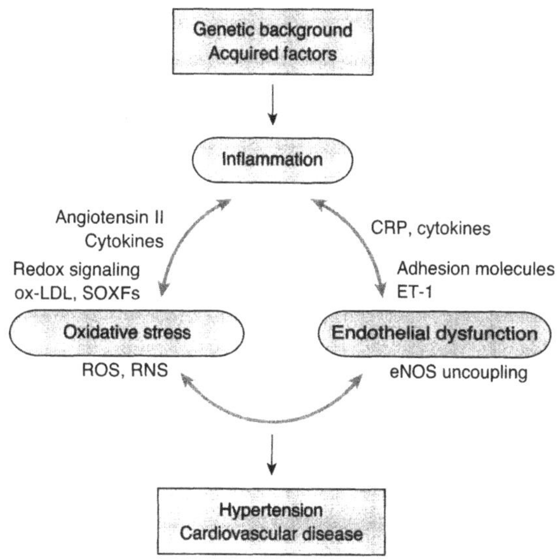

Figure 35.1 Inflammation, oxidative stress and endothelial dysfunction in the pathogenesis of hypertension and cardiovascular disease. Genetic background (e.g. single nucleotide polymorphisms (SNPs)) and acquired factors (e.g. hypertension, hyperlipidemia, diabetes, and systemic inflammation) promote inflammation, oxidative stress, and endothelial dysfunction in the vascular wall, which feed back positively on each other through specific mechanisms as noted. Finally, chronic vascular dysfunction leads to structural changes in the vascular wall, establishing hypertension and augmenting cardiovascular disease. CRP, C-reactive protein, ox-LDL, oxidized low density lipoprotein; SOXFs, secreted oxidative stress-induced factors, ET-1; endothelin-1, ROS; reactive oxygen species, RNS; reactive nitrogen species, eNOS; endothelial nitric oxide synthase

MECHANISMS OF INFLAMMATION IN SPECIFIC CARDIOVASCULAR DISEASES

Hypertension

The renin-angiotensin-aldosterone system (RAAS) is one of the most important mediators of blood volume and blood pressure in mammalians. Although RAAS inhibition by angiotensin converting enzyme (ACE) inhibitors or angiotensin receptor blockers (ARBs) is recognized as a standard therapy for hypertension, it is still unclear to what extent activation of the systemic RAAS plays a causative role in essential hypertension. Importantly, RAAS components found locally in various tissues including the vessel wall may contribute to hypertension. Angiotensin (Ang) II not only causes contraction of VSMCs, but also activates extracellular signal regulated kinases (ERK1/2) that stimulate proliferation and migration of VSMCs to promote vascular remodeling and hypertrophy. Another important effect of Ang II is activation of NAD(P)H oxidases (e.g. NOX1 and NOX4) to increase superoxide, which acts as a messenger to activate p38 mitogen-activated protein kinase (MAPK), c-Jun N-terminal kinases (JNK), and downstream transcription factors such as nuclear factor-κB (NF-κB)[1] that regulate inflammatory genes. Endothelin-1 (ET-1) is another pathological mediator that links hypertension and inflammation. ET-1 is a 21-amino acid peptide that is produced from endothelial cells and found to be elevated in many patients with essential hypertension. ET-1 possesses strong vasoconstrictive properties and, in part through production of ROS, activates protein kinases and downstream inflammatory signals including NF-κB in VSMCs.[1]

Hyperlipidemia

In early atherosclerotic lesions (fatty streaks), accumulation of lipoproteins is found within the subendothelial matrix, where oxidative modification may generate oxidized low-density lipoprotein (ox-LDL) followed by migration and phagocytosis by monocytes/macrophages to create foam cells. Ox-LDL is very proinflammatory by inducing oxidative stress (by up-regulating NAD(P)H oxidase expression in vascular cells,[2] and by activating phagocytes to produce ROS) and by stimulating expression of inflammatory cytokines such as interleukin (IL)-6. Also, ox-LDL binds to the ox-LDL receptor-1 (LOX1) in endothelial cells, which increases ROS production and activates NF-κB[3] that regulates expression of inflammatory genes including adhesion molecules and cytokines causing endothelial dysfunction. The expression of LOX-1 is enhanced by C-reactive protein (CRP) in endothelial cells.[4] The relationship between hyperlipidemia and hypertension is complex, but clearly synergistic in terms of oxidative stress.

Diabetes

Diabetes is an important risk factor for coronary artery disease that contributes to inflammation in the vascular wall. Elevated blood glucose in diabetes contributes to inflammation in several ways. 1) Glucose causes modification of macromolecules to form advanced glycation end products (AGEs). In atherosclerotic plaques from diabetic patients who underwent carotid endarterectomy, plaque was characterized by increased expression of receptor for AGEs (RAGE), cyclooxygenase (COX)-2 and matrix metalloproteinases, and activated NF-κB.[5] AGE activates RAGE to enhance expression of adhesion molecules such as vascular cell adhesion molecule-1 (VCAM-1), intercellular adhesion molecule-1 (ICAM-1), and E-selectin,[6] accelerating vascular inflammation. Of interest, AGEs activate NAD(P)H oxidase to increase superoxide production in endothelial cells, which provides a link between diabetes and oxidative stress.[7] 2) Hyperglycemia increases mitochondrial production of ROS in endothelial cells, stimulating NF-κB and expression of ICAM-1 and VCAM-1.[8] 3) High glucose enhances Ang II-mediated proinflammatory events by up-regulating angiotensin type 1 receptor expression and by increasing transactivation of the epidermal growth factor receptor.[9]

Turbulent blood flow

As frequently observed in human carotid artery bifurcation, atherosclerosis preferentially occurs in areas of turbulent flow and low shear stress. This phenomenon can be explained by the anti-inflammatory effect of steady laminar blood flow with appropriate shear stress on endothelial cells. In our experimental model, steady laminar flow inhibited tumor necrosis factor-α (TNF-α)-induced activation of JNK and subsequent expression of adhesion molecules in endothelial cells on perfused blood vessels ex vivo.[10] In addition, turbulent and oscillatory flow patterns increase ROS production.[11]

Infection

Infection is a common cause of inflammation in humans. Among several pathogens, epidemiological studies have shown increased risk of cardiovascular disease in individuals with prior infection by *Chlamydia pneumoniae*, *Helicobacter pylori*, cytomegalovirus, herpes simplex virus, hepatitis A virus, and other organisms. Heat shock protein (HSP)-60 derived from *Chlamydia pneumoniae* activates toll-like receptor (TLR)-4 and downstream NF-κB in endothelial cells and macrophages[12] causing inflammatory responses. Infection of cytomegalovirus causes expression of tissue factor and cytokines in cultured endothelial cells. Rather than specific pathogens, accumulation of antibody responses to multiple pathogens ('pathogen burden') appears to be a predictor for cardiovascular risk.[13]

Systemic inflammatory diseases

Finally, systemic inflammatory diseases such as rheumatoid arthritis and systemic lupus erythematosus are known to be a risk for atherosclerosis and cardiovascular diseases.[14,15] Thus, systemic inflammation that arises either primarily or secondarily appears to promote vascular inflammation and cardiovascular disease through oxidative stress and endothelial dysfunction as discussed below.

INFLAMMATION, OXIDATIVE STRESS AND ENDOTHELIAL DYSFUNCTION

ROS and reactive nitrogen species (RNS) pathways

Vascular cells and leukocytes possess numerous sources of ROS including endothelial nitric oxide (NO) synthase (eNOS), xanthine oxidase, NAD(P)H oxidase, COX, lipoxygenase, cytochrome P-450 enzymes, and mitochondria. Reaction of NO with ROS forms reactive nitrogen species (RNS) including NO_2^-, $\bullet NO_2$, N_2O_3 and $ONOO^-$, which cause secondary reactions including protein modification. Myeloperoxidase (MPO) is exclusively expressed in leukocytes and forms hypochlorous acid (HOCl) that leads to oxidative reactions including chlorination of LDL and L-arginine.[16] MPO also catalyzes oxidation of NO_2^- to $\bullet NO_2$ causing protein tyrosine nitration.[17] Importantly, elevated serum levels of MPO have been shown to predict future cardiovascular events in patients with chest pain.[18] The most important pathological roles of ROS and RNS are 1) impairment of endothelial function, 2) post-translational modification of proteins, and 3) activation of redox-sensitive signaling that regulates inflammatory genes. It is important to note that the biological effects of ROS and RNS may not simply be generalized because specific molecules, concentration and localization, interactions with endogenous antioxidants, and specific targets (lipids, proteins and nucleic acids) may affect the resulting biological responses.

Endothelial dysfunction

Endothelial dysfunction is an important hallmark of hypertension and cardiovascular disease. It is well established that coronary risk factors including hypertension cause endothelial dysfunction in humans and experimental animals, and endothelial dysfunction frequently precedes structural changes in the vessel wall. In humans, endothelial function is evaluated in coronary or forearm arteries as vasodilating responses to pharmacological or physical stimuli that increase endothelial production of endothelium-derived relaxing factors (EDRFs) including NO, prostacyclin and endothelium-derived hyperpolarizing factor. Endothelial dysfunction is explained by decreased production of EDRFs and/or increased production of endothelium-derived contracting factors such as ET-1 and superoxide. Based on our current knowledge, decreased bioavailability of NO through either eNOS uncoupling or inactivation by ROS has greatest impact on vascular homeostasis. In hypertensive animals, increased superoxide derived from NAD(P)H oxidase reacts with NO to form $ONOO^-$, which in turn causes oxidation of eNOS cofactor tetrahydrobiopterin resulting in uncoupling of eNOS in endothelial cells.[19] Monocyte-derived HOCl chlorinates L-arginine also causing eNOS uncoupling or may consume NO directly.[16] NO suppresses vascular inflammation by down-regulating adhesion molecule expression and chemokines including MCP-1 that are key mediators of inflammation.[20] NO also down-regulates plasminogen activator inhibitor-1 so that NO deficiency may promote thrombotic events. Thus, endothelial dysfunction means not only impairment of vasodilation in particular vascular beds, but a systemic pathogenic state that initiates local vascular inflammation through adhesiveness of leukocytes and/or platelets.

Post-translational modifications of proteins

Oxidative modification of proteins is evolving as an important molecular mechanism for regulation of redox-sensitive signaling pathways. For example, S-glutathionylation of small GTPase Ras mediates Ang II-induced phosphorylation of p38 and Akt in VSMCs, which is inhibited by overexpression of catalase, Grx-1 or dominant-negative p47phox, a NAD(P)H oxidase component.[21] S-glutathionylation mediated by $ONOO^-$ activates sarco/endoplasmic reticulum Ca^{2+}-ATPase in VSMCs, whereas tyrosine nitration inhibits NO-induced activation. These mechanisms explain NO-mediated arterial relaxation as well as decreased relaxation in hyperlipidemia.[22]

Redox signaling

ROS, especially superoxide and H_2O_2, act as second messengers activating various signaling molecules including tyrosine kinase receptors, Ras, MAPKs and Akt (see elsewhere for review[23]). Oxidative modification of proteins may in part account for the redox sensitivity of signaling molecules. Endogenous antioxidants modulate redox-sensitive signaling by both scavenging ROS and directly interacting with signaling molecules. Superoxide dismutase (SOD), catalase and glutathione peroxidase (GPX) are the major defenses against superoxide and H_2O_2. Recently, erythrocyte GPX-1 activity was shown to be inversely associated with risk of cardiovascular events in humans.[24] The thioredoxin (TRX) antioxidant system that comprises TRX, TRX reductase and TRX peroxidase is a ubiquitous thiol oxidoreductase system, which is capable of reducing disulfide cysteine groups. In addition, reduced TRX suppresses activity of apoptosis signal-regulating kinase 1 (ASK1) through direct binding. The interaction of TRX and ASK1 is sensitive to oxidation of TRX itself, which presents another form of redox-sensitive mechanism. Interestingly, our group found that physiological laminar flow decreases expression of TRX interacting protein (TXNIP, also termed VDUP-1), an endogenous inhibitor of TRX, and thereby decreased TNF-α-induced ASK1 activation and VCAM-1 expression in endothelial cells.[25]

Our laboratory also found that oxidative stress causes secretion of a class of molecules termed secreted oxidative stress-induced factors (SOXFs) including cyclophilin A, cyclophilin B, and HSP-90.[26] Among SOXFs, cyclophilin A appears to activate JNK, p38, and NF-κB to increase expression of VCAM-1 and E-selectin in endothelial cells.[27] This novel redox-sensitive signaling pathway provides another link between oxidative stress and inflammation in the vascular wall.

INFLAMMATORY MARKERS AS PREDICTORS OF CARDIOVASCULAR DISEASE

C-reactive protein (CRP)

CRP is an acute-phase reactant protein, termed a pentraxin, produced primarily by the liver in response to cytokines such as IL-1, IL-6 and TNF-α. Among several biomarkers for inflammation, CRP is one of those most used in clinical practice. Berk et al. reported in 1990 that plasma CRP was higher in patients with unstable angina than in those with stable coronary artery disease.[28] As the involvement of inflammation has been appreciated in development of cardiovascular diseases in recent years, more than 10 epidemiological studies have shown the predictive value of CRP as an independent risk factor for future cardiovascular events even in apparently healthy men and women.[29,30] Recent reports suggest that CRP itself acts as a mediator of inflammatory signaling in vascular cells and leukocytes. In cultured human endothelial cells, CRP induces expression of ICAM-1, VCAM-1, E-selectin, and monocyte chemoattractant protein 1 (MCP-1).[31,32] In human monocytes, CRP up-regulates expression of CC-chemokine receptor 2 (CCR2) that is a primary receptor for MCP-1 and regulates monocyte/macrophage chemotaxis. Since VSMCs and monocytes express CRP in human atherosclerotic plaques,[33] CRP itself may play a role in regulation of local inflammatory responses in the vascular wall during atherogenesis.

IL-6

IL-6 is a versatile cytokine that is produced by several cell types including vascular cells and leukocytes during inflammatory responses. IL-6 is recognized as a primary regulator of CRP production and also regulates inflammatory genes including TNF-α, IL-1β and adhesion molecules through the JAK/STAT and MAPKs pathway. Ridker et al. showed a significant correlation of plasma IL-6 and CRP levels, and the positive predictive value of plasma IL-6 level for the risk of future myocardial infarction in apparently healthy men.[34]

IL-10

IL-10, a potent anti-inflammatory cytokine, is expressed in a substantial number of advanced human atherosclerotic plaques.[35] IL-10-deficient mice fed an atherogenic diet exhibit a significant increase in lipid accumulation.[36] Elevated IL-10 serum levels are associated with improved endothelial vasoreactivity in patients with coronary artery disease.[37] These observations emphasize the importance of the balance between anti-inflammatory and proinflammatory mechanisms in cardiovascular disease.

Single nucleotide polymorphisms of inflammatory genes and the risk of cardiovascular diseases

Cardiovascular disease is obviously a multifactorial disease resulting from genetic factors and acquired factors. Susceptibility to acquired risk factors such as hypertension or diabetes might also be affected by genetic background. Whereas any two humans are approximately 99.9% identical in their DNA sequences, single nucleotide polymorphisms (SNPs) are the most common DNA sequence variations among individuals and may have an impact on the difference in susceptibility to diseases including atherosclerosis. At the time of writing, over 10 million human SNPs are registered in dbSNP (http://www.ncbi.nih.gov/SNP). SNPs are the subject of gene–disease association studies in order to identify genes whose function has an influence on susceptibility to specific disease. For example, comparison of cDNA sequences from SHRSP rats, a stroke-prone substrain of spontaneously hypertensive rats (SHRs), and reference WKY rats identified 478 SNP candidates, which may include genes that explain

Table 35.1 SNPs of inflammatory genes associated with cardiovascular diseases

Gene	*SNP*	*Intermediate phenotype*	*Primary phenotype*	*Reference*
CRP	+1059G/C		↓ CRP	40
		↓ CRP	No association with arterial thrombosis	41
	+1444C/T		↑ CRP after CABG	42
IL-1β	−511C/T	↓ monocyte responsiveness	↓ risk of MI	43
IL-6	−174G/C	↑ BP, ↑ CRP	↑ risk of CAD	44
		↑ IL-6, ↑ IL-10, ↑ TNF-α	↑ bilateral carotid atherosclerosis in old subjects	45
RANTES	−403G/A		↑ risk of CAD	46
TLR4	299D/G	↓ IL-6, ↓ fibrinogen, ↓ soluble VCAM-1	↓ carotid atherosclerosis	47
		↓ fibrinogen, ↓ soluble VCAM-1	Low probability in CAD patients	48
			No association with MI or stroke	49
CD14	−159C/T		↑ carotid atherosclerosis	50
COX-2	−765G/C	↓ COX-2 expression	↓ CRP	51
CYP2J2	−50T/G	↓ plasma EETs	High probability in CAD patients	52

SNP, single nucleotide polymorphism; CRP, C-reactive protein; IL, interleukin; TNF, tumor necrosis factor; RANTES, regulated upon activation, normal T-cell expressed and secreted; VCAM, vascular cell adhesion molecule; COX, cyclooxygenase; CYP, cytochrome P450; EETs, epoxyeicosatrienoic acids; BP, blood pressure; CABG, coronary artery bypass graft surgery; CAD, coronary artery disease; MI, myocardial infarction.

the susceptibility of the SHRSP strain to stroke, although the functional consequence of each SNP (if any) remains to be validated.[38]

Recent advances in DNA array technology allow us to screen known SNPs in a large-scale manner.[39] Currently available DNA chips provide for screening of over 100 000 human SNPs in 2 chips. The HapMap project (http://www.hapmap.org) is an international effort to gather information on SNP genotypes from 270 individuals among several populations in the world. Identification of haplotype, variation in clusters of SNPs that are inherited together, and 'tag' SNPs that uniquely identify these haplotypes, as planned in the HapMap project, will greatly enhance the efficiency to identify haplotypes and SNPs in each individual since the number of 'tag' SNPs is estimated to be about 300 000–600 000, which is far fewer than the 10 million common SNPs. Thus, large-scale SNP screening appears to be an affordable strategy for disease–gene association studies in the near future, and to potentially identify either inflammatory genes or new classes of genes that are currently not recognized to be associated with inflammation or cardiovascular disease, and help to identify potential target genes for the treatment of cardiovascular disease.

On the other hand, the conventional approach to identify significant SNPs is to sequence and genotype SNPs of candidate genes in patients and healthy individuals. Candidate genes for cardiovascular disease include genes related to inflammation and coagulation. Indeed, a number of studies have shown the association of SNPs in inflammatory genes with increased risk of cardiovascular events as summarized in Table 35.1.[40–52] These observations further strengthen the involvement of inflammation in the development of cardiovascular disease.

ANTI-INFLAMMATORY THERAPIES FOR HYPERTENSION AND CARDIOVASCULAR DISEASE

Established therapeutic pathways

As involvement of inflammation has been appreciated in hypertension and atherosclerosis, anti-inflammatory therapy has been highlighted as an additional effect of established medicines such as hydroxymethylglutaryl coenzyme A inhibitors (statins), RAAS inhibitors, activators of nuclear receptor/transcription factor peroxisome proliferator-activated receptor-α (PPAR-α), and aspirin. Statins not only inhibit cholesterol synthesis, but also increase expression and activity of eNOS through activation of Akt and inhibition of small G protein Rho geranylgeranylation and downstream Rho-kinase. Since Rho-kinase also mediates Ang II-induced up-regulation of MCP-1 in VSMC,[53] statins may suppress inflammation and oxidative stress through multiple pathways and improve endothelial function. In a clinical study, lovastatin and pravastatin decreased plasma CRP in patients with hypercholesterolemia.[54,55]

Although RAAS inhibition by ACE-inhibitors and ARBs is an established therapy for hypertension, recent clinical trials have shown that ARBs may have additional beneficial effects on cardiovascular disease beyond lowering blood pressure.[56] This beneficial effect may be explained by the ability to inhibit proinflammatory properties of Ang II that include increases in TNF, IL-6, and ICAM-1. PPAR-α agonists have been used for diabetic patients with insulin resistance and have been shown to lower plasma concentrations of IL-6 in patients with atherosclerosis. PPAR-α agonists suppress NF-κB and AP-1 transcriptional activity by interference of p65 and c-Jun that are key regulators of inflammatory genes.[57] COX catalyzes arachidonic acid to form prostaglandin (PG)H_2 that is a precursor of more than 30 bioactive prostanoids including proinflammatory PGE_2, prothrombotic thromboxane A_2, and vasodilator PGI_2. Aspirin is a classic COX inhibitor that inhibits both constitutive COX-1 and inducible COX-2, and has been used for secondary prevention of myocardial infarction. A primary prevention study using 325 mg aspirin on alternative days showed that aspirin decreased risk for future myocardial infarction and that the beneficial effect of aspirin was more profound in patients with higher plasma CRP.[29] By contrast, COX-2 specific inhibitor rofecoxib has been used for inflammatory disorders, and shown to lower CRP and IL-6 levels in patients with acute coronary syndromes;[58] however, rofecoxib increases the risk of myocardial infarction and was withdrawn from the market in 2004. Further information is needed for each COX inhibitor regarding its potential effects on targets other than COX, and its effect on both pro- and anti-atherogenic prostanoids.

NF-κB/MCP-1/macrophage pathway

Signaling pathways that activate the transcription factor NF-κB appear to be feasible therapeutic targets to control inflammation since NF-κB regulates expression of adhesion molecules such as ICAM-1 and VCAM-1 and inflammatory cytokines including MCP-1, IL-6, and TNF-α. MCP-1 in turn induces proliferation and IL-6 production in human smooth muscle cells through activation of NF-κB.[59] Activation of the NF-κB/MCP-1/macrophage pathway appears to maintain inflammatory process within the vascular wall. Indeed, MCP-1 deletion in LDL receptor null mice[60] or MCP-1 receptor CCR2 deletion in ApoE null mice[61] ameliorates atherosclerosis development. Thus, inactivation of NF-κB appears to be an promising approach as supported by the finding that 'NF-κB decoy' oligonucleotide transfection inhibits angioplasty-induced neointima formation in animals.[62]

CONCLUSION

Recent advances have identified molecular mechanisms and acquired factors that stimulate inflammation, oxidative stress, and endothelial dysfunction in the vasculature. This inflammatory state promotes chronic changes in gene expression and vessel wall architecture that contribute to hypertension, atherosclerosis, and cardiovascular events. Clinical studies employing inflammatory markers and SNPs support a role for inflammation in cardiovascular disease in humans. Genomics may identify novel genes that accelerate atherogenesis by stimulating inflammation as well as genes that retard atherosclerosis by inhibiting inflammation. Knowledge of disease-related SNPs may enable us to provide customized therapies for individuals even in a preventive manner. Therapeutics targeting inflammation, oxidative stress, and endothelial dysfunction represent attractive new approaches to prevent diseases including hypertension and atherosclerosis.

REFERENCES

1. Touyz RM, Yao G, Viel E et al. Angiotensin II and endothelin-1 regulate MAP kinases through different redox-dependent mechanisms in human vascular smooth muscle cells. J Hypertens 2004; 22: 1141–9.
2. Rueckschloss U, Galle J, Holtz J et al. Induction of NAD(P)H oxidase by oxidized low-density lipoprotein in human endothelial cells: antioxidative potential of hydroxymethylglutaryl coenzyme A reductase inhibitor therapy. Circulation 2001; 104: 1767–72.
3. Cominacini L, Pasini AF, Garbin U et al. Oxidized low density lipoprotein (ox-LDL) binding to ox-LDL receptor-1 in endothelial cells induces the activation of NF-kappaB through an increased production of intracellular reactive oxygen species. J Biol Chem 2000; 275: 12633–8.
4. Li L, Roumeliotis N, Sawamura T et al. C-reactive protein enhances LOX-1 expression in human aortic endothelial cells: relevance of LOX-1 to C-reactive protein-induced endothelial dysfunction. Circ Res 2004; 95: 877–83.

5. Cipollone F, Fazia M, Iezzi A et al. Blockade of the angiotensin II type 1 receptor stabilizes atherosclerotic plaques in humans by inhibiting prostaglandin E2-dependent matrix metalloproteinase activity. Circulation 2004; 109: 1482–8.
6. Basta G, Lazzerini G, Massaro M et al. Advanced glycation end products activate endothelium through signal-transduction receptor RAGE: a mechanism for amplification of inflammatory responses. Circulation 2002; 105: 816–22.
7. Wautier MP, Chappey O, Corda S et al. Activation of NADPH oxidase by AGE links oxidant stress to altered gene expression via RAGE. Am J Physiol Endocrinol Metab 2001; 280: E685–E694.
8. Nishikawa T, Edelstein D, Du XL et al. Normalizing mitochondrial superoxide production blocks three pathways of hyperglycemic damage. Nature 2000; 404: 787–90.
9. Konishi A, Berk BC, Epidermal growth factor receptor transactivation is regulated by glucose in vascular smooth muscle cells. J Biol Chem 2003; 278: 35049–56.
10. Yamawaki H, Lehoux S, Berk BC. Chronic physiological shear stress inhibits tumor necrosis factor-induced proinflammatory responses in rabbit aorta perfused ex vivo. Circulation 2003; 108: 1619–25.
11. Silacci P, Desgeorges A, Mazzolai L et al. Flow pulsatility is a critical determinant of oxidative stress in endothelial cells. Hypertension 2001; 38: 1162–6.
12. Bulut Y, Faure E, Thomas L et al. Chlamydial heat shock protein 60 activates macrophages and endothelial cells through Toll-like receptor 4 and MD2 in a MyD88-dependent pathway. J Immunol 2002; 168: 1435–40.
13. Prasad A, Zhu J, Halcox JP et al. Predisposition to atherosclerosis by infections: role of endothelial dysfunction. Circulation 2002; 106: 184–90.
14. Wallberg-Jonsson S, Ohman ML, Dahlqvist SR. Cardiovascular morbidity and mortality in patients with seropositive rheumatoid arthritis in Northern Sweden. J Rheumatol 1997; 24: 445–51.
15. Roman MJ, Shanker BA, Davis A et al. Prevalence and correlates of accelerated atherosclerosis in systemic lupus erythematosus. N Engl J Med 2003; 349: 2399–406.
16. Vita JA, Brennan ML, Gokce N et al. Serum myeloperoxidase levels independently predict endothelial dysfunction in humans. Circulation 2004; 110: 1134–9.
17. Baldus S, Eiserich JP, Mani A et al. Endothelial transcytosis of myeloperoxidase confers specificity to vascular ECM proteins as targets of tyrosine nitration. J Clin Invest 2001; 108: 1759–70.
18. Brennan ML, Penn MS, Van Lente F et al. Prognostic value of myeloperoxidase in patients with chest pain. N Engl J Med 2003; 349: 1595–604.
19. Landmesser U, Dikalov S, Price SR et al. Oxidation of tetrahydrobiopterin leads to uncoupling of endothelial cell nitric oxide synthase in hypertension. J Clin Invest 2003; 111: 1201–9.
20. De Caterina R, Libby P, Peng HB et al. Nitric oxide decreases cytokine-induced endothelial activation. Nitric oxide selectively reduces endothelial expression of adhesion molecules and proinflammatory cytokines. J Clin Invest 1995; 96: 60–8.
21. Adachi T, Pimentel DR, Heibeck T et al. S-glutathiolation of Ras mediates redox-sensitive signaling by angiotensin II in vascular smooth muscle cells. J Biol Chem 2004; 279: 29857–62.
22. Adachi T, Weisbrod RM, Pimentel DR et al. S-Glutathiolation by peroxynitrite activates SERCA during arterial relaxation by nitric oxide. Nat Med 2004; 10: 1200–7.
23. Griendling KK, Sorescu D, Lassegue B et al. Modulation of protein kinase activity and gene expression by reactive oxygen species and their role in vascular physiology and pathophysiology. Arterioscler Thromb Vasc Biol 2000; 20: 2175–83.
24. Blankenberg S, Rupprecht HJ, Bickel C et al. Glutathione peroxidase 1 activity and cardiovascular events in patients with coronary artery disease. N Engl J Med 2003; 349: 1605–13.
25. Yamawaki H, Pan S, Lee RT et al. Fluid shear stress is anti-inflammatory by decreasing thioredoxin-interacting protein in endothelial cells. J Clin Invest 2005; 115: 733–8.
26. Liao D-F, Jin Z-G, Baas AS et al. Purification and identification of secreted oxidative stress-induced factors from vascular smooth muscle cells. J Biol Chem 2000; 275: 189–96.
27. Jin ZG, Lungu AO, Xie L et al. Cyclophilin A is a proinflammatory cytokine that activates endothelial cells. Arterioscler Thromb Vasc Biol 2004; 24: 1186–91.
28. Berk BC, Weintraub WS, Alexander RW. Elevation of C-reactive protein in 'active' coronary artery disease. Am J Cardiol 1990; 65: 168–72.
29. Ridker PM, Cushman M, Stampfer MJ et al. Inflammation, aspirin, and the risk of cardiovascular disease in apparently healthy men. N Engl J Med 1997; 336: 973–9.
30. Ridker PM, Hennekens CH, Buring JE et al. C-reactive protein and other markers of inflammation in the prediction of cardiovascular disease in women. N Engl J Med 2000; 342: 836–43.
31. Pasceri V, Willerson JT, Yeh ET, Direct proinflammatory effect of C-reactive protein on human endothelial cells. Circulation 2000; 102: 2165–8.
32. Pasceri V, Cheng JS, Willerson JT et al. Modulation of C-reactive protein-mediated monocyte chemoattractant protein-1 induction in human endothelial cells by anti-atherosclerosis drugs. Circulation 2001; 103: 2531–4.
33. Yasojima K, Schwab C, McGeer EG et al. Generation of C-reactive protein and complement components in atherosclerotic plaques. Am J Pathol 2001; 158: 1039–51.
34. Ridker PM, Rifai N, Stampfer MJ et al. Plasma concentration of interleukin-6 and the risk of future myocardial infarction among apparently healthy men. Circulation 2000; 101: 1767–72.
35. Mallat Z, Heymes C, Ohan J et al. Expression of interleukin-10 in advanced human atherosclerotic plaques: relation to inducible nitric oxide synthase expression and cell death. Arterioscler Thromb Vasc Biol 1999; 19: 611–16.
36. Mallat Z, Besnard S, Duriez M et al. Protective role of interleukin-10 in atherosclerosis. Circ Res 1999; 85: e17–24.
37. Fichtlscherer S, Breuer S, Heeschen C et al. Interleukin-10 serum levels and systemic endothelial vasoreactivity in patients with coronary artery disease. J Am Coll Cardiol 2004; 44: 44–9.
38. Zimdahl H, Nyakatura G, Brandt P et al. A SNP map of the rat genome generated from cDNA sequences. Science 2004; 303: 807.
39. Wang DG, Fan JB, Siao CJ et al. Large-scale identification, mapping, and genotyping of single-nucleotide polymorphisms in the human genome. Science 1998; 280: 1077–82.
40. Suk HJ, Ridker PM, Cook NR et al. Relation of polymorphism within the C-reactive protein gene and plasma CRP levels. Atherosclerosis 2005; 178: 139–45.
41. Zee RY, Ridker PM, Polymorphism in the human C-reactive protein (CRP) gene, plasma concentrations of CRP, and the risk of future arterial thrombosis. Atherosclerosis 2002; 162: 217–19.
42. Brull DJ, Serrano N, Zito F et al. Human CRP gene polymorphism influences CRP levels: implications for the prediction and pathogenesis of coronary heart disease. Arterioscler Thromb Vasc Biol 2003; 23: 2063–9.
43. Iacoviello L, Di Castelnuovo A, Gattone M et al. Polymorphisms of the interleukin-1 beta gene affect the risk of myocardial infarction and ischemic stroke at young age and the response of mononuclear cells to stimulation in vitro. Arterioscler Thromb Vasc Biol 2005; 25: 222–7.
44. Humphries SE, Luong LA, Ogg MS et al. The interleukin-6 -174 G/C promoter polymorphism is associated with risk of coronary

heart disease and systolic blood pressure in healthy men. Eur Heart J 2001; 22: 2243–52.

45. Giacconi R, Cipriano C, Albanese F et al. The -174G/C polymorphism of IL-6 is useful to screen old subjects at risk for atherosclerosis or to reach successful ageing. Exp Gerontol 2004; 39: 621–8.
46. Simeoni E, Winkelmann BR, Hoffmann MM et al. Association of RANTES G-403A gene polymorphism with increased risk of coronary arteriosclerosis. Eur Heart J 2004; 25: 1438–46.
47. Kiechl S, Lorenz E, Reindl M et al. Toll-like receptor 4 polymorphisms and atherogenesis. N Engl J Med 2002; 347: 185–92.
48. Ameziane N, Beillat T, Verpillat P et al. Association of the Toll-like receptor 4 gene Asp299Gly polymorphism with acute coronary events. Arterioscler Thromb Vasc Biol 2003; 23: e61–4.
49. Zee RY, Hegener HH, Gould J et al. Toll-like receptor 4 Asp299Gly gene polymorphism and risk of atherothrombosis. Stroke 2005; 36: 154–7.
50. Funakoshi Y, Ichiki T, Shimokawa H et al. Rho-kinase mediates angiotensin II-induced monocyte chemoattractant protein-1 expression in rat vascular smooth muscle cells. Hypertension 2001; 38: 100–4.
51. Ridker PM, Rifai N, Clearfield M et al. Measurement of C-reactive protein for the targeting of statin therapy in the primary prevention of acute coronary events. N Engl J Med 2001; 344: 1959–65.
52. Albert MA, Danielson E, Rifai N et al. Effect of statin therapy on C-reactive protein levels: the pravastatin inflammation/CRP evaluation (PRINCE): a randomized trial and cohort study. JAMA 2001; 286: 64–70.
53. Risley P, Jerrard-Dunne P, Sitzer M et al. Promoter polymorphism in the endotoxin receptor (CD14) is associated with increased carotid atherosclerosis only in smokers: the Carotid Atherosclerosis Progression Study (CAPS). Stroke 2003; 34: 600–4.
54. Papafili A, Hill MR, Brull DJ et al. Common promoter variant in cyclooxygenase-2 represses gene expression: evidence of role in acute-phase inflammatory response. Arterioscler Thromb Vasc Biol 2002; 22: 1631–6.
55. Spiecker M, Darius H, Hankeln T et al. Risk of coronary artery disease associated with polymorphism of the cytochrome P450 epoxygenase CYP2J2. Circulation 2004; 110: 2132–6.
56. Dahlof B, Devereux RB, Kjeldsen SE et al. Cardiovascular morbidity and mortality in the Losartan Intervention For Endpoint reduction in hypertension study (LIFE): a randomised trial against atenolol. Lancet 2002; 359: 995–1003.
57. Delerive P, De Bosscher K, Besnard S et al. Peroxisome proliferator-activated receptor alpha negatively regulates the vascular inflammatory gene response by negative cross-talk with transcription factors NF-kappaB and AP-1. J Biol Chem 1999; 274: 32048–54.
58. Monakier D, Mates M, Klutstein MW et al. Rofecoxib, a COX-2 inhibitor, lowers C-reactive protein and interleukin-6 levels in patients with acute coronary syndromes. Chest 2004; 125: 1610–15.
59. Viedt C, Vogel J, Athanasiou T et al. Monocyte chemoattractant protein-1 induces proliferation and interleukin-6 production in human smooth muscle cells by differential activation of nuclear factor-kappaB and activator protein-1. Arterioscler Thromb Vasc Biol 2002; 22: 914–20.
60. Gu L, Okada Y, Clinton SK et al. Absence of monocyte chemoattractant protein-1 reduces atherosclerosis in low density lipoprotein receptor-deficient mice. Mol Cell 1998; 2: 275–81.
61. Boring L, Gosling J, Cleary M et al. Decreased lesion formation in CCR2–/– mice reveals a role for chemokines in the initiation of atherosclerosis. Nature 1998; 394: 894–7.
62. Yamasaki K, Asai T, Shimizu M et al. Inhibition of NFkappaB activation using cis-element 'decoy' of NFkappaB binding site reduces neointimal formation in porcine balloon-injured coronary artery model. Gene Ther 2003; 10: 356–64.

36

Biological effects of salt loading

Edward D Frohlich and Jasmina Varagic

INTRODUCTION

Over the millennia, tremendous interest has been generated regarding the role of salt in society and in social intercourse.[1] Salt and its linguistic derivatives have become a part of the daily parlance in various societies and cultures (Box 36.1). Indeed, the various positive and negative attitudes about salt have been inculcated in social practices, perception, and stature (social position, payment for services, etc.).

Box 36.1 Examples of salt in daily parlance in the English language

Commonly used words	Commonly used phrases
• Salary	• ... not worth his salt
• Salute	• worth his weight in salt
• Salutary	• with a grain of salt
• Salutatorian	• salt of the sea
• Salutation	• salt of the earth
• Salvation	• at the table, to sit above the salt

Salt excess and salt sensitivity

In more recent generations, clinical and laboratory scientists have been concerned about the biological effects of dietary sodium excess or salt loading in large numbers of experimental types of hypertension as well as in the various clinical expressions of disease.[2–4] For the most part, clinical reports have related sodium or salt excess to its effects on blood pressure; and relatively little attention has been focused on its effects on the major target organs of hypertensive disease (e.g. brain, heart, vessels, and kidneys). Thus, there is little wonder that the primary attention of dietary salt excess has been related chiefly to studies of large population groups of normotensive and hypertensive individuals. For this reason, most of the studies have confirmed and re-confirmed the relationship of dietary sodium (or salt) intake with the prevalence of hypertension in that specific population.[5,6] The obvious conclusion from these observational population studies with measured blood pressures and prevalence of hypertension: not all of the subjects were 'sodium-sensitive'. The natural clinical question arising from these studies was how to detect sodium sensitivity and how to prevent associated morbidity or mortality. Of course, this has been determined by the effects of salt (or sodium) loading and the response of blood pressure in the subjects studied. From these efforts a large number of reports have related salt or sodium loading to blood pressure elevation in the 'sensitive' patients. This continues to remain an area of much study, greater controversy, and unsatisfying resolution. But, as has been stated by some wise clinicians, the best way to detect sodium or salt sensitivity is by demonstrating an incontrovertible rise in pressure in the 'sensitive' subject with salt (or sodium) loading and, thereby, proving the existence of that sensitivity when arterial pressure is reduced following salt withdrawal.

Salt excess and hypertensive disease

However, hypertension is more than a persistent elevation of arterial pressure; it is a disease state that it is also manifested by the associated evidence of structural and functional impairment of the target organs of the disease. It was because of this fundamental concept that we focused not only on the effects of salt loading on arterial pressure but, primarily, on the assessment of structural and functional alterations of the heart, circulation, aorta, and kidneys. This is not to suggest that others have not focused their attention on this issue, but they are few in number. In this chapter, we shall focus on their contributions as well. At this juncture in our work, it seems fair to conclude that dietary salt or sodium excess does not solely elevate blood pressure: it is importantly expressed on significantly impaired target organs structurally and functionally. Indeed, it is our conviction that salt loading has far more widespread deleterious effects than simply its effects on arterial pressure.[7]

EXPERIMENTAL MODEL: OUR EXPERIENCE

The SHR

The spontaneously hypertensive rat (SHR) and its normotensive Wistar Kyoto (WKY) control strain have been employed for over four decades as the best experimental model available for its most common clinical counterpart, essential hypertension in man.[8] The SHR is a model of naturally occurring genetic hypertension that requires no surgical extirpation of organs and no co-treatment with steroidal or other chemical substances to exacerbate the disease. Moreover, the effect of persistent blood pressure elevation (appearing within days of birth) produces pathophysiological alterations and complications of the target organs of the disease.[9] Indeed, the heart[10,11] and kidney[12] are very similarly involved, and they mimic very closely the changes that occur in patients with essential hypertension.

Laboratory methods

To assess the physiological alterations produced naturally by the disease in the SHR, we have adapted established experimental or clinical techniques to quantify the hemodynamic alterations which occur over time.[13–19] Of specific interest, similar to findings in man, the arterial pressure increases with time into early adulthood and left ventricular hypertrophy is initially adaptive; and we have developed several interventions to assess its effects on cardiac function.[18–20] Furthermore, at this stage of early adulthood, renal function also appears normal but, as with cardiac involvement, it becomes naturally impaired later in adulthood.[12] On the other hand, both SHR and essential hypertension can be exacerbated earlier in adult life by induction of endothelial dysfunction; and this can be accomplished with prolonged treatment with N -nitro-L-arginine methyl ester (L-NAME), an inhibitor of the endothelial enzyme nitric oxide synthase. Thus, each of the pathophysiological alterations that occur naturally with more prolonged disease may, therefore, be induced earlier in life with this substance.[21] All this is pertinent, but as with any hereditable induced abnormality, other genetically produced aberrations may also occur; and, in the SHR and the WKY rat, biventricular hypertrophy may occur due to a congenital arteriovenous abnormality (usually a ventricular septal defect).[22–24] Of particular importance, as with essential hypertension, associated with the hypertensive cardiac and renal alterations are evidence of ischemia and impaired blood flow reserve,[25,26] fibrosis,[25,27] and apoptosis.[28]

Salt loading

Target organ changes become more evident in older adulthood and, when they do occur, functional consequences may be evident without additional experimental interventions.[11,12] This discussion concerns the deleterious effects of salt loading primarily on heart, although some early findings on aorta, organ circulations, and renal function will be discussed less extensively. Before leaving the subject of our experimental model, it is important to clarify the importance of the terms 'salt loading' and 'sodium loading'. In the studies to which we refer, we specifically mean salt (NaCl) loading. It must be appreciated that in the human being, only one-half of the dietary intake of sodium is in the form of sodium chloride; and confusion and controversy also exist as to the potential pathogenetic role of the chloride ion in salt loading.

SALT LOADING

Initial studies

Our earliest studies of salt loading in the SHR began in the 1970s when most workers were of the opinion that experimental salt-induced hypertension required specific experimental models of hypertension that were 'salt-sensitive' by: addition of exogenously administered steroid with salt loading (e.g. desoxycorticosterone acetate – DOCA); extirpation of five-sixth renal mass in addition to sodium loading; or exogenously administered agents together with the salt excess. Our first efforts were designed to determine whether the SHR could develop an exacerbated expression of hypertension with co-administration of salt and DOCA. Indeed, these studies demonstrated that the SHR was most vulnerable to this maneuver and, in fact, malignant hypertension was thereby induced.[29] We then set out to determine whether increasing amounts of dietary salt excess would also produce an exacerbated form of SHR hypertension.[30,31] Several important consequences were observed. First, the salt excess did induce a progressive rise in arterial pressure but, even more intriguing, it promoted an increased left ventricular mass even before arterial pressure or total peripheral resistance increased.[31] In these early studies, a 4% salt loading (in drinking water) was sufficient to produce these effects, although other investigators later produced exacerbated cardiac and renal alterations with a greater degree of salt loading (8%) in the SHR.[32–35]

Salt loading protocols

Because 8% salt loading was so uniformly successful in studies by others,[32–35] we continued our work with this amount of salt loading, although our present studies are, once again, focusing on 4% loading (a daily dietary intake which is more comparable to the daily sodium intake that not infrequently occurs in many patients with essential hypertension). Because our early experiences dealing with cardiac pathophysiology in SHR hypertension demonstrated that the factor of age was exquisitely important with respect to the extent of ischemia, coronary and renal blood flow reserve, and on collagen (i.e. hydroxyproline) content which was deposited perivascularly as well as within the ventricular extracellular matrix, our initial efforts involved administration of 8% salt diet to two groups of adult SHRs. The younger adult group was salt loaded for 8 weeks (from 8 to 16 weeks of age) when their studies were conducted; the older adult group of SHRs was salt loaded for 32 weeks (from 20 to 52 weeks of age) when similar studies were conducted.[36]

FINDINGS

Age-related cardiac data

Of great interest were our findings dealing with the overall effect of salt loading in the foregoing two groups of adult SHRs. Contrary to what might be expected, all of the older adult SHRs were able to withstand the prolonged period of salt loading without any further adverse effects than a statistically significant (but less than dramatic) rise in arterial pressure associated with impaired diastolic ventricular functions and renal functional impairment. On the other hand, approximately 25% of the younger adult SHRs developed overt systolic ventricular malfunction manifested by severe ventricular failure, pulmonary edema or death.[36] The remaining 75% of these younger SHR adults demonstrated only impaired diastolic ventricular function and a rise in arterial pressure (Table 36.1). By the diastolic dysfunction produced we mean that they exhibited a number of abnormal diastolic functional indices in the presence of preserved systolic function. In order to validate our techniques

Table 36.1 Systolic arterial pressure (SAP), left ventricular (LV) mass index and hydroxyproline concentration, and LV ECHO-derived parameters of systolic and diastolic functions

	Young adult SHR			*Old SHR*	
Parameter	*Control*	*Salt without CHF*	*Salt with CHF*	*Control*	*Salt*
SAP (mm Hg)	206±9	243±8*	164±14*+	207±6	242±7*
LV mass index (mg/g)	2.5±0.1	4.7±0.2*	6.8±0.4*+	3.2±0.1	4.0±0.02*
LV hydroxyproline (mg/g)	4.53±0.16	5.59±0.16*	6.84±0.57*+	4.68±0.25	5.89±0.46*
Fractional shortening (%)	41±1	44±1	35±1*+	41±1	44±1
IVRT (msec)	4.0±0.1	5.5±0.2*	4.7±0.2*+	4.3±0.1	5.1±0.1*
E/A	2.6±0.1	1.5±0.1*	2.5±0.2+	2.6±0.1	2.2±0.1
DTE (msec)	4.5±0.1	4.0±0.2*	3.6±0.2*	4.6±0.2	4.2±0.2
E/Vp	0.030±0.001	0.031±0.001	0.039±0.002*+	0.032±0.001	0.034±0.001

Data are presented as mean value ± 1 SEM. SALT with CHF indicates salt-loaded young adults with congestive heart failure (CHF). IVRT, isovolumic relaxation time; E, peak early filling velocity; A, peak velocity of late filling; DTE, deceleration time of E; E/V_p, index of LV filling pressure.

*$p < 0.05$ versus respective control group, +$p < 0.05$ versus salt-loaded young adults without congestive heart failure (salt without CHF).

for determining systolic and diastolic ventricular functions in the same rat over an extended period of time, we adapted and validated accepted clinical and larger animal echocardiographic techniques to the rat.[19,20] Thus, 8% salt loading did, in fact, further increase arterial pressure and ventricular mass, but it also impaired left ventricular function in both the younger and older SHRs – although, as already stated, more severe left ventricular failure was produced in the younger SHRs.[36]

Other organ responses

It is also of importance to recognize that the increased left ventricular mass and impaired function was associated with increased aortic mass and reduced distensibility as well as increased pulse wave velocity (Table 36.2). In addition, these profound hemodynamic derangements also included impaired coronary and renal blood flow and flow reserves, although these circulatory alterations were not uniformly distributed throughout all of the organ circulations.[37] And, further, the impaired renal hemodynamics were associated with reduced glomerular filtration rate and massive proteinuria (Table 36.3).

Table 36.2 Aortic distensibility and pulse wave velocity in young adult salt-loaded SHRs

Parameter	*Control SHRs*	*Salt-loaded SHRs*
PP (mm Hg)	61±6	75±3*
Aortic distensibility (mm Hg^{-1})	4.67±0.04	2.49±0.02*
PWV (cm/s)	491±13	651±34*

PP, pulse pressure; PWV, pulse wave velocity.

*$p<0.05$ vs control.

Remodeling

Having demonstrated that 8% salt loading produced severe structural and functional changes in heart, aorta, and kidney it was of further importance to determine whether these changes could be prevented with specific therapy. A large body of literature has become available in recent years that has demonstrated prevention of left ventricular remodeling experimentally and in patients with recent myocardial infarction or cardiac failure.[38–50] Additionally, ventricular structural remodeling was associated with increased extracellular matrix fibrosis and perivascular fibrosis of the coronary vasculature which was prevented by agents that inhibit the renin-angiotensin system (RAS) (i.e. angiotensin converting enzyme (ACE) inhibitors and/or type-1 angiotensin II receptor blockers).[51–53] Therefore, it seemed eminently reasonable to hypothesize that these very same therapeutic agents might be of value in preventing the ventricular fibrosis induced by salt loading.

Angiotensin receptor blockade with salt loading

The angiotensin (Ang) II (type 1) receptor blocker candesartan was shown to be efficacious in preventing ventricular remodeling in a recently reported large clinical trial.[48–50] Therefore, we administered this agent in two doses to two separate SHR groups receiving the 8% salt loading maneuver for a period of 8 weeks. Under these conditions of salt loading, we found that the Ang II receptor blocker (ARB) failed to reduce arterial pressure[54] (Table 36.4). However, we also found that there was a profound and significant reduction in left ventricular mass and wall thickness that was associated with a significant decrease in left ventricular hydroxyproline concentration and collagen volume fraction.[54] Furthermore, none of

Table 36.3 Systemic and renal hemodynamics, and urinary albumin (UAE) and protein (UPE) excretions after 8 weeks of 8% NaCl diet in SHRs

	MAP mm Hg	*ERBF ml/min/g*	*GFR ml/min/g*	*RVR U*	*UAE mg/day*	*UPE mg/day*
Control	207±3	6.42±0.43	1.12±0.08	33±0.9	0.9±0.1	27±0.1
Salt loaded	189±8*	2.75±0.68*	0.48±0.11*	161±56*	77±22*	156±36*

MAP, mean arterial pressure; ERBF, renal blood flow; GFR, glomerular filtration rate; RVR, renal vascular resistance.

*$p<0.05$ vs control.

Table 36.4 The effects of angiotensin receptor blocker (ARB – candesartan) on mean arterial pressure (MAP), left ventricular mass index (LVMI) and hydroxyproline concentration, and urinary protein excretion in young adult salt-loaded SHRs

Parameter	*Control*	*Salt without CHF*	*Salt with CHF*	*Salt with ARB (1 mg/kg/day)*	*Salt with ARB (10 mg/kg/day)*
MAP (mm Hg)	184±5	225±6*	150±23*+	220±5*	219±4*
LVMI (mg/g)	2.85±0.03	4.7±0.2*	6.96±0.33*+	3.16±0.06+	3.26±0.04+
LV hydroxyproline (mg/g)	4.32±0.22	5.37±0.21*	6.1±0.38*+	4.60±0.21+	4.51±0.20+
Urinary protein excretion (mg/day/100 g body weight)	7±0.2	49±6*	104±22*+	11±1+	10±1+

CHF, congestive heart failure.

*$p<0.05$ vs control; +$p<0.05$ vs salt without CHF.

the younger adult SHRs developed overt systolic ventricular failure and they also demonstrated preserved left ventricular diastolic function. In contrast to these recent findings, 25% of younger SHRs given 8% salt died of cardiac failure in our earlier study.[36] Thus, it seems reasonable to conclude that local inhibition of the cardiac RAS was dramatically effective in preventing the adverse structural changes of ventricular remodeling as well as in maintaining normal left ventricular systolic and diastolic functions. In addition, aortic distensibility was not preserved, but the proteinuria was (Table 36.4).

SIGNIFICANCE

The significance of these changes challenges current thinking about physiological responses to sodium loading. First and foremost, we confirmed in the SHR the long-standing concept that severe salt loading elevates arterial pressure in normotensive subjects, and it markedly increases arterial pressure in those who already have hypertension. Secondly, the cardiovascular events associated with salt loading in this experimental model of naturally occurring hypertension that mimics essential hypertension, depend upon the age of the adult SHR. Thus, 25% of younger adult SHRs developed overt cardiac (i.e. systolic) failure, although the remaining number (75%) of younger and all of the older SHRs developed left ventricular diastolic dysfunction (with preserved systolic function). Thirdly, the abnormal left ventricular function was associated with structural changes that were identical with those changes associated with cardiac remodeling in patients. These changes were manifested histologically and biochemically by an increase in hydroxyproline, collagen volume fraction, and fibrous deposition in the left ventricular extracellular matrix as well as perivascularly. Fourthly, these structural and functional changes induced by salt excess were prevented by the concomitant administration of a type-1 Ang II receptor blocking agent. And, finally, the sodium loading-induced cardiac changes described above were associated with functional changes in the large arteries and kidney that were manifested by reduced aortic distensibility and increased pulse wave velocity and impaired renal function and proteinuria, respectively. Thus, strong evidence is now appearing to demonstrate that salt loading stimulated the local cardiac (and, perhaps, renal) RAS[55–59] as well as the converse – suppression of the systemic (or endocrine) RAS.

It would be premature to suggest that the salt loading described in this report only primarily stimulated the local cardiac and renal systems while concurrently inhibiting the systemic RAS.[60–63] Although these effects seem reasonable, additional biological systems and functions may also be involved. Thus, evidence is at hand that confirms the existence of a local cardiac aldosterone system[64] which may operate independently of the adrenal aldosterone systems; however, at this time, it is not possible to support this suggestion. It is possible that the stimulation of cardiac aldosterone[65] may be provoked directly by the sodium excess state or, by the same token, it may be secondarily stimulated by locally produced Ang II in the heart (or both). These possibilities must be resolved carefully by future studies. Of interest, is the possibility of dual RAS in the kidney, one at the level of the macula densa and the other at the distal tubular collecting duct.[66]

Other workers have suggested participation of other physiological adaptations or alterations produced by sodium loading: enhancement of adrenergic responses;[67] participation of the adrenergic system or catecholamines;[33,68,69] induction of other humoral or growth factors;[70] the direct effect of sodium *per se*[71] and, even more intriguing, by involvement of yet undescribed biological responses to sodium loading. Thus, the findings presented herein provide evidence that salt excess does far more than elevate arterial pressure or expand extracellular and intravascular volumes; it directly affects the target organs of hypertensive cardiovascular and renal disease by adversely promoting organ remodeling and other structural and functional impairments.

CONCLUSIONS

Salt loading has been said to have strongly positive cultural and social implications and other major negative effects on the health of man. Over the years, strong epidemiological evidence has incriminated salt loading as an important modality that increases blood pressure. In fact, many studies have demonstrated that the prevalence of hypertension in many societies is directly related to this daily dietary sodium or salt intake of those populations. It is disturbing to conclude with this rather simplistic thinking that sodium loading only increases arterial pressure. Moreover, arterial pressure is not uniformly increased in all individuals (whether normotensive or hypertensive) of those populations studied epidemiologically. In fact, an increased arterial pressure occurs in only a minority of individuals with essential hypertension in acculturated societies. However, to conclude that failure of salt loading to increase arterial pressure does not necessarily imply that the salt loading has no effect on the overall manifestations of hypertensive cardiovascular and renal disease. The results of the recent studies in our laboratory with the SHR (an excellent model of essential hypertension in men) strongly suggest that salt loading, while not always responsible for major increases in arterial pressure, does promote severe adverse structural and functional changes in the target organs of hypertensive disease. Thus, even in the absence of small further elevations in arterial pressure, salt excess may promote severe extracellular matrix and perivascular fibrotic structural changes in heart, aorta, and kidney which, in turn, are responsible for impaired function of those organs. Hence, the age-old mystery concerning the role of salt goes on.

REFERENCES

1. Kurlansky M. SALT: a world history. New York: Penguin Books, 2003.
2. Ambard L, Beaujard S. Causes de l'hypertension centenelle. Arch Gen Med 1904; 1: 520–533.
3. Dahl LK. Salt intake and salt need. N Engl J Med 1958; 258: 1152–1157, 1205–1208.
4. Meneely GR, Dahl LK. Electrolytes in hypertension: the effects of sodium chloride. Med Clin North Am 1961; 45: 271–283.
5. Elliot P, Stamler J, Nichols R et al. Intersalt revisited: further analysis of 24 hour sodium excretion and blood pressure within and across populations: Intersalt Cooperative Research Group. Br Med J 1996; 312: 1249–53.
6. Stamler J. The INTERSALT Study: background, methods, findings, and implications. Am J Clin Nutr 1997; 65 (Suppl): 626–42.
7. Frohlich ED, Varagic J. The role of sodium in hypertension is more complex than simply elevating arterial pressure. Nature Clinical Practice Cardiovascular Medicine 2004; 1: 24–30.
8. Trippodo NC, Frohlich ED. Controversies in cardiovascular research: similarities of genetic (spontaneous) hypertension. Man and rat. Circ Res 1981; 48: 309–19.
9. Trippodo NC, Walsh GM, Frohlich ED. Fluid volumes during onset of spontaneous hypertension in rats. Am J Physiol 1978; 235: H52–H55.
10. Frohlich ED, Apstein C, Chobanian AV et al. The heart in hypertension. N Engl J Med 1992; 327: 998–1008.
11. Frohlich ED. Risk mechanisms in hypertensive heart disease. Hypertension 1999; 34: 782–9.
12. Frohlich ED. Arthur C. Corcoran Memorial Lecture: Influence of nitric oxide and angiotensin II on renal involvement in hypertension. Hypertension 1997; 29: 188–93.
13. Pfeffer JM, Pfeffer MA, Frohlich ED. Validity of an indirect tail-cuff method for determining systolic arterial pressure in unanesthetized normotensive and spontaneously hypertensive rats. J Lab Clin Med 1971; 78: 957–62.
14. Pfeffer MA, Frohlich ED. Electromagnetic flowmetry in anesthetized rats. J Appl Physiol 1972; 33: 137–40.
15. Nishiyama K, Nishiyama A, Frohlich ED. Regional blood flow in normotensive and spontaneously hypertensive rats. Am J Physiol 1976; 230: 691–8.
16. Dunn FG, Pfeffer MA, Frohlich ED. ECG alterations with progressive left ventricular hypertrophy in spontaneous hypertension. Clin Exp Hypertens 1978; 1: 67–86.
17. Ishise S, Pegram BL, Yamamoto J, Kitamura Y, Frohlich ED. Reference sample microsphere method: cardiac output and blood flows in conscious rats. Am J Physiol 1980; 239: H443–H449.
18. Pfeffer MA, Pfeffer JM, Frohlich ED. Pumping ability of the hypertrophying left ventricle of the spontaneously hypertensive rat. Circ Res 1976; 38: 423–9.
19. Slama M, Susic D, Varagic J, Ahn J, Frohlich ED. Echocardiographic measurement of cardiac output in rats. Am J Physiol 2003; 284: H7692–H697.
20. Slama M, Ahn J, Varagic J, Susic D, Frohlich ED. Long-term left ventricular echocardiographic follow-up of SHR and WKY rats: effects of hypertension and age. Am J Physiol 2004; 286: H181–H185.
21. Ono H, Ono Y, Frohlich ED. Nitric oxide synthase inhibition in spontaneously hypertensive rats. Hypertension 1995; 26: 249–55.
22. Pfeffer MA, Pfeffer JM, Dunn FG, Nishiyama K, Tsuchiya M, Frohlich ED. Natural biventricular hypertrophy in normotensive rats. I. Physical and hemodynamic characteristics. Am J Physiol 1979; 236: H640–H643.

23. Sesoko S, Pegram BL, Kuwajima I, Frohlich ED. Hemodynamic studies in spontaneously hypertensive rats with congenital arteriovenous shunts. Am J Physiol 1982; 242: H722–H725.
24. Slama M, Susic D, Varagic J Frohlich ED. High rate of ventricular septal defect in WKY rats. Hypertension 2002; 40: 175–8.
25. Susic D, Nunez E, Hosoya K, Frohlich ED. Coronary hemodynamics in aging spontaneously hypertensive and normotensive Wistar-Kyoto rats. J Hypertens 1998; 16: 231–237.
26. Susic D, Varagic J, Frohlich ED. Abnormal renal vascular response to dipyridamole-induced vasodilation in SHR. Hypertension 2001; 37: 894–7.
27. Varagic J, Susic D, Frohlich ED. Clinidipine improves SHR coronary hemodynamics without altering cardiovascular mass and collagen. J Hypertens 2002; 20: 317–22.
28. Ono Y, Ono H, Matsuoka H, Fujimori T, Frohlich ED. Apoptosis, coronary arterial remodeling, and myocardial infarction after nitric oxide inhibition in SHR. Hypertension 1999; 34: 609–16.
29. Chrysant SG, Walsh GM, Frohlich ED. Hemodynamic changes induced by prolonged NaCl and DOCA administration in spontaneously hypertensive rats (SHR). Angiology 1978; 29: 303–9.
30. Chrysant SG, Walsh GM, Kern DC, Frohlich ED. Hemodynamic and metabolic evidence of salt sensitivity in spontaneously hypertensive rats. Kidney Int 1979; 15: 68–74.
31. Frohlich ED, Chien Y, Sesoko S, Pegram B. Relationship between dietary sodium intake, hemodynamics and cardiac mass in SHR and WKY rats. Am J Physiol 1993; 264: R30–R34.
32. Yu HC, Burrell LM, Black MJ et al. Salt induces myocardial and renal fibrosis in normotensive and hypertensive rats. Circulation 1998; 98: 2621–8.
33. Leenen FHH, Yuan B. Dietary-sodium-induced cardiac remodeling in spontaneously hypertensive rat versus Wistar-Kyoto rat. J Hypertens 1998; 16: 885–92.
34. Partovian C, Benetos A, Pommies JP, Mischler W, Safar ME. Effects of chronic high-salt diet on large artery structure: role of endogenous bradykinin. Am J Physiol 1998; 274: H1423–H1428.
35. Labat C, Lacolley P, Lamemi M, de Gasparo M, Safar ME, Benetos A. Effects of valsartan on mechanical properties of the carotid artery in spontaneously hypertensive rats under high-salt diet. Hypertension 2001; 38: 439–43.
36. Ahn J, Varagic J, Slama M, Susic D, Frohlich ED. Cardiac structural and functional responses to salt loading in SHR. Am J Physiol 2004; 287: H767–H772.
37. Varagic J, Ahn J, Susic D, Frohlich ED. Altered coronary hemodynamics and enhanced myocardial fibrosis are associated with biventricular dysfunction in salt-loaded SHR. Circulation 2004; 110 (Suppl): III-199 (abstract).
38. Pfeffer JM, Pfeffer MA, Fletcher PJ, Fishbein MC, Braunwald E. Favorable effects of therapy on cardiac performance in spontaneously hypertensive rats. Am J Physiol 1982; 242: H766–H784.
39. Pfeffer JM, Pfeffer MA, Mirsky I, Braunwald E. Regression of left ventricular hypertrophy and prevention of ventricular dysfunction by captopril in the spontaneously hypertensive rat. Proc Natl Acad Sci U S A 1982; 79: 3310–14.
40. Pfeffer JM, Pfeffer MA, Fletcher PJ, Braunwald E. Progressive ventricular remodeling in the rat with myocardial infarction. Am J Physiol 1991; 260: H1406–H1414.
41. Pfeffer MA, Braunwald E, Moyé LA et al., on behalf of the SAVE investigators. Effect of captopril on mortality and morbidity in patients with left ventricular dysfunction after myocardial infarction. Results of the Survival and Ventricuar Enlargement Trial. N Engl J Med 1992; 2327: 669–677.
42. Moyé LA, Pfeffer MA, Wun C-C et al., for the SAVE investigators. Uniformity of captopril benefit in the SAVE study: subgroup analysis. Eur Heart J 1994; 15 (Suppl B): 2–8.
43. Hunt SA, Baker DW, Chin MH et al. ACC/AHA guidelines for the evaluation and management of chronic heart failure in the adult. J Am Coll Cardiol 2001; 38: 2101–113.
44. The SOLVD Investigators. Effect of enalapril on survival in patients with reduced left ventricular ejection fractions and congestive heart failure. N Engl J Med 1991; 325: 293–301.
45. The Acute Infarction Ramipril Efficacy (AIRE) Study Investigators. Effects of ramipril on mortality and morbidity of survivors of acute myocardial infarction with clinical evidence of heart failure. Lancet 1993; 342: 821–8.
46. Kober L, Torp-Pedersen C, Carlsen JE et al., for Trandolapril Cardiac Evaluation (TRACE) Study Group. A clinical trial of the angiotensin-converting-enzyme inhibitor trandolapril in patients with left ventricular dysfunction after myocardial infarction. N Engl J Med 1995; 333: 1670–6.
47. Cohn JN, Tognoni G. A randomized trial of the angiotensin-receptor blocker valsartan in chronic heart failure. N Engl J Med 2001; 345: 1667–75.
48. Pfeffer MA, Swedberg K, Granger CB et al. CHARM Investigators and Committees. Effects of candesartan on mortality and morbidity in patients with chronic heart failure: the CHARM-Overall programme. Lancet 2003; 362: 759–66.
49. McMurray JJ, Ostergren J, Swedberg K et al. CHARM Investigators and Committees. Effects of candesartan in patients with chronic heart failure and reduced left-ventricular systolic function taking angiotensin-converting-enzyme inhibitors: the CHARM-Added trial. Lancet 2003; 362: 767–71.
50. Granger CB, McMurray JJ, Yusuf S et al. CHARM Investigators and Committees. Effects of candesartan in patients with chronic heart failure and reduced left ventricular systolic function intolerant to angiotensin-converting-enzyme inhibitors: the CHARM-Alternative trial. Lancet 2003; 362: 772–6.
51. Pitt B, Zannad F, Remme WJ et al., for Randomized Aldactone Evaluation Study Investigators. The effect of spiranolactone on morbidity and mortality in patients with severe heart failure. N Engl J Med 1999; 341: 709–17.
52. Brilla CG, Funck RC, Rupp H. Lisinopril-mediated regression of myocardial fibrosis in patients with hypertensive heart disease. Circulation 2000; 102: 1388–93.
53. Lopez B, Querejeta R, Varo N et al. Usefulness of serum carboxy-terminal propeptide of procollagen type I in assessment of the cardioreparative ability of antihypertensive treatment in hypertensive patients. Circulation 2001; 104: 286–91.
54. Varagic J. Salt loading: a paradigm for a local cardiac renin-angiotensin-aldosterone system. Monograph Springer; in press.
55. Kreutz R, Fernandez-Alfonso MS, Liu Y, Ganten D, Paul M. Induction of cardiac angiotensin I-converting enzyme with dietary NaC1-loading in genetically hypertensive and normotensive rats. J Mol Med 1995; 73: 243–8.
56. Zhao X, White R, Van Huysse J, Leenen FH. Cardiac hypertrophy and cardiac renin-angiotensin system in Dahl rats on high salt intake. J Hypertens 2000; 18: 1319–26.
57. Zhu Z, Zhu S, Wu Z et al. Effect of sodium on blood pressure, cardiac hypertrophy, and angiotensin receptor expression in rats. Am J Hypertens 2004; 17: 21–4.
58. Nishiyama A, Yoshizumi M, Rahman M et al. Effects of AT_1 receptor blockade on renal injury and mitogen-activated protein activity in Dahl salt-sensitive rats. Kidney Int 2004; 65: 972–81.
59. Kobori H, Nishiyama A, Abe Y, Navar GL. Enhancement of intrarenal angiotensinogen in Dahl salt-sensitive rats on high salt diet. Hypertension 2003; 41: 592–7.
60. Re RN. The implications of intracrine hormone action for physiology and medicine. Am J Physiol 2003; 284: H751–H757.
61. Re RN. Intracellular renin and the nature of intracrine enzymes. Hypertension 2003; 42: 117–22.

62. Re RN. Tissue renin angiotensin systems. Med Clin North Am 2004; 88: 19–38.
63. Re RN. Local renin-angiotensin-aldosterone systems and the pathogenesis and treatment of cardiovascular disease. Nature Clinical Practice. Cardiovascular Medicine 2004; 1: 42–7.
64. Slight SH, Joseph J, Ganjam VK, Weber KT. Extra-adrenal mineralocorticoids and cardiovascular tissue. J Mol Cell Cardiol 1999; 31: 1175–84.
65. Takeda Y, Yoneda T, Demura M, Furukawa K, Miyamori I, Mabuchi H. Effects of high sodium intake on cardiovascular aldosterone synthesis in stroke-prone spontaneously hypertensive rats. J Hypertens 2001; 19: 635–9.
66. Prieto-Carrasquero MC, Harrison-Bernard LM, Kobori H et al. Enhancement of collecting duct renin in angiotensin II-dependent hypertensive rats. Hypertension 2004; 44: 223–9.
67. Skraabal F, Aubock J, Hortnagl H. Low sodium/high potassium diet for prevention of hypertension: possible mechanisms of action. Lancet 1981; 2: 895–900.
68. Limas C, Limas CJ. Cardiac beta-adrenergic receptors in salt-dependent genetic hypertension. Hypertension 1985; 7: 760–6.
69. MacPhee AA, Blakesley HL, Graci KA, Frohlich ED, Cole FE. Altered cardiac beta-adrenoreceptors in spontaneously hypertensive rats receiving salt excess. Clin Sci 1980; 59: 169s-170s.
70. Feron O, Salomone S, Godfraind T. Influence of salt loading on the cardiac and renal preproendothelin-1 mRNA expression in stroke-prone spontaneously hypertensive rats. Biochem Biophys Res Commun 1995; 209: 161–6.
71. Gu J-W, Anand V, Shek EW et al. Sodium induces hypertrophy of cultured myocardial myoblasts and vascular smooth muscle cells. Hypertension 1998; 31: 1083–7.

37

The renal dopamine system: paracrine regulator of salt sensitivity and blood pressure

Robert M Carey, Robin A Felder and Pedro A Jose

INTRODUCTION

The kidney is the principal organ responsible for the long-term regulation of blood pressure (BP) through control of sodium (Na^+) excretion.[1] Sodium chloride balance and BP are the result of the interaction among many factors bearing on renal tubule Na^+ transport, such as the sympathetic nervous system, the renin-angiotensin system (RAS), the kallekrein-kinin system and the nitric oxide (NO)-cyclic GMP system. Many of these hormonal systems have been demonstrated to act in a cell-to-cell or paracrine/autacrine manner at the local tissue level without influence from the systemic circulation. Because the kidney is critical to long-term BP regulation, studies have focused on the abnormal transport of Na^+ in the pathophysiology of primary hypertension, wherein there is increased Na^+ reabsorption in the proximal tubule and the medullary thick ascending limb of Henle.[2,3] Two of the principal pathways of Na^+ transport control, the RAS and the dopaminergic system, are responsible for increasing or decreasing proximal tubule Na^+ reabsorption, respectively. These pathways may be augmented or retarded by the influence of other systems, such as NO, kinins, prostaglandins, and endothelin. This chapter will discuss the renal dopaminergic system, including the evidence for the autacrine and paracrine actions of dopamine (DA) formed within the kidney, their cell signaling pathways, the finding of a D_1 receptor coupling defect in hypertension and its relationship to G protein-related kinase 4, and the potential role of renal dopaminergic mechanisms in the pathogenesis of salt sensitivity and primary hypertension.

RENAL DA FORMATION AND SECRETION

The classic pathway for DA biosynthesis occurs in neurons, but in the kidney DA is synthesized independently of neruronal activity. Renal DA originates almost exclusively from proximal tubule cells (PTCs) as a result of the cellular uptake of filtered L-dihydroxyphenylalanine (L-DOPA) via a Na^+ transporter in the brush border membrane.[4] Within the proximal tubule cell, L-DOPA is rapidly decarboxylated to DA by the ubiquitous and constitutively expressed enzyme L-aromatic amino acid decarboxylase (L-AAAD), the activity of which is accelerated by high Na^+ intake and diminished by low Na^+ intake.[5] In the PTC, DA is not converted to norepinephrine, as it is in neurons, because renal tubules do not express DA-β-hydroxylase. Little is known concerning the mechanisms by which DA is stored in the PTC, but DA is catabolized within the kidney by catechol-o-methyl-transferase (COMT) and monamine oxidase (MAO) A.[6,7] DA is secreted from the PTC either across the apical surface into the lumen, the preferred pathway, or via the basolateral surface into the renal interstitium.[8] The basolateral outward transporter is dependent upon Na^+ and pH and is regulated developmentally, but little is known about apical DA secretion.[9] Once in the tubule lumen, DA acts as an autacrine/paracrine substance to regulate Na^+ transport in the PTC, the thick ascending limb of Henle, and the cortical collecting duct.

RENAL DA RECEPTORS

DA receptors are members of the G protein-coupled superfamily of hepta-helical cell membrane receptors.[10–13] At least five distinct DA receptors have been identified, which are divided pharmacologically into two subfamilies, the D_1-like and D_2-like receptor groups. Both of the cloned members of the D_1-like receptor group (D_1 and D_5) are coupled to the stimulating G protein $G_{s\alpha}$ and stimulate adenylyl cyclase. All three of the cloned D_2-like receptors (D_2, D_3 and D_4) are linked to the inhibitory G protein G_i/G_o and inhibit adenylyl cyclase. All of the central nervous system DA receptors are expressed in peripheral tissues, including the kidney.[11]

Both the D_1-like and D_2-like receptor families are expressed in the kidney at post-junctional neuron sites. Pre-junctional nerves are endowed with D_4 receptors.[14] In the renal arterioles, the D_2, D_3 and D_4 receptors are localized in the adventitia and the adventitia/media junction, while the D_1 and D_3 receptors are expressed in the media.[15–18] D_3 and D_4, but not D_1 and D_5, receptors are expressed in glomeruli.[15–18] PTCs express D_1, D_2, D_3 and D_4 receptors.[14–21] The medullary but not the cortical thick ascending limb of Henle expresses D_1, D_5 and D_3 receptors.[17,18,22] The cortical and medullary collecting ducts express D_1, D_5, D_3 and D_4 receptors.[15–18,23,24] The juxtaglomerular (JG) and macula densa cells express D_1 and D_3 receptors.[23,25] However, the D_1 receptor is not expressed in human JG cells.[20]

DA inhibits Na^+ transport at multiple sites along the nephron. Within each nephron segment, DA acts on several Na^+ transporters, including the Na^+-hydrogen exchangers (NHE-1 and NHE3), the Na^+-phosphate co-transporter (Na/Pi), the Na^+-bicarbonate exchanger (Na^+/HCO_3^-), the chloride-bicarbonate exchanger (Cl/HCO_3^-) and the basolateral membrane Na^+ pump ($Na^+/K^+ATPase$).[26–46] The action of DA to inhibit Na^+ transport is dependent upon the intracellular concentrations of Na^+ and calcium. DA's ability to inhibit $Na^+/K^+ATPase$ is augmented by intracellular Na^+ concentrations greater than 20 mM and calcium concentrations less than 120 mM.[28,34]

DA REGULATION OF RENAL Na^+ EXCRETION

The D_1-like receptor family plays a major role in the regulation of Na^+ excretion. Exogenous DA induces a large increase in Na^+ excretion that depends on both renal hemodynamic and tubular mechanisms. D_1-like receptor-mediated natriuresis was first demonstrated using the selective D_1-like receptor agonist fenoldopam, which decreases Na^+ reabsorption.[47–49] The natriuretic action of intrarenal DA was first observed following administration of the DA prodrug, gludopa, which is converted to DA in PTCs. Earlier studies employing pharmacological quantities of gludopa showed natriuresis via both hemodynamic and tubule effects.[50–52] However, the administration of physiological quantities of gludopa engendered natriuresis by only a tubule effect.[8]

During conditions of normal Na^+ balance, endogenous intrarenal DA is a major physiological regulator of Na^+ excretion. Indeed, about 50% of basal Na^+ excretion is controlled by DA.[53–55] Conclusive evidence that DA synthesized within the kidney controls Na^+ excretion by exclusively inhibiting tubule Na^+ reabsorption has been provided by the direct intrarenal administration of D_1-like receptor antagonist SCH-23390.[54] Thus, the autacrine/paracrine dopaminergic regulation of Na^+ excretion is *mediated by tubular but not by hemodynamic mechanisms.*[54] The regulation of Na^+ excretion by renal D_1-like receptors is depicted schematically in Figure 37.1.

Molecular evidence for a natriuretic action of endogenous renal DA also has been provided.[55] Selective reduction in the expression of D_1 receptors in the rat kidney using antisense oligodeoxynucleotides resulted in significant antinatriuresis during both normal and high Na^+ intake.[54]

EFECTIVE RENAL DA MECHANISMS IN HYPERTENSION

Increased renal PTC reabsorption of Na^+ is both an initiating and sustaining mechanism in human primary hypertension.[2,3] Subjects with hypertension have increased difficulty in excreting a salt load.[2,3] D_1-like receptors are critical to the maintenance of a normal BP because BP is increased when these receptors are absent (D_1 or D_5 receptor knockout mice) or chronically blocked with specific pharmacological antagonists.[55,56] However, a mutation in the coding region of the D_1 or D_5 receptor has not been found either in spontaneously hypertensive rats (SHRs) or in human essential hypertension.[57–60]

Disruption of the D_2 receptor also generates hypertension, but the increased BP is due to increased noradrenergic discharge and is not associated with antinatriuresis.[61] Disruption of the D_3 receptor gene produces a renin-angiotensin-dependent form of hypertension and the mice are not able to excrete a Na^+ load.[62] While the whole body, DA receptor knockout for the lifetime of the animal is informative,

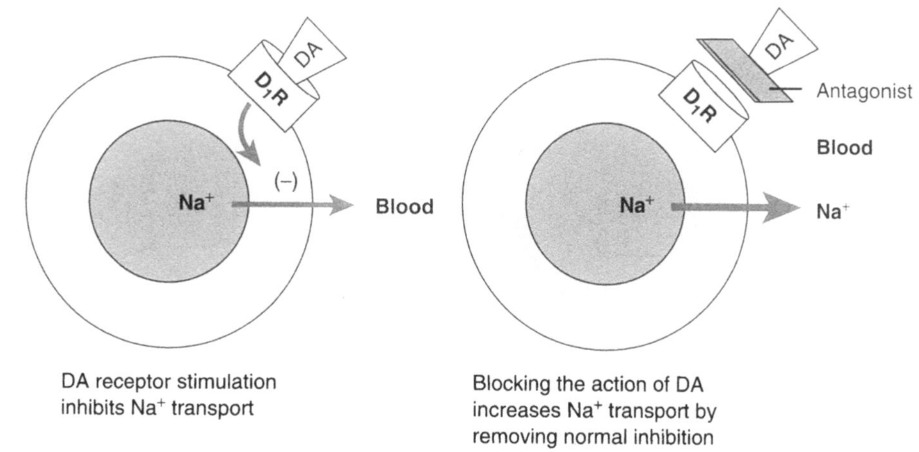
DA
D_1R
(−)
Na^+
Blood
DA receptor stimulation inhibits Na^+ transport
DA
D_1R
Antagonist
Blood
Na^+
Na^+
Blocking the action of DA increases Na^+ transport by removing normal inhibition

Figure 37.1 Schematic representation of the action of dopamine (DA) on Na^+ transport via D_1-like receptors on renal proximal tubule cells

compensatory physiological mechanisms alter the phenotype. A better method of determining the role of the individual DA receptors in hypertension would be to perform a selective renal receptor knockout in adulthood.

Two independent defects in the renal dopaminergic system have been described in hypertension: (1) a deficiency in renal DA production due to reduced PTC uptake and/or decarboxylation of L-DOPA[63,64] and (2) defective D_1-like receptor-G protein-coupling rendering the renal DA signal ineffective to inhibit Na^+ excretion.[65] Each of these defects results in increased renal Na^+ reabsorption and hypertension.

Reduced renal synthesis of DA may be involved in some human subjects with salt sensitivity and hypertension.[63,64,66,67] However, in many cases renal DA production is normal or increased in humans[68–70] and rodents.[71–73] Indeed, increasing renal DA production in SHR did not increase the ability of D_1-like receptor agonists to enhance Na^+ excretion to the level observed in WKY rats.[74]

The major dopaminergic defect in primary hypertension is the failure of D_1-like receptors to stimulate cAMP production in the renal PTC and the thick ascending limb of Henle in face of normal downstream signaling pathways, including G protein subunits, adenylyl cyclase, phospholipase C, Na^+/K^+/ATPase and NHE-3.[10,58,65,75–92] This defect, in which there is reduced D_1-like receptor-mediated inhibition of renal tubule Na^+ transport due to an uncoupling from its G protein/effector complex, has been demonstrated consistently in Dahl salt-sensitive rats, SHRs and humans with primary hypertension. The uncoupling of the renal D_1-like receptor from its second messenger cAMP is specific because other adenylyl cyclase-associated receptors function normally.[20,65,93–95] Importantly, the D_1-like receptor coupling defect in hypertension is organ-specific to the kidney and small intestinal transporting epithelia, and is not present in other organs such as the brain.[75] The defect is also nephron segment-specific because it is confined to the proximal tubule and thick ascending limb of Henle and is not present in the cortical collecting duct.[96] Thus, D_1-like receptor agonist administration to individuals with primary hypertension may induce natriuresis by activating D_1-like receptors in the cortical collecting duct.

The uncoupling of D_1-like receptors in primary hypertension is likely to be genetic in origin because the defect precedes onset of hypertension in a variety of rodent models of genetic hypertension.[38,65,75,81,97] Polymorphisms in the D_1 and D_5 receptors have been described in humans[98,99] and a polymorphism of the non-coding region of the D_1 receptor has been associated with hypertension in a single study.[98] No polymorphisms of the D_1 or D_5 receptors have been found in SHRs but D_5 receptor expression is decreased in the renal cortex of SHRs.[99]

In primary hypertension in humans, the uncoupling of the D_1-like receptor from its G protein/effector complex is due to activating mutations of G protein receptor kinase type 4 (GRK4).[76] Activating mutations of GRK4 hyper-phosphorylate the D_1 receptor causing the receptor to be internalized into the cytosol. Internalization occurs via arrestin and clathrin-coated pit-dependent mechanisms. Inside the cell, the receptor

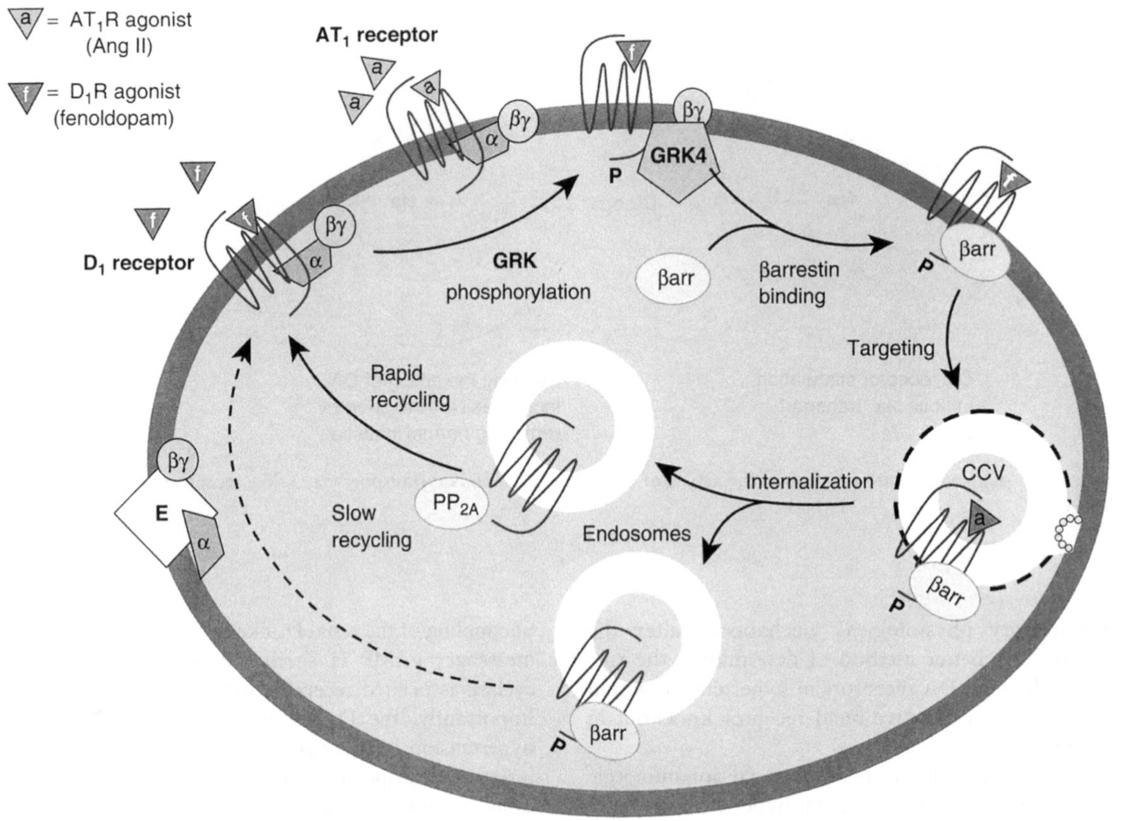

Figure 37.2 Schematic depiction of the interaction of dopamine D_1 receptors and angiotensin AT_1 receptors demonstrating the action of G-protein-related kinase-4 (GRK4) on D_1 receptor internalization and desensitization

can be sequestered in endosomes, where it can be degraded by lysosomes or proteosomes. Alternatively the receptor can be dephosphorylated by phosphatases to be recycled to the plasma membrane.[100,101] Dephosphorylation can also occur directly at the plasma membrane[102] and receptor desensitization also may be clathrin-independent.[92] The regulation of D_1 receptor phosphorylation, internalization, desensitization, and re-insertion into the plasma membrane of PTCs are shown schematically in Figure 37.2.

The uncoupling of the D_1-like receptor in primary human hypertension involves the D_1 receptor exclusively and specifically does not involve the D_5 receptor.[103,104] The renal tubule D_1 receptor is hyper-serine phosphorylated and is removed from the plasma membrane.[20,91] A reduction in GRK4 expression in the PTCs from hypertensive subjects normalizes the action of D_1-like receptor agonists to stimulate adenylyl cyclase to form cAMP.[76]

Although seven members of the GRK family exist, in the renal PTC GRK4 is the most important GRK in phosphorylating and desensitizing D_1 receptors.[104] GRK4 activity is increased in PTCs from hypertensive humans and molecular inhibition of GRK4 normalizes the ability of D_1 receptors to increase cAMP generation. In humans with primary hypertension, the desensitization of D_1 receptors is a result of three GRK4 variants (R65L, A142V, and A486V).[76] A schematic illustration of the human GRK4 gene and its described polmorphisms is presented in Figure 37.3. Although there are no differences in the GRK4 nucleotide sequence between WKY and SHR, GRK4 activity is increased in SHR kidneys and chronic renal interstitial infusion of antisense oligodeoxynucleotides reduces GRK4 expression and prevents the increase in BP with advancing age.[105] A schematic depiction of the renal effects of GRK4 over- and under-expression is shown in Figure 37.4. The D_1 receptor functional defect in

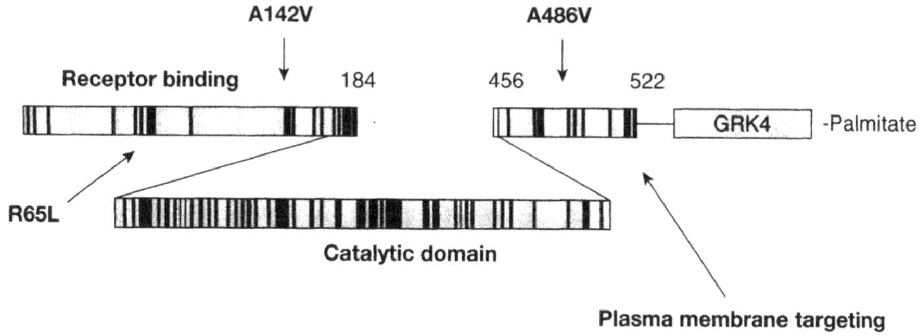

Figure 37.3 Structure of the gene for G-protein-related kinase-4 (GRK4) showing three single nucleotide polymorphisms in humans

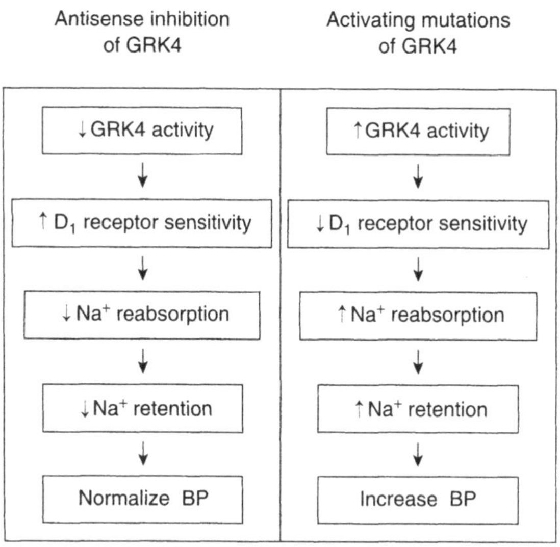

Figure 37.4 Schematic diagram showing the effects of G-protein-kinase-4 (GRK4) inhibition (left) and activation (right) on renal Na^+ transport and blood pressure

hypertension can be replicated by transfection of GRK4 gene variants into Chinese hamster ovary (CHO) cells and is reversed by prevention of GRK4 expression using antisense oligodeoxynucleotides. In mice, overexpression of GRK4 142V inhibits D_1-like receptor agonist-induced natriuresis and induces hypertension.[76] Whereas GRK4 142V transgenic mice have hypertension independently of Na^+ intake, GRK4 486V transgenic mice only become hypertensive following a salt load.[106]

GRK4 GENE POLYMORPHISM AND HYPERTENSION

Box 37.1 summarizes the relationship of GRK4 gene variants to primary hypertension in humans. Genetic association and linkage studies confirm that the GRK4 locus (4p16.3) is linked to hypertension.[107,108] GRK4 486V is associated with salt-sensitive hypertension in Caucasians.[109,110] In the Japanese population, the presence of all three GRK4 gene variants (65L, 142V, 486V) predicts the expression of salt-sensitive hypertension with 94% accuracy.[111] The ability to excrete a

Box 37.1 GRK4 and Hypertension

- GRK4 locus linked with essential hypertension
- GRK4 single nucleotide polymorphisms (SNPs) – associated with hypertension in Caucasian, Ghanian, Italian, and Japanese populations
- D1 receptor functional defect noted in renal proximal tubule and medullary thick ascending limb of Henle in hypertension:
  - replicated by GRK4 in cell lines (CHO, HEK cells)
  - rectified by the prevention of GRK4 expression
- GRK4 SNPs impair renal tubular function and produce hypertension in transgenic mice

Na^+ load in hypertensive subjects is directly proportional to the number of GRK4 alleles with a correlation coefficient (r^2) of 0.99, establishing a gene dose effect. Even in normotensive subjects, the presence of all three GRK4 gene variants reduces natriuretic responses to D_1-like receptor agonist administration. Therefore, GRK4 gene variants may be crucial to the pathogenesis of salt sensitivity.

In a Ghanian population, the hypertension prediction rate was 70% for subjects with gene variants in angiotensin converting enzyme (ACE) and GRK4 in combination.[112] More work needs to be performed on gene–gene interactions, particularly those of the renin-angiotensin and dopaminergic systems, in the pathophysiology of primary hypertension.

CONCLUSION

The renal dopaminergic system is crucial to the long-term control of Na^+ balance by acting primarily at the proximal tubule and the thick ascending limb of Henle to reduce Na^+ reabsorption. The renal dopaminergic system is an autacrine/paracrine system that is responsible for the maintenance of approximately 50% of baseline Na^+ excretion. While exogeneous DA engenders natriuresis by both hemodynamic and tubular mechanisms, endogenous renal DA does so only via tubule actions.

In primary hypertension, two renal dopaminergic defects have been described: decreased renal DA production and a defect in DA action via D_1-like receptors in the nephron. The major defect in hypertension is a D_1 receptor coupling defect in the proximal tubule and the thick ascending limb of Henle, whereby D_1-like receptor agonists do not stimulate adenylyl cyclase normally. This dopaminergic defect is due to the presence of activating mutations of GRK4, by which the D_1 receptor is hyper-phosphorylated, internalized, and desensitized. Initial studies indicate that GRK4 activating mutations predict clinical salt sensitivity with a high degree of accuracy. Studies also suggest that GRK4 polymorphisms may be important in the development of primary hypertension, possibly in the presence of gene variants of the RAS, such as the ACE I/D polymorphism. Future studies should target the interaction between the renal dopaminergic and renin-angiotensin systems, which hold great promise for understanding the pathophysiology of the complex polygeneic disorder of primary (essential) hypertension.

REFERENCES

1. Guyton AC, Coleman TG, Young DB, Lohmeier TE, DeClue JW. Salt balance and long-term blood pressure control. Annu Rev Med 1980; 31: 15–27.
2. Barba G, Cappuccio FP, Russo L, Stinga F, Iacone R, Strazzullo P. Renal function and blood pressure response to dietary salt restriction in normotensive men. Hypertension 1996; 27: 1160–4.
3. Chiolero A, Maillard M, Nussberger J, Brunner HR, Burnier M. Proximal sodium reabsorption: an independent determinant of blood pressure response to salt. Hypertension 2000; 36: 631–7.
4. Soares-da-Silva P, Fernandes MH, Pinto-do OP. Cell inward transport of L-DOPA and 3-O-methyl-L-DOPA in rat renal tubules. Br J Pharmacol 1994; 112: 611–15.
5. Seri I, Kone BC, Gullans SR, Aperia A, Brenner BM, Ballermann BJ. Influence of Na^+ intake on dopamine-induced inhibition of renal cortical Na(+)-K(+)-ATPase. Am J Physiol 1990; 258: F52–F60.
6. Eklof AC, Holtback U, Sundelof M, Chen S, Aperia A. Inhibition of COMT induces dopamine-dependent natriuresis and inhibition of proximal tubular Na^+, K^+-ATPase. Kidney Int 1997; 52: 742–7.
7. Guimaraes JT, Soares-da-Silva P. The activity of MAO A and B in rat renal cells and tubules. Life Sci 1998; 62: 727–37.
8. Wang ZQ, Siragy HM, Felder RA, Carey RM. Intrarenal dopamine production and distribution in the rat. Physiological control of sodium excretion. Hypertension 1997; 29: 228–34.
9. Soares-Da-Silva P, Serrao MP, Vieira-Coelho MA. Apical and basolateral uptake and intracellular fate of dopamine precursor L-dopa in LLC-PK1 cells. Am J Physiol 1998; 274: F243–F251.
10. Carey RM. Theodore Cooper Lecture: Renal dopamine system: paracrine regulator of sodium homeostasis and blood pressure. Hypertension 2001; 38: 297–302.
11. Jose PA, Eisner GM, Felder RA. Renal dopamine receptors in health and hypertension. Pharmacol Ther 1998; 80: 149–82.
12. Jose PA, Eisner GM, Felder RA. Dopamine receptor-coupling defect in hypertension. Curr Hypertens Rep 2002; 4: 237–44.
13. Jose PA, Eisner GM, Felder RA. Dopamine and the kidney: a role in. hypertension? Curr Opin Nephrol Hypertens 2003; 12: 189–94.
14. Ricci A, Marchal-Victorion S, Bronzetti E, Parini A, Amenta F, Tayebati SK. Dopamine D4 receptor expression in rat kidney: evidence for pre- and postjunctional localization. J Histochem Cytochem 2002; 50: 1091–6.
15. Amenta F, Barili P, Bronzetti E, Felici L, Mignini F, Ricci A. Localization of dopamine receptor subtypes in systemic arteries. Clin Exp Hypertens 2000; 22: 277–88.
16. O'Connell DP, Botkin SJ, Ramos SI et al. Localization of dopamine D1A receptor protein in rat kidneys. Am J Physiol 1995; 268: F1185–F1197.
17. O'Connell DP, Vaughan CJ, Aherne AM et al. Expression of the dopamine D3 receptor protein in the rat kidney. Hypertension 1998; 32: 886–95.
18. O'Connell DP, Aherne AM, Lane E, Felder RA, Carey RM. Detection of dopamine receptor D1A subtype-specific mRNA in rat kidney by in situ amplification. Am J Physiol 1998; 274: F232–F241.
19. Nash SR, Godinot N, Caron MG. Cloning and characterization of the opossum kidney cell D1 dopamine receptor: expression of identical D1A and D1B dopamine receptor mRNAs in opossum kidney and brain. Mol Pharmacol 1993; 44: 918–25.
20. Ozono R, O'Connell DP, Wang ZQ et al. Localization of the dopamine D1 receptor protein in the human heart and kidney. Hypertension 1997; 30: 725–9.

21. Yamaguchi I, Jose PA, Mouradian MM et al. Expression of dopamine D1A receptor gene in proximal tubule of rat kidneys. Am J Physiol 1993; 264: F280–F285.
22. Aoki Y, Albrecht FE, Bergman KR, Jose PA. Stimulation of Na(+)-K(+)-2Cl- cotransport in rat medullary thick ascending limb by dopamine. Am J Physiol 1996; 271: R1561–R1567.
23. Sanada H, Yao L, Jose PA, Carey RM, Felder RA. Dopamine D3 receptors in rat juxtaglomerular cells. Clin Exp Hypertens 1997; 19: 93–105.
24. Sun D, Wilborn TW, Schafer JA. Dopamine D4 receptor isoform mRNA and protein are expressed in the rat cortical collecting duct. Am J Physiol 1998; 275: F742–F751.
25. Yamaguchi I, Yao L, Sanada H et al. Dopamine D1A receptors and renin release in rat juxtaglomerular cells. Hypertension 1997; 29: 962–8.
26. Bertorello A, Aperia A. Na+-K+-ATPase is an effector protein for protein kinase C in renal proximal tubule cells. Am J Physiol 1989; 256: F370–F373.
27. Bertuccio CA, Cheng SX, Arrizurieta EE, Martin RS, Ibarra FR. Mechanisms of Na+-K+-ATPase phosphorylation by PKC in the medullary thick ascending limb of Henle in the rat. Pflugers Arch 2003; 447: 87–96.
28. Budu CE, Efendiev R, Cinelli AM, Bertorello AM, Pedemonte CH. Hormonal-dependent recruitment of Na+, K+-ATPase to the plasmalemma is mediated by PKC beta and modulated by [Na+]i. Br J Pharmacol 2002; 137: 1380–6.
29. Cheng SX, Aizman O, Nairn AC, Greengard P, Aperia A. [Ca2+]i determines the effects of protein kinases A and C on activity of rat renal Na+,K+-ATPase. J Physiol 1999; 518 (Pt 1): 37–46.
30. Chibalin AV, Zierath JR, Katz AI, Berggren PO, Bertorello AM. Phosphatidylinositol 3-kinase-mediated endocytosis of renal Na+, K+-ATPase alpha subunit in response to dopamine. Mol Biol Cell 1998; 9: 1209–20.
31. Debska-Slizien A, Ho P, Drangova R, Baines AD. Endogenous dopamine regulates phosphate reabsorption but not NaK-ATPase in spontaneously hypertensive rat kidneys. J Am Soc Nephrol 1994; 5: 1125–32.
32. de Toledo FG, Thompson MA, Bolliger C, Tyce GM, Dousa TP. Gamma-L-glutamyl-L-DOPA inhibits Na(+)-phosphate cotransport across renal brush border membranes and increases renal excretion of phosphate. Kidney Int 1999; 55: 1832–42.
33. Efendiev R, Bertorello AM, Pedemonte CH. PKC-beta and PKC-zeta mediate opposing effects on proximal tubule Na+, K+-ATPase activity. FEBS Lett 1999; 456: 45–8.
34. Efendiev R, Bertorello AM, Zandomeni R, Cinelli AR, Pedemonte CH. Agonist-dependent regulation of renal Na+, K+-ATPase activity is modulated by intracellular sodium concentration. J Biol Chem 2002; 277: 11489–96.
35. Gesek FA, Schoolwerth AC. Hormone responses of proximal Na(+)-H+ exchanger in spontaneously hypertensive rats. Am J Physiol 1991; 261: F526–F536.
36. Glahn RP, Onsgard MJ, Tyce GM, Chinnow SL, Knox FG, Dousa TP. Autocrine/paracrine regulation of renal Na(+)-phosphate cotransport by dopamine. Am J Physiol 1993; 264: F618–F622.
37. Gomes P, Soares-da-Silva P. Dopamine acutely decreases type 3 Na(+)/H(+) exchanger activity in renal OK cells through the activation of protein kinases A and C signalling cascades. Eur J Pharmacol 2004; 488: 51–9.
38. Horiuchi A, Albrecht FE, Eisner GM, Jose PA, Felder RA. Renal dopamine receptors and pre- and post-cAMP-mediated Na+ transport defect in spontaneously hypertensive rats. Am J Physiol 1992; 263: F1105–F1111.
39. Hu MC, Fan L, Crowder LA, Karim-Jimenez Z, Murer H, Moe OW. Dopamine acutely stimulates Na+/H+ exchanger (NHE3) endocytosis via clathrin-coated vesicles: dependence on protein kinase A-mediated NHE3 phosphorylation. J Biol Chem 2001; 276: 26906–15.
40. Hussain T, Lokhandwala MF. Altered arachidonic acid metabolism contributes to the failure of dopamine to inhibit Na+, K(+)-ATPase in kidney of spontaneously hypertensive rats. Clin Exp Hypertens 1996; 18: 963–74.
41. Ibarra F, Aperia A, Svensson LB, Eklof AC, Greengard P. Bidirectional regulation of Na+, K(+)-ATPase activity by dopamine and an alpha-adrenergic agonist. Proc Natl Acad Sci U S A 1993; 90: 21–4.
42. Khundmiri SJ, Lederer E. PTH and DA regulate Na-K ATPase through divergent pathways. Am J Physiol Renal Physiol 2002; 282: F512–F522.
43. Li XX, Albrecht FE, Robillard JE, Eisner GM, Jose PA. Gbeta regulation of Na/H exchanger-3 activity in rat renal proximal tubules during development. Am J Physiol Regul Integr Comp Physiol 2000; 278: R931–R936.
44. Nowicki S, Chen SL, Aizman O et al. 20-Hydroxyeicosa-tetraenoic acid (20 HETE) activates protein kinase C. Role in regulation of rat renal Na+, K+-ATPase. J Clin Invest 1997; 99: 1224–30.
45. Wiederkehr MR, Di Sole F, Collazo R et al. Characterization of acute inhibition of Na/H exchanger NHE-3 by dopamine in opossum kidney cells. Kidney Int 2001; 59: 197–209.
46. Xu J, Li XX, Albrecht FE, Hopfer U, Carey RM, Jose PA. Dopamine(1) receptor, G(salpha), and Na(+)-H(+) exchanger interactions in the kidney in hypertension. Hypertension 2000; 36: 395–9.
47. Hughes JM, Beck TR, Rose CE Jr, Carey RM. The effect of selective dopamine-1 receptor stimulation on renal and adrenal function in man. J Clin Endocrinol Metab 1988; 66: 518–25.
48. Hughes JM, Ragsdale NV, Felder RA, Chevalier RL, King B, Carey RM. Diuresis and natriuresis during continuous dopamine-1 receptor stimulation. Hypertension 1988; 11: I69–74.
49. Ragsdale NV, Lynd M, Chevalier RL, Felder RA, Peach MJ, Carey RM. Selective peripheral dopamine-1 receptor stimulation. Differential responses to sodium loading and depletion in humans. Hypertension 1990; 15: 914–21.
50. Worth DP, Harvey JN, Brown J, Lee MR. Gamma-L-glutamyl-L-dopa is a dopamine pro-drug, relatively specific for the kidney in normal subjects. Clin Sci (Lond) 1985; 69: 207–14.
51. Barthelmebs M, Caillette A, Ehrhardt JD, Velly J, Imbs JL. Metabolism and vascular effects of gamma-L-glutamyl-L-dopa on the isolated rat kidney. Kidney Int 1990; 37: 1414–22.
52. Wang ZQ, Way D, Shimizu K, Fong F, Trigg L, McGrath BP. Beneficial acute effects of selective modulation of renal dopamine system by gamma-L-glutamyl-L-dopa in rabbits with congestive heart failure. J Cardiovasc Pharmacol 1993; 21: 1004–11.
53. Pelayo JC, Fildes RD, Eisner GM, Jose PA. Effects of dopamine blockade on renal sodium excretion. Am J Physiol 1983; 245: F247–F253.
54. Siragy HM, Felder RA, Howell NL, Chevalier RL, Peach MJ, Carey RM. Evidence that intrarenal dopamine acts as a paracrine substance at the renal tubule. Am J Physiol 1989; 257: F469–F477.
55. Hegde SS, Jadhav AL, Lokhandwala MF. Role of kidney dopamine in the natriuretic response to volume expansion in rats. Hypertension 1989; 13: 828–34.
56. Yang Z, Sibley DR, Jose PA. D5 dopamine receptor knockout mice and hypertension. J Recept Signal Transduct Res 2004; 24: 149–64.
57. Albrecht FE, Xu J, Moe OW et al. Regulation of NHE3 activity by G protein subunits in renal brush-border membranes. Am J Physiol Regul Integr Comp Physiol 2000; 278: R1064–R1073.

58. Albrecht FE, Drago J, Felder RA et al. Role of the D1A dopamine receptor in the pathogenesis of genetic hypertension. J Clin Invest 1996; 97: 2283–8.
59. Kren V, Pravenec M, Lu S et al. Genetic isolation of a region of chromosome 8 that exerts major effects on blood pressure and cardiac mass in the spontaneously hypertensive rat. J Clin Invest 1997; 99: 577–81.
60. Matsumoto T, Ozono R, Sasaki N et al. Type 1A dopamine receptor expression in the heart is not altered in spontaneously hypertensive rats. Am J Hypertens 2000; 13: 673–7.
61. Li XX, Bek M, Asico LD et al. Adrenergic and endothelin B receptor-dependent hypertension in dopamine receptor type-2 knockout mice. Hypertension 2001; 38: 303–8.
62. Asico LD, Ladines C, Fuchs S et al. Disruption of the dopamine D3 receptor gene produces renin-dependent hypertension. J Clin Invest 1998; 102: 493–8.
63. Gill JR Jr, Gullner G, Lake CR, Lakatua DJ, Lan G. Plasma and urinary catecholamines in salt-sensitive idiopathic hypertension. Hypertension 1988; 11: 312–19.
64. Gill JR, Jr, Grossman E, Goldstein DS. High urinary dopa and low urinary dopamine-to-dopa ratio in salt-sensitive hypertension. Hypertension 1991; 18: 614–21.
65. Kinoshita S, Sidhu A, Felder RA. Defective dopamine-1 receptor adenylate cyclase coupling in the proximal convoluted tubule from the spontaneously hypertensive rat. J Clin Invest 1989; 84: 1849–56.
66. Clark BA, Rosa RM, Epstein FH, Young JB, Landsberg L. Altered dopaminergic responses in hypertension. Hypertension 1992; 19: 589–94.
67. Damasceno A, Santos A, Serrao P, Caupers P, Soares-da-Silva P, Polonia J. Deficiency of renal dopaminergic-dependent natriuretic response to acute sodium load in black salt-sensitive subjects in contrast to salt-resistant subjects. J Hypertens 1999; 17: 1995–2001.
68. Kuchel OG, Kuchel GA. Peripheral dopamine in pathophysiology of hypertension. Interaction with aging and lifestyle. Hypertension 1991; 18: 709–21.
69. Saito I, Itsuji S, Takeshita E et al. Increased urinary dopamine excretion in young patients with essential hypertension. Clin Exp Hypertens 1994; 16: 29–39.
70. Saito I, Takeshita E, Saruta T, Nagano S, Sekihara T. Urinary dopamine excretion in normotensive subjects with or without family history of hypertension. J Hypertens 1986; 4: 57–60.
71. Pinho MJ, Gomes P, Serrao MP, Bonifacio MJ, Soares-da-Silva P. Organ-specific overexpression of renal LAT2 and enhanced tubular L-DOPA uptake precede the onset of hypertension. Hypertension 2003; 42: 613–18.
72. Grossman E, Hoffman A, Tamrat M, Armando I, Keiser HR, Goldstein DS. Endogenous dopa and dopamine responses to dietary salt loading in salt-sensitive rats. J Hypertens 1991; 9: 259–63.
73. Racz K, Kuchel O, Buu NT, Tenneson S. Peripheral dopamine synthesis and metabolism in spontaneously hypertensive rats. Circ Res 1996; 57: 889–97.
74. Jose PA, Eisner GM, Drago J, Carey RM, Felder RA. Dopamine receptor signaling defects in spontaneous hypertension. Am J Hypertens 1996; 9: 400–5.
75. Felder RA, Kinoshita S, Ohbu K et al. Organ specificity of the dopamine1 receptor/adenylyl cyclase coupling defect in spontaneously hypertensive rats. Am J Physiol 1993; 264: R726–R732.
76. Felder RA, Sanada H, Xu J et al. G protein-coupled receptor kinase 4 gene variants in human essential hypertension. Proc Natl Acad Sci U S A 2002; 99: 3872–7.
77. Kunimi M, Seki G, Hara C et al. Dopamine inhibits renal Na+: HCO3- cotransporter in rabbits and normotensive rats but not in spontaneously hypertensive rats. Kidney Int 2000; 57: 534–43.
78. Li XX, Xu J, Zheng S et al. D(1) dopamine receptor regulation of NHE3 during development in spontaneously hypertensive rats. Am J Physiol Regul Integr Comp Physiol 2001; 280: R1650–R1656.
79. Nishi A, Eklof AC, Bertorello AM, Aperia A. Dopamine regulation of renal Na+, K(+)-ATPase activity is lacking in Dahl salt-sensitive rats. Hypertension 1993; 21: 767–71.
80. Ohbu K, Hendley ED, Yamaguchi I, Felder RA. Renal dopamine-1 receptors in hypertensive inbred rat strains with and without hyperactivity. Hypertension 1993; 21: 485–90.
81. Ohbu K, Kaskel FJ, Kinoshita S, Felder RA. Dopamine-1 receptors in the proximal convoluted tubule of Dahl rats: defective coupling to adenylate cyclase. Am J Physiol 1995; 268: R231–R235.
82. Pedrosa R, Gomes P, Zeng C, Hopfer U, Jose PA, Soares-da-Silva P. Dopamine D3 receptor-mediated inhibition of Na+/H+ exchanger activity in normotensive and spontaneously hypertensive rat proximal tubular epithelial cells. Br J Pharmacol 2004; 142: 1343–53.
83. Pedrosa R, Jose PA, Soares-da-Silva P. Defective D1-like receptor-mediated inhibition of the Cl-/HCO3- exchanger in immortalized SHR proximal tubular epithelial cells. Am J Physiol Renal Physiol 2004; 286: F1120–F1126.
84. Sidhu A, Vachvanichsanong P, Jose PA, Felder RA. Persistent defective coupling of dopamine-1 receptors to G proteins after solubilization from kidney proximal tubules of hypertensive rats. J Clin Invest 1992; 89: 789–93.
85. Uh M, White BH, Sidhu A. Alteration of association of agonist-activated renal D1(A) dopamine receptors with G proteins in proximal tubules of the spontaneously hypertensive rat. J Hypertens 1998; 16: 1307–13.
86. Chen C, Beach RE, Lokhandwala MF. Dopamine fails to inhibit renal tubular sodium pump in hypertensive rats. Hypertension 1993; 21: 364–72.
87. Hussain T, Lokhandwala MF. Renal dopamine DA1 receptor coupling with G(S) and G(q/11) proteins in spontaneously hypertensive rats. Am J Physiol 1997; 272: F339–F346.
88. Sela S, White BH, Uh M, Kimura K, Patel S, Sidhu A. Dysfunctional D1A receptor-G-protein coupling in proximal tubules of spontaneously hypertensive rats is not due to abnormal G-proteins. J Hypertens 1997; 15: 259–67.
89. Yao LP, Li XX, Yu PY, Xu J, Asico LD, Jose PA. Dopamine D1 receptor and protein kinase C isoforms in spontaneously hypertensive rats. Hypertension 1998; 32: 1049–53.
90. Yu P, Asico LD, Eisner GM, Hopfer U, Felder RA, Jose PA. Renal protein phosphatase 2A activity and spontaneous hypertension in rats. Hypertension 2000; 36: 1053–8.
91. Yu PY Hopfer U, Felder RA, Jose PA. Increased serine-phosphorylation of the D_1 receptor in renal proximal tubule cells in hypertension. Am J Hypertens 2000; 13: 12A–13A.
92. Yu P, Yang Z, Jones JE et al. D1 dopamine receptor signaling involves caveolin-2 in HEK-293 cells. Kidney Int 2004; 66: 2167–80.
93. Ladines CA, Zeng C, Asico LD et al. Impaired renal D(1)-like and D(2)-like dopamine receptor interaction in the spontaneously hypertensive rat. Am J Physiol Regul Integr Comp Physiol 2001; 281: R1071–R1078.
94. Michel MC, Jager S, Casto R et al. On the role of renal alpha-adrenergic receptors in spontaneously hypertensive rats. Hypertension 1992; 19: 365–70.

95. Onsgard-Meyer MJ, Berndt TJ, Khraibi AA, Knox FG. Phosphaturic effect of parathyroid hormone in the spontaneously hypertensive rat. Am J Physiol 1994; 267: R78–R83.
96. Ohbu K, Felder RA. Nephron specificity of dopamine receptor-adenylyl cyclase defect in spontaneous hypertension. Am J Physiol 1993; 264: F274–F279.
97. Lee MR. Dopamine, the kidney and essential hypertension studies with gludopa. Clin Exp Hypertens A 1987; 9: 977–86.
98. Cravchik A, Gejman PV. Functional analysis of the human D5 dopamine receptor missense and nonsense variants: differences in dopamine binding affinities. Pharmacogenetics 1999; 9: 199–206.
99. Sato M, Soma M, Nakayama T, Kanmatsuse K. Dopamine D1 receptor gene polymorphism is associated with essential hypertension. Hypertension 2000; 36: 183–6.
100. Wu KD, Chen YM, Chu TS et al. Dopaminergic modulation of aldosterone secretions on changes of sodium intake in aldosterone-producing adenoma. Am J Hypertens 2002; 15: 609–14.
101. Efendiev R, Yudowski GA, Zwiller J et al. Relevance of dopamine signals anchoring dynamin-2 to the plasma membrane during Na+, K+-ATPase endocytosis. J Biol Chem 2002; 277: 44108–14.
102. Gardner B, Liu ZF, Jiang D, Sibley DR. The role of phosphorylation/dephosphorylation in agonist-induced desensitization of D1 dopamine receptor function: evidence for a novel pathway for receptor dephosphorylation. Mol Pharmacol 2001; 59: 310–21.
103. Wang X GJ, Bengra C, Sasaki M et al. Human renal angiotensin type 1 receptor regulation by the D1 dopamine receptor. Am Heart Assoc 2003: 85.
104. Zeng C, Luo Y, Asico LD, Hopfer U, Eisner GM, Felder RA, Jose PA. Perturbation of D1 dopamine and AT_1 receptor interaction in spontaneously hypertensive rats. Hypertension 2003; 42: 787–92.
105. Sanada HYJ, Yoneda M, Hashimoto S et al. In vivo targeting of the renal G protein-coupled receptor kinase type 4 (GRK4) with antisense oligonucleotides induces natriuresis in spontaneously hypertensive rats. Circulation 2002; 106: II–234.
106. Wang ZAL, Felder RA, Robillard JE, Jose PA. Human GRK4y A142V variant produces hypertension in transgeneic mice. FASEB J 2004; 18: A353.
107. Allayee H, de Bruin TW, Michelle Dominguez K et al. Genome scan for blood pressure in Dutch dyslipidemic families reveals linkage to a locus on chromosome 4p. Hypertension 2001; 38: 773–8.
108. Casari G, Barlassina C, Cusi D et al. Association of the alpha-adducin locus with essential hypertension. Hypertension 1995; 25: 320–6.
109. Bengra C, Mifflin TE, Khripin Y et al. Genotyping of essential hypertension single-nucleotide polymorphisms by a homogeneous PCR method with universal energy transfer primers. Clin Chem 2002; 48: 2131–40.
110. Speirs HJ, Katyk K, Kumar NN, Benjafield AV, Wang WY, Morris BJ. Association of G-protein-coupled receptor kinase 4 haplotypes, but not HSD3B1 or PTP1B polymorphisms, with essential hypertension. J Hypertens 2004; 22: 931–6.
111. Williams SM, Addy JH, Phillips JA 3rd et al. Combinations of variations in multiple genes are associated with hypertension. Hypertension 2000; 36: 2–6.
112. Williams SM, Ritchie MD, Phillips JA 3rd et al. Identification of multilocus analysis of hypertension: a hierarchical approach. Hum Hered 2004; 57: 28–38.

38

Hypertension and diabetes mellitus

Brian S Pavey, John Palmer, James R Sowers and Craig S Stump

INTRODUCTION

The prevalence of diagnosed diabetes mellitus (DM) has increased dramatically over the past 40 years both in the United States and worldwide. In 1985, there were approximately 30 million people with DM worldwide.[1] By the year 1995, this number had increased to 135 million. According to current projections, the worldwide incidence of DM in 2025 is expected to increase by 42%, bringing the total number of patients affected by DM to over 300 million. In the United States, at least 18 million people have been diagnosed with DM, and another 5.9 million are unaware they have the disease. Based on national trends from 1980 to 1998, that number is expected to swell to 29 million by 2050.[2]

While the number of cases of diabetes increases, the burden it will place on society and our economy will increase as well. In 2002, the American Diabetes Association calculated the total economic cost of diabetes to be $132 billion, or one out of every ten health care dollars spent in the United States. Direct medical expenditures totaled $92 billion and comprised $23.2 billion for diabetes care, $24.6 billion for chronic diabetes-related complications, and $44.1 billion for excess prevalence of general medical conditions. Indirect costs resulting from lost work days, restricted activity days, mortality, and permanent disability due to DM totaled $40.8 billion.

Several factors are thought to be at the core of this explosion in the number of diagnosed patients. Increased awareness of the disease, better diagnostic testing, increased availability of health care, and advances in technology are likely contributors. The worldwide increase in the incidence of DM over the past 20 years has been seen in both industrialized and developing nations. While public health measures have seen a great number of advances in this period in regards to treating infectious diseases that once cut short the normal lifespan, it has ironically added to the global burden of DM by increasing average lifespan.[3]

This rapid advancement in technology has been seen in the shift in dietary and occupational habits. As human societies have progressed, our occupations and lifestyles have shifted from active to more sedentary forms. Despite our less active way of life, we still have the metabolism and physiology of Paleolithic hunter-gatherers, and our fundamental nutritional needs have probably changed little over the course of the past two million years.[4]

Though our dietary physiology has changed little through the course of time, the majority of people living in the United States today consume a diet considerably different in nutrient content from that of their genetic ancestors. For example, the US diet provides the highest amount of calories for the lowest cost worldwide, and the US is the leading nation in refined and processed food products.[4] Nevertheless, the explosion in obesity and related metabolic diseases is probably more related to decreases in physical activity than changes in food intake, since caloric consumption does not seem to have changed significantly over the past 40 years.[5] The ramifications of adopting a lifestyle of relative caloric excess to decreased physical activity is seen in ethnic groups residing within the US, who are from geographic regions with historically low rates of DM. In one study that compared seven ethnic groups residing in the US with their countries of origin, a consistent theme of elevated prevalence of type 2 DM mellitus was observed.[6] The commonalities in these diverse groups lie within their shared dietary habits, which include increased total calories and fat with decreased intake in fiber, superimposed on lifestyle, which requires less need to expend energy. Adding to this increased prevalence is the fact that some of these groups also have a genotype selected for survival in less plentiful environments.[7] While these ancestral genes allowed for increased storage of fat, providing a survival advantage during periods of famine, these genetic arrangements appear to be maladaptive by promoting obesity when food is always plentiful.[6,7] Moreover, the increased prevalence of obesity in these ethnic populations has contributed to the greater incidence of DM and hypertension.[8,9]

The end result of this shift in energy balance can be seen directly in the striking prevalence of overweight children and adults in the US. When comparing the years 1988–1994 and 1999–2000, the prevalence of overweight in the age groups of 2–5, 6–11, and 12–19 years increased from 7.2%, 11.3%, and 10.5% to 10.4%, 15.3%, and 15.5%, respectively.[10] Among adults during the same period, the prevalence of overweight increased from 55.9% to 64.5%, obesity from 22.9% to 30.5%, and extreme obesity from 2.9% to 4.7%.[11] And, while these trends are contributing to the diabetes epidemic in the US, they are not only limited to the US. As the other geographic regions continue to develop such that even subtle shifts in energy balance occur, the number of worldwide cases will increase. By 2050, India and China are projected to be the leading nations in DM prevalence,[12] and the incidence of type 2 DM has increased 1.5 times annually between 1975 and 1990 in Japanese schoolchildren.[13]

Hypertension and diabetes

Currently, at least 18 million people in the United States have been diagnosed with DM, and an additional 60 million people are known to have hypertension. Both of these diseases have been proven to be important predisposing risk factors for the development of cardiovascular disease (CVD) and renal disease.[14] Hypertension frequently coexists with DM, as the prevalence of hypertension in patients with type 2 DM is up to three times greater than in age- and sex-matched patients without DM.[8,15,16] Likewise, those patients with documented hypertension are 2.5 times more prone to have DM than are their normotensive counterparts.[17] It is the combination of the two diseases that, when coexisting together, acts as a powerful promoter in the development of CVD and renal disease.[18]

When hypertension coexists with DM, the risk for CVD is increased by 75%, which further contributes to the overall morbidity and mortality of an already high-risk population.[18] Even relatively small increases in blood pressure (BP) are detrimental in the diabetic population, as a 10 mm Hg increase in systolic blood pressure (SBP) leads to a 15% increase in death related to DM, 11% increase in myocardial infarctions, 19% increase in strokes, and 12% increase in episodes of congestive heart failure.[15,19] In addition, when these two conditions coexist, the risk for developing end-stage renal disease is increased five to six times compared with those patients who are hypertensive without DM.[15]

Several factors are seen in the development of hypertension in the diabetic population. Increasing age, obesity, and the onset of renal disease are all factors that increase the likelihood of the development of hypertension in patients with DM.[8,15,16] Generally, hypertension in type 2 diabetic persons clusters with other components of the metabolic syndrome, such as microalbuminuria, central obesity, insulin resistance, dyslipidemia, hypercoagulation, increased inflammation, and left ventricular hypertrophy.[18] It is the combination of all these detrimental conditions that ultimately results in the development of CVD, which is the major cause of premature mortality in patients with type 2 DM.[15]

Cardiometabolic syndrome

The National Cholesterol Education Program (NCEP) Adult Treatment Panel III (ATP III) defines the metabolic syndrome as the presence of any three or more of the following: BP ≥130/85 mm Hg, waist circumference >40 inches in men and >35 inches in women, triglycerides ≥150 mg/dl, HDL <40 mg/dl in men and <50 mg/dl in women, fasting glucose ≥110 mg/dl. The American Diabetes Association (ADA) has recently lowered the impaired fasting glucose threshold from 110 mg/dl to 100 mg/dl. While these groups have minor variations in the definition, it is not by coincidence that both impaired glucose tolerance and elevated BP are listed as contributing factors.

This syndrome comprises a group of risk factors that not only warn of future DM, but also warn of impending CVD (Box 38.1). Hence, it is our preference to use the term cardiometabolic syndrome. Currently, the overall prevalence of the metabolic syndrome in the US is 26.7% in men and women older than 20 years of age, up from 23.1% in NHANES III (1988–1994). Furthermore, prevalence increases to 31.7% for ages 40–59 years and 42.5% for ages greater than 60.[20] Obesity, specifically central obesity, seems to be the common causative factor in the individual components of the metabolic syndrome. Obesity, when conveyed as body mass index (BMI), is associated with a linear increase in SBP, diastolic blood pressure (DBP), and pulse pressure.[21] In addition, central obesity as measured by waist circumference is a risk factor for type 2 DM as well as CVD.[22] Lastly, triglyceride levels are generally higher in obese persons than in lean persons.[23]

Insulin resistance is likely a primary contributor in the pathophysiology of the cardiometabolic syndrome.[21] Patients with hypertension have a high prevalence of

Box 38.1 Cardiometabolic syndrome manifestations associated with increased risk for cardiovascular and renal disease

- Insulin resistance/hyperinsulinemia
- Impaired glucose tolerance
- Visceral obesity
- Microalbuminuria
- Low serum HDL-cholesterol levels
- High serum triglyceride levels
- Increased serum apolipoprotein B levels
- Small, dense LDL-cholesterol particles
- Increased PAI/PA ratio
- Increased serum fibrinogen levels
- Increased serum C-reactive protein
- Increased production of TNF-α
- Increased production of interleukin-6
- Increased blood viscosity
- Increased systolic and pulse pressure
- Left ventricular hypertrophy
- Premature atherosclerosis
- Enhanced tissue RAAS
- Absent nocturnal dipping of blood pressure and heart rate
- Salt sensitivity
- Endothelial dysfunction

HDL, high-density lipoprotein; LDL, low-density lipoprotein; PAI/PA, plasminogen activator inhibitor/plasminogen activator; TNF-α, tumor necrosis factor-α; RAAS, renin-angiotensin-aldosterone system.

Box 38.2 Mechanisms of insulin resistance in hypertension

Decreased skeletal muscle non-oxidative glucose metabolism

- Post insulin receptor defect
  - Decreased signaling through PI3K-Akt pathway
  - Decreased GLUT-4 content and translocation to the plasma membrane
  - Decreased glycogen synthase activity
  - Increased oxidative stress
  - Increased intramyocellular lipid
- Altered skeletal muscle fiber type
  - Decreased insulin-sensitive slow-twitch skeletal muscle fibers
  - Decreased mitochondrial content

Decreased delivery of insulin and glucose to skeletal muscle

- Increased reactive oxygen species
- Reduced generation of nitric oxide
- Vascular rarefaction
- Vascular hypertrophy
- Increased vasoconstriction

PI3K, phophatidylinositol 3-kinase; Akt, protein kinase B; GLUT, glucose transporter.

insulin resistance,[24] and are at a greater risk of developing type 2 DM.[25] Factors contributing to the development of insulin resistance in patients with hypertension include altered composition of skeletal muscle, decreased blood flow and delivery of insulin to skeletal muscle, and post insulin receptor abnormalities in metabolic signaling (Box 38.2). Aging and a sedentary lifestyle predispose to decreased slow-twitch insulin-sensitive fibers as increased fat deposition in skeletal muscle.[24]

The CVD risk factors that comprise the metabolic syndrome have been documented in clinical trials as causative factors in mediating CVD events.[26] The Framingham Heart Study demonstrated the synergistic action of CVD risk factors in predicting poor CVD morbidity and mortality endpoints.[27] Even with mild impaired glucose tolerance, CVD mortality is significantly increased when the intolerance coexists with moderate hypertension (SBP 140–149).[28]

Cardiovascular end points

Both hypertension and DM greatly increase the risk of CVD events. The age-adjusted relative risk of death due to CVD events in DM is threefold higher than that of the general population.[15,29] In addition, hypertension substantially increases the risks of coronary heart disease, stroke, nephropathy, and retinopathy.[18]

Sudden cardiac death (SCD), defined as death occurring suddenly or unexpectedly within 1 hour of onset of symptoms, is a major problem in industrialized nations, and has been found to be more prevalent in the diabetic population.[30] In addition, hypertension, obesity, and dyslipidemia, all components of the cardiometabolic syndrome, are also predictive of SCD.[31,32] The role DM plays in SCD is multifactorial. This population is more prone to macrovascular complications in the form of coronary atherosclerosis and thrombosis, microvascular disease, especially in the form of cardiac autonomic neuropathy, affecting the electrical conduction system of the heart, and predisposing the patient to premature death by enhancing fatal ventricular arrhythmias.[33]

CVD, including stroke and congestive heart failure, accounts for up to 80% of excess deaths in people with type 2 DM.[34] Middle-aged individuals with type 2 DM who have yet to develop CVD events have been reported to have the same risk of fatal or nonfatal myocardial infarction as those without DM who have already experienced CVD events.[35] The major risk factors for CVD in patients with type 2 DM are hypertension, dyslipidemia, and smoking,[36–43] but the presence of type 2 DM markedly accentuates these risk factors.[39–43]

These findings have been substantiated in multiple clinical trials. The Multiple Risk Factor Intervention Trial (MRFIT) followed more than 5000 patients with DM and 350 000 nondiabetic people for 12 years to evaluate the impact of various CVD risk factors. The study confirmed that hypertension, elevated cholesterol levels, and cigarette smoking were independent CVD risk factors in men with DM and had greater impact than in nondiabetic patients.[39] In the Hypertension Optimal Treatment (HOT) Trial, the diabetic subgroup that was studied was found to have a decrease in major CVD events by 51% in those randomized to a diastolic BP of <80 mm Hg compared to a DBP goal of <90 mm Hg.[44] In the United Kingdom Prospective Diabetes Study (UKPDS), the subset of patients that were assigned to tighter BP control (144/82 mm Hg), were found to have significant reductions in DM-related end points, in death-related end points due to DM, in strokes, and in microvascular end points.[43]

Hypertension appears to play an important role in the development and progression of renal damage in type 2 DM,[45,46] and diabetic nephropathy has become the leading cause of ESRD in the United States.[47,48] Moreover, if current trends continue, approximately 175 000 new cases of ESRD will be diagnosed in 2010, at a cost expected to exceed $28 billion by 2010.[49]

PATHOPHYSIOLOGY OF HYPERTENSION IN THE DIABETIC PATIENT

Individuals with type 2 DM are 2.5 times more likely to develop hypertension than normotensive individuals[50] and hypertension is more common in persons with type 2 DM.[51] These epidemiologic reports provide evidence for a common genetic factor or mechanism between DM and hypertension.

Research into the molecular and physiologic mechanisms in DM has also yielded clues to the pathophysiology of hypertension in diabetic patients. Insulin resistance, increased cytokine and reactive oxygen species (ROS) production resulting in endothelial dysfunction, increased tissue renin-angiotensin-aldosterone system (RAAS), and increased sympathetic discharge have all been implicated in promoting elevated BP in the diabetic patient (Figure 38.1).

Insulin resistance

It has been well documented that resistance to the action of insulin is related to elevated BP. Clinical studies have shown that improved insulin sensitivity lowers BP.[52,53] Multiple mechanisms have been proposed to account for the relationship between insulin resistance and hypertension in a variety of tissues.[24]

When patients with untreated essential hypertension were compared with normotensive controls, fasting and postprandial insulin levels were found to be higher in the hypertensive group regardless of patient BMI. Additionally, there was a direct correlation between plasma insulin concentrations and BP.[18] In rat studies, insulin resistance and hyperinsulinemia exist in rats with genetic hypertension[54,55] but not in rats with secondary hypertension.[56] Insulin resistance and hyperinsulinemia have been documented in normotensive offspring of hypertensive parents.[57,58] These studies suggest that there is a common genetic linkage between essential hypertension and insulin resistance.

Insulin resistance and the resultant hyperinsulinemia have several mechanisms that contribute to elevated BP. Hyperinsulinemia enhances sympathetic nervous system activity that can activate the tissue RAAS.[59] Moreover, insulin directly stimulates renal absorption of sodium in the proximal tubule.[60] Both of these mechanisms lead to volume expansion, increased cardiac output, and elevated BP. Another mechanism is the up-regulation of angiotensin type 1 receptors (AT_1Rs) by post-transcriptional mechanisms enhancing the vasoconstrictive and volume-expanding actions of the RAAS.[61] Interestingly, there is also evidence that angiotensin II (Ang II) interferes with the insulin-stimulated glucose transport and GLUT-4 glucose transporter content in skeletal muscle.[62,63] This further contributes to hyperglycemia and hyperinsulinemia and potentiates the mechanisms outlined above.[18]

Endothelial dysfunction

Endothelial dysfunction has long been identified as an important component in the development of pathology in those with DM. The integrity of the endothelium is needed to maintain the balance between vasodilation and vasoconstriction, and to preserve a sufficient vascular diameter for the satisfactory perfusion of the cardiovascular system.[64] Both insulin resistance and chronic hyperglycemia have been shown to cause endothelial dysfunction, which contributes to subsequent development of hypertension and nephropathy.[60]

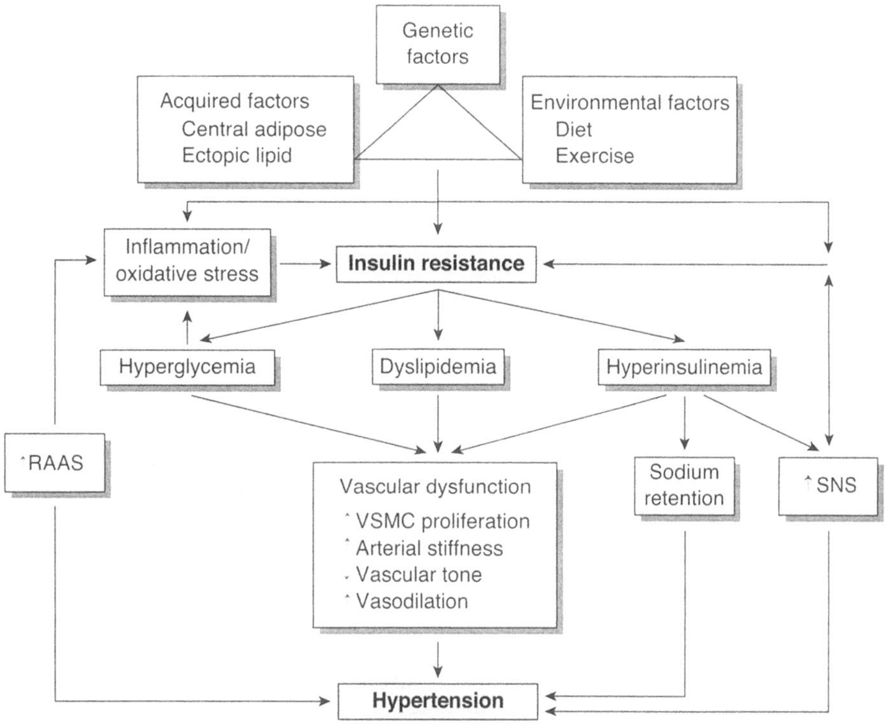

Figure 38.1 Summary of putative pathophysiologic mechanisms in the development of hypertension in diabetes mellitus. RAAS, renin-angiotensin-aldosterone system; SNS, sympathetic nervous system; VSMC, vascular smooth muscle cells

Several factors are present in the normal functioning endothelium that act to promote vasodilation. Nitric oxide (NO) is produced in response to a variety of stimuli by the oxidation of L-arginine by the NADPH-dependent enzyme, NO synthase (NOS).[65] Its production leads to physiological vasodilation and the relaxation of smooth muscle cells. NO acts on smooth muscle cells by stimulating guanylate cyclase and by increasing the intracellular concentration of cyclic guanosine monophosphate (cGMP). The cGMP decreases the intracellular Ca^{2+} concentration causing vascular relaxation. In addition to its vasodilating properties, NO further aids in the prevention of atherogenic phenomena as it inhibits platelet aggregation by a mechanism dependent on cGMP, and also inhibits the proliferation of smooth muscle cells.[66]

In the normally functioning endothelium, insulin stimulates NO production through the phosphatidylinositol 3-kinase (PI3K) and protein kinase B (Akt) pathways,[67] while it stimulates migration and growth of vascular smooth muscle cells (VSMCs) via the mitogen-activated protein kinase (MAPK) pathway.[68] In the diabetic patient, there is a selective defect in the PI3K/Akt pathway, which may ultimately result in the development of hypertension, left ventricular hypertrophy, and glomerulosclerosis.[24]

Superoxide production by vascular tissues and its affect on NO also plays a role in vascular pathophysiology[69] and has been shown to be elevated during episodes of hyperglycemia.[70] Superoxide is a highly reactive compound produced when oxygen is reduced by a single electron, and may be generated during the normal catalytic function of a number of enzymes. Potential vascular sources in humans include NADPH-dependent oxidases,[71,72] xanthine oxidase,[73] lipoxygenase, mitochondrial oxidases, and NO synthases.[74] When superoxide is produced, it reacts rapidly with NO, reducing NO bioactivity.[75] Increased ROS also decreases NOS activity in endothelial cells, resulting in decreased production of NO.[76] In addition to its effects on NO, increased ROS causes further endothelial damage through proatherogenic actions on smooth muscle cell proliferation, and through the recruitment of inflammatory modulators.[77]

To further complicate vascular function, superoxide dismutase (SOD), an antioxidant enzyme that acts to seek out potentially harmful free radicals of oxygen, is suppressed in hypertension associated with DM. Moreover, plasma levels of asymmetric dimethylarginine (ADMA), an endogenous competitive inhibitor of NOS, are significantly increased in hypertension associated with DM.[78] Endothelial dysfunction occurs as a result of this combination of increased production of free radicals, with the decreased ability for their removal, creating an environment of increased oxidative stress that ultimately contributes to the development of hypertension.

Several other mechanisms of endothelial dysfunction in DM have also been proposed, and all seem to center around hyperglycemia. One such proposal focuses on protein kinase C (PKC). In the face of hyperglycemia, there is increased production of diacylglycerol (DAG) through the process of glycolysis, which in turn increases the level of PKC activation. PKC activity leads to reduced levels of NOS, as well as producing vasoconstrictive substances such as endothelin-1 (ET-1).[79] In addition, PKC increases the production of growth factors by the endothelium, such as vascular endothelial growth factor (VEGF), epidermal growth factor (EGF), and transforming growth factor (TGF) as well, which contributes to the migration and proliferation of VSMCs.[80]

Another proposal has focused on hyperglycemia-induced formation of nonenzymatic advanced glycosylation products (AGEs) that tend to accumulate in vascular tissue.[81] These products act to neutralize NO and increase the susceptibility of LDL (low-denisty lipoprotein) to oxidation. The binding of the AGEs to their receptors (RAGE), also activates the receptors for the cytokines interleukin-1 (IL-1), tumor necrosis factor-α (TNF-α) and growth factors, leading to the migration and proliferation of VSMCs.[82]

Lastly, increased activity of the polyol pathway resulting in the formation of sorbitol has been studied as well. In this pathway, glucose is reduced into sorbitol by aldose reductase, leading to depletion of NADPH. NADPH co-enzyme is essential for the regeneration of antioxidant molecules.[82] Reduced NADPH is required for the functioning of many endothelial enzymes, including eNOS and cytochrome P450, as well as for the antioxidant activity of glutathione reductase. Alternatively, a high polyol pathway flux consumes large quantities of ATP and may thus compromise the energy supply required for endothelium-derived relaxation factor (EDRF) production.[83]

Increased sympathetic nervous system activity

Increased sympathetic nervous system (SNS) activity has been implicated in hypertension in the diabetic patient. Hyperleptinemia and hyperinsulinemia have been proposed to play a role in this increased SNS activity.[84]

Leptin is the product of the 'obese' gene and is primarily produced by adipose tissue. It functions to regulate energy balance by stimulating thermogenesis and decreasing appetite. While people with type 2 DM are resistant to this action of leptin and develop hyperleptinemia, leptin's ability to activate the SNS appears to be preserved.[84] Leptin has been reported to act in the hypothalamus to increase sympathetic discharge and increase BP.[85] Leptin has also been reported to increase SNS activity in brown adipose tissue, hindlimbs, and kidneys of rats.[86] Furthermore, leptin infusion into carotid arteries of rats increases heart rate and BP.[87] Leptin overexpression in transgenic mice increased arterial pressure that was attenuated by SNS blockade.[25] Studies in humans have demonstrated that increased plasma leptin in hypertensive individuals is associated with increased heart rate, elevated plasma renin activity, angiotensinogen, Ang II, and aldosterone levels, and hyperinsulinemia.[60,88–91]

Hyperinsulinemia may also contribute to hypertension, especially in obese patients who exhibit increased muscle SNS activity.[92] Hyperinsulinemia in a rat model produced a PI3K and mitogen-activated protein kinase (MAP kinase)-mediated increase in sympathetic outflow to the hindlimb, brown adipose tissue, adrenal gland, and kidney.[93]

Whether initiated by hyperinsulinemia, hyperleptinemia or other mechanism, increased SNS discharge leads to increased sodium and water retention by the kidney. Increased SNS activity appears to affect BP through other mechanisms as well. Specifically, it increases endothelin-1, decreases NO and increases Ang II and aldosterone, which all contribute to vasoconstriction.[84]

RAAS

Hypertension has been reported as a risk factor for developing type 2 DM.[17] Two recent large studies have shown that therapy with angiotensin converting enzyme (ACE) inhibitors decreases the progression to type 2 DM in high-risk patients. In the Captopril Prevention Project (CAPPP) and Heart Outcomes Prevention Evaluation (HOPE) randomized trials, subjects taking ACE inhibitors were less likely to progress to type 2 DM mellitus than control subjects.[94,95] Thus, these studies suggest that ACE inhibitors may play a role in increasing sensitivity to insulin.[96]

The RAAS is typically activated by a decrease in BP and/or decreased renal perfusion. The kidney responds by releasing renin from juxtoglomerular cells. However, renin release is also stimulated by β-agonists

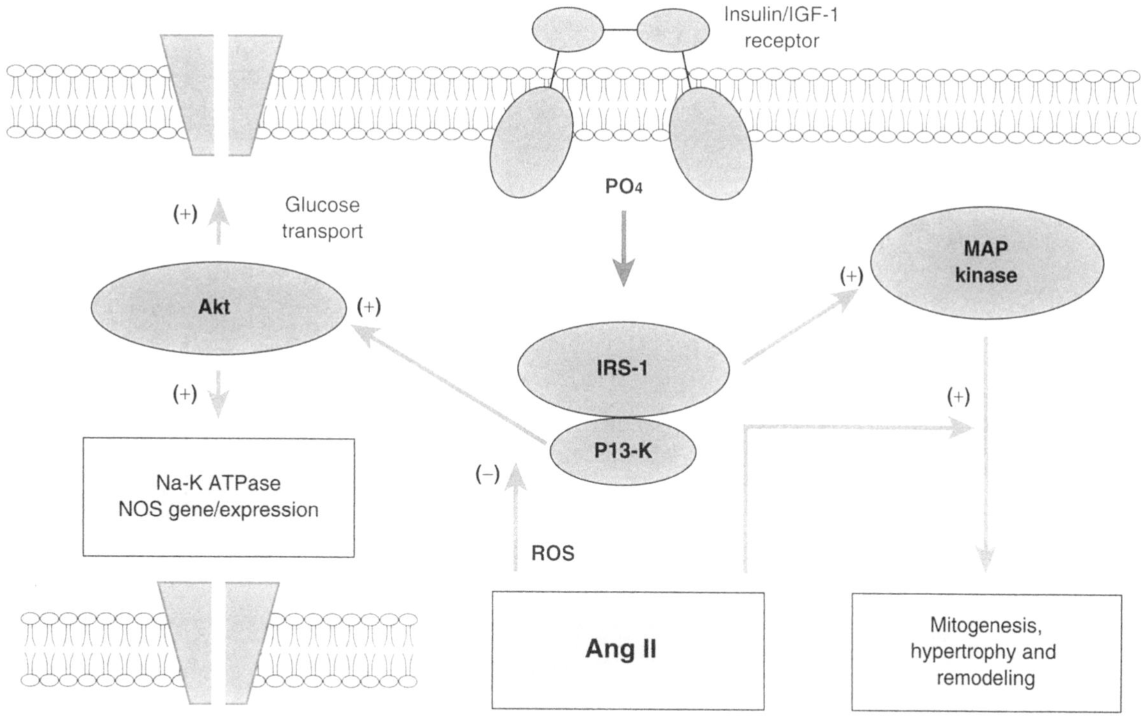

Figure 38.2 Insulin and insulin-like growth factor-1 (IGF-1) effects on cardiovascular tissue as well as conventional insulin-sensitive tissues such as skeletal muscle. Many of the metabolic and vasomotor effects of insulin and IGF-1 are mediated by activation of the phosphatidylinositol 3-kinase (PI3K) and downstream signaling pathways, including protein kinase B (Akt)

and activation of the SNS. In plasma, renin catalyzes the conversion of angiotensinogen to Ang I, a precursor to the more biologically active Ang II. ACE and other enzymes (chymase) cleave Ang I to form Ang II primarily in liver and kidney. Ang II has three specific functions. First, it stimulates zona glomerulosa cells of the adrenal gland to synthesize and secrete aldosterone into the blood. Aldosterone causes sodium reabsorption at the principal cells of the distal tubules of the nephron. This causes an increased extracellular volume and volume expansion leading to increased BP. Second, Ang II acts on the AT_1R at the arterioles to cause vasoconstriction. Third, Ang II can directly stimulate Na^+-H^+ exchange in the proximal tubule of the nephron yielding an increase in the reabsorption sodium. This again results in volume expansion.

Ang II appears to play a role in insulin resistance and may provide an explanation for the relationship between DM and hypertension (Figure 38.2). Ang II has been shown to inhibit the PI3K system. PI3K is activated by insulin binding to the insulin receptor which in turn stimulates NOS-mediated NO production and vascular relaxation. Insulin activates the PI3K system in skeletal muscle, adipose and myocardial tissues and initiates translocation of GLUT-4 glucose receptor to the cell membrane.[21] Thus, Ang II likely contributes to higher postprandial and fasting insulin levels by inhibiting glucose transport into skeletal muscle and contributes to hypertension by suppressing NO production in vascular tissue.[56]

Insulin and insulin-like growth factor-1 (IGF-1) promote vasodilation, in part, by increased production of NO. This vasodilation is mediated by binding to the insulin receptor, which initiates a cascade of cellular signaling resulting in activation of PI3K-dependent Akt. Activated Akt, in turn, phosphorylates endothelial NOS yielding an increased production of the vasodilator NO.[24] Additionally, insulin and IGF-1 cause a decrease in intracellular calcium concentrations in VSMCs by stimulating the Na^+-K^+-ATPase pump and inhibiting membrane-bound and intracellular organelle Ca^{2+} channels.[25] Another mechanism responsible for the vascular relaxation by insulin and IGF is Ca^{2+}-myosin light chain desensitization.[18]

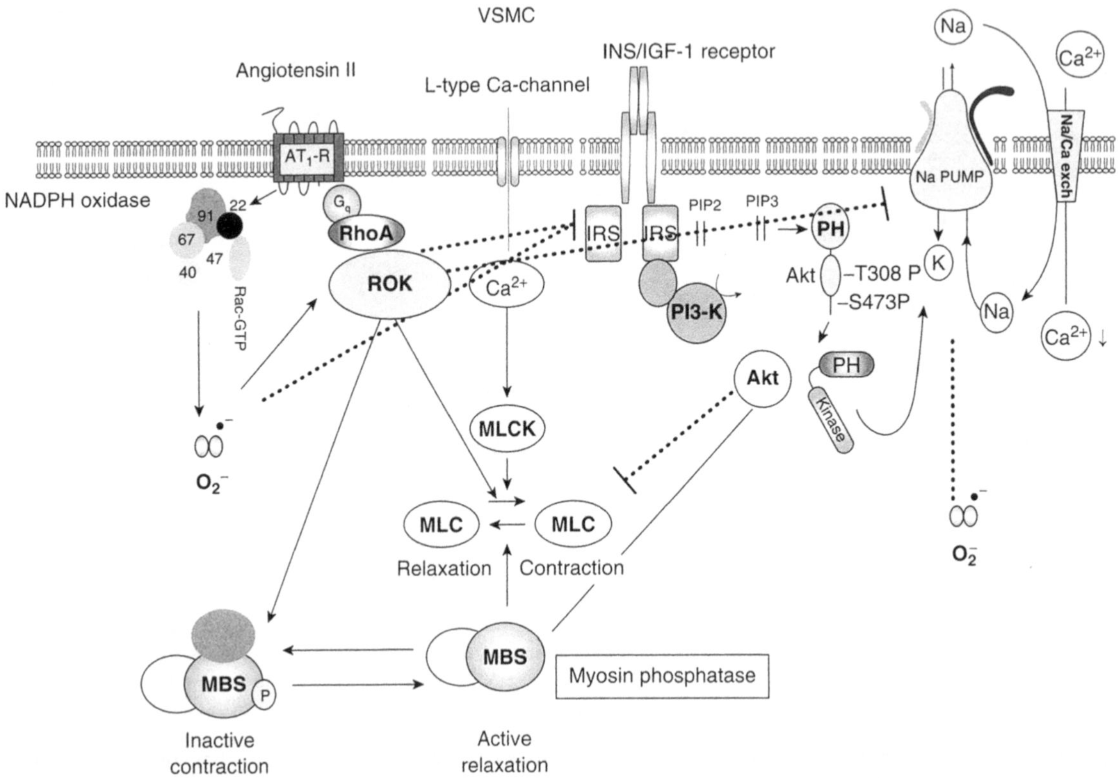

Figure 38.3 Angiotensin II and insulin/IGF-1 counterregulatory actions in vascular smooth muscle cells (VSMC). Insulin and IGF-1 reduce VSMC intracellular Ca^{2+} by inhibiting agonist-induced inward Ca^{2+} currents, intracellular organelle release of Ca^{2+}, and by reducing Ca^{2+}-myosin light chain (MLC) sensitization. Insulin and IGF-1 also reduce intracellular Ca^{2+} by stimulating the activity of the Na^+-K^+-ATPase pump in VSMCs, a process that is dependent on PI3K/Akt signaling. ANG II antagonizes the vasodilatory actions of insulin/IGF-1 via activation of low molecular weight G proteins such as Rho A, and generation of reactive oxygen species (ROS) through NADPH oxidase. MBS, myosin-bound serine. (Reproduced from Sowers JR. Am J Physiol Heart Circ Physiol 2004; 286: H1597–H1602.[24])

Ang II binding to AT_1R results in production of ROS through activation of NAD(P)H oxidase and low molecular weight G proteins. These ROS and G proteins inhibit PI3K/Akt signaling, thus impairing the vascular relaxing mechanisms of insulin (Figure 38.3). ROS can also degrade/inactivate NO that has already been produced,[24] further compromising vascular relaxation (Figure 38.4). Similar RAAS-mediated increases in oxidative stress likely contribute to insulin resistance in skeletal muscles.[62,63] This is supported by findings that ROS are increased in skeletal muscle from Ren-2 rats that overexpress tissue Ang II,[62] and that this effect is abolished when the animals are treated with an AT_1R blocker (Figure 38.5). Furthermore, when ROS production is abrogated or superoxide scavenged, skeletal muscle insulin-stimulated glucose uptake is normalized (Figure 38.6).

Activation of the RAAS also results in increased aldosterone secretion from the adrenal glands. Aldosterone causes sodium reabsorption at the principal cells of the distal tubules of the nephron and increased release of renin from the juxtogomerular cells. These responses increase extracellular volume leading to elevated BP. Aldosterone also contributes to hypertension by enhancing sympathetic activity, decreasing parasympathetic activity and reducing baroreceptor sensitivity.[34] Aldosterone affects the kidney by increasing extracellular matrix deposition by glomerular cells, leading to glomerulosclerosis and hypertension.[34]

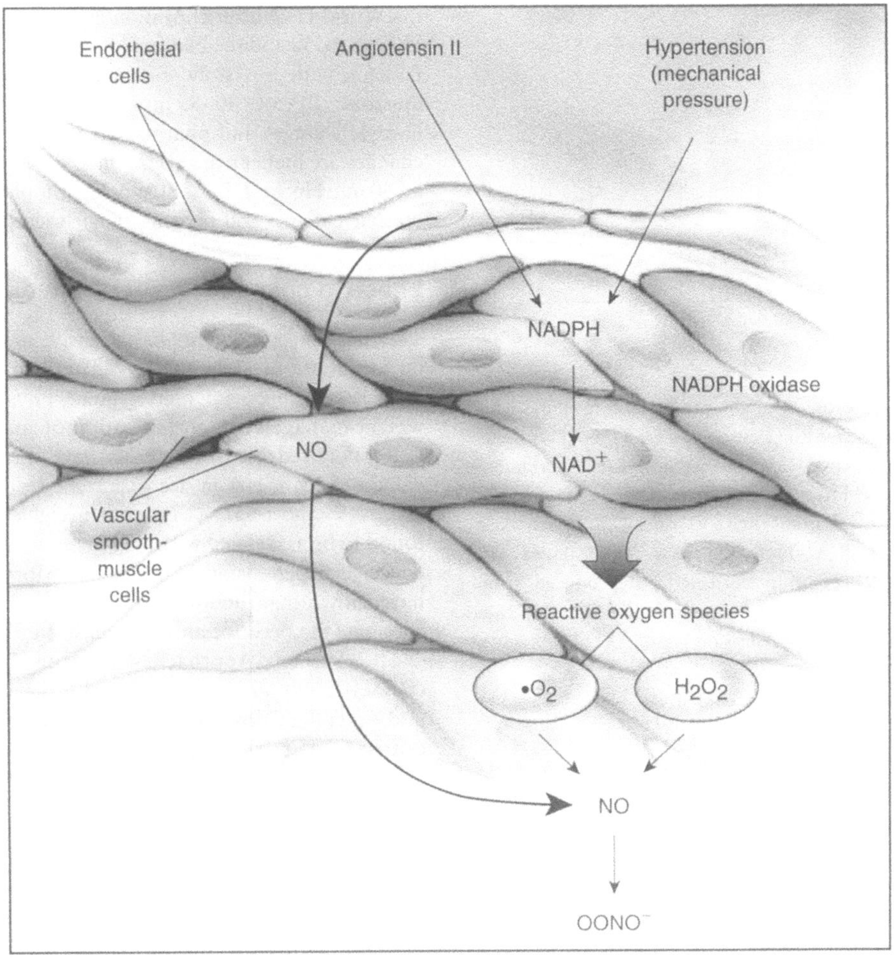

Figure 38.4 Angiotensin II stimulated increases in reactive oxygen species (ROS) by NADPH oxidase in vascular smooth muscle cells. Nitric oxide (NO) produced by endothelial cells is inactivated by conversion to peroxynitrite in the presence of excess ROS. (Reproduced from Sowers JR. N Engl J Med 2002; 346: 1999–2001. © Massachusetts Medical Society)

In vascular tissues aldosterone interferes with endothelial NO production and promotes remodeling. In part, these effects are mediated at the level of gene transcription and translation leading to increased protein synthesis, inflammation and fibrosis. Aldosterone effects are also regulated through various physiologic mechanisms including enhancement of tyrosine phosphorylation, increased Na^+/H^+ exchange and alkalinization of VSMCs, and inositol phosphate activation.[34] In the Randomized Aldactone Evaluation Study (RALES), it was reported that coadministration of the aldosterone receptor antagonist spironolactone with an ACE inhibitor in patients with severe congestive heart failure substantially reduced mortality.[97] Additionally, aldosterone receptor antagonist eplerenone has been reported to enhance the effects of enalapril in reducing albuminuria in hypertensive, type 2 diabetic patients with proteinuria.[98]

MANAGEMENT

A complete review of the management of hypertension is beyond the scope of this chapter. However, understanding the mechanisms associated with hypertension in the type 2 diabetic will help one to better manage the patient with the cardiometabolic syndrome.

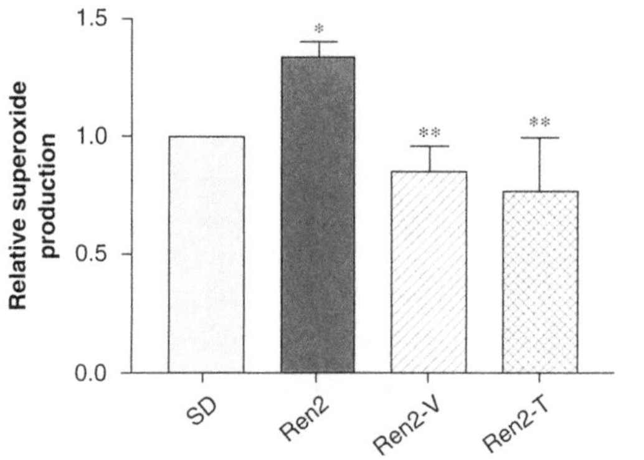

Figure 38.5 Superoxide anion production in the soleus muscle in hypertensive Ren2 rats which are a model for tissue angiotensin II compared with Sprague-Dawley (SD) normotensive control rats. Effect of treatment with the angiotensin receptor blocker valsartan (Ren2-V) or superoxide/catalase mimetic tempol (Ren2-T) for 21 days. $*p<0.05$ vs SD, $**p<0.05$ vs Ren2 group untreated. (Reproduced from Blendea et al. Am J Physiol Endocrinol Metab 2005; 288: E353–E359.[62] Used with permission.)

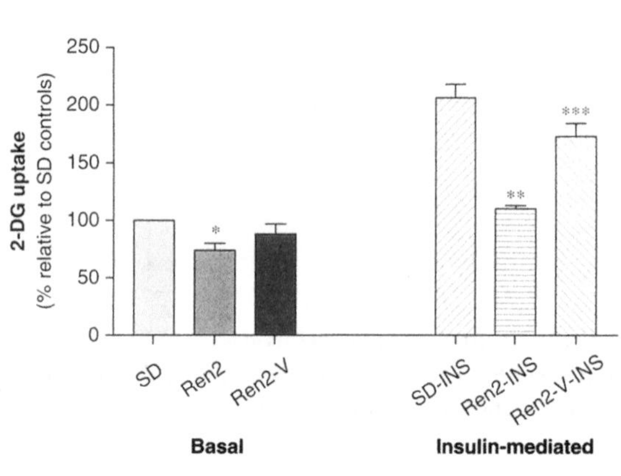

Figure 38.6 Basal and insulin-mediated 2-deoxyglucose (2-DG) uptake into *ex vivo* soleus muscle preparations from Sprague-Dawley (SD) and Ren2 rats. Effect of treatment with the angiotensin receptor blocker valsartan (Ren2-V) or superoxide/catalase mimetic tempol (Ren2-T) for 21 days. $*p<0.05$ vs SD in basal conditions, $**p<0.05$ vs SD-INS, $***p<0.05$ vs INS-stimulated Ren2. (Reproduced from Blendea et al. Am J Physiol Endocrinol Metab 2005; 288: E353–E359.[62] Used with permission.)

In patients with DM, the Joint National Committee on the Detection, Evaluation, and Treatment of High Blood Pressure (JNC 7) recommends a goal BP of <130/80. This goal is also supported by the ADA, the World Health Organization/International Society of Hypertension and the National Kidney Foundation.[99–102] Patients with a systolic BP of 130–139 mm Hg or a diastolic BP of 80–89 mm Hg should incorporate lifestyle changes and pharmacologic therapy if lifestyle changes are ineffective at 3 months. Patients with a SBP ≥140 mm Hg or DBP ≥90 mm Hg should incorporate lifestyle changes and pharmacologic therapy.[103]

Lifestyle changes

The first objective in any hypertensive diabetic should be to initiate lifestyle changes. These changes should include an improved diet, regular physical activity, weight management, and cessation of smoking.

Randomized controlled trials have documented the value of weight loss in decreasing the risk of hypertension.[104–107] Short-term (18-month) weight loss has been found to be associated with a 77% reduction in the incidence of hypertension at 7 years.[107] Moreover, studies have shown that modest weight loss can lower or even eliminate the need for antihypertensive medication.[108]

The Dietary Approaches to Stop Hypertension (DASH) Study group investigated a diet rich in fruits and vegetables, low-fat dairy products, with or without sodium restriction. They reported a substantially reduced BP, significantly more in hypertensive than in normotensive individuals.[109] A diet that is high in fiber and potassium and lower in saturated refined carbohydrates and salt can improve the lipid profile, improve glycemic control, and significantly lower BP.[110]

Studies have linked physical activity to lowering BP and improving insulin sensitivity. The Finnish Diabetes Prevention Study investigated diet and a minimum of 30 minutes of daily exercise in overweight subjects with glucose intolerance and reported a significant drop in BP (4 mm Hg for SBP and 2 mm Hg for diastolic BP compared with control subjects) and decrease in the risk of developing type 2 DM.[111] Other studies report similar results.[112,113]

Pharmacotherapy

Patients with DM and hypertension should be treated to a SBP of <130 mm Hg and a DBP of <80 mm Hg. Persons who are found to be hypertensive on BP screening should have their BP rechecked within 1 month to confirm the presence of hypertension. Patients with a SBP of 130–139 mm Hg or a DBP of 80–89 mm Hg should be given a maximum of 3 months to reduce BP through lifestyle changes. If unsuccessful in reducing BP in 3 months, pharmacologic therapy should be instituted. Patients with a SBP ≥140 mm Hg or a DBP ≥90 mm Hg should be given lifestyle changes and drug therapy. Individuals with a SBP ≥ 160 mm Hg or a DBP ≥ 100 mm Hg should begin immediate pharmacologic therapy.[114]

Drug therapy for hypertension in diabetics is typically required to achieve goal BP. First-line drug therapy should be an ACE inhibitor or an angiotensin receptor blocker (ARB) to block the RAAS, during which serum potassium and renal function should be monitored. ACE inhibitors and ARBs have been shown to delay progression to macroalbuminuria in type 2 DM.[94,95,115] In type 2 DM with hypertension, renal insufficiency, and macroalbuminuria, ARBs have reported to delay the progression to nephropathy. Other agents that have been shown to decrease CVD events in patients with DM include beta-blockers, diuretics, and calcium channel blockers. Furthermore, insulin sensitizers have been shown to reduce BP[53,116] and decrease cardiac SNS activity.[117]

A BP goal of 110–129/65–79 mm Hg is recommended in the pregnant diabetic patient. ACE inhibitors and ARBs are contraindicated during pregnancy. Antihypertensive agents known to be safe in pregnancy include methyldopa, labetolol, diltiazem, clonidine, and prazosin. Elderly hypertensive diabetic persons should have their BPs gradually lowered and orthostatic measurements should be performed to look for dysautonomia if clinically indicated. Lastly, patients who are resistant to multiple drug therapy should be referred to a specialist in hypertension.

CONCLUSION

Insulin resistance, hyperinsulinemia, and type 2 DM mellitus may represent a genetic predisposition to hypertension rather than a result of hypertension. Combined with obesity and dyslipidemia, the cardiometabolic syndrome ensues resulting in an increased risk of coronary artery disease. Proper management of these patients requires recommending lifestyle changes along with pharmacologic intervention. Additionally, insight into the pathophysiologic mechanisms underlying hypertension in the diabetic patient aids the clinician in appropriate management to help prevent or reduce progression of DM, hypertension, and the risk of coronary artery disease and other complications.

REFERENCES

1. International Diabetes Federation Task Force on Diabetes Health Economics: facts, figures and forecasts. Brussels: International Diabetes Federation, 1997.
2. Weiner N, Sowers JR. Epidemiology of diabetes. J Clin Pharmacol 2004; 44: 397–405.
3. Zimmet P, Albertie KGMM, Shaw J. Global and societal implications of the diabetes epidemic. Nature 2001; 13: 782–7.
4. Broadhurst CL. Nutrition and non-insulin dependent diabetes mellitus from an anthropological perspective. Alternative Medicine Review 1997; 2: 378–99.
5. Blair SN, Nichaman MZ. The public health problem of increasing prevalence rates of obesity and what should be done about it. Mayo Clinic Proc 2002; 77: 109–13.
6. Carter JS, Pugh JA, Monterrosa A. Non-insulin dependent diabetes mellitus in minorities in the United States. Ann Intern Med 1996; 125: 221–32.
7. Neel JV. Diabetes mellitus: a thrifty genotype rendered detrimental by 'progress'? Am J Hum Genet 1962; 14: 353–62.
8. Bakris GL, William M, Dworkin L et al. National Kidney Foundation Hypertension and Diabetes Executive Committees Working Group. Preserving renal function in adults with hypertension and diabetes: a consensus approach. Am J Kidney Dis 2000; 36: 646–61.
9. The Diabetes Control and Complications Trial. Epidemiology of diabetes interventions and complications research group. N Engl J Med 2003; 348: 2294–303.
10. Ogden CL, Flegal KM, Carroll MD, Johnson CL. Prevalence and trends in obesity in overweight among US children and adolescents. 1999–2000. JAMA 2002; 288: 1728–32.
11. Stratton IM, Adler AI, Neil HA et al. Association of glycaemia with macrovascular and microvascular complications of type 2 diabetes (UKPDS 35): prospective observational study. BMJ 2000; 321: 405–12.
12. King H, Aubert RE, Herman WH. Global burden of diabetes, 1995–2025. Prevalence, numerical estimates, and projections. Diabetes Care 1998; 21: 1414–31.
13. Kitagawa T, Owada M, Urakami T, Tajima N. Epidemiology of type 1 (insulin-dependent) and type 2 (non-insulin-dependent) diabetes mellitus in Japanese children. Diabetes Res Clin Pract 1994; 24 (Suppl): S7–S13.
14. Sowers JR. Treatment of hypertension in patients with diabetes. Arch Intern Med 2004; 164: 1850–7.
15. Sowers JR, Epstein M, Frolich ED. Diabetes, hypertension, and cardiovascular disease: an update. Hypertension 2001; 37: 1053–9.
16. Sowers JR, Williams M, Epstein M, Bakris G. Hypertension in patients with diabetes: strategies for drug therapy to reduce complications. Postgrad Med 2000; 107: 47–54.
17. Gress TW, Nieto FJ, Shahar E, Wofford MR, Brancati FL. Hypertension and antihypertensive therapy as risk factors for type 2 diabetes mellitus. N Engl J Med 2000; 342: 905–12.
18. El-Atat F, McFarlane SI, Sowers JR. Diabetes, hypertension, and cardiovascular derangements: pathophysiology and management. Curr Hypertens Rep 2004; 6: 215–23.
19. Adler AI, Stratton IM, Neil HA et al. Association of systolic blood pressure with macrovascular and microvascular complications of type 2 diabetes (UKPDS 36): prospective observational study. BMJ 2000; 321: 412–19.
20. Ford ES, Giles WH, Mokdad AH. Increasing prevalence of the metabolic syndrome among U.S. adults. Diabetes Care 2004; 27: 2444–9.
21. Mcfarlane SI, Banerji M, Sowers JR. Insulin resistance and cardiovascular disease. J Clin Endocrinol Metab 2001; 86: 713–18.
22. Wang Y, Rimm EB, Stampfer MJ et al. Comparison of abdominal adiposity and overall obesity in predicting risk of type 2 diabetes among men. Am J Clin Nutr 2005; 81: 555–63.
23. Pi-Sunyer FX. Medical hazards of obesity. Ann Intern Med 1993; 119 (7 Pt 2): 655–60.
24. Sowers JR. Insulin resistance and hypertension. Am J Physiol Heart Circ Physiol 2004; 286: H1597–H1602.

25. Sowers JR, Bakris GL. Antihypertensive therapy and the risk of type 2 diabetes mellitus. N Engl J Med 2000; 342: 969–70.
26. Tan AS, Kuppuswamy S, Whaley-Connell AT et al. Recommendations for special sopulations: the treatment of hypertension in diabetes mellitus. Endocrinologist 2004; 14: 368–81.
27. Schunkert H. Obesity and target organ damage: the heart. Int J Obesity 2002; 4 (Suppl): S15–S20.
28. Henry P, Thomas F, Benetos A et al. Impaired fasting glucose, blood pressure and cardiovascular disease mortality. Hypertension 2002; 40: 458–63.
29. Sowers JR, Haffner S. Treatment of cardiovascular and renal risk factors in the diabetic hypertensive. Hypertension 2002; 40: 781–8.
30. Center for Disease Control and Prevention (CDC). State-specific mortality from sudden cardiac death – United States, 1999. MMWR Morb Mortal Wkly Rep 2002; 51: 123–6.
31. Kannel WB, Schatzkin A. Sudden death: lessons from subsets in population studies. J Am Coll Cardiol 1985; 5 (Suppl 6): 141B.
32. Jouven X, Desnos M, Guerot C, Ducimetiere P. Predicting sudden death in the population: the Paris Prospective Study I. Circulation 1999; 99: 1978–83.
33. El-Atat F, McFarlane SI, Sowers JR et al. Sudden cardiac death in patients with diabetes. Curr Diab Rep 2004; 4: 187–93.
34. McFarlane SI, Sowers JR. Aldosterone function in diabetes mellitus: effects on cardiovascular and renal disease. J Clin Endocrinol Metab 2003; 88: 516–23.
35. Haffner SM, Lehto S, Ronnemaa T, Pyorala K, Laakso M. Mortality from coronary heart disease in subjects with type 2 diabetes and in nondiabetic subjects with and without prior myocardial infarction. N Engl J Med 1998; 339: 229–34.
36. Grundy SM, Benjamin IJ, Burke GL et al. Diabetes and cardiovascular disease: a statement for healthcare professionals from the American Heart Association. Circulation 1999; 100: 1134–46.
37. Sowers JR, Lester MA. Diabetes and cardiovascular disease. Diabetes Care 1999; 22 (Suppl 3): C14–C20.
38. Haffner SM, Alexander CM, Cook TJ et al. Reduced coronary events in simvastatin-treated patients with coronary heart disease and diabetes or impaired fasting glucose levels: subgroup analyses in the Scandinavian Simvastatin Survival Study. Arch Intern Med 1999; 159: 2661–7.
39. Stamler J, Vaccaro O, Neaton JD, Wentworth D. Diabetes, other risk factors, and 12-yr cardiovascular mortality for men screened in the Multiple Risk Factor Intervention Trial. Diabetes Care 1993; 16: 434–44.
40. Kassab E, McFarlane SI, Sowers JR. Vascular complications in diabetes and their prevention. Vasc Med 2001; 6: 249–55.
41. Davis TM, Millns H, Stratton IM, Holman RR, Turner RC. Risk factors for stroke in type 2 diabetes mellitus: United Kingdom Prospective Diabetes Study (UKPDS) 29. Arch Intern Med 1999; 159: 1097–103.
42. Fagan TC, Sowers J. Type 2 diabetes mellitus: greater cardiovascular risks and greater benefits of therapy. Arch Intern Med 1999; 159: 1033–4.
43. UK Prospective Diabetes Study Group. Tight blood pressure control and risk of macrovascular and microvascular complications in type 2 diabetes: UKPDS 38. BMJ 1998; 317: 703–13.
44. Hansson L, Zanchetti A, Carruthers SG et al. Effects of intensive blood-pressure lowering and low-dose aspirin in patients with hypertension: principal results of the Hypertension Optimal Treatment (HOT) randomised trial. Lancet 1998; 351: 1755–62.
45. Parving HH, Osterby R, Ritz E. Diabetic nephropathy. In: Brenner BM (ed). The kidney. Philadelphia: WB Saunders, 2000, pp 1731–73.
46. Viberti GC, Walker JD, Pinto J. Diabetic nephropathy. In: Alberti KGMM, DeFronzo RA, Keen H, Zimmet P (eds). International textbook of diabetes mellitus. New York: John Wiley & Sons, 1992, pp 1267–328.
47. Tuomilehto J, Lindstrom J, Eriksson JG et al. Finnish Diabetes Prevention Study among subjects with impaired glucose tolerance. N Engl J Med 2001; 344: 1343–50.
48. Sacks FM, Svetkey LP, Vollmer WM et al. DASH Sodium Collaborative Research Group. Effects on blood pressure of reduced dietary sodium and the Dietary Approaches to Stop Hypertension (DASH) diet. N Engl J Med 2001; 344: 3–10.
49. Ruddy M. Angiotensin II receptor blockade in diabetic nephropathy. Am J Hypertens 2002; 15: 468–71.
50. Gress TW, Nieto FJ, Shahar E et al. Hypertension and antihypertensive therapy as risk factors for type 2 diabetes mellitus. Atherosclerosis Risk in Communities Study. N Engl J Med 2000; 342: 905–12.
51. Sowers JR, Epstein M. Diabetes mellitus and associated hypertension, vascular disease, and nephropathy: an update. Hypertension 1995; 26: 869–79.
52. Dengel DR, Hagberg JM, Pratley RE, Rogus EM, Goldberg AP. Improvements in blood pressure, glucose metabolism, and lipoprotein lipids after aerobic exercise plus weight loss in obese, hypertensive middle-aged men. Metabolism 1998; 47: 1075–82.
53. Ogihara T, Rakugi H, Ikegami H, Mikami H, Masuo K. Enhancement of insulin sensitivity by troglitazone lowers blood pressure in diabetic hypertensives. Am J Hypertens 1995; 8: 316–20.
54. Kotchen TA, Zhang HY, Covelli M, Blehschmidt N. Insulin resistance and blood pressure in Dahl rats and in one-kidney, one-clip hypertensive rats. Am J Physiol 1991; 261 (6 Pt 1): E692–E697.
55. Reaven GM, Chang H. Relationship between blood pressure, plasma insulin and triglyceride concentration, and insulin action in spontaneous hypertensive and Wistar-Kyoto rats. Am J Hypertens 1991; 4 (1 Pt 1): 34–8.
56. Sechi LA, Melis A, Tedde R. Insulin hypersecretion: a distinctive feature between essential and secondary hypertension. Metabolism 1992; 4: 1261–6.
57. Beatty OL, Harper R, Sheridan B, Atkinson AB, Bell PM. Insulin resistance in offspring of hypertensive parents. BMJ 1993; 307: 92–6.
58. Grunfeld B, Balzareti M, Romo M, Gimenez M, Gutman R. Hyperinsulinemia in normotensive offspring of hypertensive parents. Hypertension 1994; 23 (1 Suppl): I12–15.
59. Castro JP, El-Atat FA, McFarlane SI, Aneja A, Sowers JR. Cardiometabolic syndrome: pathophysiology and treatment. Curr Hypertens Rep 2003; 5: 393–401.
60. Epstein M, Sowers JR. Insulin resistance in hypertension – a focused review. Am J Med Sci 1993; 306: 345–7.
61. Nickenig G, Roling J, Strehlow K, Schnabel P, Bohm M. Insulin induces upregulation of vascular AT1 receptor gene expression by posttranscriptional mechanisms. Circulation 1998; 98: 2453–60.
62. Blendea MC, Jacobs D, Stump CS et al. Abrogation of oxidative stress improves insulin sensitivity in the Ren-2 rat model of tissue angiotensin II overexpression. Am J Physiol Endocrinol Metab 2005; 288: E353–E359.
63. Henriksen EJ, Saengsirisuwan V. Exercise training and antioxidants: relief from oxidative stress and insulin resistance. Exerc Sport Sci Rev 2003; 31: 79–84.
64. Moncada S, Higgs A. The L-arginine-nitric oxidase pathway. N Engl J Med 1993; 329: 2002–12.
65. Guerci B, Kearney-Schwartz A, Zannad F et al. Endothelial dysfunction and type 2 diabetes (Part 1). Diabetes Metab (Paris) 2001; 27: 425–34.
66. Garg UC, Hassid A. Nitric oxide-generating vasodailators and 8-bromo-cyclic guanosine monophosphate inhibit mitogenesis

and proliferation of cultured rat vascular smooth muscle cells. J Clin Invest 1989; 83: 1774–7.
67. Kuboki K, Jiang ZY, Takahara N et al. Regulation of endothelial constitutive nitric oxide synthase gene expression in endothelial cells in vivo: a specific vascular action of insulin. Circulation 2000; 101: 676–81.
68. Hsueh WA, Quinones M. Role of endothelial dysfunction in insulin resistance. Am J Cardiol 2003; 92 (Suppl): 10J-17J.
69. Guzik TJ, Mussa S, Gastaldi D et al. Mechanisms of increased vascular superoxide production in human diabetes mellitus. Circulation 2002; 105: 1656.
70. Cosentino F, Hishikawa K, Katusic ZS et al. High glucose increases nitric oxide synthase expression and superoxide anion generation in human aortic endothelial cells. Circulation 1997; 86: 25–8.
71. Rajagopalan S, Kurz S, Munzel T et al. Angiotesin II-mediated hypertension in the rat increases vascular superoxide production via membrane NAD/NAD(P)H oxidase activation. J Clin Invest 1996; 97: 1916–23.
72. Ushio-Fukai M, Zafari AM, Fukui T et al. p22phox is a critical component of the superoxide-generating NADH/NAD(P)H oxidase system and regulates angiotensin II-induced hypertrophy in vascular smooth muscle cells. J Biol Chem 1996; 271: 23317–21.
73. White CR, Darley-Usmar V, Berrington WR et al. Circulation plasma xanthine oxidase contributes to vascular dysfunction in hypercholesterolemic rabbits. Proc Natl Acad Sci U S A 1996; 93: 8745–9.
74. Vasquez-Vivar J, Kalyanaraman B, Martasek P et al. Superoxide generation by endothelial nitric oxide synthase: the influence of cofactors. Proc Natl Acad Sci U S A 1998; 95: 9220–5.
75. Gryglewski RJ, Palmer RM, Moncada S. Superoxide anion is involved in the breakdown of endothelium-derived vascular relaxing factor. Nature 1986; 320: 454–6.
76. Peterson TE, Poppa V, Ueba H et al. Opposing effects of reactive oxygen species and cholesterol on endothelial nitric oxide synthase and endothelial cell caveolae. Circ Res 1999; 85: 29–37.
77. Wolin MS. Interactions of oxidants with vascular signaling systems. Arterioscler Thromb Vasc Biol 2000; 20: 1430–42.
78. Williams SB, Cusco JA, Roddy MA, Johnstone MT, Creager MA. Impaired nitric oxide-mediated vasodilation in patients with non-insulin-dependent diabetes mellitus. J Am Coll Cardiol 1996; 27: 567–74.
79. Tesfamariam B, Brown ML, Cohen RA. Elevated glucose impairs endothelium-dependent relaxation by activating protein kinase. Clin Invest 1991; 87: 1643–8.
80. Williams B. Factors regulating the expression of vascular permeability/vascular endothelial growth human vascular tissues. Diabetologia 1997; 40: S118–S120.
81. Vlassara H. Recent progress on the biologic and clinical significance of advanced glycosylation end products. J Lab Clin Med 1994; 124: 19–30.
82. Guerci B, Bohme P, Kearney-Schwartz A et al. Endothelial dysfunction and type 2 diabetes (II). Diabetes Metab (Paris) 2001; 27: 436–47.
83. De Vriese AS, Verbeuren TJ, Van de Voorde J et al. Endothelial dysfunction in diabetes. Br J Pharmacol 2000; 130: 963–74.
84. Rahmouni K, Correia ML, Haynes WG, Mark AL. Obesity-associated hypertension: new insights into mechanisms. Hypertension 2005; 45: 9–14.
85. Carlyle M, Jones OB, Kuo JJ, Hall JE. Chronic cardiovascular and renal actions of leptin: role of adrenergic activity. Hypertension 2002; 39 (2 Pt 2): 496–501.
86. Edelson GW, Sowers JR. Treatment of hypertension in selected patient groups: an emphasis on diabetes mellitus and hypertension. Endocrinologist 1994; 4: 205–11.
87. Lind L, Berne C, Lithell H. Prevalence of insulin resistance in essential hypertension. J Hypertens 1995; 13: 1457–62.
88. Facchini F, Chen Y-DI, Clinkingbeard C et al. Insulin resistance, hyperinsulinemia, and dyslipidemia in nonobese individuals with a family history of hypertension. Am J Hypertens 1992; 5: 694–9.
89. Reaven GM, Lithell H, Landsberg L. Hypertension and associated metabolic abnormalities: the role of insulin resistance and the sympathoadrenal system. N Engl J Med 1996; 334: 374–82.
90. Sawicki PT, Heinemann L, Starke A et al. Hyperinsulinaemia is not linked with blood pressure evaluation in patients with insulinoma. Diabetologia 1992; 35: 649–52.
91. Heise, T, Magnusson K, Heinemann L et al. Insulin resistance and the effect of insulin on blood pressure in essential hypertension. Hypertension 1998; 32: 243–8.
92. Grassi G, Seravalle G, Columbo M et al. Body weight reduction sympathetic nerve traffic and arterial baroreflex in obese normotensive humans. Circulation 1998; 97: 2037–42 .
93. Rahmouni K, Morgan DA, Morgan GM et al. Hypothalamic PI3K and MAPK differentially mediate regional sympathetic activation to insulin. J Clin Invest 2004; 114: 652–8.
94. Hansson L, Lindholm LH, Niskanen L et al., for the Captopril Prevention Project (CAPPP) study group. Effect of angiotensin-converting-enzyme inhibition compared with conventional morbidity and mortality in hypertension: the Captopril Prevention Project (CAPPP) randomised trial. Lancet 1999; 353: 611–16.
95. The Heart Outcomes Prevention Evaluation Study Investigators. Effects of an angiotensin-converting-enzyme inhibitor, ramipril, on cardiovascular events in high-risk patients. N Engl J Med 2000; 342: 145–53.
96. Sowers JR. Hypertension in type II diabetes: update on therapy. J Clin Hypertens (Greenwich) 1999; 1: 41–7.
97. Pitt B, Zannad F, Remme WJ et al. The effect of spironolactone on morbidity and mortality in patients with severe heart failure. N Engl J Med 1999; 341: 709–17.
98. Epstein M, Buckalew Jr V, Martinez F et al., the Eplerenone 021 Investigators. Antiproteinuric efficacy of eplerenone, enalapril, and eplerenone/enalapril combination therapy in diabetic hypertensives with microalbuminuria. Am J Hypertens 2002; 15: OR–54.
99. Whelton SP, Chin A, Xin X et al. Effect of aerobic exercise on blood pressure: a meta-analysis of randomized, controlled trials. Ann Intern Med 2002; 136: 493–503.
100. Bakris GL, Williams M, Dworkin L et al. Preserving renal function in adults with hypertension and diabetes: a consensus approach. National Kidney Foundation Hypertension and Diabetes Executive Committees Working Group. Am J Kidney Dis 2000; 36: 646–61.
101. Hansson L, Zanchetti A, Carruthers SG et al. Effects of intensive blood-pressure lowering and low-dose aspirin in patients with hypertension: principal results of the Hypertension Optimal Treatment (HOT) randomised trial. HOT Study Group. Lancet 1998; 351: 1755–62.
102. Whitworth JA. 2003 World Health Organization (WHO)/ International Society of Hypertension (ISH) statement on management of hypertension. J Hypertens 2003; 21: 1983–92.
103. Chobanian AV, Bakris GL, Black HR et al. The Seventh Report of the Joint National Committee on Prevention, Detection, Evaluation, and Treatment of High Blood Pressure: the JNC 7 report. JAMA 2003; 289: 2560–72.
104. The effects of nonpharmacologic interventions on blood pressure of persons with high normal levels. Results of the Trials of Hypertension Prevention, Phase I. JAMA 1992; 267: 1213–20.

105. Effects of weight loss and sodium reduction intervention on blood pressure and hypertension incidence in overweight people with high-normal blood pressure. The Trials of Hypertension Prevention, phase II. The Trials of Hypertension Prevention Collaborative Research Group. Arch Intern Med 1997; 157: 657–67.
106. The Hypertension Prevention Trial: three-year effects of dietary changes on blood pressure. Hypertension Prevention Trial Research Group. Arch Intern Med 1990; 150: 153–62.
107. He J, Whelton PK, Appel LJ et al. Long-term effects of weight loss and dietary sodium reduction on incidence of hypertension. Hypertension 2000; 35: 544–9.
108. Wassertheil-Smoller S, Blaufox MD, Oberman AS et al. The Trial of Antihypertensive Interventions and Management (TAIM) study. Adequate weight loss, alone and combined with drug therapy in the treatment of mild hypertension. Arch Intern Med 1992; 152: 131–6.
109. Sacks FM, Svetkey LP, Vollmer WM et al. Effects on blood pressure of reduced dietary sodium and the Dietary Approaches to Stop Hypertension (DASH) diet. DASH-Sodium Collaborative Research Group. N Engl J Med 2001; 344: 3–10.
110. Stewart KJ. Exercise training and the cardiovascular consequences of type 2 diabetes and hypertension: plausible mechanisms for improving cardiovascular health. JAMA 2002; 288: 1622–31.
111. Tuomilehto J, Lindstrom J, Eriksson JG et al. Prevention of type 2 diabetes mellitus by changes in lifestyle among subjects with impaired glucose tolerance. N Engl J Med 2001; 344: 1343–50.
112. Hu G, Barengo NC, Tuomilehto J et al. Relationship of physical activity and body mass index to the risk of hypertension: a prospective study in Finland. Hypertension 2004; 43: 25–30.
113. Whelton SP, Cin A, Xin X et al. Effect of aerobic exercise on blood pressure: a meta-analysis of randomized, controlled trials. Ann Intern Med 2002; 136: 493–503.
114. American Diabetes Association. Standards of medical care in diabetes (Position Statement). Diabetes Care 2005; 28 (Suppl 1): S4–S36.
115. Effects of ramipril on cardiovascular and microvascular outcomes in people with diabetes mellitus: results of the HOPE study and MICRO-HOPE substudy. Heart Outcomes Prevention Evaluation Study Investigators. Lancet 2000; 355: 253–9.
116. Raji A, Seely EW, Bekins SA et al. Rosiglitazone improves insulin sensitivity and lowers blood pressure in hypertensive patients. Diabetes Care 2003; 26: 172–8.
117. Watanabe K, Komatsu J, Kurata M et al. Improvement of insulin resistance by troglitazone ameliorates cardiac sympathetic nervous dysfunction in patients with essential hypertension. J Hypertens 2004; 22: 1761–8.

39

Critical role of dyslipidemia and angiotensin II in atherogenesis

Jawahar L Mehta

INTRODUCTION

Hyperlipidemia and hypertension are major risk factors for atherosclerosis. These conditions are often present in the same patient. It has been proposed that an interaction between hyperlipidemia and neurohumoral systems, such as the renin-angiotensin system (RAS), explains the co-existence of hypertension and dyslipidemia in the same patient. Data from various studies have suggested that the effects of the RAS and hyperlipidemia are not independent and the underlying mechanisms, which both initiate and accelerate atherosclerosis, overlap. Treatment directed at lowering total cholesterol, low-density lipoprotein (LDL)-cholesterol, and triglycerides, and raising high-density lipoprotein (HDL)-cholesterol levels has resulted in a reduction of cardiovascular events. Treatment directed at inhibiting angiotensin converting enzyme (ACE) and angiotensin type 1 (AT_1) receptors has also been shown to reduce cardiovascular events in patients with vascular disease. There is a suggestion that treatment directed at lowering cholesterol along with agents that modulate the RAS may have added benefits in the prevention, progression and treatment of hypertension and atherogenesis.

This chapter discusses the pathways by which the RAS may facilitate the adverse effects of dyslipidemia, how dyslipidemia stimulates the RAS, and how conjunctive therapy with statins and RAS blockers may have an additive beneficial effect in atherosclerosis.

FACILITATIVE ROLE OF RAS ON THE UPTAKE OF LDL-CHOLESTEROL IN THE VESSEL WALL

Oxidized LDL (ox-LDL) is more important than native LDL-cholesterol in atherogenesis.[1] Cholesterol accumulation in the macrophages and their transformation into foam cells are major events in the development of atherosclerosis. This process results from an increased uptake of ox-LDL[2] and enhanced macrophage cholesterol synthesis. Angiotensin II (Ang II) has been shown to increase macrophage cellular cholesterol biosynthesis with no significant effect on blood pressure or plasma cholesterol levels.[3] This effect of Ang II has been shown to be reversed by ACE inhibitors like fosinopril and the AT_1 receptor blocker losartan. Nickenig et al.[4] have shown that LDL-cholesterol accumulates in cultured vascular smooth muscle cells via AT_1 receptor activation. The relevance of AT_1 receptors became evident in experiments wherein Ang II was unable to increase cholesterol synthesis in macrophages that lacked the AT_1 receptors.

Ang II facilitates macrophage cholesterol influx, perhaps by enhancing LDL oxidation in arterial wall components.[5] Ang II can bind to LDL and form a modified lipoprotein, which is taken up by the scavenger receptors on the macrophages, leading to cellular cholesterol accumulation.[6] We examined the kinetics of ox-LDL uptake in endothelial cells and observed that Ang II enhanced the uptake of ox-LDL in these cells.[7] This effect was blocked by the AT_1 receptor blocker losartan, but not by the AT_2 receptor blocker PD 123319.

Ang II has also been shown to up-regulate macrophage messenger RNA (mRNA) for 3-hydroxy-3-methylglutaryl coenzyme A (HMG-CoA) reductase. In one study, fluvastatin, a competitive inhibitor of HMG-CoA reductase, blocked the stimulatory effect of Ang II on macrophage cholesterol biosynthesis.[8] This demonstrates that the probable biochemical site for the action of Ang II along the cholesterol biosynthesis pathway is HMG-CoA reductase, the rate-limiting enzyme in cholesterol biosynthesis. Further, the stimulation of cholesterol biosynthesis in macrophages and ox-LDL uptake in smooth muscle cells, macrophages and endothelial cells requires or is at least facilitated by AT_1 receptor activation. HMG-CoA reductase expression may play an important role in this process.

ACTIVATION OF RAS BY DYSLIPIDEMIA

Hypercholesterolemia has been shown to increase the expression of ACE and AT_1 receptors in the atherosclerotic lesions in experimental animals.[9,10] Studies in human atherosclerotic tissues have confirmed the up-regulation of RAS, particularly in the regions prone to plaque rupture.[11,12] Importantly, these same areas show extensive deposits of inflammatory cells, macrophages, and apoptosis.

Incubation of vascular smooth muscle cells with LDL-cholesterol has been shown to increase AT_1 receptor expression.[13] Li et al.[14] in our laboratory observed that ox-LDL increases mRNA and protein for AT_1 but not AT_2, receptors in the human coronary artery endothelial cells, implying that AT_1 expression is amplified at the transcriptional level. Activation of the redox-sensitive transcription factor NF-κB (nuclear factor kappa B) plays an important role in the process. To define the relationship of the RAS and lipids in humans, Nickenig et al.[4] administered Ang II to normocholesterolemic and hypercholesterolemic men and found that the increase in blood pressure was exaggerated in the latter group and was blunted by LDL-cholesterol-lowering agents. A linear relationship between AT_1 receptor density on platelets and LDL-cholesterol concentration in the plasma was observed. Down-regulation of AT_1 receptor expression with statins has also been shown in vascular smooth muscle and endothelial cells.[15,16]

The expression of genes for chymases, enzymes by which Ang II can be formed independently of ACE activation, has been shown to be increased in aortic atherosclerotic lesions of monkeys fed a high-cholesterol diet.[17] The functional significance of chymases in the development of atherosclerosis, however, remains uncertain. These observations nonetheless suggest a close interaction of dyslipidemia and RAS.

As will be discussed later, oxidative stress plays a major role in atherosclerosis,[18] and Ang II enhances oxidative stress at least in part by oxidation of native LDL.

ANGIOTENSIN II, DYSLIPIDEMIA AND LOX-1

Atherosclerotic plaques are rich in ox-LDL, and patients with acute coronary syndrome have increased plasma levels of ox-LDL, while the serum total cholesterol levels in these patients are not significantly different from control subjects.[19] We have identified LOX-1, high-affinity lectin-like receptors for ox-LDL, in cultured human coronary artery endothelial cells.[20] Native LDL does not bind to this receptor. Endothelial cells in vitro and in vivo internalize and degrade ox-LDL through this putative receptor-mediated pathway that does not seem to involve the classic macrophage scavenger receptor. Cytokine tumor necrosis factor-α (TNF-α)[21] and fluid shear stress[22] have also been shown to up-regulate LOX-1 gene expression. LOX-1 expression is involved in the occurrence of apoptosis (programmed cell death) in response to ox-LDL,[23,24] the activation of mitogen-activated protein kinases (MAPKs), and the expression of adhesion molecules and attachment of monocytes to activated endothelial cells.[25] NF-κB plays a critical role in these effects of ox-LDL on endothelial cells.[20] The pro-apoptotic effect of Ang II in human coronary artery endothelial cells and the role of AT_1 receptors and protein kinase C activation in the process have also been shown by our group.[26]

We showed that Ang II up-regulates LOX-1 expression and this effect can be blocked by the AT_1, but not AT_2, receptor blockers. On the other hand, ox-LDL up-regulates AT_1, but not the AT_2, receptor expression in human coronary artery endothelial cells.[27]

These observations suggest a cross-talk between dyslipidemia and Ang II. The two systems act synergistically in inducing cell injury and initiating an inflammatory state, a prelude to atherosclerosis (Figure 39.1).

We showed intense immunostaining for and up-regulation of the gene for LOX-1 in the atherosclerotic tissue of rabbits fed a high-cholesterol diet.[28] In addition to reducing atherosclerosis, losartan blocked LOX-1 up-regulation. Previous studies from our laboratory showed marked up-regulation of AT_1 receptors in the aortas of hypercholesterolemic rabbits.[10] In more recent studies, we showed marked up-regulation of LOX-1 in concert with apoptosis in human atherosclerotic plaques, particularly in the regions that are prone to rupture.[29] These reports together emphasize the importance of the cross-talk between ox-LDL and RAS.

Statins have been shown to reduce atherosclerotic plaque formation,[30] attenuate the reduction in endothelial nitric oxide synthase (eNOS) expression,[31] and reduce the expression of leukocyte adhesion molecules.[32] Statins have also been shown to reduce the transcription of LOX-1 as well as reduce the binding of ox-LDL to human coronary endothelial cells.[32]

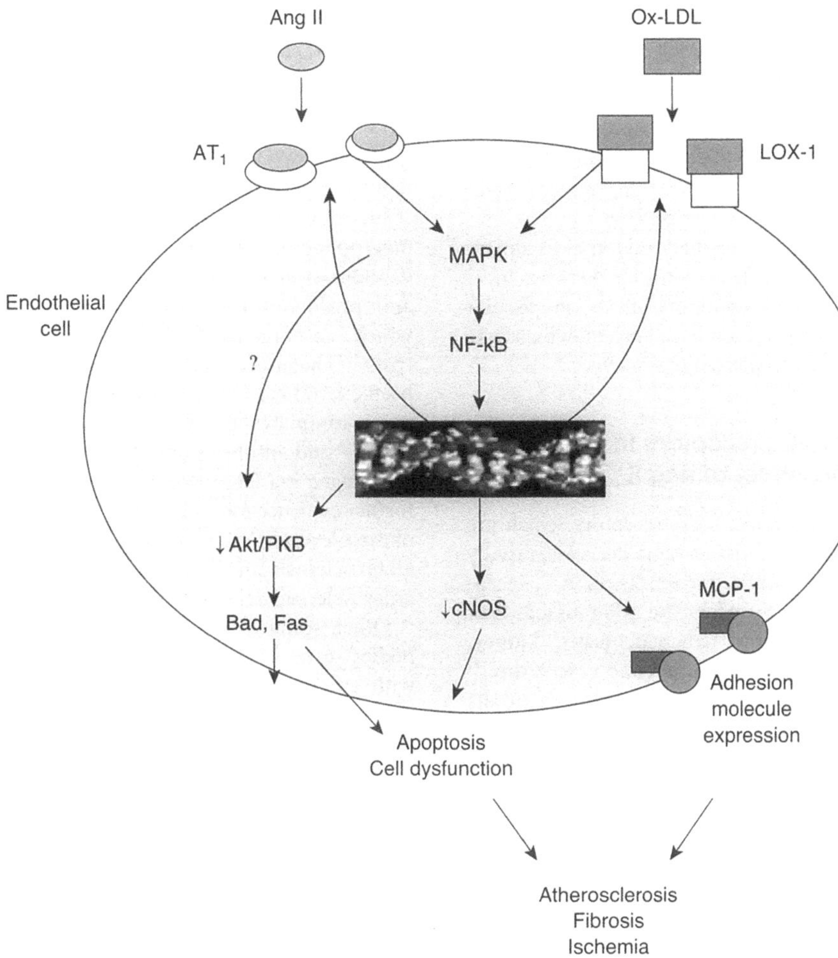

Figure 39.1 Up-regulation of AT_1 receptors by ox-LDL and of LOX-1 by angiotensin II (Ang II)

INHIBITORY EFFECT OF RAS INHIBITORS ON ATHEROGENESIS

Both ACE inhibitors and AT_1 receptor blockers have been shown to reduce the progression of atherosclerosis.[28,33,34] Therapy with the AT_1 receptor blocker losartan has been shown to suppress the expression of adhesion molecules and NF-κB by activating its regulatory protein IκBα in rabbits fed a high cholesterol diet.[28] To determine the specific role of RAS inhibitors (vs the blood pressure-lowering effect), Hayek et al.[35] conducted a study with low doses of fosinopril or losartan. Control animals were given either a placebo or a dose of hydralazine that lowered blood pressure. LDL oxidation, as measured by thiobarbituric acid reactive substances or by formation of conjugated dienes, was suppressed by low-dose fosinopril, suppressed only modestly by losartan, and unaffected by placebo or hydralazine hydrochloride. Atherosclerosis was inhibited by fosinopril and losartan, but not by hydralazine, suggesting that the anti-atherosclerotic effects of RAS inhibitors may be due, at least in part, to direct inhibition of LDL oxidation and other actions of Ang II in the vessel wall, and not to the lowering of blood pressure.

Bavry et al.[36] showed that the ACE inhibitor quinapril decreased intra-arterial thrombus formation, whereas the AT_1 receptor blocker losartan had a minimal effect. The inhibitory effect of ACE inhibitors on the generation of plasminogen activator inhibitor (PAI-1) may be relevant in this differential effect.

Endothelial dysfunction (a surrogate for atherosclerosis) in hypercholesterolemic animals has been shown to be improved by ACE inhibitors.[37] Bradykinin antagonists can diminish some of this effect, suggesting that the inhibition of bradykinin breakdown rather than Ang II formation may be important in this effect.[38] Inhibition of Ang II-sensitive, NADH-dependent, superoxide-producing enzymes may be another mechanism responsible for the improvement in the reduction of NO inactivation.[39]

Lauren et al.[40] have suggested that the treatment with ACE inhibitor and AT_1 receptor blockers has independent additive anti-inflammatory effects on vascular endothelium and smooth muscle cell layers, which may contribute to their anti-atherosclerosis effect.

Role of AT_1 and AT_2 receptors in the pro-atherogenic effect of ang II

Besides AT_1, Ang II activates AT_2 receptors which are highly expressed in fetal tissues and decrease rapidly after birth.[41] Under normal circumstances AT_2 receptors are minimally expressed in the adult tissues, but are still detectable in the pancreas, heart, kidney, adrenals, myometrium, ovary, brain, and vasculature.[41] However, these receptors are re-expressed in adults after vascular and cardiac injury and during wound healing, suggesting a potential role for AT_2 receptors in tissue remodeling. The functional role of these receptors is unclear, but may relate to antagonism of AT_1 receptor activity. Although most studies have focused on the protective effects of AT_2 receptor activation against cardiac ischemia-reperfusion injury and hypertension, there is a suggestion that AT_2 receptor activation triggers an anti-growth effect and prevents extracellular matrix accumulation.[42] Further AT_1 receptor blockers may enhance the expression and activity of AT_2 receptors, a potential mechanism of the cardioprotective effects of the AT_1 receptor blockers against ischemia-reperfusion injury.[43]

MECHANISM OF PRO-ATHEROGENIC EFFECTS OF OX-LDL

Ox-LDL induces endothelial dysfunction.[44] This endothelial dysfunction involves a decreased expression/activity of eNOS; an increased expression of adhesion molecules, such as intercellular adhesion molecule-1 (ICAM-1), vascular cell adhesion molecule-1 (VCAM-1), and monocyte chemoattractant protein-1 (MCP-1), which are responsible for the adhesion of monocytes to endothelial cells; an increased expression of inflammatory mediators such as matrix metalloproteinase-1 (MMP-1) and CD40L/CD40; increased platelet aggregation and increased apoptosis. In endothelial cells, many of the pro-atherosclerotic effects of ox-LDL are mediated via LOX-1, whose activation induces the generation of intracellular reactive oxygen species (ROS),[20] which in turn stimulate mitogen MAPK and transcription factor NF-κB activation, leading to the regulated gene expression.

In addition to endothelial cells and monocytes/macrophages, ox-LDL affects the biology of other vascular components. Ox-LDL induces the migration and proliferation of vascular smooth muscle cells, which is a hallmark in the pathogenesis of atherosclerosis.[45] The effects of ox-LDL on fibroblasts have also been examined. One study showed that ox-LDL treatment stimulates the proliferation of vascular fibroblasts,[46] and another study showed increased formation of collagen in LDL- or ox-LDL-treated fibroblasts.[47] As further evidence for a role of ox-LDL in atherosclerosis, plasma levels of ox-LDL are increased in patients with atherosclerosis and in those at high risk of developing atherosclerosis-related events.[48]

Other studies have shown that a number of antibodies to ox-LDL are increased in plasma in patients with atherosclerosis. Recent studies from our laboratory show that Cu-LDL-IgG antibody levels parallel the progression as well as regression of atherosclerosis.[49]

COMMON MODES OF PRO-ATHEROGENIC EFFECTS OF DYSLIPIDEMIA AND HYPERTENSION

Dyslipidemia and large amounts of Ang II exert very similar pro-atherogenic effects on the arterial wall, many of which have been discussed earlier. One of the major features of atherosclerosis is oxidative stress, more than can be neutralized by endogenous antioxidants,[18] and both dyslipidemia and hypertension enhance oxidative stress.

The adverse effects of RAS on vessel walls are exacerbated by the presence of dyslipidemia. Daugherty and Cassis[50] in an elegant study demonstrated aneurysm formation in the aorta in rodents given Ang II infusion, and this effect of Ang II was particularly marked in the presence of hypercholesterolemia.

In our laboratory, we fed New Zealand White rabbits high cholesterol diets for 10 weeks, which resulted in extensive plaque formation. There was intense up-regulation of AT_1 receptors. Importantly, therapy with losartan concurrent with high cholesterol diets decreased plaque formation, and most importantly, blocked many of the pro-atherogenic signals associated with atherosclerosis without affecting plasma cholesterol levels (Figure 39.2).[28,51]

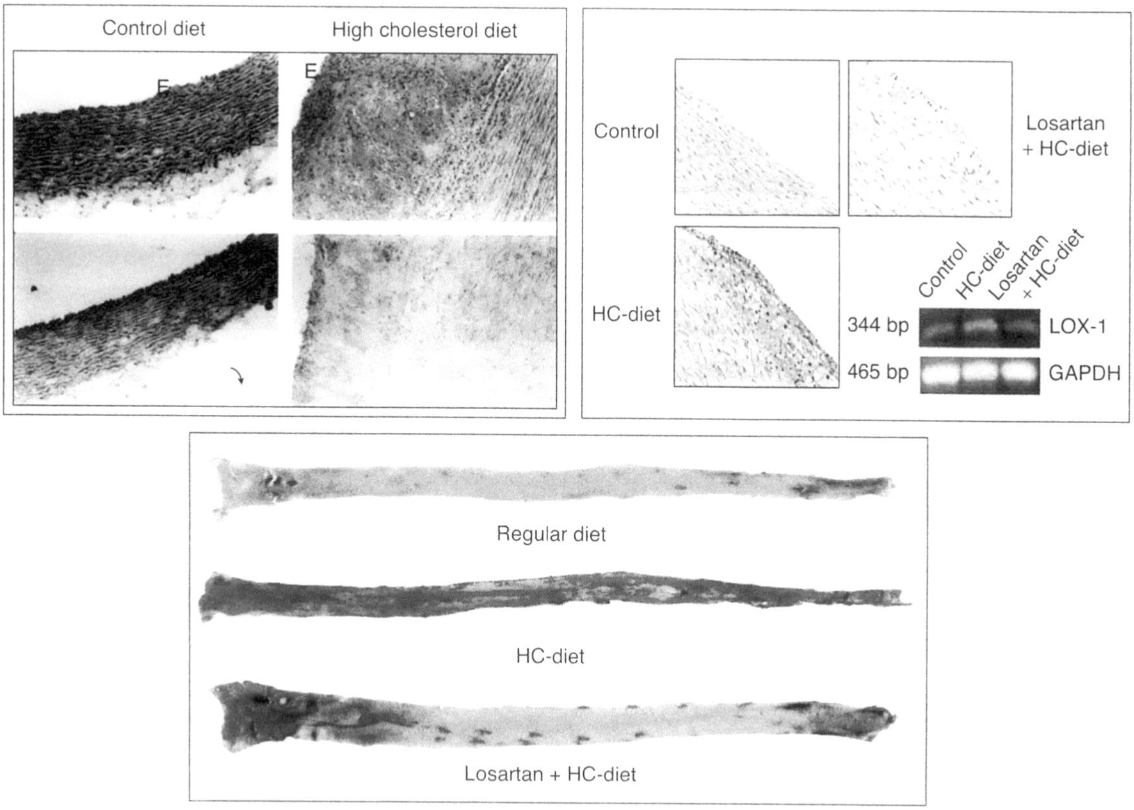

Figure 39.2 The atherosclerotic regions in the high cholesterol diet-fed rabbits exhibit intense immunostaining for Ang II AT_1receptors (top left) and LOX-1 (top right). Concurrent therapy with AT_1 receptor blocker losartan decreases LOX-1 expression, as determined by immunostaining and RT-PCR (inset upper right). This therapy reduces sudanophilic areas in the aorta (lower panel)

ANIMAL STUDIES ON THE FACILITATIVE INTERACTION BETWEEN DYSLIPIDEMIA AND RAS IN ATHEROSCLEROSIS

Since hyperlipidemia and RAS activation are two well-known interrelated risk factors for atherogenesis, the simultaneous blockades of hyperlipidemia and RAS (with statins) and AT_1 receptor blockers may have synergistic anti-atherosclerotic effects. Both these groups of agents are independently effective in preventing atherosclerosis-related events.

In recent studies, we observed that the concurrent treatment of hyperlipidemia and inhibition of RAS had a synergistic anti-atherogenic effect in apo-E-deficient mice. Apo-E-deficient mice were given regular chow supplemented with 1% cholesterol (high cholesterol diet) or rosuvastatin (a member of the HMG-CoA reductase inhibitor family, 1 mg/kg/day) in addition to a high cholesterol diet or the AT_1 receptor blocker candesartan (1 mg/kg/day) in addition to a high cholesterol diet. For the 'concurrent therapy' group, the mice were administered the two therapies concurrently along with the high cholesterol diet. All mice were treated for 12 weeks, and the extent of aortic atherosclerosis was measured by Sudan IV staining. We found that the aortic atherosclerosis induced by the high cholesterol diet was attenuated by rosuvastatin or candesartan given alone, but interestingly, the concurrent therapy had a synergistic anti-atherogenic effect (Figure 39.3).

We also examined the potential mechanisms for the synergistic anti-atherogenic effects of concurrent therapy. First, we observed the expression of LOX-1 in mice aorta from each group and found that both rosuvastatin and candesartan each decreased the expression of high cholesterol diet-induced LOX-1 expression (Figure 39.3). However, the concurrent therapy with rosuvastatin and candesartan decreased LOX-1 expression to a level even

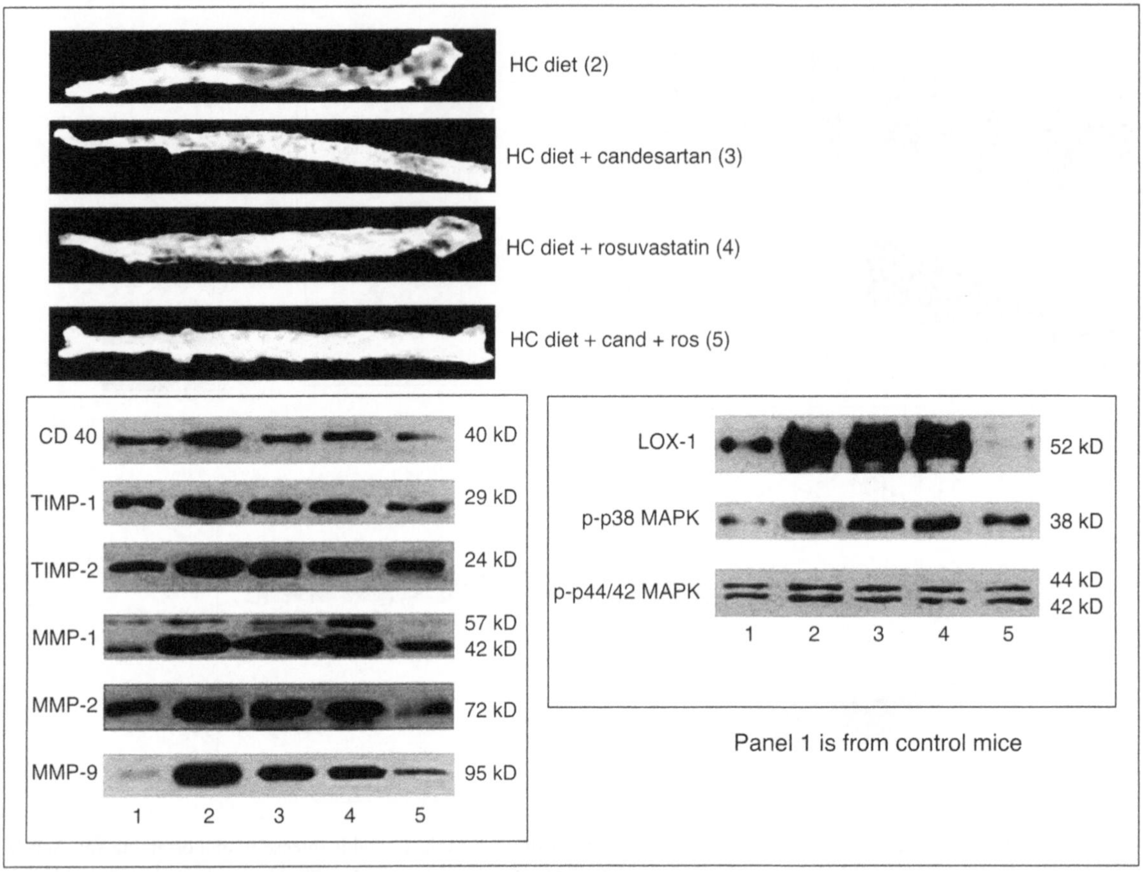

Figure 39.3 The sudanophilic areas in representative ApoE knockout mice given high cholesterol diet alone, or with rosuvastatin, candesartan, or both. Note that rosuvastatin and candesartan alone decrease the expression of CD40, MMPs, TIMPs, LOX-1 and p38 MAPK, whereas the combination therapy reduces the expression of all parameters to control levels

lower than the untreated negative control mice. Based on these observations, it is safe to state that LOX-1 is a critical player in atherogenesis, and it is targeted by anti-hyperlipidemia therapy as well as anti-RAS therapy, leading to potent anti-atherosclerotic effects. These observations gain support from preliminary observations that deletion of LOX-1 almost entirely blocks the evolution of atherosclerosis in LDL-receptor-deficient mice (unpublished data).

A number of studies support the idea that atherosclerosis is a chronic inflammatory disease. Considerable evidence implicates inflammatory mediators such as CD40,[52] MMPs,[53] and their endogenous tissue inhibitors TIMPs[54] as being involved in the development of atherosclerosis. CD40 expression has been shown to be inhibited by AT_1 receptor blockers[55] and statins.[56] The expression of MMPs has also been reduced by both AT_1 receptor blockers[51] and statins.[57] We looked at the expression of these inflammatory mediators in the mice aortas from each group in our study. We found that all these pro-atherogenic inflammatory mediators were markedly up-regulated in the apo-E-deficient mice after a 12-week period of feeding on a high cholesterol diet. Although these hyperlipidemia-induced effects were modestly attenuated by rosuvastatin or candesartan alone, the combination therapy showed total blockade of these pro-atherogenic mediators (Figure 39.3).

We also studied the signal transduction pathway involved in the regulated expression of LOX-1 and CD40 as well as MMPs in the mice aortas. We focused on MAPKs, because it has been shown that the oxidative stress-sensitive p38 subtype is involved in hyperlipidemia-induced atherosclerosis.[58] We identified that p38 MAPK (expression as well as phosphorylation) was up-regulated in apo-E-deficient mice fed a high cholesterol diet, compared with the control mice on a regular diet. Rosuvastatin and candesartan each had a moderate inhibitory effect on p38 MAPK expression and phosphorylation. However, the concurrent therapy dramatically reduced the expression as well as the phosphorylation of p38 MAPK back to the control level. We also checked the expression and phosphorylation of p44/42 MAPK, but did not find any changes among the different groups.

This study confirms the interaction between hyperlipidemia and RAS activation, and also implies that LOX-1 and inflammatory mediators MMPs and TIMPs as well as p38 MAPK play a critical role in atherogenesis. More importantly, this study has suggested a novel combination therapeutic strategy against atherosclerosis.

SUGGESTIVE EVIDENCE OF CROSS-TALK BETWEEN DYSLIPIDEMIA AND RAS IN HUMANS

Hypertension is found to be most prevalent in populations with high levels of serum cholesterol. Dyslipidemia may be another metabolic factor influencing blood pressure. These two entities are frequently associated, even when current rigorous definitions are used. Hypertensive individuals are more likely to become dyslipidemic over time.

Lloyd-Jones et al.[59] evaluated patients from the Framingham Heart Offspring Study and noted that on average more than 40% of men and 33% of women with blood pressures of 145/90 mm Hg or higher were also dyslipidemic. Sung et al.[60] examined the blood pressure responses to a standard mental arithmetic test in healthy, normotensive patients with hypercholesterolemia (mean total cholesterol, 263 mg/dl) and 33 normotensive, normocholesterolemic patients. None of the hypercholesterolemic patients were receiving lipid-lowering therapy. They noted that the blood pressure response during the arithmetic test was significantly higher in the hypercholesterolemic group compared with the normocholesterolemic group (18 vs 10 mm Hg, respectively, $p < 0.005$). In a double-blind crossover design, hypercholesterolemic patients were then divided into two subgroups and received 6 weeks of either lovastatin or placebo. Treatment with statins reduced total cholesterol and LDL-cholesterol levels and was associated with lower mean systolic blood pressure. Diastolic blood pressure changes did not significantly correlate with lipid-lowering, suggesting that hypercholesterolemic patients have exaggerated systolic blood pressure and that lipid-lowering therapy improves the patients' responses to stress.

Nazzaro et al.[61] examined the effects of lipid-lowering on blood pressure in hypertensive and hypercholesterolemic patients. Subjects were given a placebo for 4 weeks and then divided into two groups. Each group of 15 patients subsequently received simvastatin (10 mg) or enalapril (20 mg) for 14 weeks, and a combination of both drugs for an additional 14 weeks. Blood pressure was then measured during stressful stimuli such as the Stroop color test and the cold pressor forehead test. Enalapril lowered blood pressure, but interestingly, simvastatin also had a blood pressure-lowering effect, although to a lesser extent. The combination treatment had a much higher impact.

Several human studies have shown that lipid-lowering therapy with statins may have blood pressure-lowering effect.[62–68] Other clinical trials have also suggested an interaction between the RAS and dyslipidemia.[69–72] In the TREND (Trial on Reversing Endothelial Dysfunction), quinapril hydrochloride was shown to improve endothelial dysfunction in patients with elevated LDL-cholesterol levels of ≥130 mg/dl.[69] QUIET (Quinapril Ischemic Events Trial) studied the effect of ACE inhibition on coronary artery disease and showed less progression of disease in patients with LDL-cholesterol of ≥130 mg/dl.[70] In the LCAS (Lipoprotein and Coronary Atherosclerosis Study), the change in lumen diameter as assessed by quantitative coronary angiography was noted in patients randomized to fluvastatin sodium. LDL-cholesterol reduction was also analyzed by Marian et al.[71] according to the ACE insertion/deletion (I/D) phenotype. ELITE (Evaluation of Losartan In The Elderly) studied the effect of captopril and losartan in elderly patients with CHF and found a greater survival benefit in patients taking statins in addition to captopril and losartan.

CONCLUSIONS

Hypertension and dyslipidemia, the two major risk factors for atherosclerotic disease, are frequently associated in patients with coronary atherosclerosis. Data from clinical studies suggest the existence of lipoprotein–neurohormonal interactions that may adversely affect vascular ultrastructure and function. On the other hand, data from preclinical studies suggest up-regulation of RAS by dyslipidemia, most likely from increased ox-LDL production. Activation of RAS leads to the release of superoxide anions, transcriptional up-regulation of LDL and increased ox-LDL uptake in macrophages, smooth muscle cells, and endothelial cells. These findings broaden our vision regarding the interplay among different risk factors for atherosclerosis which can act synergistically to increase cardiovascular risk. It also extends our knowledge of the reduction of cardiovascular risk by the anti-atherosclerotic effects of local ACE inhibition. Trials aimed at modifying the RAS along with the drugs that reduce total cholesterol and LDL-cholesterol levels will address the clinical relevance of this biological interaction. In conclusion, findings from cellular, animal, and human experiments suggest a cross-talk between dyslipidemia and the RAS relative to vascular dynamics.

REFERENCES

1. Witztum JL, Steinberg D. Role of oxidized low-density lipoprotein in atherogenesis. J Clin Invest 1991; 88: 1785–92.
2. Aviram M. Modified forms of low-density lipoprotein and atherosclerosis. Atherosclerosis 1993; 98: 1–9.
3. Keidar A, Attias J, Heinrich R, Coleman R, Aviram M. Angiotensin II atherogenicity in apolipoprotein E deficient mice is associated with increased cellular biosynthesis. Atherosclerosis 1999; 146: 249–57.
4. Nickenig G, Baumer AT, Temur Y et al. Distinct and combined vascular effects of ACE blockade HMG-CoA reductase inhibition in hypertensive subjects. Hypertension 1999; 33: 719–25.
5. Keidar S. Angiotensin, LDL peroxidation and atherosclerosis. Life Sci 1998; 63: 1–11.
6. Keidar S, Kaplan M, Aviram M. Angiotensin II-modified LDL is taken up by macrophages via the scavenger receptor, leading to cellular cholesterol accumulation. Arterioscler Thromb Vasc Biol 1996; 16: 97–105.
7. Li DY, Zhang YC, Philips MI, Sawamura T, Mehta JL. Upregulation of endothelial receptor for oxidized low-density lipoprotein (LOX-1) in cultured human coronary artery endothelial cells by angiotensin II type 1 receptor activation. Circ Res 1999; 84: 1043–9.
8. Keidar A, Attias J, Heinrich R, Coleman R, Aviram M. Angiotensin II atherogenicity in apolipoprotein E deficient mice is associated with increased cellular biosynthesis. Atherosclerosis 1999; 146: 249–57.
9. Mitanchi H, Bandoh T, Kumura M, Totsuka T, Hayashi S. Increased activity of vascular ACE related to atherosclerosis lesions in hyperlipidemic rabbits. Am J Physiol 1996; 271: H1065–H1071.
10. Yang BC, Phillips MI, Mohuczy D et al. Increased angiotensin II type 1 receptor expression in hypercholesterolemic atherosclerosis in rabbits. Arterioscler Thromb Vasc Biol 1998; 18: 1433–9.
11. Schieffer B, Schieffer E, Hilfiker-Kleiner D et al. Expression of angiotensin II and interleukin 6 in human coronary atherosclerotic plaques: potential implications for inflammation and plaque instability. Circulation 2000; 101: 1372–8.
12. Gross CM, Gerbaulet, S, Quensel C et al. Angiotensin II type 1 receptor expression in human coronary arteries with variable degrees of atherosclerosis. Basic Res Cardiol 2002; 97: 327–33.
13. Nickenig G, Sachinidis A, Seewald S, Bohm M, Vetter H. Influence of oxidized low-density lipoprotein on vascular angiotensin II receptor expression. J Hypertens 1997; 15 (Suppl 6): S27–S30.
14. Li D, Saldeen T, Romeo F, Mehta JL. Oxidized LDL upregulates angiotensin II type 1 receptor expression in cultured human coronary artery endothelial cells: the potential role of transcription factor NF-kappa B. Circulation 2000; 102: 1970–6.
15. Wassman S, Nickenig G, Bohm M. HMG-CoA reductase inhibitor atorvastatin downregulates AT1 receptor gene expression and cell proliferation in vascular smooth muscle cells. Kidney Blood Press Res 1999; 21: 392–3.
16. Nickenig G, Baumer AT, Temur Y, Kebben D, Jockenhovel F, Bohm M. Statin-sensitive dysregulated AT1 receptor function and density in hypercholesterolemic men. Circulation 1999; 100: 2131–4.
17. Takai S, Shiota N, Kobayashi S, Matsumura E, Miyasaki M. Induction of chymase that forms angiotensin II in the monkey atherosclerotic aorta. FEBS Lett 1997; 412: 86–90.
18. Chen J, Mehta JL. Role of oxidative stress in coronary heart disease. Indian Heart J 2004; 56: 163–73.
19. Ehara S, Ueda M, Naruka T et al. Elevated levels of oxidized low-density lipoprotein show a positive relationship with the severity of acute coronary syndromes. Circulation 2001; 103: 1955–60.
20. Mehta JL, Li D. Identification, regulation and function of a novel lectin like oxidized low-density lipoprotein receptor. J Am Coll Cardiol 2002; 39: 1429–35.
21. Moriwakitt H, Kume N, Kataoka H et al. Expression of lectin-like oxidized low density lipoprotein receptor-1 in human and murine macrophages: upregulated expression by TNF-alpha. FEBS Lett 1998; 440: 29–32.
22. Murase T, Kume N, Korenaga R et al. Fluid shear stress transcriptionally induces lectin-like oxidized LDL receptor-1 in vascular endothelial cells. Circ Res 1998; 83: 329–33.
23. Li DY, Yang BC, Mehta JL. Ox-LDL induces apoptosis in cultured human coronary artery endothelial cells: role of PKC, PTK, bcl-2, and Fas. Am J Physiol 1998; 275: H568–H576.
24. Li D, Mehta JL. Upregulation of endothelial receptor for oxidized LDL (LOX-1) by oxidized LDL and implications in apoptosis of human coronary artery endothelial cells: evidence from use of antisense LOX-1 mRNA and chemical inhibitors. Arterioscler Thromb Vasc Biol 2000; 20: 1116–22.
25. Li D, Mehta JL. Antisense to LOX-1 inhibits oxidized-mediated upregulation of monocyte chemoattractant protein-1 and monocyte adhesion to human coronary artery endothelial cells. Circulation 2000; 101: 2889–95.
26. Li D, Yang B, Philips MI, Mehta JL. Pro-apoptotic effects of angiotensin II in human coronary artery endothelial cells: role of AT1 receptor and PKC activation. Am J Physiol 1999; 276: H786–H792.
27. Mehta JL, Li D. Facilitative interaction between angiotensin II and oxidized LDL in cultured human coronary artery endothelial cells. J Renin Angiotensin Aldosterone Syst 2001; 2: D70–S76.
28. Chen H, Li D, Sawamura T, Inoue K, Mehta JL. Upregulation of LOX-1 expression in aorta of hypercholesterolemic rabbits: modulation by losartan. Biochem Biophys Res Commun 2000; 276: 1100–4.
29. Li DY, Chen HJ, Staples ED et al. Oxidized LDL receptor LOX-1 and apoptosis in human atherosclerotic lesions. J Cardiovasc Pharmacol Ther 2002; 7: 147–53.
30. Chen LY, Haught WH, Yang BC et al. Preservation of endogenous antioxidant activity and inhibition of lipid peroxidation as common mechanisms of anti-atherosclerotic effect of vitamin E, lovastatin and amlodipine. J Am Coll Cardiol 1997; 30: 569–75.
31. Mehta JL, Li D, Chen HJ et al. Inhibition of LOX-1 by statins may relate to upregulation of eNOS. Biochem Biophys Res Commun 2001; 289: 857–61.

32. Li D, Chen H, Romeo F et al. Statins modulate oxidized low-density lipoprotein-mediated adhesion molecule expression in human coronary artery endothelial cells: role of LOX-1. J Pharmacol Exp Ther 2002; 302: 601–5.
33. Hayek T, Attias J, Coleman R et al. The angiotensin-converting enzyme inhibitor, fosinopril, and the angiotensin II receptor antagonist, losartan, inhibit LDL oxidation and attenuate atherosclerosis independent of lowering blood pressure in apolipoprotein E deficient mice. Cardiovasc Res 1999; 44: 579–87.
34. Leif SJ, Karin P, Gunnar A, Rolf GGA, Bengt EK, Anders GO. Antiatherosclerotic effects of the angiotensin-converting enzyme inhibitors captopril and fosinopril in hypercholesterolemic minipigs. J Cardiovasc Pharmacol 1994; 24: 670–7.
35. Hayek T, Attias J, Coleman R et al. The angiotensin-converting enzyme inhibitor, fosinopril, and the angiotensin II receptor antagonist, losartan, inhibit LDL oxidation and attenuate atherosclerosis independent of lowering blood pressure in apolipoprotein E deficient mice. Cardiovasc Res 1999; 44: 579–87.
36. Bavry AA, Li D, Zander DS, Phillips MI, Mehta JL. Inhibition of arterial thrombogenesis by quinapril but not losartan. J Cardiovasc Pharmacol Ther 2000; 5: 121–7.
37. Becker RH, Wiemer G, Linz W. Preservation of endothelial function by ramipril in rabbits on a long-term atherogenic diet. J Cardiovasc Pharmacol 1991; 18: S110–S115.
38. Farhy RD, Carretro OA, Ho KL, Scicli AG. Role of kinins and nitric oxide in the effects of angiotensin converting enzyme inhibitors on neointima formation. Circ Res 1993; 72: 1202–10.
39. Chen K, Chen J, Li D, Zhang X, Mehta JL. Angiotensin II regulation of collagen type I expression in cardiac fibroblasts: modulation by PPAR-gamma ligand pioglitazone. Hypertension 2004; 44: 655–61.
40. Lauren WB, Khan QA, Rajagopalan S et al. Usefulness of quinapril and irbesartan to improve the anti-inflammatory response of atorvastatin and aspirin in patients with coronary heart disease. Am J Cardiol 2003; 91: 1116–19.
41. Touyz RM, Berry C. Recent advances in angiotensin II signaling. Braz J Med Biol Res 2002; 35: 1001–15.
42. Ohkubo N, Matsubara H, Nozawa Y et al. Angiotensin type 2 receptors are reexpressed by cardiac fibroblasts from failing myopathic hamster hearts and inhibit cell growth and fibrillar collagen metabolism. Circulation 1997; 96: 3954–62.
43. Jugdutt BI, Xu Y, Balghith M, Moudgil R, Menon V. Cardioprotection induced by AT1R blockade after reperfused myocardial infarction: association with regional increase in AT2R, IP3R and PKCepsilon proteins and cGMP. J Cardiovasc Pharmacol Ther 2000; 5: 301–11.
44. Li D, Mehta JL. 3-hydroxy-3-methylglutaryl coenzyme A reductase inhibitors protect against oxidized low-density lipoprotein-induced endothelial dysfunction. Endothelium 2003; 10: 17–21.
45. Chatterjee S. Role of oxidized human plasma low density lipoproteins in atherosclerosis: effects on smooth muscle cell proliferation. Mol Cell Biochem 1992; 111: 143–7.
46. Bjorkerud B, Bjorkerud S. Contrary effects of lightly and strongly oxidized LDL with potent promotion of growth versus apoptosis on arterial smooth muscle cells, macrophages, and fibroblasts. Arterioscler Thromb Vasc Biol 1996; 16: 416–24.
47. Joseph J, Ranganathan S, Mehta JL. Low-density lipoproteins modulate collagen metabolism in fibroblasts. J Cardiovasc Pharmacol Ther 2003; 8: 161–6.
48. Ridker PM, Brown NJ, Harrison DG, Mehta JL, Vaughn DE. Established and emerging plasma biomarkers in the prediction of first atherothrombotic event. Circulation 2004: 109 (25 Suppl 1): IV6–IV19.
49. Chen J, Li D, Witztum J, Miller E, Mehta JL. A specific antibody against ox-LDL, Cu-LDL-IgG, may serve as a marker for predictor of atherosclerosis. Circulation 2004; in press.
50. Daugherty A, Cassis LA. Mechanisms of abdominal aortic aneurysm formation. Curr Atheroscler Rep 2002; 4: 222–7.
51. Chen H, Mehta JL. Modulation of matrix metalloproteinase-1, its tissue inhibitor, and nuclear factor-kappa B by losartan in hypercholesterolemia rabbits. J Cardiovasc Pharmacol 2002; 39: 332–9.
52. Schonbeck U, Libby P. CD40 signaling and plaque instability. Circ Res 2001; 89: 1092–103.
53. Beaudeux JL, Giral P, Bruckert E, Foglietti MJ, Chapman MJ. Matrix metalloproteinases and atherosclerosis. Ann Biol Clin 2003; 61: 147–58.
54. Noji Y, Kajinami K, Kawashiri MA et al. Circulating matrix metalloproteinases and their inhibitors in premature coronary atherosclerosis. Clin Chem Lab Med 2001; 39: 380–4.
55. Nahmod KA, Vermeulen ME, Raiden S, Nahmod V, Giordano M, Geffner JR. Control of dendritic cell differentiation by angiotensin II. FASEB J 2003; 17: 491–3.
56. Schonbeck U, Gerdes N, Ganz P, Kinlay S, Libby P. Oxidized low-density lipoprotein augments and 3-hydroxy-3-methylglutaryl coenzyme A reductase inhibitors limit CD40 and CD40L expression in human vascular cells. Circulation 2002; 106: 2888–93.
57. Bellosta S, Via D, Canavesi M, Bernini F. HMG-CoA reductase inhibitors reduce MMP-9 secretion by macrophages. Arterioscler Thromb Vasc Biol 1998; 18: 1671–8.
58. Werle M, Schmal U, Hanna K et al. MCP-1 induces activation of MAP-kinases ERK, JNK, and p38 MAPK in human endothelial cells. Cardiovasc Res 2002; 56: 284–92.
59. Lloyd-Jones DM, Evans JC, Larson MG, O'Donnell CJ, Wilson PWF, Levy D. Cross-classification of JNC VI blood pressure stages and risk groups in the Framingham Heart Study. Arch Intern Med 1999; 159: 2206–12.
60. Sung BH, Izzo JI, Wilson MF. Effects of cholesterol reduction on BP response to mental stress in patients with high cholesterol. Am J Hypertens 1997; 10: 592–9.
61. Nazzaro P, Manzari M, Merlo M et al. Distinct and combined vascular effects of ACE blockade and HMG-CoA reductase inhibition in hypertensive subjects. Hypertension 1999; 33: 719–25.
62. O'Callaghan CJ, Krum H, Conway EL et al. Short-term effects of pravastatin on blood pressure in hypercholesterolaemic hypertensive patients. Blood Press 1994; 3: 404–6.
63. Abetel G, Poget PN, Bonnabry JP. Hypotensive effect of an inhibitor of cholesterol synthesis (fluvastatin): a pilot study. Schweiz Med Wochenschr 1998; 128: 272–7.
64. Glorioso N, Troffa C, Filigheddu F et al. Effect of the HMG-CoA reductase inhibitors on blood pressure in patients with essential hypertension and primary hypercholesterolemia. Hypertension 2000; 36: E1–E2.
65. Sposito AC, Mansur AP, Coelho OR, Nicolau JC, Ramirez JA. Additional reduction in blood pressure after cholesterol-lowering treatment by statins (lovastatin or pravastatin) in hypercholesterolemic patients using angiotensin-converting enzyme inhibitors (enalapril or lisinopril). Am J Cardiol 1999; 83: 1497–9.
66. Borghi C, Prandin MG, Costa FV, Baccheli S, Degli Esposti D, Ambrosioni E. Use of statins and blood pressure control in treated hypertensive patients with hypercholesterolemia. J Cardiovasc Pharmacol 2000; 35: 549–55.
67. Tonolo G, Melis MG, Formato M et al. Additive effects of simvastatin beyond its effects on LDL cholesterol in hypertensive type 2 diabetic patients. Eur J Clin Invest 2000; 30: 980–7.

68. Jonkers IJ, de Man FH, van der Laarse A et al. Bezafibrate reduces heart rate and blood pressure in patients with hypertriglyceridemia. J Hypertens 2001; 19: 749–55.
69. Mancini GB, Henry GC, Macaya C et al. Angiotensin-converting enzyme inhibition with quinapril improves endothelial vasomotor dysfunction in patients with coronary artery disease: the TREND (Trial on Reversing Endothelial Dysfunction). Circulation 1996; 94: 258–65.
70. Pitt B, O'Neill B, Feldman R et al. The Quinapril Ischemic Event Trial (QUIET): evaluation of chronic ACE inhibitor therapy in patients with ischemic heart disease and preserved left ventricular function. Am J Cardiol 2001; 87: 1058–63.
71. Marian AJ, Safavi F, Ferlic L, Dunn JK, Gotto AM, Ballantyne CM. Interactions between angiotensin-I converting enzyme insertion/deletion polymorphism and response of plasma lipids and coronary atherosclerosis to treatment with fluvastatin: the lipoprotein and coronary atherosclerosis study. J Am Coll Cardiol 2000; 35: 89–95.
72. Pitt B, Poole-Wilson PA, Segal R et al. Effect of losartan compared with captopril on mortality in patients with symptomatic heart failure: randomized trial, the Losartan Heart Failure Survival Study ELITE II. Lancet 2000; 355: 1582–7.

40

Molecular mechanisms in obesity hypertension: focus on the renin-angiotensin system and the sympathetic nervous system

Dalila B Corry and Michael L Tuck

INTRODUCTION

There has been a marked increase in the prevalence of overweight and obesity across the world in both industrialized and non-industrialized countries. In the US, 64% of the adult population is overweight and about 30% are obese (body mass index, BMI>30). Also in Europe more than 50% of the population between 35 and 65 years of age is overweight or obese. Obesity and especially visceral obesity is strongly associated with arterial hypertension documented throughout different racial groups, ethnic groups, age levels, gender, and socioeconomic status. In most industrialized countries there is an almost linear relationship between body weight and blood pressure (BP) level; in fact just examining the general cause of hypertension shows that 78% of its risk in men is associated with obesity and this same figure reaches almost 65% in women. The therapeutic value of weight reduction in controlling BP is documented in almost every study examining this relationship.

There are numerous different regulatory systems that participate in the mechanism for hypertension in obesity including central mechanisms, renal sodium handling, the renin-angiotensin-aldosterone system (RAAS), the sympathetic nervous system (SNS), the adipocyte and the various adipocytokine products it produces and hormones such as insulin, leptin, adinopectin, atrial natriuretic hormones and several new candidate factors. Most of the knowledge in these areas connecting obesity and hypertension is based on epidemiologic or physiologic studies, with a dearth of knowledge on the molecular basis of obesity hypertension. The present chapter will address several abnormalities in these regulatory systems and the knowledge available in the molecular area to explain the tight relation between BP and BMI.

THE RENIN-ANGIOTENSIN-ALDOSTERONE SYSTEM

Tuck and Sowers and colleagues[1–3] showed in 1981 that levels of plasma renin activity (PRA) were elevated in obese individuals. Additionally, with severe caloric restriction over 12 weeks a highly significant fall in blood pressure was accompanied by a fall in PRA levels to normal. Interestingly, to attain normal BP and PRA, the obese individuals did not need to reach ideal body weight; in fact, they only lost 5–10% of their initial body weight. Later studies from our laboratory showed that other components of the RAAS including angiotensinogen, angiotensin I, and angiotensin II (Ang II) also were elevated in obesity hypertension and fell with weight loss.[3,4] Since these studies numerous investigators have found that both the circulating and the tissue RAAS are high in obesity hypertension.[5–16] Given that obesity is generally associated with some degree of sodium and water retention, even normal activity of the RAAS would be surprising as the system should be suppressed unless the RAAS elevation is connected to the fluid retention in obesity; an observation that has never been well established. There may be a molecular explanation for the elevation in the RAAS in obesity.[5–7] A large amount of data now shows that most components of the RAAS are present in the adipocyte

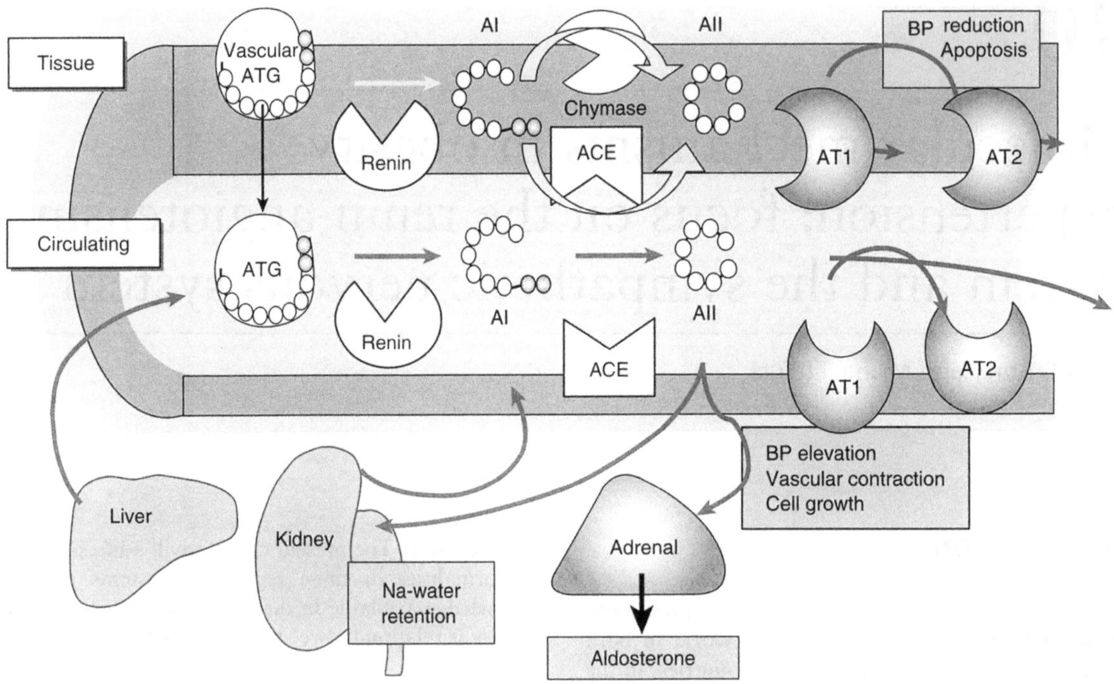

Figure 40.1 Components of the RAAS as depicted in a blood vessel

and there is a correlation with adipocyte mass and levels of RAAS components.[5–11] In fact, adipose tissue especially in obesity may be an important site for production of angiotensinogen (AGT). Studies have shown a positive correlation between adipocyte AGT, blood pressure, and body weight.[8–12] Further observations now reveal that obese subjects have higher levels of circulating AGT and some have concluded that the main source for circulating AGT in obesity is not the liver but is from the adipocyte and that this rise in AGT could contribute to body size, gonadal hormones and nutritional status.[12–19]

In animal models of obesity such as the obese Zucker rat, AGT mRNA expression is substantially elevated in adipose tissue when compared with the lean Zucker control rats.[19] Overexpression of AGT in adipose tissue in an AGT knockout mouse can restore AGT levels and this correction raises BP due to increased sodium retention.[20–22] These high levels of AGT in obesity could imply a high level of Ang II as the active end-product acting on renal sodium balance and vascular tone in obesity.[23,24] Ang II mRNA expression levels are also higher in cultured adipocytes,[23–25] and there are higher circulating levels of Ang II in obese subjects.[5–7] Locally produced Ang II has been shown to increase leptin production[8,25] and activate prostaglandin I_2 that, in turn, stimulates adipocyte differentiation from pre-adipocytes into mature adipocytes.[26] These observations raise the possibility that local RAAS might also further enhance the increase in fat mass seen in obesity. In mouse and human adipocytes in culture, Ang II also elevates triglyceride content.

High levels of AGT mRNA are found in rat brown and white tissues; AGT levels were as much as 60% of those found in liver, the primary source of AGT.[25,27] In the 3T3L1 white adipocyte cell line, AGT mRNA expression was correlated to adipocyte differentiation.[28] Thus, AGT expression is closely correlated with adipocyte phenotype. AGT in adipocytes can be regulated by many factors such as fatty acids,[29] glucocorticoids,[30] insulin,[31] and other factors. In fact, food intake during a fasting period produces a decrease in AGT production in epidermal white fat and feeding increases its production.[32] Also, Ang II production is increased by feeding in the epididymal fat pad from ob/ob mice compared with C57 controls. However, in the Zucker fa/fa mRNA expression of Ang II in adipose tissue is decreased by feeding.[19] These findings suggest a role for

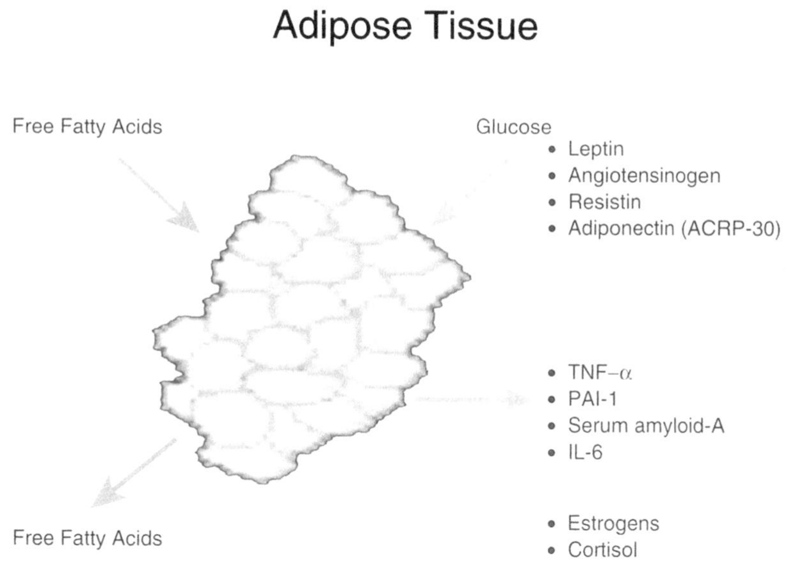

Figure 40.2 Adipocytes are endocrine glands that secrete important hormones, cytokines, vasoactive substances and other peptides

the adipocyte RAAS in the control of food intake as well as in adipocyte differentiation. Most evidence shows that Ang II can be processed to other angiotensin peptides in brown adipose tissue, white adipocyte cell lines (3T3L1, 3T3–F442A),[28,33] and human adipose tissue.[28,33] The exact processing enzymes are not well understood, as renin is found in low quantity in fat cells and alternate serine peptidase enzymes such as chymase and chemothepsins may be important. However, mostly the renin and angiotensin converting enzyme (ACE) have been localized in human white adipose tissue.[34] Intrascapular brown adipose tissue (ISBAT) can also form Ang II and other angiotensins, suggesting the presence of other processing enzymes RAAS.

Alternative processing enzymes such as chymases may function instead of ACE in adipose tissue. Additionally, subtypes of the Ang II receptor such as the AT_2 receptor have been localized in brown and white adipose tissue.[35] These AT_2 receptors are of high affinity to Ang II with kinetics similar to the AT_1 receptors in other Ang II target tissues sites such as heart, kidneys and adrenal glands.[35] As some of the effects of Ang II are blocked by a specific antagonist of the AT_2 receptor subtype in adipose tissue, the AT_2 receptor may also be functional in the regulation of fat differentiation and distribution.[35]

There may be several potential functions for Ang II in fat cells. Ang II can activate sympathetic nervous system (SNS) activity by facilitating the release of norepinephrine (NE) in slices of fat brown.[36] Ang II may also be involved in cold thermogenesis in brown adipose tissue.[37] It could be proposed that the RAAS system has an effect on body weight with low RAAS components favoring obesity as seen in the Zucker obese rat. The opposite might also pertain that high activity of the RAAS system in fat cells would favor a more normal body weight. Chronic infusion of Ang II has been shown to cause a reduction in food intake and body weight in rats in a dose-dependent fashion. Infusion of Ang II also lowers plasma leptin levels and reduces adipose tissue mass.[38] A most likely explanation for the effect of Ang II on food intake and body weight would be its normal augmentation of NE release with activation of brown adipose tissue metabolism and increased energy expenditure. Thus, Ang II might act to both reduce energy intake through unknown mechanisms and increase energy expenditure by activating the SNS. Ang II may also regulate the fat cell cycle progression, as studies show that it has an effect on differentiation of the fat cell phenotype.[38] Ang II may also control adiposity by regulating free fatty acid metabolism, as it can increase triglyceride content by activating lipogenic enzymes such as fatty acid synthetase and glycerol-3-phosphate dehydrogenase.[27] These observations also point towards a strong role for adipose-derived Ang II in the genesis of obesity-related hypertension. Studies show that there is a strong correlation between Ang II levels, BMI, and plasma leptin levels.[39] Plasma Ang II levels show a positive correlation to blood pressure, especially in subjects with a family history of hypertension.[5-7] Thus, the adipocyte itself may play a key molecular role through its highly active tissue RAAS expression, in control of body weight through actions on SNS activity, regulation of adipose tissue mass and differentiation, regulation of fatty acid metabolism, and finally by effects on food intake. It is of recent interest that blockade of the RAAS increases adiponectin concentration in patients with essential hypertension that would improve insulin sensitivity and obesity.[40] Also, blockade of the RAAS reduces adipocyte size and improves insulin sensitivity.[41]

Polymorphisms in the Ang II converting enzyme (ACE) have been described in obesity and hypertension. In Caucasian subjects, the insertion/deletion (I/D) polymorphism of the ACE gene is associated with coronary artery disease (CAD) and fatal myocardial infarction. On the other hand, Pima Indians have a low incidence of CAD despite a high prevalence of diabetes. This discrepancy has been proposed to be due to a lower frequency of the D allele in Pima Indians compared with Caucasians.[42] Yet findings show that the ACE gene I/D polymorphism is not likely to be a major determinant of CAD in Pima Indians. Plasma ACE levels, but not ACE genotype, correlated with plasma glucose and BP, suggesting that elevated plasma ACE levels may contribute to the link between insulin resistance and CAD in this population.[42]

Overweight and obesity have been described as associated with increased levels of aldosterone[1,43] that might contribute to hypertension in obesity. Investigators[44] have proposed that the adipocyte directly stimulates adrenocortical aldosterone release, as in a recent study where secretory products from the human adipocyte stimulated steroidogenesis in human adrenocortical cells (NCI-H295R).[43] These data suggest that excess expression of aldosterone, as well as Ang II, may play a big role in the pathogenesis of obesity.

THE SYMPATHETIC NERVOUS SYSTEM AND ADRENORECEPTOR POLYMORPHISMS

Excess sympathetic nervous activity (SNA) as reflected by elevated plasma NE levels has been described in very obese individuals both in the basal state and after upright posture stimulation.[2] Moreover, during weight loss there is a significant fall in plasma NE levels that is highly correlated with reductions in body weight and blood pressure.[2] Although these studies point to a heightened level of SNA in obesity, they do not identify the source of sympathetic overdrive. Other investigators using direct measurement of SNA with the microneurography method, have found a several fold increase in sympathetic discharge in young, very obese subjects who were normotensive.[45] Studies from other laboratories[46] using the NE spillover technique identified regional NE excess in the kidneys of obese subjects, suggesting a renal source for neurogenic overdrive in obesity leading to Na and water retention. Hall et al.[47] have shown that blockade of both α- and β-adrenoceptors blunts the increases in arterial BP that occurs in fat-fed obese dogs.[47] Increased SNA in obesity could also result from circulating humoral factors such as increased expression of insulin and leptin exerting central and peripheral actions on SNA. It should be noted that there are experimental studies that have not found heightened SNA in obesity.[48]

Obesity results from an imbalance between caloric intake and energy expenditure and the adrenergic system could play a major role in the control of energy expenditure. Catecholamines mobilize energy-rich lipids by stimulating lipolysis in fat cells and producing thermogenesis in brown fat and skeletal muscle. These effects are mediated through the β-adrenergic system and mainly the β3-adrenergic receptor, although some effects are transmitted by the β1- and β2-adrenoceptors. The β3-adrenoceptor differs from the other receptors in that it has a lower affinity for catecholamines and is more resistant to desensitization or down-regulation.[49] Low β3-adrenergic activity could promote obesity through decreased thermogenesis in brown adipose tissue, decreased function of the β receptor in white adipose tissue with slowing of lipolysis causing retention of lipids in fat cells.[49]

Studies of candidate genes show that most of the genes that associate with obesity control important functions of adipose tissue. Structural variation in these genes may alter adipose tissue function in a way that promotes obesity. Genes that are functional in human adipose tissue include hormone-sensitive lipase, α2-adrenoceptors, β2-adrenoceptors and β3-adrenoceptors, uncoupling protein-1 (UCP-1), peroxisome proliferator activating receptor gamma (PPARγ), tumor necrosis factor-α (TNF-α), and low density lipoprotein receptor. These genes contribute to obesity by gene–gene interactions (β3-adrenoceptor and uncoupling protein-1) or by gene–environmental interactions (β2-adrenoceptors and physical activity).

The pathophysiology of the β3-adrenoceptor in obesity is being actively investigated. The β3-adrenergic receptor, expressed mainly in brown and white adipose tissue in rodents and in visceral fat in humans, is actively involved in the regulation of lipolysis and thermogenesis.[50] A pathological role for the visceral fat β3-adrenergic receptor in humans was investigated by Lonnquist et al.[51] who found that obese subjects have higher fat cell volume, and a several-fold higher rate of fatty acid production and glycerol response to NE. They also found a 50 times higher sensitivity of the β3-adrenergic receptor along with greater coupling efficiency of the β3-adrenoceptor and a six fold reduction in sensitivity to the α2-adrenoceptor. This group also noticed that only β3-adrenoceptor activities correlated with NE-induced lipolysis and fat cell volume. It was concluded that elevated rates of lipolysis in obesity are mainly due to an increased rate of β3-adrenoceptor function along with a reduced α2-adrenoceptor function. Another investigative group examined the relation of the β3-adrenoceptor in the visceral fat in subjects with the metabolic syndrome finding that increased visceral fat β3-adrenoceptor sensitivity was associated with metabolic complications.[52] Thus, β3-adrenoceptor sensitivity may be best related to upper body visceral obesity as seen in the metabolic syndrome.

As it plays a crucial role in regulating the storage and mobilization of energy, adipose tissue has been a strong focus in efforts to identify candidate genes for obesity such as the β3-adrenoreceptor gene[53] as it is the main receptor involved in the regulation of thermogenesis and lipolysis in brown and white adipose tissue, especially in rodents.[54] Krief et al.[55] noted that the β3-adrenoceptor in humans is expressed predominantly in fat and adipocytes lining the gastrointestinal tract. The receptor's primary role is thought to be in the regulation of the resting metabolic rate and lipolysis.[56] Thus, the β3-adrenergic receptor, located mainly in adipose tissue, is involved in the sympathetic control of body fat mass by regulating utilization of fat stores. This receptor also regulates the rate of lipid assimilation during the digestive process that affects lipolysis and thermogenesis.[55] In animal models of obesity and type 2 diabetes, selective β3-adrenoceptor agonists produce significant weight loss and improve glucose homeostasis.[56] However, these compounds are less selective for the human β3-adrenoceptor and induce β1- and β2-adrenoceptor side effects because of their poor selectivity in humans.[57] Numerous pharmacological studies using highly selective β3-adrenergic agonists have confirmed the involvement of β3-adrenoceptors in both adipocyte lipolysis and thermogenic activity. In vivo studies using the microdialysis technique have revealed a weak role for β3- compared with β1- and β2-adrenoceptors in control of both lipolysis and nutritive blood in human subcutaneous adipose tissue.[38] However, it has also been proposed that increased β3-adrenoceptor components in adipose tissue could be responsible for the enhanced delivery of free fatty acids into the portal vein; a process that could be involved in the formation of abdominal obesity.[51] Thus, an abnormality in the β3-adrenergic receptor could potentially represent a link between abdominal obesity and insulin resistance through the free fatty acid pathway.

Studies in Pima Indians, Finnish subjects and Mexican Americans have shown a missense mutation in the β3-adrenoceptor gene, resulting in the replacement of tryptophan by arginine at position 64 (Trp64Arg) associated with early onset of type 2 diabetes (DM), a decreased resting metabolic rate, insulin resistance, and weight gain.[58] The findings imply that the genotype of the β3-adrenoceptor is one of the genetic determinants of body weight and a predisposing factor for DM. Not all investigators have found a relationship between the Try64Arg missense and obesity and these discrepancies could be due to ethnic differences, as the frequency of the Arg64 allele is quite different between racial groups.[59] The Arg64 mutation has been reported to be more frequent in Japanese than other ethnic groups (0.37 in Japanese versus 0.04 in Swedish subjects).[59] The Trp64Arg mutation of the β3-adrenoceptor gene had no effect on obesity in the Quebec Family Study and in Swedish obese cohorts.[59] In the Finnish population, the Try64Arg mutation is associated with weight gain, abdominal obesity and insulin resistance.[60] However, in some ethnic groups, this mutation may have a protective effect against metabolic disorders.[61] The Pima Indians may represent the best manifestation of the Arg64 allele as studied in 642 Pima Indians (390 with DM and 252 non-diabetic subjects), where this mutation may accelerate the onset of type 2 diabetes by altering the balance of energy metabolism in visceral fat tissue. Walston et al.[62] reported that the Pima Indian individuals homozygous for the Arg 64 mutation and Arg/Try heterozygotes expend an average of 82 and 36 Kcal/day, respectively, less than normal Pima Indian homozygotes due to a decreased resting metabolic rate. It is also possible that the β3-adrenoceptor mutation exerts an energy-saving effect during limited food intake. In this sense, Yoshida et al.[63] reported that obese women with the Trp64Arg mutation were more resistant to weight loss during a low calorie diet than matched subjects with the wild-type genotype (Trp/Trp).

Most major investigations suggest that the Trp64 Arg mutation relates to obesity, insulin resistance, weight gain, and hypertension. Individuals who are homozygous for the Arg64 allele have decreases in acute insulin release to glucose and lower glucose effectiveness. There is a decreased ability of glucose to influence its own uptake in the Arg64 homozygous subject as a second mechanism where the Trp64Arg variant may affect glucose homeostasis.[64] The frequency of the Trp64Arg allele is similar in the morbid obese and normal weight subjects. However, subjects with morbid obesity who are heterozygous for the Trp64Arg mutation have an increased capacity to gain weight.[65] It was also postulated that mutational defects in the β3-adrenoceptor in very obese subjects may affect binding, signal transduction or regulatory mechanisms, so their defect may be caused by functional differences in the Trp64Arg mutation. Any of these defects could result in diminished lipolytic responses in adipose tissue with exacerbation of obesity.[66,67]

In a large Japanese cohort study of 1685 subjects (935 women and 750 men), the genotype Arg/Arg but not Trp/Arg was associated with type 2 diabetes but very few subjects were carrying the Arg/Arg genotype ($n=44$).[68] They compared the frequency of obesity and type 2 diabetes between Arg/Arg and Trp/Trp ($n=1155$) and Arg/Arg had a higher frequency of obesity and type 2 diabetes (13.6% vs 3.29%, $p<0.001$, 13.6% vs 4.16%, $p<0.007$, respectively). In a Finnish population, the ability of visceral obesity to predict the mutation in the β3-adrenoceptor was studied by the gene encoding the β3-adrenoceptor (Trp64Arg) in visceral fat.[60] In this study, Finnish subjects ($n=355$, 207 non-diabetics and 128 type 2 diabetic subjects) were studied. The Try64Arg allele was associated with abdominal obesity and insulin resistance and there was a suggestion that it contributed to early-onset diabetes in this population.[60] Another investigative team showed that BMI was higher in subjects carrying the Arg allele than in those who were homozygous for Trp and that there was no association of the Arg haplotype with blood pressure and metabolic parameters. They administered a β3-adrenoceptor agonist (CGP12177) in visceral adipocytes and found that its sensitivity was decreased 10-fold in Arg compared with Trp subjects. It was concluded that a well-conserved β3-Arg haplotype was associated with moderate overweight and decreased receptor function.[66] Arner[67] has reviewed the importance of polymorphisms in catecholamine signaling pathways for lipolysis. A Trp64Arg polymorphism of the β3-receptor that is associated with obesity is accompanied by changes in lipolytic sensitivity of the receptor in human fat cells. Similarly, a Gln16Glu and an Arg164Ile variation in the β2-receptor causes marked variations in the lipolytic sensitivity of this receptor in human adipocytes.

Not all population studies have found that the Trp64 Arg mutation in the β3-adrenoceptor relates to obesity, insulin resistance, and hypertension. Shiwaku et al.[68,69] found in Japanese men and women that the Trp64Arg mutation is not a major determinant of obesity but it may relate especially in women to more difficulty in losing weight. In addition, in the Japanese population, the Trp64Arg mutation does not play a role in susceptibility to essential hypertension, insulin resistance or basal adrenergic state.[70] In another study from Japan, Azuma et al.[71] showed that the Trp64Arg allele may contribute to insulin resistance in individuals with a moderate BMI. In a longitudinal analysis, it was also shown in Japanese subjects that the Arg64 alleles of the Trp64Arg mutation of the β3-receptor do not contribute to obesity of type 2 diabetes.[72] However, Japanese people with a western lifestyle (Japanese-American men with impaired glucose tolerance) have an association between the Trp64Arg and insulin resistance, suggesting a strong effect of lifestyle in association with disorders of the β3-adrenoceptor in its metabolic effects.

In young healthy Danish subjects (mean age 25 years) a homozygous mutation (Arg/Arg) can affect growth and body weight gain during childhood to adolescence rather than during adulthood, although the results were obtained from only three homozygous subjects, so the result must be interpreted with caution. However, their results are the first to suggest that age may be an important factor in studying the relation of the Trp64Arg mutation in its role in weight gain and metabolic disorders.[73] In a large population-based Caucasian cohort from Germany ($n=6450$) the Arg64 allele of the Trp64 Arg had no significant association with metabolic disorder.[74] Furthermore, in 200 Caucasian subjects (137 with and 63 without diabetes), there was no association between the β3-adrenoceptor polymorphism and gender, obesity, blood pressure and HbA1c.[75] Additionally, in the Quebec Family Study and the Swedish Obese Subjects studies, no association was found between the Trp64Arg mutation and BMI, body fat, visceral fat, resting metabolic rate and other metabolic parameters.[59] The insulin receptor substrate (IRS-1) has been linked to the β3-adrenergic receptor in the pathogenesis of obesity related to increased insulin resistance and there might be synergy between the polymorphisms of the Trp64Arg and the Gly972Arg mutation of the IRS-1 gene as found in obese German women who had difficulty in weight loss.[76]

Thus, a large number of studies have shown either an association between obesity and the β3-adrenoceptor or a lack thereof. The explanation for such discrepant findings is not entirely clear. It is not small number of subjects studied, gender, age or consistent differences in ethnic background. There seem to be discrepancies even in similar ethnic groups. Maybe there is truly only a weak influence of the Arg allele on obesity and hypertension. On the other hand, the gene polymorphism might only affect a fraction of subjects; thus the differences in the proportion of the fraction among the studies might have led to different results.

Studies of the β2-adrenergic receptor polymorphisms have identified the Arg16Gly and the Gln27Glu polymorphisms; both having some association with obesity and hypertension, mainly through an effect on physical exercise. One group found that the Gln27/Gln27 variants were associated with obesity (abdominal) in men who did not take physical activity, whereas no effect of the Gln27/Gln27 polymorphism was found in men who did exercise regularly.[77] Thus, physical exercise may counterbalance the effect of a genetic predisposition to increased body weight and body fat, and obese individuals with the Gln27/Gln27 genotype of the β2-adrenergic receptor might especially benefit from exercise. Corbalan et al.[78] reported that obese women who are carriers of the Glu27 allele do not benefit equally from physical activity compared with noncarriers. These subjects may show resistance to weight loss by diet and exercise.

In a 5-year longitudinal study, Masuo and colleagues[79] examined the β2-adrenoreceptor polymorphisms Arg16Gly and Gln27Glu during a highly controlled weight loss program by diet and exercise in Japanese men by separating them into three groups: those who lost and retained a significant amount of the weight loss; those who were weight loss resistant during the entire study; and those who had initial successful weight loss but by 6 months had rebound weight gain. The important findings were that the weight rebound group had higher levels of sympathetic activity as determined by plasma NE levels related to polymorphisms in the Arg16Gly and Gln27Glu of the β2-adrenoceptor. Thus, failure to be able to retain weight loss may relate to genetic abnormalities in the β2-adrenergic receptor, resulting in increased sympathetic activity. As all study individuals were monitored and remained on exactly the same diet and exercise program as the other two groups, variation in diet or exercise could not account for the weight rebound or the weight resistant groups.

Polymorphisms in the α2-adrenoceptor have also been investigated in obesity. The α2-adrenergic receptor inhibits lipolysis in fat so could have some potential to modulate obesity and hypertension. The Lys198Asn polymorphism of the α2-adrenoceptor in the endothelin-1 gene has been described in abdominal obesity, insulin resistance, and hypertension.[80]

MISCELLANEOUS POLYMORPHISMS IN OBESITY AND HYPERTENSION

Neuropeptide Y-Y1 polymorphism (NYP Y-1)

β2-Adrenoceptors and neuropeptide-Y (NPY) are coexpressed within adipose tissue, liver, and pancreas and act together in regulation of several fundamental metabolic functions. NPY secreted from sympathetic fibers innervating adipocytes controls β-agonist-regulated lipolysis, affecting overall energy balance, lipid mobilization and circulating concentrations of several lipid factors. However, it has not been clarified whether the metabolic effect of β2-adrenoceptors and NPY are dependent on genetic variation.[81] An investigative team reported that the β2-adrenoceptor gene and NPY gene have epistatic interaction in determination of LDL-cholesterol in hypertensive patients,[81] whereas others have found that the NPY Y1 receptor gene polymorphism does not associate with hypertension or obesity.[82]

Endothelin-1 gene polymorphism (198G/T, Lys198Asn)

Endothelin-1 (ET-1) is a powerful vasoconstrictor peptide produced by vascular endothelial and smooth muscle cells. Some severely hypertensive subjects exhibit enhanced endothelial expression of ET-1 gene.[83] Three large population studies have shown that ET-1 gene interacts with BMI in association with BP.[83,84] The Lys198Asn polymorphism of ET-1 is involved in determination of BP levels in obese subjects as shown in the Ohasama study.[85] In addition, the K198N (G/T) polymorphism and BMI are associated with hypertension.[86] On the other hand, a novel ET-1 gene polymorphism G862T/Ala288Ser found in exon 5 was not associated with hypertension in a Japanese cohort.[87]

Adiponectin receptor polymorphisms (I164T, G276T)

Adiponectin is one of the key molecules derived primarily from the adipocyte and has a major role in the metabolic control. The concentration of adiponectin is decreased in obesity, type 2 diabetes and coronary artery disease. The two polymorphisms (I164T, G276T) related to adiponectin are determinants of the onset of obesity and diabetes. In subjects carrying the TC genotype of the I164T polymorphism, adiponectin concentration was significantly lower and most of the subjects had hypertension, suggesting that the polymorphism of the TC genotype is associated with obesity hypertension. In contrast, the G276T polymorphism was not associated with adiponectin concentration or hypertension. These findings show that the I164T but not the G276T polymorphism is associated with low adiponectin concentrations and obesity-related hypertension.[88]

Natriuretic peptide clearance receptor polymorphism

Natriuretic peptide clearance receptor (NPRC) polymorphism, the C (-55), is associated with obesity but not hypertension, as shown in the Olivetti Heart Study with cross-sectional and longitudinal studies. Subjects carrying the AA genotype of C9-55A polymorphism might have stronger lipolytic and lipomobilizing activity of the natriuretic peptide.[89] The Leu554Phe polymorphism in the E-selectin gene is associated with elevated BP in overweight subjects and E-selectin was implicated in hypertension in a French cohort in a longitudinal study.[90]

Glucocorticoid receptor gene polymorphism (GR)

The role of endogenous glucocorticoids such as cortisol is of great interest in the pathogenesis of the metabolic syndrome but the topic needs clarification, as many proposedgene defects could lead to cortisol excess in the metabolic syndrome as recently reviewed.[91]

Insulin receptor substrate-1 Gly972Arg polymorphism

In a Caucasian Dutch population, the insulin receptor substrate-1 (IRS-1) Gly972Arg variant does not increase the risk of type 2 diabetes in obese subjects.[92] On the other hand, the insulin gene NsiI RFLP is associated with diastolic BP as studied in Chinese subjects.[93]

Uncoupling protein 2 polymorphism (UCP2)

A functional polymorphism in the UCP2 promoter has been reported to be associated with obesity in Caucasians. Polymorphism (-866G/A) of the UCP2 gene is associated with hypertension.[94]

G protein β3-subunit gene polymorphism (GNB3, C825T)

Heterotrimic guanine nucleotide-binding protein (G proteins) mediate pathways including the β-adrenergic signal pathways. The C825T polymorphisms in the gene coding for the β3-subunit of G protein has been shown to be associated with hypertension, obesity, and DM as part of the metabolic syndrome. The T825 allele of the G protein β3-subunit was found to be associated with essential hypertension and obesity in cross-sectional studies.[95] The investigators studied 737 Caucasian men and 735 women as a part of a Belgian population study and concluded that the male TT genotype of the C825G has higher BP, more obesity and more insulin resistance than the C allele.[96] In a large cohort of Japanese subjects, the C825T polymorphism was significantly associated with clustering of the metabolic syndrome (obesity, hypertension, hypertriglyceridemia, and diabetes). Although the individual effect of this polymorphism on each phenotype was weak, the combined effect of the C825T polymorphism on the various risk factors strengthens the association.[97] In young mild hypertensive subjects, carrying the 825T allele of the C825T is associated with a progressive rise in BP levels to more severe hypertension.[98] The T allele of the C825T is associated with reduced insulin sensitivity, abdominal obesity, and more advanced carotid atherosclerosis in men and women.[99] In the Heritage Family study, the investigators failed to show that the GNB3 polymorphism is a major modifier of body composition, heart rate, body fat, or fat regulation.[100] The 825 allele of the GNB3 may also be related to insulin resistance in hypertensive patients independently of BMI.[101] The TC genotype is not associated with a primary defect in insulin secretion or sensitivity, suggesting that obesity and hypertension in carriers of 825T do not result from primary alterations in glucose and insulin homeostasis.[102] Finally, the 825 allele of the GNB3 polymorphism is associated with an impairment of the β-adrenergic control of lipolysis.[103]

REFERENCES

1. Tuck M, Sowers JR, Dornfeld L Kletzig, Maxwell M. Weight reduction lowers plasma renin activity and aldosterone in obese subjects. N Engl J Med 1981; 304: 930–8.
2. Tuck ML, Sowers JR, Dornfeld L, Whitefield L, Maxwell M. Reductions in plasma catecholamines and blood pressure during weight loss in obese subjects. Acta Endocrinol 1983; 102: 252–60.
3. Tuck ML, Golub MG, Eggena P, Sowers JR, Maxwell M. Hypertension symposium on normal and abnormal blood pressure regulatory mechanisms. Western J Med 1983; 139: 190–202.

4. Mikhail N, Golub M, Tuck ML. Obesity and hypertension. Prog Cardiovasc Dis 1999; 42: 39–58.
5. Sharma AM, Engeli S, Pischon T. New developments in mechanisms of obesity induced hypertension: role of adipose tissue. Curr Hypertens Rep 2001; 3: 152–6.
6. Sharma AM. Is there a rationale for angiotensin blockade in the management of obesity hypertension? Hypertension 2004; 44: 12–19.
7. Engeli S, Schling P, Gorzelniak K et al. The adipose-tissue renin-angiotensin-aldosterone system: role in the metabolic syndrome. Int J Biochem Cell Biol 2003; 35: 807–25.
8. Schoor U, Blaschkem K, Turan S et al. Relationship between angiotensinogen, leptin and blood pressure levels in young normotensive men. J Hypertens 1998; 16: 1475–80.
9. Cooper R, McFarlane N, Bennet FL et al. ACE, angiotensinogen and obesity: a potential pathway leading to hypertension. J Hum Hypertens 1997; 11: 107–11.
10. Cooper R, Forrester T, Ogumbuyi O, Muffinda A. Angiotensinogen levels and obesity in four black populations. ICSHIB Investigators. J Hypertens 1998; 16: 571–5.
11. Bloemw LJ, Manatunga AK, Tewksbury DA, Pratt JH. The serum angiotensinogen concentration and variants of the angiotensinogen gene in white and black children. J Clin Invest 1995; 99: 948–52.
12. Umemura S, Nyui N, Tamura K et al. Plasma angiotensinogen concentration in obese patients. Am J Hypertens 1997; 10: 629–33.
13. Uckaya G, Ozata M, Sonmez A et al. Plasma leptin levels strongly correlate with plasma renin activity in patients with essential hypertension. Horm Metab Res 1999; 31: 435–8.
14. Licata G, Scaglione R, Ganguzza A et al. Central obesity and hypertension: relationship between fasting serum insulin, plasma renin activity and diastolic blood pressure in young obese subjects. Am J Hypertens 1994; 7: 314–20.
15. Engeli S, Bohnke J, Gorzelniak K et al. Weight loss and the renin-angiotensin-aldosterone system. Hypertension 2005; 45: 1–7.
16. Cassis LA, Saye J, Peach MJ. Location and regulation of rat angiotensinogen messenger RNA. Hypertension 1998; 11: 591–6.
17. Pratt JH, Ambrosius WT, Tewksbury DA, Wagner MA, Zhou L, Hanna MP. Serum angiotensinogen concentration in relation to gonadal hormones, body size, and genotype in growing young people. Hypertension 1998; 32: 875–9.
18. Jones BH, Standridge MK, Taylor JW, Moustaid N. Angiotensinogen gene expression in adipose tissue: analysis of obese models and hormonal and nutritional control. Am J Physiol 1997; 273: R236–R242.
19. Ailhaud G, Fukamizi A, Massiera F, Negrel R, Saint-Mark, Teboul M. Angiotensinogen, angiotensin II, and adipose tissue development. Obes Relat Metab Disord 2000; 24: S33–S35.
20. Massiera F, Bloch-Faure M, Ceiler D et al. Adipose angiotensinogen is involved in adipose tissue growth and blood pressure regulation. FASEB J 2001; 15: 2727–9.
21. Mazuraki H, Yamomoto H, Kenyon CJ et al. Transgenic amplification of glucocorticoid action in adipose tissue causes high blood pressure in mice. J Clin Invest 2003; 112: 83–90.
22. Tsai YS, Kim HJ, Takahashi N et al. Hypertension and abnormal fat distribution but not insulin resistance in mice with P465LPPARγ. J Clin Invest 2004; 114: 240–9.
23. Schling P, Schafer T. Human adipose tissue cells keep tight control on the angiotensin II levels in their vicinity. J Biol Chem 2002; 227: 48006–75.
24. Ailhaud G. Cross talk between adipocytes and their precursors: relationships with adipose tissue development and blood pressure. Ann N Y Acad Sci 1999; 892: 127–33.
25. Cassis LA, English VL, Bharadwaj K, Boustany CM. Differential effects of local versus systemic angiotensin II in the regulation of leptin release from adipocytes. Endocrinology 2004; 145: 174–96.
26. Darimont C, Vassaux, Gaillard G, Ailhaud G, Negrel R. In situ microdialysis of prostaglandins in adipose tissue: stimulation of prostacyclin release by angiotensin II. Int J Obes Relat Metab Disord 1994; 18: 783–8.
27. Cassis LA. Fat cell metabolism: insulin, fatty acids and renin. Curr Hypertens Rep 2000; 2: 132–8.
28. Saye J, Ragsdale V, Carey R, Peach M. Localization of angiotensin peptide-forming enzymes of 3T3-F442A adipocytes. Am J Physiol 1993; 264: C1570–C1576.
29. Safanova J, Aubert J, Negrel R, Ailhaud G. Regulation by fatty acids of angiotensinogen gene expression in preadipose cells. Biochem J 1997; 322 (Suppl 1): 235–9.
30. Aubert J, Darimont C, Safanova I et al. Regulation by glucocorticoids of angiotensingen gene expression and secretion in adipose cells. Biochem J 1997; 328: 701–6.
31. Aubert J, Safanova I, Negrel R, Ailhaud G. Insulin downregulates angiotensinogen gene expression and angiotensinogen secretion in cultured adipose cells. Biochem Biophys Res Commun 1998; 250 (Suppl 1): 77–82.
32. Frederich R, Kahn B, Peach M, Flier J. Tissue-specific nutritional regulation of angiotensinogen in adipose tissue. Hypertension 1992; 19: 339–44.
33. Shenoy U, Cassis L. Characterization of renin activity in brown adipose tissue. Am J Physiol 1997; 272: 989–99.
34. Schiling P, Mallow H, Trindl A, Loffler G. Evidence for a local renin-angiotensin system in primary cultured human preadipocytes. Int J Obes Metab Disord 1999; 23: 336–41.
35. Crandall DL, Armellino DC, Busler DE et al. Angiotensin II receptors in human preadipocytes: role of cell cycle regulation. Endocrinology 1999; 140 (Suppl 1): 154–8.
36. English V, Cassis L. Facilitation of sympathetic neurotransmission contributes to angiotensin regulation of body weight. J Neural Transm 1999; 106: 631–44.
37. Cassis L. Role of angiotensin II in brown adipose tissue thermogenesis during cold acclimation. Am J Physiol 1993; 265: E860–E865.
38. Cassis LA, Marshall DE, Fettinger MJ et al. Mechanisms contributing to angiotensin II regulation of body weight. Am J Physiol 1998; 247: E867–E876.
39. Schorr U, Blaschke K, Distler TS, Sharma AM. Relationship between angiotensinogen, leptin and blood pressure in young normotensive men. J Hypertens 1998; 16: 1475–80.
40. Furuhashi M, Ura N, Higashiura K et al. Blockade of the renin angiotensin system increases adiponectin concentrations in patients with essential hypertension. Hypertension 2003; 42: 76–81.
41. Furuhashi M, Ura N, Takizawa H et al. Blockade of the renin angiotensin system decreases adipocyte size with improvement in insulin sensitivity. J Hypertens 2004; 22: 1977–82.
42. Nagi DK, Foy CA, Mohamed-Ali V, Yudkin JS, Grant PJ, Knowler WC. Angiotensin-1-converting enzyme (ACE) gene polymorphism, plasma ACE levels, and their association with the metabolic syndrome and electrocardiographic coronary artery disease in Pima Indians. Metabolism 1998; 47: 622–6.
43. Goodfriend TL, Ball DL, Egan BM, Campbell WB, Nithipatikom K. Epoxy-keto derivative of linoleic acid stimulates aldosterone secretion. Hypertension 2004; 43: 358–63.
44. Ehrhart-Bornstein M, Arakelyan K, Krug AW, Scherbaum WA, Bornst SR. Fat cells may be the obesity-hypertension link: human adipogen factors stimulate aldosterone secretion from adrenocortical cells. Endocr Res 2004; 30: 865–70.

45. Grassi G, Servalle G, Colombo M et al. Body weight reduction, sympathetic nerve traffic, and arterial baroreflex in obese normotensive humans. Circulation 1998; 97: 2037–42.
46. Esler M, Lambert G, Brunner-La Roca et al. Sympathetic nerve activity and neurotransmitter release in humans: translation from pathophysiology to clinical practice. Acta Physiol Scand 2003; 177: 275–84.
47. Hall J, Jones DW, Kuo JJ, da Silva A, Tallum LS, Liu J. Impact of the obesity epidemic on hypertension and renal disease. Curr Hypertens Rep 2003; 5: 386–92.
48. Bray GA. Obesity is a chronic, relapsing neurochemical disease. Int J Obes 2004; 28: 34–8.
49. Arner P. The beta3-adrenergic receptor – a cause and cure of obesity? N Engl J Med 1995; 333: 382–3.
50. Emorine LJ, Marullo S, Briend-Sutren MM et al. Molecular characterization of the beta3-adrenergic receptor. Science 1989; 245: 1118–21.
51. Lonnqvist F, Thome A, Nisell K, Hoffsedt J, Arner P. A pathogenic role of visceral fat beta3-adrenoreceptors in obesity. J Clin Invest 1995; 95: 1109–16.
52. Hoffsedt J, Warhrenberg H, Thorne A, Lonnqvist E. The metabolic syndrome is related to beta3-aderenoreceptor sensitivity in visceral adipose tissue. Diabetologia 1996; 39: 838–44.
53. Nahmias C, Blin N, Elalouf JM, Mattei MG, Strosberg AD, Emorine LJ. Molecular characterization of the mouse beta3-adrenergic receptor. Relationship with the atypical receptor of adipocytes. EMBO J 1991; 10: 3721–7.
54. Atgie C, D'Allaire F, Bukowiecki LJ. Role of beta1- and beta3-adrenoceptors in the regulation of lipolysis and thermogenesis in rat brown adipocytes. Am J Physiol 1997; 273: C1136–42.
55. Krief S, Lonqvist F, Raimbault S et al. Tissue distribution of beta3-adrenergic receptor mRNA in man. J Clin Invest 1993; 91: 344–9.
56. Emorine L, Blin N, Strosberg AD. The human beta3-receptor: the search for a physiological function. Trends Pharmacol Sci 1994; 15: 3–7.
57. Enocksson S, Shimizu M, Sjostedt SM, Lonnqvist F, Nordenstrom J, Arner P. Demonstration of an in vivo functional beta3-adrenoreceptor in man. J Clin Invest 1995; 95: 2239–45.
58. Silver K, Mitchell BD, Waltson J et al. TRP64ARG beta3-adrenergic receptor and obesity in Mexican Americans. Hum Genet 1997; 101: 306–11.
59. Gagnon G, Mauriege P, Roy S et al. The Trp64Arg mutation of the beta3-adrenergic receptor gene has no effect on obesity phenotypes in the Quebec Family Study and Swedish Obese Subjects cohorts. J Clin Invest 1996; 98: 2086–93.
60. Widen E, Letho M, Kanninen T, Walston J, Shuldiner AR, Groop LC. Association of a polymorphism in the beta3-adrenergic receptor gene with features of the insulin resistance syndrome in Finns. N Engl J Med 1995; 333: 348–51.
61. Kim-Motoyama H, Yasuda K, Yamaguchi T et al. A mutation of the beta3-adrenergic receptor is associated with visceral obesity but decreased serum triglyceride. Diabetologia 1997; 40: 469–72.
62. Walston J, Silver K, Bogardus C et al. Time of onset of non-insulin-dependent diabetes mellitus and genetic variation in the beta3-adrenergic-receptor gene. N Engl J Med 1995; 333: 343–7.
63. Yoshida T, Sakane N, Umekawa T, Sakai M, Takahashi T, Kondo M. Mutation of beta3-adrenergic-receptor gene and response to treatment of obesity. Lancet 1995; 346: 1433–4.
64. Walston J, Silver K, Hilfiker H et al. Insulin response to glucose is lower in individuals homozygous for the Arg 64 variant of the beta-3-adrenergic receptor. J Clin Endocrinol Metab 2000; 85: 4019–22.
65. Clement K, Vaisse C, Manning BS et al. Genetic variation in the beta3-adrenergic receptor and an increased capacity to gain weight in patients with morbid obesity. N Engl J Med 1995; 333: 382–3.
66. Hoffstedt J, Poirier O, Thorne A et al. Polymorphism of the human beta3-adrenoceptor gene forms a well-conserved haplotype that is associated with moderate obesity and altered receptor function. Diabetes 1999; 48: 203–5.
67. Arner P. Genetic variance and lipolysis regulation: implications for obesity. Ann Med 2001; 33: 542–6.
68. Shiwaku K, Gao TQ, Isobe A, Fukushima T, Yamane Y. A Trp 64 Arg mutation in the beta3-adrenergic receptor gene is not associated with moderate overweight in Japanese workers. Metabolism 1998; 47: 1528–30.
69. Shiwaku K, Nogi A, Anuurad E et al. Difficulty in losing weight by behavioral intervention for women with Trp64Arg polymorphism of the beta3-adrenergic receptor gene. Int J Obes Relat Metab Disord 2003; 27: 1028–36.
70. Fujisawa T, Ikegami H, Yamato E et al. Trp64Arg mutation of beta3-adrenergic receptor in essential hypertension: insulin resistance and the adrenergic system. Am J Hypertens 1997; 10: 101–5.
71. Azuma N, Yoshimasa Y, Nishimura H et al. The significance of the Trp 64 Arg mutation of the beta3-adrenergic receptor gene in impaired glucose tolerance, non-insulin-dependent diabetes mellitus, and insulin resistance in Japanese subjects. Metabolism 1998; 47: 456–60.
72. Nagase T, Aoki A, Yamamoto M et al. Lack of association between the Trp64 Arg mutation in the beta3-adrenergic receptor gene and obesity in Japanese men: a longitudinal analysis. J Clin Endocrinol Metab 1997; 82: 1284–7.
73. Urhammer SA, Clausen JO, Hansen T, Pedersen O. Insulin insensitivity and body weight changes in young white carriers of the codon 64 amino acid polymorphism of the beta3-adrenergic receptor gene. Diabetes 1996; 45: 1115–20.
74. Buettner R, Schaffler A, Arndt H et al. The Trp64Arg polymorphism of the beta3-adrenergic receptor gene is not associated with obesity or type 2 diabetes mellitus in a large population-based Caucasian cohort. J Clin Endocrinol Metab 1998; 83: 2892–7.
75. Oeveren van-Dybicz AM, Vonkeman HE, Bon MA, van den Bergh FA, Vermes I. Beta3-adrenergic receptor gene polymorphism and type 2 diabetes in a Caucasian population. Diabetes Obes Metab 2001; 3: 47–51.
76. Benecke H, Topak H, von zur Muhlen A, Schuppert F. A study on the genetics of obesity: influence of polymorphisms of the beta-3-adrenergic receptor and insulin receptor substrate 1 in relation to weight loss, waist to hip ratio and frequencies of common cardiovascular risk factors. Exp Clin Endocrinol Diabetes 2000; 108: 86–92.
77. Meirhaeghe A, Helbecque N, Cottel D, Amouyel P. Beta2-adrenoceptor gene polymorphism, body weight, and physical activity. Lancet 1999; 353: 896.
78. Corbalan MS. The 27Glu polymorphism of the beta2-adrenergic receptor gene interacts with physical activity influencing obesity risk among female subjects. Clin Genet 2002; 61: 305–7.
79. Masuo K, Katsuya T, Fu Y et al. Beta2- and beta3-adrenergic receptor polymorphisms are related to the onset of weight gain and blood pressure elevation over 5 years. Circulation 2005; 111: 3429–34.
80. Tiret L, Poirier O, Hallet V et al. The Lys198Asn polymorphism in the endothelin-1 gene is associated with blood pressure in overweight people. Hypertension 1999; 33: 1169–74.
81. Tomaszewski M, Charchar FJ, Lacka B et al. Epistatic interaction between beta2-adrenergic receptor and neuropeptide Y

genes influences LDL-cholesterol in hypertension. Hypertension 2004; 44: 689–94.
82. Herzog H, Selbie LA, Zee RY, Morris BJ, Shine J. Neuropeptide-Y Y1 receptor gene polymorphism: cross-sectional analyses in essential hypertension and obesity. Biochem Biophys Res Commun 1993; 196: 902–6.
83. Schiffrin EL, Deng LY, Sventek P, Day R. Enhanced expression of endothelin-1 gene in resistance arteries in severe human essential hypertension. J Hypertens 1997; 15: 57–63.
84. Herrmann SM, Nicaud V, Tiret L et al. Polymorphisms of the beta2-adrenoceptor (ADRB2) gene and essential hypertension: the ECTIM and PEGASE studies. J Hypertens 2002; 20: 229–35.
85. Asai T, Ohkubo T, Katsuya T et al. Endothelin-1 gene variant associates with blood pressure in obese Japanese subjects: the Ohasama Study. Hypertension 2001; 38: 1321–4.
86. Jin JJ, Nakura J, Wu Z et al. Association of endothelin-1 gene variant with hypertension. Hypertension 2003; 41: 163–7.
87. Kaetsu A, Kishimoto T, Osaki Y, Okamoto M, Fukumoto S, Kurozawa Y. The lack of relationship between an endothelin-1 gene polymorphism (Ala288ser) and incidence of hypertension: a retrospective cohort study among Japanese workers. J Epidemiol 2004; 14: 129–36.
88. Iwashima Y, Katsuya T, Ishikawa K et al. Hypoadiponectinemia is an independent risk factor for hypertension. Hypertension 2004; 43: 1318–23.
89. Sarzani R, Strazzullo P, Salvi F et al. Natriuretic peptide clearance receptor alleles and susceptibility to abdominal adiposity. Obes Res 2004; 12: 351–6.
90. Marteau JB, Sass C, Pfister M, Lambert D, Noyer-Weidner M, Visvikis S. The Leu554Phe polymorphism in the E-selectin gene is associated with blood pressure in overweight people. J Hypertens 2004; 22: 305–11.
91. Rosmond R. The glucocorticoid receptor gene and its association to metabolic syndrome. Obes Res 2002; 10: 1078–86.
92. van Dam RM, Hoebee B, Seidell JC, Schaap MM, Blaak EE, Feskens EJ. The insulin receptor substrate-1 Gly972Arg polymorphism is not associated with Type 2 diabetes mellitus in two population-based studies. Diabetic Med 2004; 21: 752–8.
93. Thomas GN, Tomlinson B, Chan JC, Lee ZS, Cockran CS, Critchley JA. An insulin receptor gene polymorphism is associated with diastolic blood pressure in Chinese subjects with components of the metabolic syndrome. Am J Hypertens 2000; 13: 745–52.
94. Ji Q, Ikegami H, Fujisawa T et al. A common polymorphism of uncoupling protein 2 gene is associated with hypertension. J Hypertens 2004; 22: 97–102.
95. Brand E, Wang JG, Herrmann SM, Staessen JA. An epidemiological study of pressure and metabolic phenotypes in relation to the Gbeta3 C825T polymorphism. J Hypertens 2003; 21: 729–37.
96. Siffert W. G-protein beta3 subunit 825T allele and hypertension. Curr Hypertens Rep 2003; 5: 47–53.
97. Yamamoto M, Abe M, Jin JJ et al. Association of GNB3 gene with pulse pressure and clustering of risk factors for cardiovascular disease in Japanese. Biochem Biophys Res Commun 2004; 316: 744–8.
98. Sartori M, Semplicini A, Siffert W et al. G-protein beta3-subunit gene 825T allele and hypertension: a longitudinal study in young grade I hypertensives. Hypertension 2003; 42: 909–14.
99. Wascher TC, Paulweber B, Malaimare L et al. Associations of a human G protein beta3 subunit dimorphism with insulin resistance and carotid atherosclerosis. Stroke 2003; 34: 605–9.
100. Rankinen T, Rice T, Leon AS et al. G protein beta3 polymorphism and hemodynamic and body composition phenotypes in the HERITAGE Family Study. Physiol Genomics 2002; 8: 151–7.
101. Poch E, Giner V, Gonzalez-Nunez D, Coll E, Oriola J, de la Sierra A. Association of the G protein beta3 subunit T allele with insulin resistance in essential hypertension. Clin Exp Hypertens 2002; 24: 345–53.
102. Saller B, Nemesszeghy P, Mann K, Siffert W, Rosskopf D. Glucose and lipid metabolism in young lean normotensive males with the G protein beta3 825T-allele. Eur J Med Res 2003; 8: 91–7.
103. Hauner H, Rohrig K, Siffert W. Effects of the G-protein beta3 subunit 825T allele on adipogenesis and lipolysis in cultured human preadipocytes and adipocytes. Horm Metab Res 2002; 34: 475–80.

41

Obesity and hypertension: a clinical update

Gurushankar Govindarajan, Adam Whaley-Connell and James R Sowers

INTRODUCTION

The prevalence of obesity is rapidly increasing in developing as well as in industrialized countries.[1-5] Up to 61% of Americans are either overweight or obese, according to the most recent United States Census. The increase in prevalence of obesity and overweight was observed in both men and women of all age groups and ethnicity and more so in children and adolescents.[6-8] Economic costs attributable to obesity in the United States in 2000 were estimated at $117 billion.[2,5,9,10] A study involving 80 000 women revealed that a 5-kg weight gain after age 18 was associated with a 60% higher relative risk of developing hypertension,[11] compared with those women who gained 2 kg or less. Those who gained 10 kg or more increased their risk by 2.2-fold. Similar increases have been observed in other populations and in children.[12,13]

Obesity is a state of multiple molecular variances that leads to hypertension and subsequent increased risk for cardiovascular disease (CVD). Here we will review the combined effects of chronic kidney disease, the renin-angiotensin-aldosterone system (RAAS), neurohumeral and biochemical mechanisms, the natriuretic system, and prothrombotic and proinflammatory factors that all contribute to hypertension associated with obesity.

DEFINITION

Central obesity

Overweight is defined as a body mass index (BMI) >25 (BMI is body weight in kilograms divided by the height in meters, squared, expressed as wt [in kg]/height [m^2]). Obesity is defined as a BMI > 30; morbid obesity is a BMI > 35.[2] The regional distribution of body fat has an important metabolic and CVD influence. A predominantly 'central' pattern of weight gain, as measured by a waist-to-hip ratio, is a risk factor for CVD and insulin resistance because it confers a far higher risk than that expected on the basis of BMI measurements.[14] Central obesity is often referred to as abdominal, upper body, male-type, android, or visceral obesity vs female-type or gynoid obesity, where there is preferential fat accumulation in the gluteal and femoral distribution.[3,4,15-17] Abdominal obesity is diagnosed clinically by a waist-to-hip ratio that is >0.95 in men and >0.85 in women. Measurement of waist circumference is a clinically useful indicator of obesity. This is because abdominal obesity is more closely related to metabolic risk factors.[14] The National Cholesterol Education Program (NCEP) guidelines use waist circumference as a measurement of obesity for identification of subjects with metabolic syndrome. The cut-off point for men is ≥102 cm and for women it is ≥88 cm.[18] Although clinical measures are considered acceptable in the diagnosis of true central obesity, better imaging techniques such as dual-energy X-ray absorptiometry (DEXA) or an abdominal computed tomography (CT) scan are probably required for accurate description. The pattern of obesity is important; for example, athletes such as football players often have BMIs higher than 35, making them morbidly obese by definition. A closer look may reveal a total body fat lower than 8%, quite different from the figures for those who are truly obese. So, another way of describing obesity would be in terms of percent body fat. In terms of percentage of body fat, obesity can be defined as 25% or more in men and 35% or more in women.[12] Hence, clinicians must be aware of possible misdiagnosis of obesity defined solely by BMI. The measurement of body fat percent is rarely performed in clinical practice because of inconvenience and cost.

Cardiometabolic syndrome

The cardiometabolic syndrome is a collection of metabolic and CVD risk factors including central obesity, hypertension, insulin resistance, dyslipidemia, microalbuminuria, and hypercoagulability. This collection of risk factors increases the risk of CVD end points, such as stroke, congestive heart failure, chronic kidney disease, and overall mortality.[19–21]

The Adult Treatment Panel (ATP-III) of the NCEP proposed diagnostic criteria for identification of subjects with this syndrome.[18] ATP-III identifies five diagnostic traits for this syndrome. The presence of any three of the following five factors is sufficient for diagnosis.

1. Abdominal obesity, defined as a waist circumference in men >102 cm (40 inches) and in women >88 cm (35 inches) (it was noted by ATP-III that some men with lower waist circumference (i.e. 94–102 cm) may develop insulin resistance due to genetic factors).
2. Triglycerides ≥150 mg/dl (1.7 mmol/L).
3. High-density lipoprotein (HDL)-cholesterol <40 mg/dl (1 mmol/L) in men and <50 mg/dl (1.3 mmol/L) in women.
4. Blood pressure ≥130/≥85 mm Hg.
5. Fasting glucose ≥110 mg/dl (6.1 mmol/L) (National Institutes of Health, 1998).

In 1998, a European consensus group updated a working definition for this syndrome.[22] Unlike the ATP-III criteria, their definition required the presence of insulin resistance as part of the diagnosis of this syndrome. Insulin resistance was defined as one of the following: type 2 diabetes; impaired fasting glucose (IFG); impaired glucose tolerance (IGT), or for those with normal fasting glucose values (<110 mg/dl), a glucose uptake below the lowest quartile for background population under hyperinsulinemic, euglycemic conditions. In addition to insulin resistance the presence of two additional characteristics from among the following is sufficient for the diagnosis.

1. Abdominal obesity, defined as a waist-to-hip ratio >0.90, a BMI ≥30 kg/m², or a waist girth ≥94 cm (37 inches).
2. Dyslipidemia, defined as serum triglyceride ≥150 mg/dl (1.7 mmol/L) or HDL-cholesterol <35 mg/dl (0.9 mmol/L).
3. Blood pressure ≥140/90 mm Hg or the administration of antihypertensive drugs.

ROLE OF RENAL FUNCTIONAL AND STRUCTURAL CHANGES

Obesity is related to activation of the RAAS, increased sympathetic nervous system (SNS) activity, and hyperinsulinemia, all of which contribute to sodium reabsorption and associated fluid retention.[1,3,4,10,23–33] Altered intrarenal physical forces may also play a role in sodium retention in obese patients.[34–45] Observations from animal models and human studies have shown that there is an increase in kidney weight attributable to endothelial cell proliferation, intrarenal lipid, and hyaluronate deposition in the matrix and inner medulla.[10,16,37,46] These depositions in the encapsulated kidney can lead to altered intrarenal mechanical forces. In animal models, the interstitial hydrostatic forces were elevated in obese dogs compared with lean dogs. This increased pressure leads to parenchymal collapse and urine outflow obstruction, resulting in decreased intrarenal flow and increased sodium reabsorption.[41] The increased sodium reabsorption leads to a feedback-mediated renal vasodilatation, elevation of glomerular filtration rate (GFR), and stimulation of the RAAS despite the relative volume expansion.[16] Persistent glomerular hyperfiltration, a compensatory decreased renal vascular resistance, increased renal plasma flow and elevated blood pressure that are associated with obesity are attempts to overcome sodium reabsorption. Neurohumeral factors such as the previously mentioned increased SNS activity, inflammatory cytokines, and angiotensin II (Ang II) are also involved in these compensatory mechanisms and can contribute to glomerular and vascular stress associated with obesity.

These adaptive changes, along with a combination of factors often seen in obesity (i.e. glucose intolerance, dyslipidemia, hypertension), can lead to glomerulosclerosis and chronic kidney disease. Obesity has been associated with focal glomerulosclerosis (FGS) and compared with the idiopathic variety, obesity-related FGS had lower rates of the nephrotic syndrome, fewer segmental lesions, and increased glomerular size. This was demonstrated in a large retrospective study of human kidney biopsy specimens incorporating 6800 samples. The mean BMI in this study was 41.7 and disease course in this population was thought to parallel associated comorbidities, such as dyslipidemia and hypertension.[3,42,43] A European study showed a steady increase in the presence of microalbuminuria (MAU), an early marker for renal and CVD damage. In this study, the odds ratio for development of MAU for obese individuals was not different from that for hypertensive patients. Thus, obesity may perpetuate hypertension by renal structural changes leading to nephron injury and loss, potentiating further overall vascular/endothelial dysfunction and subsequent hypertension.

ROLE OF RAAS

The RAAS is activated in obesity, despite sodium retention and a state of volume expansion. This effect is largely due to the elevated levels of serum aldosterone reported in obesity.[32,47–49] and may be due to a yet-unidentified factor (possibly a fatty acid) from adipose tissue that results in increased synthesis of aldosterone.[50,51] There are reports that suggest a relationship between BMI and plasma Ang II levels, plasma renin activity (PRA), and plasma angiotensin converting enzyme (ACE) in humans.[52–54] A report indicates a relationship between plasma leptin and Ang II levels, and then leptin and PRA. Plasma leptin levels correlate with adipose tissue mass,[55] adipose tissue may directly contribute to circulating levels of Ang II.[48]

There is evidence that adipose tissue may possess a local RAAS that carries an important role in adipose tissue function. Recent studies suggest that adipose tissue angiotensinogen (AGT) mRNA expression is higher in abdominal than in subcutaneous adipose tissue. Adipose tissue also expresses Ang II receptors, which makes them a target for the paracrine-produced Ang II.[56] It has been suggested that adipose tissue RAAS may actually govern blood pressure. Another study expressed the AGT gene in adipose tissue of AGT knockout mice, creating a transgenic-knockout mouse model in which production of AGT is limited to adipose tissue. In these animals, systemic levels of AGT increased to 20% of wild-type levels, demonstrating that AGT produced in fat cells can enter the circulation.[57] Blood pressure and sodium homeostasis were then restored in these transgenic animals, lending further credence to the theory that an increased fat cell mass may result in higher circulating AGT levels with subsequent hypertension and resultant increased cardiovascular risk.

Weight loss may also have an effect on RAAS. In a short-term study the effects of weight loss on RAAS and blood pressure in 25 obese patients placed on a 12-week weight-reducing diet was evaluated.[58] Sodium intake was either medium or low and PRA, aldosterone, and mean arterial pressure (MAP) were measured. There was a reduction in PRA but not in aldosterone that correlated with weight loss in both sodium intake groups. MAP fell significantly and to the same degree in both groups, which correlated with weight loss throughout the study. These results suggest that weight loss is accompanied by reductions in PRA and aldosterone and that PRA reduction may improve blood pressure.[49,59–61]

ROLE OF SNS, BIOCHEMICAL, NEUROCHEMICAL, AND HORMONAL MEDIATORS

Sympathetic nervous system

Obese individual are noted to have elevated adrenergic activity, measured directly and indirectly.[3,24,58,62–64] Several mechanisms and mediators have been hypothesized for the genesis of this adrenergic overactivity noted in the obese.[3,26,62–67] Few plausible hypotheses include hyperinsulinemia with its consequent insulin resistance, plasma free fatty acids (FFAs), RAAS and central nervous system (CNS) activation, and impaired cardiopulmonary and arterial baroreflex sensitivity.

Several studies in both humans and animal models have shown that this CNS and RAAS activation contribute to the obesity-hypertension syndrome.[68] Weight loss, on the other hand, reduces SNS and RAAS activity, which further supports this hypothesis. Also, medications that abolish or diminish the central sympathetic drive cause a greater blood pressure reduction in obese than in lean subjects.[27,69–71] Clonidine, which blocks central α2-receptors and thereby markedly reduces the central sympathetic drive, blunts hypertension in dogs fed a high-calorie diet.[72] Similar results have been observed in humans. One mechanism of hypertension due to increased SNS activity appears to be through the elevated renal sympathetic nerve activity,[73] resulting in salt retention. Indeed, renal denervation blunted the sodium retention and markedly attenuated the rise in blood pressure in dogs fed with a high fat diet.[74]

Insulin resistance and hyperinsulinemia

Obese subjects are noted to have elevated levels of insulin, which are required to maintain glucose and fatty acid metabolism, and they often have insulin resistance in peripheral tissues.[65,75–78] In insulin resistance state there is impaired biological and physiological response to insulin in tissue. This resistance to insulin is not uniform in all tissues. This altered response of various tissues to insulin is often accompanied by decreased insulin-mediated metabolic signaling and impaired glucose transport in skeletal muscle and fat, and impaired nitric oxide (NO)-induced vasodilatation in skeletal muscle. Thus, accentuation of some actions of insulin growth effects with concurrent resistance to other actions gives rise to diverse clinical manifestations. It is estimated that about 25–47% of subjects with hypertension have insulin resistance or impaired glucose tolerance.[79] Several mechanisms are postulated for the high prevalence of insulin resistance in patients with essential hypertension. Insulin resistance/hyperinsulinemia results in activation of the SNS, increased tissue Ang II, increased renal tubular sodium retention, elevated intracellular calcium concentration and vascular smooth muscle cell proliferation and atherosclerosis.[80–86] Therapy targeted at insulin resistance, such as aerobic exercise, or drugs like thiazolidinediones, result in decrease in blood pressure.[87,88]

Resistin

Resistin is a newly discovered cysteine-rich protein that has been proposed as an important link in the mechanism of insulin resistance in obesity.[89,90] In murine models, resistin has been shown to be elevated in both genetic and diet-induced obese mice. A recent study reported that resistin gene polymorphism is an independent factor associated with systolic and diastolic blood pressures in type 2 diabetics. Diabetics with the GG genotype were found to have a higher prevalence of hypertension in this population.[91] Other reports in Caucasian and Japanese populations found no association between resistin gene polymorphism and type 2 diabetes but the single nucleotide polymorphism (SNP) in the promoter region was a significant predictor of the insulin-sensitivity index. It was therefore hypothesized that non-coding SNPs in the resistin gene might influence insulin sensitivity in interaction with obesity. The studies in humans identifying the role of resistin in pathogenesis of insulin resistance, hypertension, and obesity have been inconsistent.[92] More studies are required to define the role of resistin in humans.

Free fatty acids (FFAs)

High FFA levels are thought to cause hypertension by increased sympathetic activity or enhanced sympathetic vascular responses or by impaired endothelium-dependent vasodilation.[93–96] Subjects with visceral obesity have increased lipolytic activity resulting in increased delivery of FFA load to the liver that, in turn, activates hepatic afferent pathways that may lead to sympathetic activation and contribute to insulin resistance.[97] An acute rise in FFA levels induced by intralipid plus heparin infusion increases vascular reactivity to α-adrenergic agonists and reflex vasoconstriction. Similar changes were also seen by direct infusion of oleic acid into the portal circulation. These effects were abolished by adrenergic blockade. Interestingly, portal vein infusion caused a greater blood pressure rise than systemic infusions, emphasizing the potential role of afferent pathways in the liver. One study reported that an elevated FFA level modulates microvascular function and may contribute to obesity-associated insulin resistance, hypertension, and microangiopathy. In that study, FFA elevation impaired capillary recruitment and acetylcholine-mediated vasodilation.[96] Another study showed that high rates of intralipid infusion caused a small (i.e. 4 mm Hg) increase in mean blood pressure.[93] It further showed that elevated FFA impairs NO-dependent vasodilation and thus results in hypertension. Studies done in animals have shown varying results. In dogs, infusion of long-chain fatty acids had no effect on blood pressure, in contrast to rats that demonstrated a rise in blood pressure and heart rate. Neither cerebral (via vertebral artery) nor systemic infusion of long-chain fatty acids in dogs has a significant effect on arterial pressure, renal function, or hemodynamic responses. Also, the long-term effect of elevated FFAs is not well understood. Therefore, the relationship between elevated FFA levels and hypertension currently is tenuous at best and merits further investigation.

Leptin

Leptin has been studied extensively in recent years for its possible role in the obesity-hypertension syndrome. Figure 41.1 illustrates the possible mechanisms via which leptin may exert its pressor effects.[98–111] Leptin's actions are mediated by binding to the long form of its receptors (Ob-Rb) in the lateral and medial regions of the hypothalamus[112] by crossing the blood-brain barrier via a saturable, transport-mediated endocytosis. The Ob-Rb is a full-length receptor with transmembrane domain and a long intracellular carboxyl-terminal tail. Ob-Ra, Ob-Rc, and Ob-Rd are leptin receptor isoforms with short intracellular tails. Ob-Re, another isomer, lacks the transmembrane domain and thus may function as a soluble receptor to bind and inactivate the circulating leptin. This binding of leptin to its receptor triggers a myriad of reactions resulting in reduced appetite and increased energy expenditure via stimulation of the adrenergic system.[113–116] Information on the action of leptin in decreasing body weight, decreasing appetite and increased energy expenditure comes from genetic studies in mice and humans. Mice that lack the ability to synthesize leptin (i.e. ob/ob mice) or that have mutations of the leptin receptor (i.e. db/db mice) develop extreme obesity. Similarly, humans with mutated leptin genes show a propensity towards extreme obesity. However, this is a rare condition and may not contribute to the current obesity epidemic. Leptin levels correlate well with the body adipose tissue stores. Levels of 5–15 μg/ml are noted in lean individuals and levels are typically elevated in most obese subjects.[117]

Studies in rodents show that intravenous and intracerebroventricular infusion of leptin results in increased sympathetic activity in kidneys, adrenals, and brown adipose tissue (BAT).[106,118] Long-term leptin infusion in rodents causes a significant and sustained rise in blood pressure.[110,119] Leptin exerts its pressor effect via the SNS, causing avid renal salt retention and hence hypertension. The rise in blood pressure with leptin infusion is slow in onset and occurs despite the other effect of leptin, namely weight loss that would tend to decrease blood pressure. These leptin-induced chronic

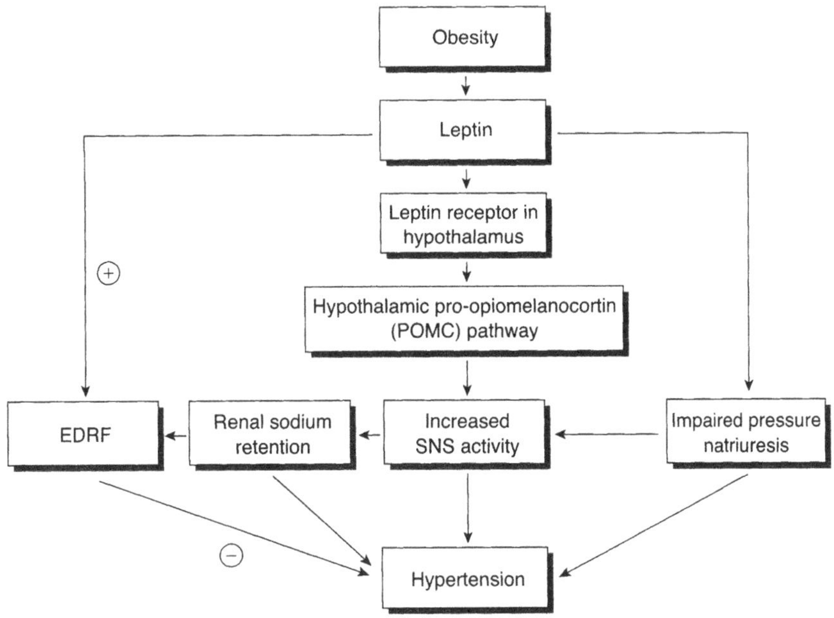

Figure 41.1 A brief outline of interactions through which leptin is thought to contribute to hypertension. EDRF, endothelium-derived relaxing factor; SNS, sympathetic nervous system

blood pressure elevations are abolished completely by α- and β-adrenergic blockade, lending credence for the action of leptin via SNS to cause hypertension.[106,120] A normally functioning leptin receptor is required for leptin-induced hypertension,[121,122] as leptin produces its effect mainly through its interaction with the receptor.

Another important concept is the presence of selective leptin resistance.[120] Obese humans continue to overeat, despite elevated circulating leptin levels, indicating a failure of feedback mechanisms on satiety; yet they develop hypertension, indicating that the effect of leptin on the sympathetic system is intact. This hypothesis of selective leptin resistance has been tested only in rodents and not in humans.[121]

ROLE OF NATRIURETIC PEPTIDE SYSTEM

The natriuretic peptide system consists of the atrial natriuretic peptide (ANP), the brain natriuretic peptide (BNP), and the C-type natriuretic peptide (CNP), each encoded by a separate gene[123–129] and synthesized predominantly in the heart, brain, and kidneys, respectively. Each peptide directs its effects via specific receptors, NPr-A, NPr-B, and NPr-C.[125,130] Collectively, the natriuretic peptides have effects on plasma volume, renal sodium handling, and blood pressure, resulting in a reduction in sympathetic tone in the peripheral vasculature. They are also known to dampen baroreceptor function and lower the activation threshold of vagal efferents, and to suppress reflex tachycardia and vasoconstriction resulting from decreased extracellular volume. In an animal model, transgenic mice that overexpress the ANP gene have lower blood pressure compared with animals with inactivated ANP gene that are prone to develop salt-sensitive hypertension.[131,132] Therefore, natriuretic peptides have a protective role in the development of hypertension due to their natriuretic and vasodilator effects as well as their inhibitory effect on the SNS and the RAAS.

ANP plasma levels are lower in the obese hypertensive than in obese normotensive subjects.[133] These obese hypertensive subjects also demonstrate a response to exogenously administered ANP, as measured by blood pressure reduction, natriuresis, and increases in urine cyclic guanylate monophosphate (cGMP) excretion.[133] The ANP response to salt load was found to be suppressed in obese subjects, compared with a potent ANP elevation in lean subjects. A recent study reported an association between a promoter variant at position -55 in the NPr-C gene, a higher blood pressure, and lower ANP plasma levels in obese hypertensive subjects.[134] Further studies are needed to understand the role of this finding as regards its possible contribution to blood pressure elevation.

PROINFLAMMATORY AND PROTHROMBOTIC CHANGES

Adipose tissue in general and central adipose tissue in states of obesity has been implicated as a tissue rich in inflammatory cytokines, such as tumor necrosis factor-α, (TNF-α) interleukin-6 (IL-6), C-reactive protein (CRP), and plasminogen activator inhibitor (PAI-1). As such, obesity has been suggested to be a low-grade inflammatory condition that is increasingly important in the causation and progression of hypertension and atherosclerosis.[135,136] It is thought that the central adipocyte synthesizes TNF-α, which in turn, stimulates IL-6, considered a major regulator in the production of acute phase reactants such as CRP, PAI-1, and fibrinogen from the hepatocyte. It is possible that the relationship between obesity and vascular disease may depend in part on the increased production and release of these inflammatory mediators from adipose tissue. However, a direct cause and effect relationship, has not been clearly established. It is not known, for example, whether long-term treatment with aspirin or other nonsteroidal anti-inflammatory drugs reduce the level of inflammatory cytokines and CVD in obese patients.

There is an increased risk for hypercoaguability and altered thrombotic mechanisms that may contribute to a higher incidence of hypertension, heart disease and stroke in obesity. Epidemiologic evidence exists that these mechanisms are related to BMI or waist-to-hip ratio. For example, obese subjects have higher levels of factor VII antigen, fibrinogen, plasminogen, and PAI-1 activity, all of which have been suggested to increase the risk for CVD.[137–139] The increased metabolism of FFAs in obesity may promote thrombosis by increasing protein C, PAI-1, and/or platelet aggregation. Adipose tissue production of leptin or inflammatory mediators have been suggested as important factors causing increased thrombosis,[140] but these aspects of the relationship between obesity and CVD are poorly understood and require additional study. Other mechanisms for platelet activation in the obese have been elucidated recently, at least in part. Another study reported that a visceral or android pattern of obesity is associated with lipid peroxidation and persistent platelet activation, both of which appear to be partially reversible with weight loss.[135] An association has been proposed between a circulating soluble CD40 ligand (CD40L) and platelet activation. CD40L is a trimeric, transmembrane protein of the TNF family that is inactive in resting platelets but is rapidly activated and expressed on the platelet surface when the platelet is stimulated. Therefore, increased levels of circulating CD40L represent an index of platelet activation. Another study addressed the relationship between central obesity and circulating levels of soluble CD40L and the effect of weight loss on this measure of platelet activation in a prospective intervention cohort study.[136] It was found that baseline levels of circulating CD40L and 8-iso-PGF2α levels (a marker of lipid peroxidation) were significantly higher in obese than in nonobese subjects. BMI levels correlated well with levels of CD40L and 8-iso-PGF2α. After a 16-week intervention period of caloric restriction and weight loss, levels of these markers went down, corresponding with a commensurate lowering of the BMI in the obese subjects.

CARDIOVASCULAR CHANGES

Obesity is a major cause of insulin resistance, hypertension, and dyslipidemia (e.g. the cardiometabolic syndrome). These disorders individually and synergistically increase CVD risk. Hypertension in lean subjects tends to produce a concentric pattern of left ventricular hypertrophy (LVH), whereas in obese subjects an eccentric pattern is predominant. Heart failure is more common in the obese subject, even when corrected for the presence of hypertension.[141] The presence of both obesity and hypertension in a patient results in a mixed pattern of cardiac hypertrophy, caused by an elevation in both cardiac preload and afterload.[142] Obesity also results in increased preload due to an expanded vascular volume, while the elevated afterload can be accounted for by the presence of hypertension and SNS activation. After adjustment for established risk factors, the risk of heart failure increases by 5% in men and 7% in women for each BMI increment of one.[143]

Since LVH itself is a major risk factor for sudden death and death due to progressive cardiac decompensation, it may partially explain the increased incidence of cardiovascular morbidity and mortality in the obese.[144] In obese individuals, LVH has been associated with mononuclear cell infiltration in and around the sinoatrial node and fat deposition all along the conduction system.[145] Lipomatous hypertrophy of the interatrial septum has also been noted in obesity.[146] These changes make the myocardium in the obese hypertensive individual an ideal substrate for cardiac arrhythmia and sudden death.[147]

Not only the does the presence of LVH promote an increased CVD risk, alterations of ions at the cellular and molecular level appear to be important in regulating vascular smooth muscle tone. In obesity, there is a state of dysregulation and resultant abnormal vascular responsiveness.[148–150] One major component of this dysregulation of ion transport is modulated by insulin, which works as a vasodilator by inhibiting voltage-gated Ca^{2+} influx. Insulin also stimulates glucose transport and phosphorylation of glucose to glucose-6-phosphate, which further activates Ca^{2+} ATP-ase transcription and increases cellular Ca^{2+} efflux. These actions result in a net decrease in intracellular Ca^{2+} and, therefore, decreased vascular resistance.[151–155] These actions result in a net decrease in intracellular Ca^{2+} and, therefore, decreased vascular resistance.[151–155] In obese person with insulin resistance these actions are blunted resulting in increased vascular resistance. An investigative group studied the effect of weight reduction on peripheral vascular resistance (PVR), reflected by forearm vascular resistance and mean arterial pressure (MAP) in obese persons. It was shown that weight loss resulted in a significant decrease in PVR and MAP.[156]

CONCLUSION

This chapter has discussed some of the mechanisms involved in the causal relation between obesity and hypertension that can lead to increased CVD risk. Obesity causes a constellation of maladaptive disorders that individually and synergistically contribute to hypertension among other aspects of cardiovascular morbidity. Well-designed, population-based studies are needed to assess the individual contribution of each of these disorders to the development of hypertension. Control of obesity may eliminate 48% of the hypertension in whites and 28% in blacks. We hope that this chapter will help scientists formulate a thorough understanding of obesity hypertension and form the basis for more research in this field.

REFERENCES

1. Mark AL, Correia M, Morgan DA et al. State-of-the-art-lecture: obesity-induced hypertension: new concepts from the emerging biology of obesity. Hypertension 1999; 33: 537–41.
2. Sowers JR. Update on the cardiometabolic syndrome. Clin Cornerstone 2001; 4: 17–23.
3. Hall JE, Hildebrandt DA, Kuo J. Obesity hypertension: role of leptin and sympathetic nervous system. Am J Hypertens 2001; 14: 103S–115S.
4. Hall JE, Crook ED, Jones DW et al. Mechanisms of obesity-associated cardiovascular and renal disease. Am J Med Sci 2002; 324: 127–37.
5. Flegal KM, Carroll MD, Kuczmarski RJ et al. Overweight and obesity in the United States: prevalence and trends, 1960–1994. Int J Obes Relat Metab Disord 1998; 22: 39–47.
6. Troiano RP, Flegal KM. Overweight children and adolescents: description, epidemiology, and demographics. Pediatrics 1998; 101: 497–504.
7. Mokdad AH, Serdula MK, Dietz WH et al. The spread of the obesity epidemic in the United States, 1991–1998. JAMA 1999; 282: 1519–22.
8. Flegal KM, Carroll MD, Ogden CL et al. Prevalence and trends in obesity among US adults, 1999–2000. JAMA 2002; 288: 1723–7.
9. Garrison RJ, Kannel WB, Stokes J 3rd et al. Incidence and precursors of hypertension in young adults: the Framingham Offspring Study. Prev Med 1987; 16: 235–51.
10. Zhang R, Reisin E. Obesity-hypertension: the effects on cardiovascular and renal systems. Am J Hypertens 2000; 13: 1308–14.
11. Huang Z, Willett WC, Manson JE et al. Body weight, weight change, and risk for hypertension in women. Ann Intern Med 1998; 128: 81–8.
12. Clinical guidelines on the identification, evaluation, and treatment of overweight and obesity in adults – the evidence report. National Institutes of Health. Obes Res 1998; 6 (Suppl 2): 51S–209S.
13. He Q, Ding ZY, Fong DY-T et al. Blood pressure is associated with body mass index in both normal and obese children. Hypertension 2000; 36: 165–70.
14. Bosello O, Zamboni M. Visceral obesity and metabolic syndrome. Obes Rev 2000; 1: 47–56.
15. Kissebah AH, Krakower GR. Regional adiposity and morbidity. Physiol Rev 1994; 74: 761–811.
16. Hall JE. Mechanisms of abnormal renal sodium handling in obesity hypertension. Am J Hypertens 1997; 10: 49S–55S.
17. Rocchini AP. Obesity hypertension. Am J Hypertens 2002; 15: 50S–52S.
18. Third Report of the National Cholesterol Education Program (NCEP) Expert Panel on Detection, Evaluation, and Treatment of High Blood Cholesterol in Adults (Adult Treatment Panel III) final report. Circulation 2002; 106: 3143–421.
19. McFarlane SI, Banerji M, Sowers JR. Insulin resistance and cardiovascular disease. J Clin Endocrinol Metab 2001; 86: 713–18.
20. Isomaa B, Almgren P, Tuomi T et al. Cardiovascular morbidity and mortality associated with the metabolic syndrome. Diabetes Care 2001; 24: 683–9.
21. Lakka HM, Laaksonen DE, Lakka TA et al. The metabolic syndrome and total and cardiovascular disease mortality in middle-aged men. JAMA 2002; 288: 2709–16.
22. Alberti KG, Zimmet PZ. Definition, diagnosis and classification of diabetes mellitus and its complications. Part 1: diagnosis and classification of diabetes mellitus provisional report of a WHO consultation. Diabetic Med 1998; 15: 539–53.
23. Tuck ML. Obesity, the sympathetic nervous system, and essential hypertension. Hypertension 1992; 19: 167–77.
24. Landsberg L, Krieger DR. Obesity, metabolism, and the sympathetic nervous system. Am J Hypertens 1989; 2: 125S–132S.
25. Carroll JF, Huang M, Hester RL et al. Hemodynamic alterations in hypertensive obese rabbits. Hypertension 1995; 26: 465–70.
26. Weyer C, Pratley RE, Snitker S et al. Ethnic differences in insulinemia and sympathetic tone as links between obesity and blood pressure. Hypertension 2000; 36: 531–7.
27. Abate NI, Mansour YH, Tuncel M et al. Overweight and sympathetic overactivity in black Americans. Hypertension 2001; 38: 379–83.

28. Reaven GM. Role of insulin resistance in human disease (syndrome X): an expanded definition. Annu Rev Med 1993; 44: 121–31.
29. Reisin E, Azar S, DeBoisblanc BP et al. Low calorie unrestricted protein diet attenuates renal injury in hypertensive rats. Hypertension 1993; 21: 971–4.
30. Burt VL, Cutler JA, Higgins M et al. Trends in the prevalence, awareness, treatment, and control of hypertension in the adult US population: data from the Health Examination Surveys, 1960 to 1991. Hypertension 1995; 26: 60–9.
31. Hall JE, Brands MW, Henegar JR. Mechanisms of hypertension and kidney disease in obesity. Ann N Y Acad Sci 1999; 892: 91–107.
32. Engeli S, Sharma AM. The renin-angiotensin system and natriuretic peptides in obesity-associated hypertension. J Mol Med 2001; 79: 21–9.
33. Stern JS, Gades MD, Wheeldon CM et al. Calorie restriction in obesity: prevention of kidney disease in rodents. J Nutr 2001; 131: 913S–917S.
34. Weisinger JR, Kempson RL, Eldridge FL et al. The nephrotic syndrome: a complication of massive obesity. Ann Intern Med 1974; 81: 440–7.
35. Wesson DE, Kurtzman NA, Frommer JP. Massive obesity and nephrotic proteinuria with a normal renal biopsy. Nephron 1985; 40: 235–7.
36. Hall JE. Louis K. Dahl Memorial Lecture. Renal and cardiovascular mechanisms of hypertension in obesity. Hypertension 1994; 23: 381–94.
37. Alonso-Galicia M, Dwyer TM, Herrera GA et al. Increased hyaluronic acid in the inner renal medulla of obese dogs. Hypertension 1995; 25: 888–92.
38. Bruzzi I, Benigni A, Remuzzi G. Role of increased glomerular protein traffic in the progression of renal failure. Kidney Int Suppl 1997; 62: S29–S31.
39. Sugerman H, Windsor A, Bessos M et al. Intra-abdominal pressure, sagittal abdominal diameter and obesity comorbidity. J Intern Med 1997; 241: 71–9.
40. Hall JE, Brands MW, Henegar JR et al. Abnormal kidney function as a cause and a consequence of obesity hypertension. Clin Exp Pharmacol Physiol 1998; 25: 58–64.
41. Bloomfield GL, Sugerman HJ, Blocher CR et al. Chronically increased intra-abdominal pressure produces systemic hypertension in dogs. Int J Obes Relat Metab Disord 2000; 24: 819–24.
42. Henegar JR, Bigler SA, Henegar LK et al. Functional and structural changes in the kidney in the early stages of obesity. J Am Soc Nephrol 2001; 12: 1211–17.
43. Kambham N, Markowitz GS, Valeri AM et al. Obesity-related glomerulopathy: an emerging epidemic. Kidney Int 2001; 59: 1498–509.
44. Okosun IS, Choi S, Dent MM et al. Abdominal obesity defined as a larger than expected waist girth is associated with racial/ethnic differences in risk of hypertension. J Hum Hypertens 2001; 15: 307–12.
45. Sundquist J, Winkleby MA, Pudaric S. Cardiovascular disease risk factors among older black, Mexican-American, and white women and men: an analysis of NHANES III, 1988–1994. Third National Health and Nutrition Examination Survey. J Am Geriatr Soc 2001; 49: 109–16.
46. Reisin E, Messerli FG, Ventura HO, Frohlich ED. Renal haemodynamic studies in obesity hypertension. J Hypertens 1987; 5: 397–400.
47. Granger JP, West D, Scott J. Abnormal pressure natriuresis in the dog model of obesity-induced hypertension. Hypertension 1994; 23: I8–11.
48. Schorr U, Blaschke K, Turan S et al. Relationship between angiotensinogen, leptin and blood pressure levels in young normotensive men. J Hypertens 1998; 16: 1475–80.
49. Engeli S, Sharma AM. Emerging concepts in the pathophysiology and treatment of obesity-associated hypertension. Curr Opin Cardiol 2002; 17: 355–9.
50. Goodfriend TL, Egan BM, Kelley DE. Aldosterone in obesity. Endocr Res 1998; 24: 789–96.
51. Goodfriend TL, Egan BM, Kelley DE. Plasma aldosterone, plasma lipoproteins, obesity and insulin resistance in humans. Prostaglandins Leukot Essent Fatty Acids 1999; 60: 401–5.
52. Licata G, Volpe M, Scaglione R et al. Salt-regulating hormones in young normotensive obese subjects. Effects of saline load. Hypertension 1994; 23: I20–4.
53. Cooper R, McFarlane-Anderson N, Bennett FI et al. ACE, angiotensinogen and obesity: a potential pathway leading to hypertension. J Hum Hypertens 1997; 11: 107–11.
54. Cooper R, Forrester T, Ogunbiyi O et al. Angiotensinogen levels and obesity in four black populations. ICSHIB Investigators. J Hypertens 1998; 16: 571–5.
55. Engeli S, Negrel R, Sharma AM. Physiology and pathophysiology of the adipose tissue renin-angiotensin system. Hypertension 2000; 35: 1270–7.
56. Giacchetti G FE, Sardu C, Mariniello B et al. Different gene expression of the RAS in human subcutaneous and visceral adipose tissue. Int J Obes Relat Metab Disord 1999; 23 (Suppl 5): S71.
57. Massiera F, Seydoux J, Geloen A et al. Angiotensinogen-deficient mice exhibit impairment of diet-induced weight gain with alteration in adipose tissue development and increased locomotor activity. Endocrinology 2001; 142: 5220–25.
58. Tuck ML, Sowers J, Dornfeld L et al. The effect of weight reduction on blood pressure, plasma renin activity, and plasma aldosterone levels in obese patients. N Engl J Med 1981; 304: 930–3.
59. Bloem LJ, Manatunga AK, Tewksbury DA et al. The serum angiotensinogen concentration and variants of the angiotensinogen gene in white and black children. J Clin Invest 1995; 95: 948–53.
60. Umemura S, Nyui N, Tamura K et al. Plasma angiotensinogen concentrations in obese patients. Am J Hypertens 1997; 10: 629–33.
61. Uckaya G, Ozata M, Sonmez A et al. Plasma leptin levels strongly correlate with plasma renin activity in patients with essential hypertension. Horm Metab Res 1999; 31: 435–8.
62. Rumantir MS, Vaz M, Jennings GL et al. Neural mechanisms in human obesity-related hypertension. J Hypertens 1999; 17: 1125–33.
63. Masuo K, Mikami H, Ogihara T et al. Weight gain-induced blood pressure elevation. Hypertension 2000; 35: 1135–40.
64. Esler M. The sympathetic system and hypertension. Am J Hypertens 2000; 13: 99S–105S.
65. Hall JE, Brands MW, Dixon WN et al. Obesity-induced hypertension. Renal function and systemic hemodynamics. Hypertension 1993; 22: 292–9.
66. Grassi G, Seravalle G, Cattaneo BM et al. Sympathetic activation in obese normotensive subjects. Hypertension 1995; 25: 560–3.
67. Grassi G, Seravalle G, Colombo M et al. Body weight reduction, sympathetic nerve traffic, and arterial baroreflex in obese normotensive humans. Circulation 1998; 97: 2037–42.
68. Hall JE, Zappe DH, Alonso-Galicia M et al. Mechanisms of obesity-induced hypertension. News Physiol Sci 1996; 11: 255–61.
69. Licata G, Scaglione R, Ganguzza A et al. Central obesity and hypertension. Relationship between fasting serum insulin, plasma renin activity, and diastolic blood pressure in young obese subjects. Am J Hypertens 1994; 7: 314–20.

70. Wofford MR, Anderson DC Jr, Brown CA et al. Antihypertensive effect of alpha- and beta-adrenergic blockade in obese and lean hypertensive subjects. Am J Hypertens 2001; 14: 694–8.
71. Antic V, Kiener-Belforti F, Tempini A et al. Role of the sympathetic nervous system during the development of obesity-induced hypertension in rabbits. Am J Hypertens 2000; 13: 556–9.
72. Rocchini AP, Mao HZ, Babu K et al. Clonidine prevents insulin resistance and hypertension in obese dogs. Hypertension 1999; 33: 548–53.
73. DiBona GF. The sympathetic nervous system and hypertension: recent developments. Hypertension 2004; 43: 147–50.
74. Kassab S, Kato T, Wilkins FC et al. Renal denervation attenuates the sodium retention and hypertension associated with obesity. Hypertension 1995; 25: 893–7.
75. DeFronzo RA, Cooke CR, Andres R et al. The effect of insulin on renal handling of sodium, potassium, calcium, and phosphate in man. J Clin Invest 1975; 55: 845–55.
76. Rocchini AP, Moorehead C, DeRemer S et al. Hyperinsulinemia and the aldosterone and pressor responses to angiotensin II. Hypertension 1990; 15: 861–6.
77. Rocchini AP, Marker P, Cervenka T. Time course of insulin resistance associated with feeding dogs a high-fat diet. Am J Physiol 1997; 272: E147–E154.
78. Bjorntorp P, Rosmond R. Neuroendocrine abnormalities in visceral obesity. Int J Obes Relat Metab Disord 2000; 24 (Suppl 2): S80–S85.
79. Lind L, Berne C, Lithell H. Prevalence of insulin resistance in essential hypertension. J Hypertens 1995; 13: 1457–62.
80. Modan M, Halkin H. Hyperinsulinemia or increased sympathetic drive as links for obesity and hypertension. Diabetes Care 1991; 14: 470–87.
81. DeFronzo RA, Ferrannini E. Insulin resistance. A multifaceted syndrome responsible for NIDDM, obesity, hypertension, dyslipidemia, and atherosclerotic cardiovascular disease. Diabetes Care 1991; 14: 173–94.
82. DeFronzo RA. The effect of insulin on renal sodium metabolism. A review with clinical implications. Diabetologia 1981; 21: 165–71.
83. Anderson EA, Hoffman RP, Balon TW et al. Hyperinsulinemia produces both sympathetic neural activation and vasodilation in normal humans. J Clin Invest 1991; 87: 2246–52.
84. Berne C, Fagius J, Pollare T et al. The sympathetic response to euglycaemic hyperinsulinaemia. Evidence from microelectrode nerve recordings in healthy subjects. Diabetologia 1992; 35: 873–9.
85. Rowe JW, Young JB, Minaker KL et al. Effect of insulin and glucose infusions on sympathetic nervous system activity in normal man. Diabetes 1981; 30: 219–25.
86. Sowers JR. Insulin resistance and hypertension. Am J Physiol Heart Circ Physiol 2004; 286: H1597–H1602.
87. Raji A, Seely EW, Bekins SA et al. Rosiglitazone improves insulin sensitivity and lowers blood pressure in hypertensive patients. Diabetes Care 2003; 26: 172–8.
88. Dengel DR, Hagberg JM, Pratley RE et al. Improvements in blood pressure, glucose metabolism, and lipoprotein lipids after aerobic exercise plus weight loss in obese, hypertensive middle-aged men. Metabolism 1998; 47: 1075–82.
89. Steppan CM, Bailey ST, Bhat S et al. The hormone resistin links obesity to diabetes. Nature 2001; 409: 307–12.
90. Rangwala SM, Rich AS, Rhoades B et al. Abnormal glucose homeostasis due to chronic hyperresistinemia. Diabetes 2004; 53: 1937–41.
91. Tan MS, Chang SY, Chang DM et al. Association of resistin gene 3′-untranslated region +62G->A polymorphism with type 2 diabetes and hypertension in a Chinese population. J Clin Endocrinol Metab 2003; 88: 1258–63.
92. Furuhashi M, Ura N, Higashiura K et al. Circulating resistin levels in essential hypertension. Clin Endocrinol 2003; 59: 507–10.
93. Steinberg HO, Tarshoby M, Monestel R et al. Elevated circulating free fatty acid levels impair endothelium-dependent vasodilation. J Clin Invest 1997; 100: 1230–9.
94. Stepniakowski KT, Goodfriend TL, Egan BM. Fatty acids enhance vascular alpha-adrenergic sensitivity. Hypertension 1995; 25: 774–8.
95. Grekin RJ, Dumont CJ, Vollmer AP et al. Mechanisms in the pressor effects of hepatic portal venous fatty acid infusion. Am J Physiol 1997; 273: R324–R330.
96. de Jongh RT, Serne EH, Ijzerman RG et al. Free fatty acid levels modulate microvascular function: relevance for obesity-associated insulin resistance, hypertension, and microangiopathy. Diabetes 2004; 53: 2873–82.
97. Bergman RN, Van Citters GW, Mittelman SD et al. Central role of the adipocyte in the metabolic syndrome. J Investig Med 2001; 49: 119–26.
98. Zhang Y, Proenca R, Maffei M et al. Positional cloning of the mouse obese gene and its human homologue. Nature 1994; 372: 425–32.
99. Pelleymounter MA, Cullen MJ, Baker MB et al. Effects of the obese gene product on body weight regulation in ob/ob mice. Science 1995; 269: 540–3.
100. Lee GH, Proenca R, Montez JM et al. Abnormal splicing of the leptin receptor in diabetic mice. Nature 1996; 379: 632–5.
101. Haynes WG, Sivitz WI, Morgan DA et al. Sympathetic and cardiorenal actions of leptin. Hypertension 1997; 30: 619–23.
102. Casto RM, VanNess JM, Overton JM. Effects of central leptin administration on blood pressure in normotensive rats. Neurosci Lett 1998; 246: 29–32.
103. Flier JS, Maratos-Flier E. Obesity and the hypothalamus: novel peptides for new pathways. Cell 1998; 92: 437–40.
104. Lu H, Duanmu Z, Houck C et al. Obesity due to high fat diet decreases the sympathetic nervous and cardiovascular responses to intracerebroventricular leptin in rats. Brain Res Bull 1998; 47: 331–5.
105. Onions KL, Hunt SC, Rutkowski MP et al. Genetic markers at the leptin (OB) locus are not significantly linked to hypertension in African Americans. Hypertension 1998; 31: 1230–4.
106. Shek EW, Brands MW, Hall JE. Chronic leptin infusion increases arterial pressure. Hypertension 1998; 31: 409–14.
107. Lembo G, Vecchione C, Fratta L et al. Leptin induces direct vasodilation through distinct endothelial mechanisms. Diabetes 2000; 49: 293–7.
108. Correia ML, Haynes WG, Rahmouni K et al. The concept of selective leptin resistance: evidence from agouti yellow obese mice. Diabetes 2002; 51: 439–42.
109. Carlyle M, Jones OB, Kuo JJ et al. Chronic cardiovascular and renal actions of leptin: role of adrenergic activity. Hypertension 2002; 39: 496–501.
110. Mark AL, Shaffer RA, Correia ML et al. Contrasting blood pressure effects of obesity in leptin-deficient ob/ob mice and agouti yellow obese mice. J Hypertens 1999; 17: 1949–53.
111. Hall J, Eugene WM, Brands MW. Does leptin contribute to obesity hypertension? Curr Opin Endocrinol Diabetes 1999; 6: 225.
112. Golden PL, Maccagnan TJ, Pardridge WM. Human blood-brain barrier leptin receptor. Binding and endocytosis in isolated human brain microvessels. J Clin Invest 1997; 99: 14–18.
113. Thornton JE, Cheung CC, Clifton DK et al. Regulation of hypothalamic proopiomelanocortin mRNA by leptin in ob/ob mice. Endocrinology 1997; 138: 5063–6.

114. Fan W, Boston BA, Kesterson RA, Hruby VJ, Cone RD. Role of melanocortinergic neurons in feeding and the agouti obesity syndrome. Nature 1997; 385: 165–8.
115. Huszar D, Lynch CA, Fairchild-Huntress V et al. Targeted disruption of the melanocortin-4 receptor results in obesity in mice. Cell 1997; 88: 131–41.
116. Haynes WG, Morgan DA, Djalali A et al. Interactions between the melanocortin system and leptin in control of sympathetic nerve traffic. Hypertension 1999; 33: 542–7.
117. Considine RV, Sinha MK, Heiman ML et al. Serum immunoreactive-leptin concentrations in normal-weight and obese humans. N Engl J Med 1996; 334: 292–5.
118. Aizawa-Abe M, Ogawa Y, Masuzaki H et al. Pathophysiological role of leptin in obesity-related hypertension. J Clin Invest 2000; 105: 1243–52.
119. Haynes WG, Morgan DA, Walsh SA et al. Cardiovascular consequences of obesity: role of leptin. Clin Exp Pharmacol Physiol 1998; 25: 65–9.
120. El-Haschimi K, Pierroz DD, Hileman SM et al. Two defects contribute to hypothalamic leptin resistance in mice with diet-induced obesity. J Clin Invest 2000; 105: 1827–32.
121. Van Heek M, Compton DS, France CF et al. Diet-induced obese mice develop peripheral, but not central, resistance to leptin. J Clin Invest 1997; 99: 385–90.
122. Ishizuka T, Ernsberger P, Liu S et al. Phenotypic consequences of a nonsense mutation in the leptin receptor gene (fak) in obese spontaneously hypertensive Koletsky rats (SHROB). J Nutr 1998; 128: 2299–306.
123. Rosenzweig A, Seidman CE. Atrial natriuretic factor and related peptide hormones. Annu Rev Biochem 1991; 60: 229–55.
124. Maack T. Receptors of atrial natriuretic factor. Annu Rev Physiol 1992; 54: 11–27.
125. Nakao K, Ogawa Y, Suga S et al. Molecular biology and biochemistry of the natriuretic peptide system. I: Natriuretic peptides. J Hypertens 1992; 10: 907–12.
126. Maoz E, Shamiss A, Peleg E et al. The role of atrial natriuretic peptide in natriuresis of fasting. J Hypertens 1992; 10: 1041–4.
127. Sarzani R, Paci VM, Dessi-Fulgheri P et al. Comparative analysis of atrial natriuretic peptide receptor expression in rat tissues. J Hypertens Suppl 1993; 11 (Suppl 5): S214–S215.
128. Sarzani R, Dessi-Fulgheri P, Paci VM et al. Expression of natriuretic peptide receptors in human adipose and other tissues. J Endocrinol Invest 1996; 19: 581–5.
129. Dessi-Fulgheri P, Sarzani R, Rappelli A. The natriuretic peptide system in obesity-related hypertension: new pathophysiological aspects. J Nephrol 1998; 11: 296–9.
130. Levin ER, Gardner DG, Samson WK. Natriuretic peptides. N Engl J Med 1998; 339: 321–8.
131. Melo LG, Steinhelper ME, Pang SC et al. ANP in regulation of arterial pressure and fluid-electrolyte balance: lessons from genetic mouse models. Physiol Genomics 2000; 3: 45–58.
132. Melo LG, Veress AT, Chong CK et al. Salt-sensitive hypertension in ANP knockout mice: potential role of abnormal plasma renin activity. Am J Physiol 1998; 274: R255–R261.
133. Dessi-Fulgheri P, Sarzani R, Serenelli M et al. Low calorie diet enhances renal, hemodynamic, and humoral effects of exogenous atrial natriuretic peptide in obese hypertensives. Hypertension 1999; 33: 658–62.
134. Sarzani R, Dessi-Fulgheri P, Salvi F et al. A novel promoter variant of the natriuretic peptide clearance receptor gene is associated with lower atrial natriuretic peptide and higher blood pressure in obese hypertensives. J Hypertens 1999; 17: 1301–5.
135. Festa A, D'Agostino R, Howard G et al. Chronic subclinical inflammation as part of the insulin resistance syndrome: The Insulin Resistance Atherosclerosis Study (IRAS). Circulation 2000; 102: 42–7.
136. Das UN. Is obesity an inflammatory condition? Nutrition 2001; 17: 953–66.
137. Alessi MC, Morange P, Juhan-Vague I. Fat cell function and fibrinolysis. Horm Metab Res 2000; 32: 504–8.
138. Chu NF, Spiegelman D, Hotamisligil GS et al. Plasma insulin, leptin, and soluble TNF receptors levels in relation to obesity-related atherogenic and thrombogenic cardiovascular disease risk factors among men. Atherosclerosis 2001; 157: 495–503.
139. Rissanen P, Vahtera E, Krusius T et al. Weight change and blood coagulability and fibrinolysis in healthy obese women. Int J Obes Relat Metab Disord 2001; 25: 212–18.
140. Konstantinides S, Schafer K, Loskutoff DJ. The prothrombotic effects of leptin: possible implications for the risk of cardiovascular disease in obesity. Ann N Y Acad Sci 2001; 947: 134–42.
141. Drenick EJ, Bale GS, Seltzer F et al. Excessive mortality and causes of death in morbidly obese men. JAMA 1980; 243: 443–5.
142. Messerli FH, Sundgaard-Riise K, Reisin ED et al. Dimorphic cardiac adaptation to obesity and arterial hypertension. Ann Intern Med 1983; 99: 757–61.
143. Kenchaiah S, Evans JC, Levy D et al. Obesity and the risk of heart failure. N Engl J Med 2002; 347: 305–13.
144. Lip GY, Gammage MD, Beevers DG. Hypertension and the heart. Br Med Bull 1994; 50: 299–321.
145. Bharati S, Lev M. Cardiac conduction system involvement in sudden death of obese young people. Am Heart J 1995; 129: 273–81.
146. Basu S, Folliguet T, Anselmo M et al. Lipomatous hypertrophy of the interatrial septum. Cardiovasc Surg 1994; 2: 229–31.
147. Duflou J, Virmani R, Rabin I et al. Sudden death as a result of heart disease in morbid obesity. Am Heart J 1995; 130: 306–13.
148. Messerli FH, Christie B, DeCarvalho JG et al. Obesity and essential hypertension. Hemodynamics, intravascular volume, sodium excretion, and plasma renin activity. Arch Intern Med 1981; 141: 81–5.
149. Frohlich ED, Messerli FH, Reisin E, Dunn FG. The problem of obesity and hypertension. Hypertension 1983; 5: III71–8.
150. Assmann G, Schulte H. The Prospective Cardiovascular Munster (PROCAM) study: prevalence of hyperlipidemia in persons with hypertension and/or diabetes mellitus and the relationship to coronary heart disease. Am Heart J 1988; 116: 1713–24.
151. Licata G, Scaglione R, Capuana G et al. Hypertension in obese subjects: distinct hypertensive subgroup. J Hum Hypertens 1990; 4: 37–41.
152. Rocchini AP, Moorehead C, Katch V et al. Forearm resistance vessel abnormalities and insulin resistance in obese adolescents. Hypertension 1992; 19: 615–20.
153. Rockstroh JK, Schmieder RE, Schachinger H et al. Stress response pattern in obesity and systemic hypertension. Am J Cardiol 1992; 70: 1035–9.
154. Schmieder RE, Messerli FH. Does obesity influence early target organ damage in hypertensive patients? Circulation 1993; 87: 1482–8.
155. Weir MR, Reisin E, Falkner B et al. Nocturnal reduction of blood pressure and the antihypertensive response to a diuretic or angiotensin converting enzyme inhibitor in obese hypertensive patients. TROPHY Study Group. Am J Hypertens 1998; 11: 914–20.
156. Jacobs DB, Sowers JR, Hmeidan A, Niyogi T, Simpson L, Standley PR. Effects of weight reduction on cellular cation metabolism and vascular resistance. Hypertension 1993; 21: 308–14.

42

Mechanisms of sex differences in hypertension

Virginia Huxley and Meredith Hay

INTRODUCTION

Sex differences in the development of hypertension and cardiovascular disease (CVD) have been well described in humans and in animal models. In general, men are at greater risk for CVD and hypertension than premenopausal women of the same age.[1,2] Ambulatory blood pressure measurements have consistently found that men have higher blood pressures than premenopausal, age-matched women.[3–5] After menopause the sex difference in the incidence of hypertension is lost.[6] In animal models of hypertension, studies have also shown males to have higher blood pressure than females. For example, in Dahl-salt hypertensive, spontaneously hypertensive rats (SHR), and reduced renal mass, high salt-fed rats, males have higher blood pressures than the females.[7–12]

While the mechanisms underlying sex differences are poorly understood, there is significant evidence for a role for both testosterone in the development of[13,14] and estrogen in the protection against[15–18] high blood pressure. Evidence supporting the hypothesis of estrogen involvement in the differential expression of CVD and hypertension between men and women has been shown by several laboratories.[1,17,19] While estrogen replacement therapy has been shown to reduce low-density lipoprotein cholesterol and increase high-density lipoproteins levels[20,21] these protective findings contrast with the findings of the Women's Health Initiative (WHI)[22,23] and Heart and Estrogen/progestin Replacement Study (HERS) I and II.[24,25] These trials failed to find a protective effect for horomone replacement therapy (HRT) against CVD. It has been suggested that the type of estrogen used in the replacement trials, and the fact that many of the women had already gone through menopause may account for these outcome discrepancies. It has been suggested that initiation of HRT in the perimenopausal period during rather than after menopause may have provided CVD protection.[26]

ION CHANNELS, SEX, AND HYPERTENSION

Both estrogen and testosterone affect vascular smooth muscle (VSM) function.[27–29] For example, acute application of 17β-estradiol in human mammary artery rings reduces the maximal contractile response to serotonin, histamine, and angiotensin (Ang) II.[30] Likewise, in aortic rings from ovariectomized rats, chronic 17β-estradiol treatment inhibits the Ang II-induced contraction.[31] Further, both acute and chronic application of estrogen components have been shown to enhance arterial endothelium-dependent vasodilatation.[32,33] While testosterone will also dilate vessels, it is a weaker vasodilator which does not appear to increase vascular nitric oxide (NO) generation.[34]

Many of the effects of estrogen on VSM are thought to be due to estrogen's effects on ion channel function. In porcine coronary arteries, 17β-estradiol results in a relaxation that is endothelium-dependent and involves activation of NO and calcium activated potassium channels (K_{Ca2+}).[35] Similar effects of estrogen on activation of K_{Ca2+} have been reported in bronchial smooth muscle.[36] Further, the estrogen analog, raloxifene, relaxes isolated rat cerebral arteries acutely, largely via an endothelium-independent mechanism, involving inhibition of Ca^{2+} influx through L-type Ca^{2+} channels.[37] Further, estrogen attenuates L- and T-type voltage-gated Ca^{2+} currents in cultured VSM cells (VSMCs).[38] Together, these studies suggest that estrogen may decrease vascular reactivity by facilitating K^+ currents and inhibiting both voltage-gated Ca^{2+} currents and ligand-induced increases in intracellular calcium ($[Ca^{2+}]$).

Genetic models have been used to analyze the role of both sex steroid receptors and sex hormones on blood pressure ion channel function. In estrogen receptor beta knockout mice, blood pressure is elevated and VSM K^+ channel activity is reduced compared with mice with normal receptor expression.[39] Thus, it appears that intact estrogen receptor function is required for normal K^+ channel distribution and blood pressure and that loss of estrogen, or its receptors, can lead to hypertension.

Testosterone may also regulate blood pressure via direct effects on VSM or via effects on central pathways regulating blood pressure control. In the SHR, the higher blood pressure of males, relative to females, is decreased following castration.[13] Similarly, low dose Ang II infusion in male mice results in hypertension that is prevented by both castration and central intracerebroventricular (i.c.v.) infusion of the androgen receptor blocker flutamide,[40] suggesting that testosterone and central testosterone receptors are involved in the development of Ang II-induced hypertension in males. The molecular mechanisms underlying these effects of testosterone are not known but are thought to include changes in ion channel function or alterations in levels of reactive oxygen species (ROS). Recent studies have shown that endogenous testosterone increases L-type Ca^{2+} channel function and activity in coronary arteries of males.[41] Further, testosterone has also been shown to increase gene expression of L-type Ca^{2+} channels and the sodium/calcium exchanger in cardiac myocytes.[42]

ROS, SEX, AND HYPERTENSION

Central and peripheral studies with estrogen and testosterone also suggest that many of the cardiovascular effects of sex steroids may be related to their role in the development of oxidative stress and their regulatory effects on the generation of ROS and nitric oxide (NO).[43–45] Estrogen is a well known antioxidant thought to protect against oxidative stress that is associated with CVD and hypertension.[46]

Molecular oxygen is reduced in mammalian cells by a number of enzyme systems involved in normal cellular metabolic processes. These systems result in the formation of ROS such as $O_2^{-}\cdot$ or hydrogen peroxide (H_2O_2), hydroxy radicals ($HO^{\bullet}$), hypochlorous acid (HOCl), and reactive nitrogen species, NO and peroxynitrite. Oxidative stress can be characterized by an imbalance between the generation and the scavenging of ROS such as $O_2^{-}\cdot$ or H_2O_2 and has been identified as a key component of the pathogenesis of hypertension, stroke, and CVD.[47] H_2O_2, superoxide and hydroxyl radicals, and peroxinitrite all induce cellular toxicity, dysfunction, and often cell death.[48] Reactive oxygen plays an important role in cell signaling in nearly all major organ systems involved in hypertension including VSMCs, endothelial cells (ECs), the central nervous system, and the kidneys. There are several sources for ROS in mammalian cells, including xanthine oxidase, cytochrome p450, NO synthase (NOS), the mitochondrial electron transport system, and NAD(P)H oxidase.

ROS generated by NAD(P)H oxidase has been localized in the brain, kidney, blood vessels, and nearly all components of the cardiovascular system. Importantly, atherosclerosis is known to involve increases in oxidative stress[48,49] and cellular toxicity, due to hydrogen peroxide, superoxide radicals, and peroxinitrite formation, is known to lead to EC and VSM dysfunction. In the brain, superoxide production, via actions of NAD(P)H oxidase, is known to be involved in neurotoxicity, stroke, and neurodegenerative diseases and has been identified throughout the brain including the thalamus, the cerebellum, the hippocampus, and the amygdala.[50–52]

Ang II is an important factor in many forms of both clinical and experimental hypertension. A growing body of evidence has shown that increases in circulating Ang II stimulate oxidative stress that participates in the peripheral and central effects of Ang II on blood pressure.[53–55] In Ang II-induced hypertension, a number of studies have shown increased oxidative stress in the circulation as well as in specific tissues.[53] In rats, the subpressor dose of Ang II that results in an increase in blood pressure is blocked by systemic administration of the superoxide dismutase (SOD) mimetic tempol.[56] Similarly, the Ang II-induced slow pressor response in mice also increases oxidative stress.[57] Importantly, recent studies have shown sex differences in the development of chronic Ang II-induced hypertension in conscious mice wherein females appear to be protected from the increases in BP.[58] Further, central i.c.v. infusion of the SOD mimetic tempol blocks systemic Ang II-induced hypertension in male mice while central i.c.v. infusion of L-NAME facilitates Ang II-induced hypertension in the females.[40] These results suggest that central sex steroid receptors modulate the development of Ang II-induced hypertension via actions on central ROS and NO systems.[40]

NO, SEX, AND HYPERTENSION

In many systems, the harmful effects of ROS are offset by NO production.[47] When these systems are out of balance, increased ROS production results in a decreased bioavailability of NO.[48] Increased production of superoxide radicals results in NO scavenging and increased peroxinitrite production.

Estrogen and testosterone have been shown to alter oxidative stress in both peripheral and central systems. In endothelial cells, estrogen has recently been shown to inhibit Ang II-induced increases in expression of NAD(P)H and (NOS).[59] In VSMC, estrogen decreases Ang II-induced free radical production and up-regulates manganese SOD (MnSOD) and ecSOD, suggesting that estrogen's cardiovascular protection against peripheral Ang II-induced oxidative stress is due to estrogen's increase in SOD activity.[60] Estrogen also appears to be an antioxidant in neuronal systems and protects against neurodegenerative disease and stroke, while testosterone may increase neurotoxicity and reperfusion injury.[61,62]

Expression of neuronal NOS has been shown to be regulated by sex steroids. Testosterone via actions on the androgen receptor (AR) and via aromatization to estrogen via actions on ER alpha decreases nNOS mRNA and activity in the hypothalamus and pre-optic area (POA).[63] On the other hand, estrogen increases NADPH-diaphorase staining, an indicator of NOS activity, and neuronal NOS mRNA and protein.[64–66] Neuronal NOS is expressed in a number of central regions involved in the regulation of sympathetic outflow and blood pressure, which also express both estrogen and androgen receptors. Within the hypothalamus, the largest population of NO-producing cells is found within the paraventricular nucleus (PVN).[67] Increases in NO within the PVN result in decreases of sympathetic outflow and blood pressure, and NO plays an important role centrally in reducing arterial pressure during recovery from psychological stress.[68] Another central area involved in blood pressure regulation that expresses high levels of neuronal NOS is the nucleus of the solitary tract (NTS). Blockade of NOS in the NTS results in increases in sympathetic outflow and blood pressure.[69,70]

There is considerable evidence to suggest that the hypertensive effects of Ang II involve central and peripheral reactive oxygen mechanisms. Further, it is known that there are sex differences in Ang II hypertension and that central androgen receptors and central estrogen receptors are involved in these sex differences. It has been hypothesized that sex and sex steroids may modulate the actions of Ang II via interactions with ROS and NO generating pathways within both peripheral tissues such as the vasculature and the kidney as well as regions of the brainstem and hypothalamus.

MICROVASCULAR REACTIVITY, PERMEABILITY, SEX, AND HYPERTENSION

Downstream of the arteries and arterioles, which are relatively constricted in hypertension, is the exchange microvasculature where materials cross from the vascular space to the tissue compartment where metabolism occurs. The role of sex differences in microvascular and exchange vessel properties has only received recent attention. With respect to the control of both blood flow and exchange, sex appears to influence basal properties separately from the responses to vasoactive substances. Several mediators of VSM function appear to influence microvascular permeability properties, presumably endothelial functions, and preliminary data suggest that the responses differ with sex. For example, in coronary venules from the hearts of sedentary pigs the permeability to albumin is independent of sex, but adenosine (ADO) increases permeability of vessels from females and decreases permeability in vessels from males.[71] This would imply that with exercise (breakdown of ATP, increases in ADO) net movement of material to cardiac myocytes would be lower in males than females. Of the multiple alterations of microvascular flow and exchange function modified by essential hypertension, differences between male and females appear to involve changes in microvascular network architecture, vessel structure, and function.

With respect to microvascular network architecture, changes in exchange surface area and total peripheral resistance occur as a consequence of vessel 'rarefaction'. In human hypertensives, without respect to sex, forearm skin capillary density is reduced (~20%) compared with normotensive subjects and correlates inversely with the blood pressure. Rarefaction of this magnitude, if present in all vascular beds, would result in a ~20% increase in peripheral resistance.[72] The contribution of sex in this process was studied in rats with reduced renal mass plus a high salt (4.0% NaCl) diet. In the males mean arterial pressure increased by 60% and skeletal muscle capillary density decreased by 30%, results similar to those observed in male normotensive and spontaneously hypertensive rats (SHR) on a high salt diet. In contrast, MAP of the females rose only slightly and no changes in microvessel density were observed.[10] These data underscore sex differences in regulation of microvascular function.

A property of larger vessels that appears to differ between males and females is vascular compliance. Reductions in the oscillatory or reflected component of the diastolic waveform (compliance) correlate with a variety of clinical conditions, including hypertension,

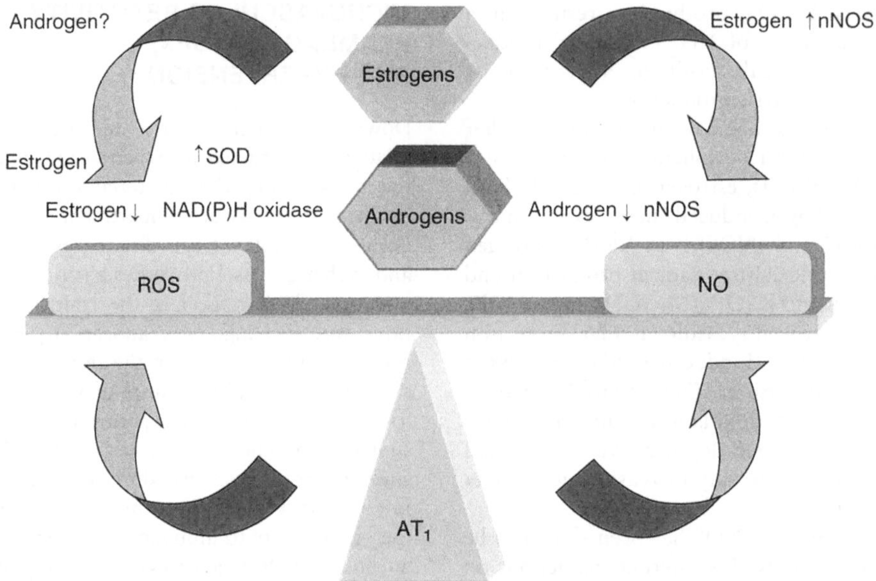

Figure 42.1 This figure illustrates this hypothesis for how sex steroids may modulate Ang II-induced hypertension. It is suggested that the physiological effects of activation of the AT_1 receptor, both centrally and peripherally, involve a balance between ROS and NO generating systems. Both estrogen and androgen receptors, which are co-localized with the AT_1 receptor, are hypothesized to modulate the activity of ROS and NOS pathways, thereby modulating the hypertensive effects of AT_1 receptor activation by Ang II

diabetes mellitus, and congestive heart failure, and may reflect endothelial dysfunction at the site of resistance vessels. Compared with men, women have reduced small vessel compliance[73] despite lower systolic blood pressure and pulse pressure and more favorable lipid and homocysteine levels, indicating unexpected negative effects of female sex hormones. In turn, this property may help to explain why premenopausal women hospitalized for myocardial infarction have higher mortality rates than men of the same age.[72]

While protective mechanisms minimize the transmission of increases in systemic blood pressure to the capillary bed in humans,[74] finger nailfold capillary pressure of women is 13% lower than men and unrelated to systolic, diastolic, or mean blood pressure.[75] Having stated these two findings, it is notable that capillary pressure of patients with essential hypertension was >60% higher than that of age- and sex-matched controls. In addition there were abnormalities in the waveforms of pulsations in capillary pressure in the group with hypertension, with an increased attenuation of high-frequency harmonics. Pulses appeared to be conducted more rapidly along the vascular tree in the hypertensive patients. The increase in capillary hydrostatic pressure in essential hypertension is in agreement with indirect evidence of capillary hyperfiltration provided by other studies, which showed a reduced plasma volume and increased transcapillary escape rate of plasma proteins.[76]

Along those lines, from Starling's Law of Filtration, elevation in capillary pressure alone would be expected to result in an increase in volume flux from the exchange microvasculature. Of interest, measures of capillary filtration coefficient (CFC) in the forearm of hypertensives average 41% of controls and the relation between CFC and arterial blood pressure values is inversely nonlinear.[77] In preliminary studies of normotensive rat skeletal muscle permeability to albumin, the anticipated difference in venular and arteriolar permeability exists only for adult males, not adult females or juveniles of either sex (unpublished data from Huxley laboratory). This result implicates testosterone in the setting of basal skeletal muscle venular permeability to protein. However, structural reorganization of the endothelial barrier with respect to volume flux does not appear to influence egress of macromolecules, as the transcapillary escape rates (TERs) of albumin and IgG in untreated subjects with essential hypertension (average MAP 193/119 mm Hg) were found to be significantly increased (50 and 57%, for albumin and IgG, respectively) compared with normal. Given that there was a significant positive correlation between MAP and TER for both proteins and the TERIgG/TERalb ratio did not differ between groups it was concluded that the transendothelial pathways of the endothelial microcirculation were not disrupted, *per se*, and that the increased flux reflected increased pressure-dependent water and solute flux.[78] In the aggregate, whether there is a net change in fluid filtration in hypertensives, relative to controls, will depend on the combination of the changes in driving force (capillary pressure), capillary area (rarefaction), and permeability properties. The mechanisms controlling these changes and the role of the sex hormones are poorly understood.

There is evidence that sex, as well as hypertension, alters resistance microvessel reactivity. Mesenteric arterioles of male SHRs are more sensitive to endothelin-1 and noradrenaline than those of female SHRs or controls of either sex.[11] Further, in DOCA rats a selective endothelin-B-receptor agonist, IRL-1620, induces marked vasoconstriction in males but only minimal changes in females. In control rats of both sexes IRL-1620 caused dilatation. Bosentan, an endothelin (ET_A/ET_B)-receptor antagonist, induced a greater decrease in mean arterial blood pressure in male than in female DOCA-salt hypertensive rats.[12] Some clues as to the mechanisms whereby male SHRs have greater hypertension than females include the finding of higher superoxide anion concentrations under basal conditions and an AT_1-dependent overexpression of the NAD(P)H-oxidase components (p22(phox), gp91(phox), p47(phox) and p67(phox)) in the microvasculature.[46]

In addition to differences in ROS there is evidence that flow-induced arteriolar dilation in male SHRs is significantly impaired, due to the absence of the NO-mediated portion of the response, resulting in an elevation of maintained wall shear stress. A further set of studies demonstrated that in female SHRs the NO-mediated portion of the flow-induced responses was preserved, consistent with the notion that estrogen's action is via NO.[79]

REFERENCES

1. Messerli FH, Garavaglia GE, Schmieder RE et al. Disparate cardiovascular findings in men and women with essential hypertension. Ann Intern Med 1987; 107: 158–61.
2. Stampher MJ, Colditz GA, Willet WC. Postmenopausal estrogen therapy and cardiovascular disease: ten year follow-up from the nurses' health study. N Engl J Med 1991; 325: 756–62.
3. Burt VL, Whelton P, Roccella EJ et al. Prevalence of hypertension in the US adult population: results from Third National Health and Nutrition Examination Survey. Hypertension 1995; 25: 305–13.
4. Khoury S, Yarows SA, O'Brien TK et al. Ambulatory blood pressure monitoring in a nonacademic setting: effects of age and sex. Am J Hypertens 1992; 5: 616–23.
5. Staessen J, Bulpitt CJ, Fagard R et al. The influence of menopause on blood pressure. J Hum Hypertens 1989; 3: 427–33.
6. Kearney PM, Whelton M, Reynolds K et al. Global burden of hypertension: analysis of worldwide data. Lancet 2005; 365: 217–23.
7. Brosnihan KB, Li P, Ganten D et al. Estrogen protects transgenic hypertensive rats by shifting the vasoconstrictor-vasodilator balance of RAS. Am J Physiol 1997; 273: R1908–R1915.
8. Chen YF. Sexual dimorphism of hypertension. Curr Opin Nephrol Hypertens 1996; 6: 181–5.
9. Rowland N, Fregly M. Role of gonadal hormones in hypertension in the Dahl salt-sensitive rat. Clin Exp Hypertens 1992; 14: 367–75.
10. Papanek PE, Rieder MJ, Lombard JH, Greene AS. Gender-specific protection from microvessel rarefaction in female hypertensive rats. Am J Hypertens 1998; 11: 998–1005.
11. Fortes ZB, Nigro D, Scivoletto R et al. Influence of sex on the reactivity to endothelin-1 and noradrenaline in spontaneously hypertensive rats. Clin Exp Hypertens 1991; 13: 807–16.
12. Tostes RC, David FL, Carvalho MH et al. Gender differences in vascular reactivity to endothelin-1 in deoxycorticosterone-salt hypertensive rats. J Cardiovasc Pharmacol 2000; 36: S99–S101.
13. Malyusz M. Effect of castration on the experimental renal hypertension in the rat. Nephron 1985; 40: 96–9.
14. Reckelhoff JF, Granger JP. Role of androgens in mediating hypertension and renal injury. Clin Exp Pharmacol Physiol 1999; 26: 127–31.
15. Pamidimukkala J, Hay M. 17 Beta-estradiol inhibits angiotensin II activation of area postrema neurons. Am J Physiol 2003; 285: H515–H520.
16. Pfeilschifter J, Fandrey J, Oschner M et al. Potentiation of angiotensin II phosphoinositide hydrolysis, calcium mobilization and contraction of renal mesangial cells upon down-regulation of protein kinase C. FEBS Lett 1990; 261: 307–11.
17. White RE, Darkow DJ, Falvo Lang JL. Estrogen relaxes coronary arteries by opening BKCa channels through a cGMP-dependent mechanism. Circ Res 1995; 71: 936–42.
18. Xue B, Pamidimukkala J, Hay M. Sex differences in the development of Angiotensin II-induced hypertension in conscious mice. Am J Physiol Heart Circ Physiol 2005; 288: H2177–H2184.
19. Hanes DS, Weir MR. Gender considerations in hypertension pathophysiology and treatment. Am J Med 1996; 101: 10S–21S.
20. Hong MK, Romm PA, Reagan K et al. Effects of estrogen replacement therapy on serum lipid values and angiographically defined coronary artery disease in postmenopausal women. Am J Cardiol 1992; 69: 176–8.
21. Walsh BW, Schiff I, Rosner B. et al. Effects of postmenopausal estrogen replacement on the concentrations and metabolism of plasma lipoproteins. N Engl J Med 1991; 325: 1196–204.
22. Manson J, Hsia J, Johnson K et al. Women's Health Institutive Investigators. Estrogen plus progestin and the risk of coronary heart disease. N Engl J Med 2003; 349: 523–34.
23. Burry KA. Risks and benefits of estrogen plus progestin in healthy postmenopausal women. Principal results from the Women's Health Initiative randomized controlled trial. Curr Women's Health Rep 2002; 2: 331–2.
24. Herrington DM. The HERS trial results: paradigms lost? Heart and Estrogen/progestin Replacement Study. Ann Intern Med 1999; 131: 463–6.
25. Grady D, Herrington D, Bittner V, Blumenthal et al. Cardiovascular disease outcomes during 6.8 years of hormone therapy: Heart and Estrogen/progestin Replacement Study follow-up (HERS II). JAMA 2002; 288: 49–57.
26. Naftolin F, Taylor H, Karas R et al. The Women's Health Initiative could not have detected cardioprotective effects of starting hormone therapy during the menopausal transition. Fertil Steril 2004; 81: 1498–501.

27. Deenadayalu VP, White RE, Stallone JN et al. Testosterone relaxes coronary arteries by opening the large-conductance, calcium-activated potassium channel. Am J Physiol 2001; 281: H1720–H1727.
28. Harder DR, Coulson PB. Estrogen receptors and effects of estrogen on membrane electrical properties of coronary vascular smooth muscle. J Cell Physiol 1979; 100: 375–82.
29. Heaps CL, Bowles DK. Gender-specific Kþ-channel contribution to adenosine-induced relaxation in coronary arterioles. J Appl Physiol 2002; 92: 550–8.
30. Mugge A, Barton M, Hans-Gerd F et al. Contractile responses to histamine, serotonin, and angiotensin II are impaired by 17β-estradiol in human internal mammary arteries in vitro. Pharmacology 1997; 54: 162–8.
31. Cheng DY, Gruetter CA. Chronic estrogen alters contractile responsiveness to angiotensin II and norepinephrine in female rat aorta. Eur J Pharmacol 1992; 215: 171–6.
32. Bell DR, Rensberger HJ, Koritnik DR et al. Estrogen pretreatment directly potentiates endothelium-dependent vasorelaxation of porcine coronary arteries. Am J Physiol 1995; 268: H377–H385.
33. Gisclard V, Miller VM, Vanhoutte PM. Effect of 17β-estradiol on endothelium-dependent responses in the rabbit. J Pharmacol ExpTher 1986; 244: 19–22.
34. Lamping KG, Nuno DW. Effects of 17β-estradiol on coronary microvascular responses to endothelin-1. Am J Physiol 1986; 271: H1117–H1124.
35. White RE, Luo L, Darkow DJ. Estrogen relaxes coronary arteries by opening BKCa channels through a cGMP-dependent mechanism. Circ Res 1995; 77: 936–42.
36. Dimitropoulou C, White RE, Ownby DR et al. Estrogen reduces carbachol-induced constriction of asthmatic airways by stimulating large conductance voltage and calcium-dependent potassium channels. Am J Respir Cell Mol Biol 2005; 32: 239–47.
37. Tsang SY, Yao X, Essin K et al. Raloxifene relaxes rat cerebral arteries in vitro and inhibits L-type voltage-sensitive Ca^{2+} channels. Stroke 2004; 35: 1709–14.
38. Zhang F, Ram J, Standley PR et al. 17β-estradiol attenuates voltage-dependent Ca^{2+} currents in A7r5 vascular smooth muscle cell line. Am J Physiol 1994; 266: C975–C980.
39. Zhu Y, Bian Z, Lu P et al. Abnormal vascular function and hypertension in mice deficient in estrogen receptor b. Science 2002; 295: 505–8.
40. Xue B, Hay M. The role of testosterone in angiotensin II dependent hypertension. FASEB J 2004; 18: Abstract 439.6.
41. Bowles DK, Maddali KK, Ganjam VK et al. Endogenous testosterone increases L-type Ca^{2+} channel expression in porcine coronary smooth muscle. Am J Physiol 2004; 287: H2091–H2098.
42. Golden KL, Marsh JD, Jiang Y. Testosterone regulates mRNA levels of calcium regulatory proteins in cardiac myocytes. Horm Metab Res 2004; 36: 197–202.
43. Barp J, Araujo AS, Fernandes TR et al. Myocardial antioxidant and oxidative stress changes due to sex hormones. Braz J Med Biol Res 2002; 35: 1075–81.
44. Gonzales RJ, Krause DN, Duckles SP. Testosterone suppresses endothelium-dependent dilation of rat middle cerebral arteries. Am J Physiol 2004; 286: H552–H560.
45. Hernandez I, Delgado JL, Diaz J et al. 17βestradiol prevents oxidative stress and decreases blood pressure in ovariectomized rats. Am J Physiol 2000; 279: R1599–R1605.
46. Dantas AP, Franco Mdo C, Silva-Antonialli MM et al. Gender differences in superoxide generation in microvessels of hypertensive rats: role of NAD(P)H-oxidase. Cardiovasc Res 2004; 61: 22–9.
47. Mates JM, Perez-Gomez C, Nunez de Castro I. Antioxidant enzymes and human diseases. Clin Biochem 1999; 32: 595–603.
48. Darley-Usmar VM, McAndrew J, Patel R et al. Nitric oxide, free radicals and cell signaling in cardiovascular disease. Biochem Soc Trans 1997; 25: 925–9.
49. Harrison DG. Endothelial function and oxidant stress. Clin Cardiol 1997; 20: II-7–II-11.
50. Dvorakova M, Hohler B, Richter E et al. Rat sensory neurons contain cytochrome b558 large subunit immunoreactivity. Neuroreport 1999; 10: 2615–17.
51. Mizuki K, Kadomatsu K, Hata K et al. Functional modules and expression of mouse p40phox and p67phox, SH3-domain-containing proteins involved in the phagocyte NDAPH oxidase complex. Eur J Biochem 1998; 251: 575–582.
52. Serrano F, Kolluri NS, Wientjes FB et al. NADPH oxidase immunoreactivity in the mouse brain. Brain Res 2003; 988: 193–8.
53. Chabrashvili T, Kitiyakara C, Blau J et al. Effects of ANG II type 1 and 2 receptors on oxidative stress, renal NADPH oxidase, and SOD expression. Am J Physiol Regul Integr Comp Physiol 2003; 285: 117–24.
54. Romero JC, Reckelhoff J. Role of angiotensin and oxidative stress in essential hypertension. Hypertension 1999; 34: 943–9.
55. Nishiyama A, Fukui T, Fujisawa Y. Systemic and regional hemodynamic responses to tempol in angiotensin II-infused hypertensive rats. Hypertension 2001; 37: 77–83.
56. Ortiz MC. Antioxidants block angiotensin II-induced increases in blood pressure and endothelin. Hypertension 2001; 38: 655–9.
57. Kawada N, Imai E, Karber A et al. A mouse model of Ang II slow pressor response: role of oxidative stress. J Am Soc Nephrol 2002; 13: 2860–8.
58. Xue B, Pamidimukkala J, Hay M. Sex differences in the development of Angiotensin II-induced hypertension in conscious mice. Am J Physiol Heart Circ Physiol 2005; 288: H2177–H2184.
59. Gragasin FS, Xu Y, Arenas IA et al. Estrogen reduces angiotensin II induced nitric oxide synthase and NADPH oxidase expression in endothelial cells. Arterioscler Thromb Vasc Biol 2003; 23: 38–44.
60. Strehlow K, Rotter S, Wassmann S et al. Modulation of antioxidant enzyme expression and function by estrogen. Circ Res 2003; 93: 170–7.
61. Hawk T, Zhang YQ, Rajakumar G et al. Testosterone increases and estradiol decreases middle cerebral artery occlusion lesion size in male rats. Brain Res 1998; 796: 296–298.
62. Ogawa S, Chester A, Hewitt SC et al. Abolition of male sexual behaviors in mice lacking estrogen receptors alpha and beta (alphaßERKO). Proc Natl Acad Sci U S A 2000; 97: 14737–41.
63. Singh M, Setalo G Jr, Frail DE et al. Estrogen-induced activation of the mitogen-activated protein kinase cascade in the cerebral cortex of estrogen receptor-gamma knock-out mice. J Neurosci 2000; 20: 1694–700.
64. Ceccatelli S, Grandison L, Scott RE et al. Estradiol regulation of nitric oxide synthase mRNAs in rat hypothalamus. Neuroendocrinology 1996; 64: 357–63.
65. Rachman IM, Unnerstall JR, Pfaff DW et al. Regulation of neuronal nitric oxide synthase mRNA in lordosis-relevant neurons of the ventromedial hypothalamus following short-term estrogen treatment. Brain Res Mol Brain Res 1998; 59: 105–8.
66. Warembourg M, Leroy D, Jolivet A. Nitric oxide synthase in the guinea pig preoptic area and hypothalamus: distribution, effect of estrogen, and co-localization with progesterone receptor. J Comp Neurol 1999; 407: 207–27.
67. Krukoff TL. Central actions of nitric oxide in regulation of autonomic functions. Brain Res Brain Res Rev 1999; 30: 52–65.

68. Cherney A, Edgell H, Krukoff TL. NO mediates effects of estrogen on central regulation of blood pressure in restrained, overiectomized rats. Am J Physiol 2003; 285: R842–R849.
69. Harada S, Tokunaga S, Momohara M et al. Inhibition of nitric oxide formation in the nucleus tractus solitarius increases renal sympathetic nerve activity in rabbits. Circ Res 1993; 72: 611–16.
70. Matsuo I, Hirooka Y, Hironaga K et al. Glutamate release via NO production evoked by NMDA in the NTS enhances hypotension and bradycardia in vivo. Am J Physiol 2001; 280: R1285–R1291.
71. Huxley VH, Wang J, Whitt SP. Sexual dimorphism in the permeability response of coronary microvessels to adenosine. Am J Physiol Heart Circ Physiol 2005; 288: H2006–H2013.
72. Prasad A, Dunnill GS, Mortimer PS et al. Capillary rarefaction in the forearm skin in essential hypertension. J Hypertens 1995; 13: 265–8.
73. Winer N, Sowers JR, Weber MA. Gender differences in vascular compliance in young, healthy subjects assessed by pulse contour analysis. J Clin Hypertens 2001; 3: 145–52.
74. Shore AC, Sandeman DD, Tooke JE. Effect of an increase in systemic blood pressure on nailfold capillary pressure in humans. Am J Physiol 1993; 265: H820–H823.
75. Shore AC, Sandeman DD, Tooke JE. Capillary pressure, pulse pressure amplitude, and pressure waveform in healthy volunteers. Am J Physiol 1995; 268: H147–H154.
76. Williams SA, Boolell M, MacGregor GA et al. Capillary hypertension and abnormal pressure dynamics in patients with essential hypertension. Clin Sci (Lond) 1990; 79: 5–8.
77. Roztocil K, Prerovsky I, Oliva I. Capillary filtration coefficient in the forearm of patients with essential hypertension. Clin Physiol 1986; 6: 77–83.
78. Parving HH, Jensen HA, Westrup M. Increased transcapillary escape rate of albumin and IgG in essential hypertension. Scand J Clin Lab Invest 1977; 37: 223–7.
79. Huang A, Sun D, Kaley G, Koller A. Estrogen preserves regulation of shear stress by nitric oxide in arterioles of female hypertensive rats. Hypertension 1998; 31: 309–14.

Index

T - #0321 - 101024 - C0 - 246/189/25 [27] - CB - 9781842143049 - Gloss Lamination